Survival Analysis

Survival Analysis

Models and Applications

Xian Liu

Uniformed Services University of the Health Sciences and Walter Reed National Military Medical Center, USA

WILEY

A John Wiley & Sons, Ltd., Publication

高等教育出版社

HIGHER EDUCATION PRESS

This edition first published 2012

Registered office
John Wiley & Sons Ltd, The Atrium, Southern Gate, Chichester, West Sussex, PO19 8SQ, United Kingdom

For details of our global editorial offices, for customer services and for information about how to apply for permission to reuse the copyright material in this book please see our website at www.wiley.com.

Library of Congress Cataloging-in-Publication Data
Liu, Xian
Survival analysis : models and applications / Xian Liu.
p. ; cm.
Includes bibliographical references and index.
ISBN 978-0-470-97715-6 (cloth)
I. Title.
[DNLM: 1. Survival Analysis. 2. Models, Statistical. WA 950]

519.5'46–dc23

2012004271

A catalogue record for this book is available from the British Library.

ISBN: 978-0-470-97715-6

Set in 10/12 pt Times Roman by Toppan Best-set Premedia Limited

Printed and bound in Singapore by Markono Print Media Pte Ltd

Contents

Preface

Survival analysis concerns sequential occurrences of events governed by probabilistic laws. Recent decades have witnessed many applications of survival analysis in various disciplines. The primary objective of this book is to provide an introduction to the many specialized facets on survival analysis. Scope-wise, this book is expected to appeal to a wide variety of disciplinary areas. Given my multidisciplinary background in training and research, this book of survival analysis covers techniques and specifications applied in medicine, biostatistics, demography, mathematical biology, sociology, and epidemiology, with practical examples associated with each of those disciplines. The celebrated Cox model, used in almost all applied areas, is paid special attention to in this book, with three chapters devoted to this innovative perspective. I also describe counting processes and the martingale theory in considerable detail, in view of their flexibility and increasing popularity in survival analysis, particularly in the field of biostatistics. Regression modeling, mathematical simulation, and computing programming, which attach to different phases of survival analysis, are described and applied extensively in this book, so scientists and professors of various disciplines can benefit from using it either as a useful reference book or as a textbook in graduate courses.

In this book, a large number of survival functions, models, and techniques are introduced, described, and discussed with empirical examples. The presentation of those survival perspectives starts with the most basic specifications and ends with some more advanced techniques in the literature of survival analysis. With a considerable volume of empirical illustrations, I attempt to make the transition from the introductory to the advanced levels as coherent and smooth as possible. Almost for every major survival method or model, step-by-step instructions are provided for leading the reader in to learning how to perform the techniques, supplemented by empirical practices, computing programs, and detailed interpretations of analytic results.

Given the focus on application and practice in this book, the audience includes professionals, academics, and graduate students who have some experience in survival analysis. A fair number of illustrations on various topics permits professionals to learn new methods or to improve their professional skills in performing survival analysis. As it covers a wide scope of survival techniques and methods, from the introductory to the advanced, this book can be used as a useful reference book for planners, researchers, and professors who are working in settings involving various lifetime events. Scientists interested in survival analysis should find it a useful guidebook for the incorporation of survival data and methods into their projects.

Graduate students of various disciplines constitute another important component of the audience. Social science students can benefit from the application of survival concepts and methods to the solution of problems in sociology, economics, psychology, geography, and political science. This book provides a useful framework and practical examples of applied social science, especially at a time when more survival-related questions are raised. The accessibility of many observational, longitudinal data in the public domain since the 1980s will facilitate interested students to practice further the methods and techniques learned from this book. Graduates students of biology, medicine, and public health, who are interested in doing research for their future careers, can learn plenty of techniques from this book for performing mathematical simulation, clinical trials, and competing risks analyses on mortality and disease. Survival analysis and some other related courses have long been recognized as essential components for graduate students training in mathematical biology, epidemiology, and some of the biomedical departments. In medical schools, for example, this book can have wide appeal among medical students who want to know how to analyze data of a clinical trial for understanding the effectiveness of a new medical treatment or of a new medicine on disease.

If the reader attempts to understand the entire body of the methods and techniques covered by this book, the prerequisites should include calculus, matrix algebra, and generalized linear modeling. For those not particularly familiar with that required knowledge, they might want to skip detailed mathematical and statistical steps, and place their focus upon empirical illustrations and computer programming skills. By doing so, they can still command how to apply various survival techniques effectively, thereby adding new dimensions to their professional, research, or teaching activities. Therefore, this book can be read selectively by the reader who is not extremely competent with high-level mathematics and statistics.

The reviewers of the proposal and an example chapter for this book were: Kenneth Land, Duke University; David Swanson, University of California, Riverside; and Jichuan Wang, George Washington University. Additionally, a number of other colleagues and friends have enriched, supported and refined the intellectual development of this book, including Lyn Albrecht, Kristie Gore, Albert I. Hermalin, James Edward McCarroll, Robert Ursano, Lois Verbrugge, Anatoli I. Yashin, and Chu Zhang. Sincere thanks are given to Paul T. Savarese of the SAS Institute for letting me use some of his personal SAS programs in Chapters 4 and 8. Part of the work in Chapter 8 was initiated at the Population Studies Center, the Institute for Social Research at the University of Michigan, and the mentorship of Albert I. Hermalin is specially acknowledged.

I owe special thanks to Charles C. Engel, whose consistent support and help has made completion of this book possible. The staff of the Deployment Health Clinical Center, Walter Reed National Military Medical Center, provides tremendous dedication, competence, and excellence in the course of the preparation of this book. Malisa Arnold's and Phoebe McCutchan's assistance in editing the text and some of the graphs was vital.

Finally, I would like to thank my wife, Ming Dong, for her support and encouragement throughout the entire period of preparing, writing, and editing this book.

Xian Liu

1

Introduction

1.1 What is survival analysis and how is it applied?

'What is survival analysis?' Before starting discussion on this topic, think about what 'survives.' In the cases considered here, we are talking about things that have a life span, those things that are 'born,' live, change status while they live, and then die. Therefore, 'survival' is the description of a life span or a living process before the occurrence of a status change or, using appropriate jargon, an *event*.

In terms of 'survival,' what we think of first are organisms like various animal species and other life forms. After birth, a living entity grows, goes through an aging process, and then decomposes gradually. All the while, they remain what they are – the same organisms. The gradual changes and developments over a life course reflect the survival process. For human beings in particular, we survive from death, disease, and functional disablement. While biology forms its primary basis, the significance of survival is largely social. At different life stages, we attend school, get married, develop a professional career, and retire when getting old. In the meantime, many of us experience family disruption, become involved in social activities, cultivate personal habits and hobbies, and make adjustments to our daily lives according to physical and mental conditions. These social facets are things that are not organisms but their life span is *like* that of a living being: things that *live*, things that have beginnings, transformations, and then *deaths*. In a larger context, survival can also include such events as an automobile breakdown, the collapse of a political system in a country, or the relocation of a working unit. In cases such as these and in others, existence dictates processes of survival and their status change, indicated by the occurrence of events.

The practice of survival analysis is the use of reason to describe, measure, and analyze features of events for making predictions about not only survival but also 'time-to-event processes' – the length of time until the change of status or the occurrence of an event – such as from living to dead, from single to married, or from healthy to sick. Because a life span, genetically, biologically, or mechanically, can be cut short by illness, violence, environment, or other factors, much research in survival analysis involves making comparisons among

Survival Analysis: Models and Applications, First Edition. Xian Liu.

groups or categories of a population, or examining the variables that influence its survival processes. As they have come to realize the importance of examining the inherent mechanisms, scientists have developed many methods and techniques seeking to capture underlying features of various survival processes. In the academic realm, survival analysis is now widely applied in a long list of applied sciences, owing considerably to the availability of longitudinal data that records histories of various survival processes and the occurrences of various events. At present, the concept of survival no longer simply refers to a biomedical or a demographic event; rather, it expands to indicate a much broader scope of phenomena characterized by time-to-event processes.

In medical research, clinical trials are regularly used to assess the effectiveness of new medicines or treatments of disease. In these settings, researchers apply survival analysis to compare the risk of death or recovery from disease between or among population groups receiving different medications or treatments. The results of such an analysis, in turn, can provide important information with policy implications.

Survival analysis is also applied in biological research. Mathematical biologists have long been interested in evolutionary perspectives of senescence for human populations and other species. By using survival analysis as the underlying means, they delineate the life history for a species' population and link its survival processes to a collection of physical attributes and behavioral characteristics for examining its responses to its environment.

Survival data are commonly collected and analyzed in social science, with topics ranging widely, from unemployment to drug use recidivism, marital disruption, occupational careers, and other social processes. In demography, in addition to the mortality analysis, researchers are concerned with such survival processes as the initiation of contraceptive use, internal and international migration, and the first live birth intervals.

In the field of public health, survival analysis can be applied to the analysis of health care utilization. Such examination is of special importance for both planners and academics because the health services system reflects the political and economic organization of a society and is concerned with fundamental philosophical issues involving life, death, and the quality of life.

Survival analysis has also seen wide applications in some other disciplines such as engineering, political science, business management, and economics. For example, in engineering, scientists apply survival analysis to perform life tests on the durability of mechanical or electric products. Specifically, they might track a sample of products over their life course for assessing characteristics and materials of the product's designed life and for predicting product reliability. Results of such studies can be used for the quality improvement of the products.

1.2 The history of survival analysis and its progress

Originally, survival analysis was used solely for investigations of mortality and morbidity on vital registration statistics. The earliest arithmetical analysis of human survival processes can be traced back to the 17th century, when the English statistician John Graunt published the first life table in 1662 (Graunt, 1939, original edition, 1662). For a long period of time, survival analysis was considered an analytic instrument, particularly in biomedical and demographical studies. At a later stage, it gradually expanded to the domain of engineering to describe/evaluate the course of industrial products. In the past forty years, the scope of survival analysis has grown tremendously as a consequence of rapid developments in computer science, particularly the advancement of powerful statistical software packages. The convenience of using computer software for creating and utilizing complex statistical models has led scientists of many disciplines to begin using survival models.

As applications of survival analysis have grown rapidly, methodological innovation has accelerated at an unprecedented pace over the past several decades. The advent of the Cox model and the partial likelihood perspective in 1972 triggered the advancement of a large number of statistical methods and techniques characterized by regression modeling in the analysis of survival data. The major contribution of the Cox model, given its capability of generating simplified estimating procedures in analyzing survival data, is the provision of a flexible statistical approach to model the complicated survival processes as associated with measurable covariates. More recently, the emergence of the counting processes theory, a unique counting system for the description of survival dynamics, highlights the dawning of a new era in survival analysis due to its tremendous inferential power and high flexibility for modeling repeated events for the same observation and some other complicated survival processes. In particular, this modern perspective combines elements in the large sample theory, the martingale theory, and the stochastic integration theory, providing a new set of statistical procedures and rules in modeling survival data. To date, the counting process system and the martingale theory have been applied by statisticians to develop new theorems and more refined statistical models, thus bringing a new direction in survival analysis.

1.3 General features of survival data structure

In essence, a survival process describes a life span from a specified starting time to the occurrence of a particular event. Therefore, the primary feature of survival data is the description of a change in status as the underlying outcome measure. More formally, a status change is the occurrence of an *event* designating the end of a life span or the termination of a survival process. For instance, a status change occurs when a person dies, gets married, or when an automobile breaks down. This feature of a status 'jump' makes survival analysis somewhat similar to some more conventional statistical perspectives on qualitative outcome data, such as the logistic or the probit model. Broadly speaking, those traditional models can also be used to examine a status change or the occurrence of a particular event by comparing the status at the beginning and the status at the end of an observation interval. Those statistical approaches, however, ignore the timing of the occurrence of this lifetime event, and thereby do not possess the capability of describing a time-to-event process. A lack of this capability can be detrimental to the quality of analytic results, thereby generating misleading conclusions. The logistic regression, for example, can be applied to estimate the probability of experiencing a particular lifetime event within a limited time period; nevertheless, it does not consider the time when the event occurs and therefore disregards the length of the survival process. Suppose that two population groups have the same rate of experiencing a particular event by the end of an observation period but members in one group are expected to experience the event significantly later than do those in the other. The former population group has an advantaged survival pattern because its average life is extended. Obviously, the logistic regression ignores this timing factor, therefore not providing precise information.

Most survival models account for the timing factor on a status jump. Given this capacity, the second feature of survival data is the description of a time-to-event process. In the literature of survival analysis, time at the occurrence of a particular event is regarded as a random variable, referred to as event time, failure time, or survival time. Compared to statistical techniques focused on structures, the vast majority of survival models are designed to describe a time course from the beginning of a specific time interval to the occurrence of a particular event. Given this feature, data used for survival analysis are also referred to as time-to-event data, which consist of information both about a discrete 'jump' in status as well as about the time passed until the occurrence of such a jump.

The third primary feature of survival data structure is censoring. Survival data are generally collected for a time interval in which the occurrences of a particular event are observed. As a result, researchers can only observe those events that occur within a surveillance window between two time limits. Consequently, complete survival times for many units under examination are not observed, with information loss taking place either before the onset or beyond the end of the study interval. Some units may be lost to observation in the middle of an investigation due to various reasons. In survival analysis, such missing status on event times is called *censoring*, which can be divided into a variety of types. For most censoring types, a section of survival times for censored observations are observable and can be utilized in calculating the risk of experiencing a particular event. In survival analysis, this portion of observed times is referred to as censored survival times. As censoring frequently occurs, the majority of survival analysis literally deals with incomplete survival data, and accordingly scientists have found ways to use such limited information for correctly analyzing the incomplete survival data based on some restrictive assumptions on the distribution of censored survival times. Given the importance of handling censoring in survival analysis, a variety of censoring types are delineated in Section 1.4.

As survival processes essentially vary massively based on basic characteristics of the observations and environmental conditions, a considerable body of survival analysis is conducted by means of censored data regression modeling involving one or more predictor variables. Given the addition of covariates, survival data structure can be viewed as consisting of information about three primary factors, otherwise referred to as a 'triple:' survival times, censoring status, and covariates. Given a random sample of n units, the data structure for survival analysis actually contains n such triples. Most survival models, as will be described extensively in later chapters, are built upon such a data structure.

Given different emphases on the variety of features, survival analysis is also known as duration analysis, time-to-event analysis, event histories analysis, or reliability data analysis. In this book, these concepts are used interchangeably.

1.4 Censoring

Methodologically, censoring is defined as the loss of observation on the lifetime variable of interest in the process of an investigation. In survival data, censoring frequently occurs for many reasons. In a clinical trial on the effectiveness of a new medical treatment for disease, for example, patients may be lost to follow-up due to migration or health problems. In a longitudinal observational survey, some baseline respondents may lose interest in participating in subsequent investigations because some of the questions in a previous questionnaire are considered too sensitive.

Censoring is generally divided into several specific types. If an individual has entered a study but is lost to follow-up, the actual event time is placed somewhere to the right of the censored time along the time axis. This type of censoring is called *right censoring*. As right censoring occurs far more frequently than do other types and its information can be included in the estimation of a survival model, the focus of this section is on the description of right censoring. For analytic convenience, descriptions of right censoring are often based on the assumption that an individual's censored time is independent of the actual survival time, thereby making right censoring noninformative. While this assumption does not always hold, the issue of informative censoring and the related estimating approaches are described in Chapter 9. Other types of censoring, including *left censoring* and *interval censoring*, are also described in this section. Additionally, I briefly discuss the impact of left truncation on survival analysis, a type of missing data that is different from censoring.

1.4.1 Mechanisms of right censoring

Right censoring is divided into several categories: Type I censoring, random censoring, and Type II censoring. In *Type I censoring*, each observation has a fixed censoring time. Type I censoring is usually related to a predetermined observation period defined according to the research design. Generally, a specific length of time is designed with a starting calendar date and an ending date. In most cases, only a portion of observations would experience a particular event of interest during this specified study interval and some others would survive to the endpoint. For those who survive the entire observation period, the only information known to the researcher is that the actual survival time is located to the right of the endpoint of the study period along the time axis, mathematically denoted by $T > C$, where T is the event time and C is a fixed censored time. Therefore, lifetimes of those survivors are viewed as right censored, with the length of the censored time equaling the length of the observation period.

Right censoring also occurs randomly at any time during a study period, referred to as *random censoring*. This type of censoring differs essentially from Type I censoring because the censored time is not fixed, but, rather, behaves as a random variable. Some respondents may enter the study after a specified starting date and then are right censored at the end of the study interval. Such observations are also listed in the category of random censoring because their *delayed entry* is random. Statistically, time for random censoring can be described by a random variable C_i (the subscript i indicates variation in C among randomly censored observations), generally assumed to be independent of survival time T_i. Mathematically, for a sample of n observations, case i ($i = 1, 2, \ldots, n$) is considered randomly censored if $C_i < T_i$ and $C_i < C$, where C is the fixed Type I censored time. The censored survival time for random censoring is measured as the time distance from the time of entry into the study to the time when random censoring occurs.

Figure 1.1 graphically displays the occurrences of Type I and random censoring. In this figure, I present data for six individuals who participate in a study of mortality at older ages, noted by, respectively, persons 1, 2, 3, 4, 5, and 6. The study specifies an observation period from 'start of study' to 'end of study.' The sign '×' denotes the occurrence of a death, whereas the sign '+' represents right censoring.

In Figure 1.1, person 1 enters the study at the beginning of the study and dies within the interval. Therefore, this case is an event, with time-to-event T_1 counted as the time elapsed from the start of the study to the time of death. Person 2 also enters the study at the beginning of the study, but at the end of the study, this person is still alive. Therefore, person 2 is a typical case of Type I right censoring, with the censored survival time equaling the full

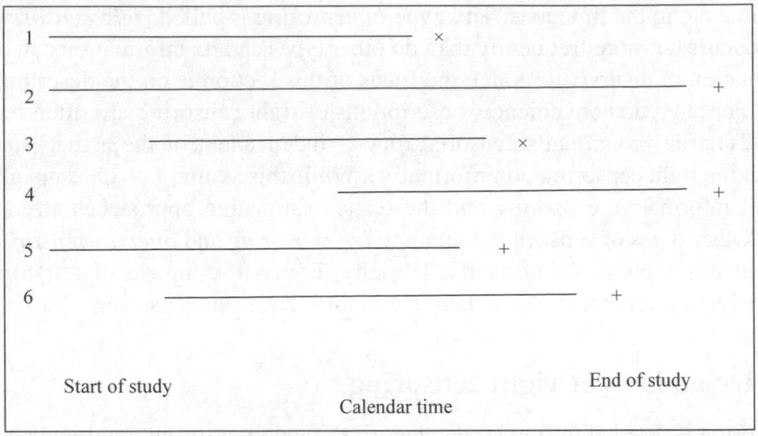

Figure 1.1 Illustration of Type I and random censoring.

length of the study interval. Persons 3 and 4 both enter the study after the start of the study, with person 3 deceased during the interval and person 4 alive throughout the rest of the interval. Consequently, person 3 has an event whose survival time is the distance from the time of the delayed entry to the time of death, whereas person 4 is a case of random censoring with the censored survival time measured as the length of time between the delayed entry and the end of the study. Entering the study later than expected, person 4 can also be considered a left truncated observation, which will be described in Subsection 1.4.2. Finally, persons 5 and 6 are lost to follow-ups before the termination of the study, with person 5 entering the investigation at the start and person 6 entering during the period of investigation. Both persons are randomly censored. Their censored times, denoted by C_5 and C_6, respectively, measured as the time elapsed between the starting date of the study and the censored time for person 5, or between the time of the delayed entry and the censored time for person 6. Unlike person 2, censored times for persons 4, 5, and 6 differ from each other and are smaller than C.

Type II right censoring refers to the situation in which a fixed number of events is targeted for a particular study. When the designed number of events is observed, a study would terminate automatically and all individuals whose survival times are beyond the time of termination are right censored. For those individuals, the censored survival time is measured as the distance from the start of observation to the time at which the study terminates. Type II right censoring is not related to a fixed ending time; rather, it is associated with a time determined by a date when a targeted number of events are observed. Given this restriction, surveys or clinical trials associated with Type II right censoring are much rarer than those with other types of right censoring.

1.4.2 Left censoring, interval censoring, and left truncation

Left censoring refers to a data point, known to be prior to a certain date but unknown about its exact location. This type of censoring frequently occurs in a study design involving two separate study stages. Individuals who enroll in the first selection process but are not eligible for the second process are viewed as left censored. For example, in a study of the initiation of first contraceptive use after marriage, if a couple marries but has already used contraceptive means prior to marriage, this couple is left censored for further analysis. Another example is a study of first marijuana use among high school students. If a respondent has used marijuana before the study, but does not remember the exact timing of the first use, this observation is left censored. In clinical trials, researchers often specify a recruitment period and a study period. If a patient is recruited into the study but has experienced an event of interest before the study period starts, the case is left censored.

Another type of censoring is *interval censoring*. In some investigations, actual event times are unknown, and the data point is only known to be located between two known time points. Demographers often use aggregate mortality data for a specific calendar year for constructing a life table and, clearly, such mortality data are interval censored. Interval censoring also occurs frequently in clinical trials and large-scale longitudinal surveys in observational studies. For example, a clinical trial on the effectiveness of a new medicine on posttraumatic stress disorder (PTSD) recruits a sample of patients diagnosed with PTSD, proposing a series of periodic follow-up investigations to examine the rate of resolution of this psychiatric disorder. Some patients with PTSD at a starting time point are observed to have recovered at the next follow-up time point. Here, the exact timing of PTSD resolution is unknown and the only information known to the researcher is the time interval in which the event occurred. As a result, the PTSD time span for those patients who have recovered is interval censored. For analytic convenience, interval-censored survival times are often assumed to be located at a fixed time point, either in the middle of a specific interval (Siegel and Swanson, 2004) or immediately prior to an exact follow-up time (Lawless, 2003; Scharfstein, Rotnitzky, and Robins, 1999). In Chapters 4 and 5, this type of censoring is further discussed and illustrated.

1.4.2.1 Left truncation

Time-to-event data are also subject to *left truncation*, a unique type of missing data. A survey respondent who enters the observation process after a given starting date is referred to as a *staggered entry* or a *delayed entry*. Such observations are left truncated, with the truncated time measured as the time distance from the time of entry to the occurrence of an event or of right censoring. Compared to various types of censoring, left truncation is a phenomenon often associated with sample selection that leaves individuals out of observation for some time. In a study of marital disruption, for example, some individuals become married after the investigation starts, so their entry into the study is delayed and their survival times are left truncated at the time of marriage. Left truncation can potentially cause serious selection bias in survival analysis because it underestimates the risk of experiencing a particular event; however, there are standard statistical techniques to handle such bias. In Chapter 5, the impact of left truncation on survival analysis and how to use certain statistical methods for handling it is illustrated.

1.5 Time scale and the origin of time

Survival processes describe the length of time measured from some specified starting time point to the occurrence of a life event. According to this specification, the measurement of an event time should start from a well-defined origin of time and ends at the time when a particular event of interest occurs. Therefore, a metric unit at which time is measured must be specified first.

In proposing a study plan, the specification of the time scale must depend on the nature of the study and the targeted length of an observation period. In observational studies, the occurrence of a behavioral event is usually a gradual process. Examples of such gradual life events are recovery from disability among older persons, changes in marital status, and discontinuation of drinking alcohol among heavy drinkers. In following up those processes, the month may be an appropriate choice as the time scale. Clinical research, on the other hand, can be linked with lifetime events, both with rapid changes in status and also with a relatively slow pace. In cancer research, for example, the survival rate within a fixed time period varies significantly for different types of cancer. A study of surgical treatment on lung cancer may examine the improvement of the survival rate for six months. In such research, a day or week is the appropriate time scale. In studies of more gradual processes such as prostate cancer, the survival rate should be observed for a substantially longer period because these patients typically live much longer than those with lung cancer. Thus, a month is a better option for the second study. In health services research, survival data with different service types can be mixed with a variety of time scales. For example, a patient admitted to a short-stay hospital stays there for only a few days, whereas the average length of stay in a nursing home generally exceeds an entire year (Liu *et al.*, 1997). Accordingly, the time scale needs to be specified based on the nature of a particular service type.

Once the metric unit is specified, the starting point (or the origin of time) of the event time must be accurately defined. Without a clear and unambiguous definition of the starting time, the event time can be severely misspecified, thereby resulting in erroneous analytic results. In different situations, the starting time can be defined in various ways. As time proceeds with ordinary calendar time, a standard scale needs to be chosen to align individuals at time 0. In general, the ideal scenario is to follow up lifetimes of one or more birth cohorts of individuals from their births to the date when the last survivor dies. This scenario, however, is utterly unrealistic because the researcher launching such a study would definitely pass away or retire long before the study is ended. In demographic and epidemiologic studies, age is often specified as the time scale, but the use of the period-specific data assumes a hypothetic birth cohort. Here, the true origin of time is actually the starting date of a specific calendar period, rather than birth.

1.5.1 Observational studies

In observational studies, survival data are usually collected from large-scale longitudinal surveys. In most cases, researchers would set a calendar date as the beginning time of the study and then draw a random sample of individuals according to a specific study plan. Those individuals' survival status would be followed up for a considerably long period of time (ten years, say). Here, the calendar date for the first interview is used as the origin of time, and all respondents should be aligned on this specific date, with the event time operationally defined as the distance between the date of the first interview and the date of an event. In practice, setting the starting calendar date as the origin of time has some advantages: it is convenient to align respondents for survival analysis and it is a straightforward method to calculate an individual's event time. This procedure, however, can encounter several selection problems. The survival process is incomplete for a targeted population and the observation is relevant only to a truncated chronological period, in which gradual processes of survival from a particular event cannot be entirely captured (Liu, 2000). Some of those limitations can be substantially mitigated by correctly specifying a causal framework. In a typical longitudinal study, the date of birth itself can be regarded as an explanatory factor, so that the cohort effect on survival processes can be incorporated into a survival model (Clayton, 1978). As age progresses with time, the age at baseline can serve as an important control variable for selection bias from left truncation.

1.5.2 Biomedical studies

In biomedical studies, survival analysis is generally performed to examine the effectiveness of a new medicine or a new treatment on reducing the rate of mortality or of disease. Given this focus, the origin of time in biomedical research is often specified as the starting date of a new treatment/medication or of exposure to disease. Consider, for example, the study of survival from prostate cancer after the surgical treatment. As the event time is defined as the time elapsed from treatment to death, the origin of time in this context should be the date of surgery performed on the patient. As a result, all patients of this study can be aligned by the time origin regardless of when the surgery is performed. Similarly, in a study of asbestos exposure and lung cancer, the date of first exposure to asbestos on a regular basis is an appropriate choice as the origin of time and all study subjects, no matter when they enter the study, should be aligned by the date of first regular exposure to asbestos. Sometimes, clinical trials use the date of randomization as the origin of time, referred to as the study time. Given a period of recruitment, patients would enter the study on different calendar dates, so that such a calendar time, referred to as the patient time, can differ considerably from the study time (Collett, 2003).

1.5.3 Health care utilization

In studies of health care utilization, some mutually exclusive service types – such as nursing home, short-stay hospital, and long-term hospital – are regularly specified for analyzing transitions from one service type to another (Liang *et al.*, 1993, 1996; Liu *et al.*, 1997). Thus, the admission date should be used as the origin of time and the time elapsed from admission to discharge is the event time. With admission episodes used as the primary unit of analysis, repeated visits within a specific observation period are common and the size of censored cases is relatively small.

There are situations in which the true origin of time is difficult to define. Consider a study of liver cirrhosis and mortality by Liestol and Andersen (2002). As is typical in biomedical research, the origin of time in this study should be the date of diagnosis. This medical condition, however, develops gradually with symptoms vague in the early stage and varying significantly among individuals, thus making the time of diagnosis a questionable time origin. Some patients with liver cirrhosis might be diagnosed with the disease later than others and some are never even diagnosed until the time of death. Consequently, patients with liver cirrhosis cannot be aligned appropriately according to the natural progression of disease, implying the origin of time to be a latent random variable representing the degree of delayed entry. Liestol and Andersen (2002) suggest the use of age or calendar time as a surrogate time 0, because age and calendar time are both well defined and serve as strong determinants of disease severity. Given strong variations in physical characteristics, genetic predisposition, and health behaviors among individuals born in the same calendar year, the use of age or calendar time still makes time a strong random effect; accordingly, more complex procedures need to be designed to account for the impact of this latent factor.

1.6 Basic lifetime functions

Survival analysis begins with a set of propositions on various aspects of a lifetime event: basic concepts, mathematical functions, and specifications generally applied in survival analysis. The focus is placed upon three most basic functions – the survival function, the probability density function, and the hazard function.

1.6.1 Continuous lifetime functions

I start by describing time as a continuous process. Let $f(t)$ be the probability density function (p.d.f.) of event time T. Then, according to probability theory, the cumulative distribution function (c.d.f.) over the time interval $(0, t)$, denoted by $F(t)$, represents the probability the random variable T takes from time 0 to time t ($t = 0, 1, \ldots, \infty$), given by

$$F(t) = \Pr(T \le t) = \int_0^t f(u)\,\mathrm{d}u. \tag{1.1}$$

Defined as the probability that no event occurs from time 0 to time t, the survival function at time t, denoted by $S(t)$, is simply the complement of the c.d.f.:

$$S(t) = \Pr(T > t) = 1 - \Pr(T \le t) = 1 - F(t). \tag{1.2}$$

By definition, given $t \to \infty$, $S(0) = 1$ and $S(\infty) = 0$. For analytic convenience, statisticians and demographers sometimes arbitrarily define a finite ending time, denoted by ω, assuming that no one survives beyond this time point. In this specification, we have $S(0) = 1$ and $S(\omega) = 0$. Empirically, the value of ω can be determined by the maximum life span ever observed, or just by a given very old age beyond which only very few have ever been found to survive, so that the very small value in $S(\omega)$ can be ignored (Liu and Witten, 1995).

The p.d.f. of T can be expressed in terms of $S(t)$, given by

$$f(t) = -\frac{\mathrm{d}S(t)}{\mathrm{d}t}. \tag{1.3}$$

Equation (1.3) indicates that the slope (the derivative) of the survival function determines the p.d.f. of T. As $S(t)$ is a nonincreasing function, this slope must take the negative sign to derive the nonnegative p.d.f. Strictly speaking, the p.d.f. is not a probability, but a probability rate, which can take values greater than one.

The hazard function at time t is defined as the instantaneous rate of failure at time t, generally denoted by $h(t)$ and mathematically defined by

$$h(t) = -\frac{1}{S(t)}\frac{\mathrm{d}S(t)}{\mathrm{d}t} = \frac{f(t)}{S(t)}, \tag{1.4}$$

or

$$h(t) = \lim_{\Delta t \to 0} \frac{\Pr\{T \in (t, t+\Delta t] \mid T \ge t\}}{\Delta t}. \tag{1.5}$$

Equation (1.4) demonstrates that the hazard rate is conceptually a standardized instantaneous rate of failure relative to the survival rate at time *t*. From another perspective, Equation (1.5) expresses the hazard rate as the ratio of the conditional probability at *t* (the probability of experiencing a particular event at time *t* given the condition $T \geq t$) over an infinitesimal time change. Because Δt tends to 0, the *hazard rate* can be literally understood as the conditional probability of failure with respect to the limit of a time interval. With this instantaneous property, the hazard rate is also referred to as the force of mortality, the intensity rate, or the instantaneous risk (Andersen *et al.*, 1993; Kalbfleisch and Prentice, 2002; Liu, 2000; Liu and Witten, 1995). Given standardization and its unique sensitivity to the change in the survival function, the hazard function is considered a preferable indicator for displaying the relative risk of experiencing a particular event in survival analysis.

Given Equation (1.3), the hazard function at time *t* can also be written by

$$h(t) = \frac{-\mathrm{d}\log S(t)}{\mathrm{d}t}. \tag{1.6}$$

By Equation (1.6), the hazard rate is mathematically defined as the derivative of the log survival probability at time *t* multiplied by −1. As a survival function is monotonically decreasing, the hazard function is nonnegative but not necessarily smaller than or equal to one. Therefore, as the standardized p.d.f., the hazard rate is a conditional probability rate. It is essential for the reader to comprehend the concept and the underlying properties of the hazard function because most survival models described in later chapters are created on the hazard rate.

The above equations highlight the intimate relationships among $f(t)$, $S(t)$, and $h(t)$. Mathematically, they reflect different profiles of a single lifetime process, with each providing a unique aspect of survival data. Therefore, each of these basic functions can be readily expressed in terms of another. For example, the survival probability $S(t)$ can be expressed as the inverse function of Equation (1.6):

$$\begin{aligned} S(t) &= \exp\left(-\int_0^t h(u)\mathrm{d}u\right) \\ &= \exp[-H(t)], \end{aligned} \tag{1.7}$$

where $H(t)$ is the integration of all hazard rates from time 0 to *t*, defined as the continuous cumulative hazard function at time *t*.

Similarly, from Equation (1.7), the cumulative hazard function $H(t)$ can be expressed in terms of $S(t)$, given by

$$H(t) = -\log S(t). \tag{1.8}$$

Furthermore, from Equations (1.4) and (1.7), the probability density function $f(t)$ can be written in terms of the hazard function:

$$f(t) = h(t)\exp\left(-\int_0^t h(u)\mathrm{d}u\right). \tag{1.9}$$

From the above basic functions, the expected life remaining at time *t*, also referred to as life expectancy at *t*, can be computed. As it represents the unit-based probability surviving at time t, $S(t)$ can be considered the intensity of expected life at t. Let $\lim_{t\to\infty} tS(t) = 0$; the expected life remaining at time 0, denoted $E(T_0)$, can be written by

$$E(T_0) = E(T|t=0) = \int_0^\infty S(u)\mathrm{d}u. \tag{1.10}$$

Likewise, the expected life remaining at time t, $E(T_t)$, is

$$E(T_t) = E(T|T \geq t) = \frac{\int_t^\infty S(u)\mathrm{d}u}{S(t)}, \tag{1.11}$$

where $S(t)$ represents exposure for the expected life remaining at time t.

The expected life between time t and time $t + \Delta t$, denoted by $E({}_{\Delta t}T_t)$, is a component in $E(T_t)$, given by

$$E({}_{\Delta t}T_t) = E\{T|T \in (t, t+\Delta t], T \geq t\} = \frac{\int_t^{t+\Delta t} S(u)\mathrm{d}u}{S(t)}. \tag{1.12}$$

In later chapters, a large number of nonparametric, parametric, and semi-parametric lifetime functions will be delineated, analyzed, and discussed. All those more complex models build upon the above basic specifications. In other words, more complicated forms of various survival models are just extensions of the basic functions. No matter how difficult an equation looks, from one function other lifetime indicators can be mathematically defined and estimated.

1.6.2 Discrete lifetime functions

If the distribution of event time T is discrete, the length of time axis t can be divided into J time intervals with unit Δt and a discrete time interval $(t, t + \Delta t)$. Given this, t becomes a discrete random variable denoted by t_j ($t_j = t_0, t_1, \ldots, t_J$). Accordingly, the discrete probability density function is defined by

$$f(t_j) = \Pr(T \in t_j), \quad i = 1, 2, \ldots, J. \tag{1.13}$$

Given Equations (1.1) and (1.2), the discrete survival function is

$$S(t) = \sum_{j|t_j > t} f(t_j). \tag{1.14}$$

Likewise, the discrete hazard function can be derived from an extension of Equation (1.4):

$$h(t_j) = \frac{f(t_j)}{S(t_j)}, \tag{1.15}$$

where $S(t_j)$ is the expectation of the survival probability with respect to the discrete time interval t_j. Conceptually, $S(t_j)$ differs from $S(t)$ because it represents the average survival probability with respect to a discrete time interval, rather than at an instantaneous time point. The deviation of $S(t_j)$ from $S(t)$ depends on the interval unit Δt. If $\Delta t \to 0$, $S(t_j) = S(t)$; if Δt does not represent an infinitesimal time unit but is small, $S(t_j) \approx S(t)$, and the difference between the continuous and discrete survival functions is ignorable. If Δt represents a considerable width, such as a week, a month, or even a year, the continuous $S(t)$ is a decreasing function within the interval, so $S(t_j) < S(t)$. Roughly, the discrete time hazard function can be considered the approximate conditional probability of failure in $(t, t + \Delta t)$. There are some conceptual problems in the specification of this approximation because the hazard rate can be greater than 1 in some extreme situations. This issue, however, is not discussed further in this text.

In the counting process theory (Andersen *et al.*, 1993; Fleming and Harrington, 1991), which will be described in Chapter 6, the continuous course of survival is restricted within a limited time interval $(0, \tau)$ where $\tau < \infty$ for a population of N where $N < \infty$ (Aalen, 1975; Andersen and Gill, 1982; Andersen *et al.*, 1993; Fleming and Harrington, 1991). Given such restrictions, it is reasonable to view the hazard rate as the conditional probability if N is large. Consequently, the hazard function and the conditional probability are used interchangeably in verifying the validity of counting processes and the martingale theory.

In demographic and epidemiologic studies, researchers often calculate the death rate within a time interval of a considerable width (one year or five years) for measuring the force of mortality for a population of interest (Keyfitz, 1985; Schoen, 1988; Siegel and Swanson, 2004). If time t is expressed as a starting exact age and Δt as the unit of an age interval, the discrete death rate in the interval $(t, t + \Delta t)$, defined as ${}_{\Delta t}M_t$, is written by

$$ {}_{\Delta t}M_t = \frac{N_t - N_{t+\Delta t}}{\pi N_t + (1-\pi)N_{t+\Delta t}} = \frac{S(t) - S(t+\Delta t)}{\pi S(t) + (1-\pi)S(t+\Delta t)}, \tag{1.16} $$

where N_t is the population at t, $N_{t+\Delta t}$ is the population at $(t + \Delta t)$, and π is some weight assigned to derive an unbiased estimate of exposure for the risk of death. Here, $S(t_j)$ is calculated as a weighted average of $S(t)$ and $S(t + \Delta t)$ because, within a wide time interval, not all individuals surviving to t are at the risk for the entire interval (Teachman, 1983b). As a result, the continuous survival probability is a decreasing function within the interval, thereby leading to the condition $S(t_j) < S(t)$. This interval-specific measure for the force of mortality can be conveniently viewed as the discrete realization of the following ratio of two integrals:

$$ {}_{\Delta t}M_t = \frac{\int_t^{t+\Delta t} S(u)h(u)\,\mathrm{d}u}{\int_t^{t+\Delta t} S(u)\,\mathrm{d}u}, \tag{1.17} $$

where the numerator is the cumulative probability densities within the interval between t and $(t + \Delta t)$ and the denominator is the exposure to the risk of dying. Then, when Δt tends to 0, ${}_{\Delta t}M_t = f(t)/S(t) = h(t)$.

From Equations (1.3) and (1.12), the interval-specific force of mortality can be written by

$$ {}_{\Delta t}M_t = \frac{{}_{\Delta t}F_t}{{}_{\Delta t}T_t \times S(t)}, \tag{1.18} $$

where ${}_{\Delta t}F_t$ is the cumulative densities in $(t, t + \Delta t)$ and ${}_{\Delta t}T_t$ is the expected life lived within this specific interval. Here, the hazard rate serves as a step function inherent in the interval with $S(u)$ decreasing due to the elimination of deaths, so that ${}_{\Delta t}M_t$ can be regarded as an average hazard rate with respect to a specific time interval (Siegel and Swanson, 2004). If $h(u)$, where $u \in (t, t + \Delta t)$, is constant throughout the entire interval, ${}_{\Delta t}M_t$ can be regarded as an estimate of $h(u)$.

1.6.3 Basic likelihood functions for right, left, and interval censoring

A likelihood function with survival data describes the probability of a set of parameter values given observed lifetime outcomes. Mathematically, it is either equal to or approximately proportional to the probability of survival data. In this subsection are several simple likelihood functions for right, left, or interval censoring. These likelihoods are basic functions that will serve as a basis for more complicated likelihood functions described in later chapters.

When right censoring occurs, the only information known to the researcher is survival time at the occurrence of censoring. Statisticians utilize this partial information of right censoring when developing a survival model. Specifically, the information of right censored survival times can be well integrated in a likelihood function of survival data.

For a specific observation i, the lifetime process can be described by three random variables: (1) a random variable of event time T_i, (2) a random variable of time t_i, given by

$$t_i = \min(T_i, C_i), \tag{1.19}$$

and (3) a random variable indicating status of surviving or right censoring for t_i, specified by

$$\begin{cases} \tilde{r}_i = 0 \text{ if } T_i = t_i \text{ or } T_i \le C_i \\ \tilde{r}_i = 1 \text{ if } T_i > t_i \text{ or } T_i > C_i, \end{cases} \tag{1.20}$$

where $\tilde{r}_i$ designates whether t_i is a lifetime ($\tilde{r}_i = 0$) or a right censored time ($\tilde{r}_i = 1$). Given these three random variables, the likelihood function for a Type I right censored sample, in which C is fixed as the time distance between the date of entry and the end of study, can be written as the probability distribution of $(t_i, \tilde{r}_i)$. The joint probability density function is given by

$$f(t_i)^{1-\tilde{r}_i} \Pr(T_i > C_i)^{\tilde{r}_i}, \tag{1.21}$$

where $f(\cdot)$ is the probability density function. It follows that, when $\tilde{r}_i = 1\,(t_i = C_i)$, Equation (1.21) reduces to $\Pr(T_i > C_i)$, which is the survival probability at time t, because the first term is 1. Likewise, when $\tilde{r}_i = 0$, Equation (1.21) yields the probability density function $f(t_i)$ because the second term is 1. Assuming the lifetimes $T_1, \ldots, T_n$ for a sample of n are statistically independent and continuous at t_i, the likelihood function for the sample is given by

$$L(\boldsymbol{\theta}) = \prod_{i=1}^{n} f(t_i)^{1-\tilde{r}_i} S(t_i)^{\tilde{r}_i}, \tag{1.22}$$

where $S(\cdot)$ is the survival function and $\boldsymbol{\theta}$ is the parameter vector to be estimated in the presence of right censoring.

For a sample of random right censoring, C is no longer fixed but behaves as a continuous random variable. As a result, there are actually two survival functions, from failure and from censoring, and two corresponding densities in the probability distribution. In this case, Equation (1.22) still applies because the survival and density functions for random right censoring are not associated with parameters in $f(t)$, so that they can basically be neglected (see Lawless, 2003, pp. 54–55).

In terms of left censored observations, the likelihood function is associated with different censoring mechanisms. As left censoring occurs before the time of observation, the random variable indicating status of surviving or left censoring at t_i is defined as

$$\begin{cases} \tilde{l}_i = 0 \text{ if } T_i > t_i \\ \tilde{l}_i = 1 \text{ if } T_i \le t_i, \end{cases} \tag{1.23}$$

where $\tilde{l}_i$ denotes whether t_i is a lifetime ($\tilde{l}_i = 0$) or a left censored time ($\tilde{l}_i = 1$). Given this, the likelihood function for left censored observations can be written as another joint probability distribution linked with $(t_i, \tilde{l}_i)$:

$$F(t_i)^{\tilde{l}_i} \Pr(T_i > t_i)^{1-\tilde{l}_i}, \tag{1.24}$$

where $F(t_i)$ is the cumulative distribution function (c.d.f.). It follows that, when $\tilde{l}_i = 0$ $(T_i > t_i)$, Equation (1.24) represents the survival probability S_i at time t_i because the first term is 1; when $\tilde{l}_i = 1$, Equation (1.24) becomes the c.d.f. $F(t_i)$ because the second term is 1. Consequently, given a series of lifetimes $T_1, \ldots, T_n$, the likelihood function for a left censored sample is given by

$$L(\boldsymbol{\theta}) = \prod_{i=1}^{n} F(t_i)^{\tilde{l}_i} S(t_i)^{1-\tilde{l}_i}. \tag{1.25}$$

As interval censoring is associated with a time range within which a particular event occurs, we have $t_{i-1} < T \le t_i$, and the contribution to the likelihood is simply $F(t_i) - F(t_{i-1})$ or $S(t_{i-1}) - S(t_i)$. Accordingly, the overall likelihood function for interval censoring is

$$L(\boldsymbol{\theta}) = \prod_{i=1}^{n} [F(t_i) - F(t_{i-1})]^{\tilde{i}_i} S(t_i)^{1-\tilde{i}_i}, \tag{1.26}$$

where $\tilde{i}_i$ is the status indicator for interval censoring (1 = interval censored; 0 = else).

If the survival data are mixed with right, left, and interval censored observations, the total likelihood function is written by

$$\begin{aligned} L(\boldsymbol{\theta}) &= \prod_{i=1}^{n} [1 - F(t_i)]^{\tilde{r}_i} F(t_i)^{\tilde{l}_i} [F(t_i) - F(t_{i-1})]^{\tilde{i}_i} \\ &= \prod_{i=1}^{n} S(t_i)^{\tilde{r}_i} F(t_i)^{\tilde{l}_i} [F(t_i) - F(t_{i-1})]^{\tilde{i}_i}. \end{aligned} \tag{1.27}$$

Mathematically, maximizing the above likelihood function yields the maximum likelihood estimate of $F(t)$. In Chapters 4 and 5, more complex likelihood functions will be described for specifying more parameters in $\boldsymbol{\theta}$.

1.7 Organization of the book and data used for illustrations

The remainder of the book is organized as follows. Chapter 2 is devoted to some descriptive approaches that are largely applied in survival analysis, including the Kaplan–Meier (product-limit) and the Nelson–Aalen estimators, calculation of the variance, the confidence interval, and the confidence bands for the survival function, the life table methods, and several testing techniques for comparing two or more group-specific survival functions. The applicability of these descriptive methods is discussed. Chapter 3 describes some popular parametric distributions of survival times with mathematical details. Chapter 4 focuses on the description of parametric regression models, with covariates involved in the analysis of survival data. General parametric regression modeling and the corresponding statistical inference are presented as a unique statistical approach combining a known parametric distribution of survival times with multivariate regression procedures. Several widely used parametric models are delineated extensively with empirical illustrations. Given its widespread applicability and flexibility, the Weibull regression model is particularly heeded to and discussed.

Chapters 5 through 7 are devoted mainly to the Cox model and its advancements. In particular, Chapter 5 describes basic specifications of the Cox model and partial likelihood. Some advances in estimating the Cox model are also presented and discussed in this chapter, such as the statistical techniques handling tied observations, the creation of a survival function without specifying an underlying hazard function, the hazard model with time-dependent covariates, the stratified proportional hazard model, modeling of left truncated survival data, and the specification of several popular coding schemes for qualitative factors and the statistical inference of local tests in the Cox model. Chapter 6 first introduces basic specifications of counting processes and the martingale theory, with particular relevance to the Cox model. Then I present, in order, five types of residuals used in the Cox model, techniques for the assessment of the proportional hazards assumption, methods of evaluating the functional form for a covariate, and approaches on identification of influential observations in the Cox model. Each of these sections is supplemented by an empirical illustration. Chapter 7 displays statistical techniques for analyzing survival data with competing risks and with repeated events. In addition to a step-by-step presentation on empirical data, the merits and limitations in various statistical techniques in those areas are discussed in this chapter.

Chapter 8 briefly discusses advantages and existing problems in the application of the structural hazard rate models. A simplified structural hazard model is specified with restrictive assumptions, with a detailed example provided for illustrating step-by-step procedures. Chapter 9 concerns several special topics in survival analysis, including informative censoring, bivariate and multivariate survival models, the frailty theory, mortality crossovers and maximum life span, survival convergence and the preceding mortality crossover, and the calculation of sample size required for survival analysis. The strengths and limitations of each of those advanced techniques are discussed. Due to consideration of coherence and conciseness of the text, some supplementary procedures, datasets, and computer programs are presented as appendices.

In this book, data from a large-scale longitudinal study is the major source for illustrating empirical examples. These data come from the Survey of Asset and Health Dynamics among the Oldest Old (AHEAD), a nationally representative investigation of older Americans. This survey, conducted by the Institute for Social Research (ISR), University of Michigan, is funded by the National Institute on Aging as a supplement to the Health and Retirement Study (HRS). The HRS Wave I survey was conducted in 1992, with a sample size of 12 652 persons including selected respondents aged between 40 and 70 years and their spouses, if married, regardless of age. Those respondents have been followed up by telephone every other year, with proxy interviews for those who have deceased prior to follow-up.

As a supplemental survey to the HRS, Wave I of the AHEAD survey was conducted between October 1993 and April 1994. Specifically, a sample of individuals aged 70 or older (born in 1923 or earlier) was identified throughout the HRS screening of an area probability sample of households in the nation. This procedure identified 9473 households and 11 965 individuals in the target area range. Like the HRS, the Wave I respondents have been followed up by telephone every second or third year, with proxy interviewing designed for those deceased between two successive surveys. At present, the AHEAD survey registers nine waves of investigation in 1993, 1995, 1998, 2000, 2002, 2004, 2006, 2008, and 2010. As a longitudinal, multidisciplinary, and US population-based study, AHEAD provides a highly representative and reliable data base for the survival analysis of older Americans aged 70 or older.

AHEAD acquires detailed information on a number of domains, including demographic characteristics, health status, health care use, housing structure, disability, retirement plans, and health and life insurance. Survival information throughout the follow-up waves has been obtained by a link to the data of the National Death Index (NDI). This book uses survival data of the AHEAD survey throughout the first six waves (1993–2004). Given the illustrative nature of using this dataset, I randomly selected 2000 persons from the baseline AHEAD sample for the analysis in the book.

While AHEAD provides a solid and reliable data source for empirical illustrations, this single dataset cannot cover the entire scope of this book. As a result, in addition to the AHEAD longitudinal data, some clinical and simulated data are used when appropriate. In performing empirical analyses, I used the SAS software package for programming a variety of statistical procedures on data management and data analysis.

1.8 Criteria for performing survival analysis

This book introduces, delineates, and summarizes a large number of survival models and techniques. Given the statistical methods and techniques presented here, the reader, after learning how to apply each one of them, might raise more questions about performing survival analysis. Given a topic of interest and the availability of a dataset, what are the criteria for performing survival analysis? In other words, what is the most appropriate perspective for conducting a survival analysis? There are four underlying criteria – relevance to theory, accurate description of data, computational tractability, and interpretability of analytic results. As the focus of this book is on application and practice, these criteria are established with specific regard to the applied phases of survival analysis.

In performing survival analysis, the first criterion is whether a statistical model builds upon an existing theory on a particular event of interest. A lifetime event usually involves complex mechanisms. Whereas one factor can influence some other factors in shaping the risk and frequency of experiencing a particular event, at the same time it may be affected by others, thus constituting a complicated structure of causal linkages in survival processes. Such complexity of causality makes it extremely difficult, if not impossible, to describe a complete set of interrelationships using a single conceptual model. Additionally, there is often a lack of suitable measures for many conceptual factors in the description of event histories. A practical approach to deal with these issues is to link a lifetime process with an explicit theoretical framework that portrays a portion of the causal effects on a particular event. The underlying conceptual framework must be based on a relevant, well-established theory or previous findings. A good theory gives rise to valid theoretical hypotheses, provides direction for specifying interrelationships of conceptual factors, and facilitates selection of measurable variables for explaining the dynamics of a lifetime phenomenon. This strategy can aid in yielding new constructive findings, in turn further solidifying the connotation of the underlying theory. In some sense, creating a survival model without relevance to theory is just like building an edifice without reference to a blueprint.

The second criterion for performing survival analysis is accurate description of data. Except for some special cases, survival models are created and applied for the generation of unbiased parameter estimates, the prediction of trajectories of survival processes, and the derivation of analytic results. Much of survival analysis is based on empirical data from various sources, such as large-scale sample surveys, clinical trials, and vital registration statistics. Given the usual representativeness of such information, it is essential for the scientist to describe the empirical data accurately, with model-based lifetime trajectories agreeable to observed patterns. Considerable deviations of model-derived trajectories from observed data generally indicate the misspecification of an underlying survival model because it fails to describe data correctly by using parameter estimates. In other words, an incorrect description of empirical data suggests failure to reflect the true set of experiences generated by the stochastic processes. Therefore, an accurate description of data is a required condition for making further inference on model fitness and the quality of various parameter estimators.

The third criterion for performing survival analysis is computational tractability. In survival analysis, a statistical model needs to be developed in such a way that the audience can follow what computational procedures are applied and how analytic results are produced, and thus understanding the rationale of the analysis. In particular, specifications of covariates, mathematical functions, and causal relationships among variables must be explicit and unambiguous, and the estimation of an underlying survival model must be based on statistical procedures and steps that are recognizable and applicable. New computational procedures, if necessary, must be fully presented, with methodological inference self-contained, for allowing the audience to understand justifications of the advancement. Exceptionally complicated link functions and reader-unfriendly mathematical expressions need to be avoided whenever possible, and the addition of model parameters should be well justified analytically. Indeed, if not computationally tractable, a survival model cannot be readily accepted by other researchers, thus failing to be disseminated in a timely fashion.

The fourth criterion is interpretability of analytic results. In survival analysis, most analysts' professional orientations are toward applied areas, and the material described in most survival analysis books is designed to demonstrate the variety of approaches in which survival models can be applied in various disciplines. This nature of applicability points to the importance of generating interpretable and substantively meaningful analytic results when performing survival analysis. Survival outcomes are generally modeled as a nonlinear function of explanatory variables, so that model parameters are sometimes not directly interpretable. Under such circumstances, the researcher needs to convert unexplainable results into interpretable ones by means of techniques of functional transformation. If hard to interpret, analytic results of a survival model cannot translate into useful explanations, in turn obstructing timely spreading of potentially valuable implications.

In all areas of applied science, statistical modeling, survival analysis being no exception, is by no means an easy task. In constructing a useful survival model, both overfitting and underfitting must be avoided while maintaining relevance to a substantive theme. By abiding by these four criteria, the difficulty in creating a good survival model can be considerably mitigated. As Box (1976) asserts, all models are wrong, and scientists cannot obtain a 'correct' one by excessive elaboration; nevertheless, if a statistical model correctly describes the essence and the trend of a phenomenon while overlooking ignorable noises, it is a useful perspective for the scientist to apply. Given this principle, many hypotheses and assumptions in statistical modeling are established just for analytic convenience and simplicity: there would rarely be a true normal distribution, there never exists an exactly linear association between two factors, and a conceptual framework can look more like an artifact than a reflection of the real world. All these steps are necessary otherwise a statistical model would become a garbage can. For survival analysis in particular, the performance of a statistical technique is a process of abstraction, rather than a course of mirroring what we see in our daily lives. If a parsimonious model with only a few parameters generates the same statistical power and the same substantive implications as does a more complicated one, the former method is the signature of a good model and the latter a mediocre one (Box, 1976).

2

Descriptive approaches of survival analysis

In this book, inferences of model parameters on survival processes are the main focus. Before proceeding with statistical procedures for such inferences, I would like to portray some descriptive approaches first. In survival analysis, such descriptive methods and techniques are used to summarize main features of raw survival data. Other than numbers, tables, graphs, and some other simple statistics, these approaches include significance tests on group differences in the survival and the hazard functions. Though generally viewed as simplistic ways for recapitulating survival data, the descriptive approaches are sometimes applied for deriving conclusions in biomedical research. In clinical trials, for example, results directly from descriptive approaches are commonly used to generate analytic results, particularly since in those studies the sample size is often too small to consider a large number of parameters and the effects on survival are partially accounted for in the process of randomization.

Many of the descriptive approaches in survival analysis are counting methods on the survival function, from which other lifetime indicators, such as the cumulative hazard function, can be easily computed. This chapter introduces some popular methods in this area used by statisticians, demographers, and other quantitative methodologists in summarizing survival data. Because they rely completely on empirical data without making assumptions on the form of the probability distribution, these approaches are also referred to as *nonparametric methods*. In particular, I start with the description of the Kaplan–Meier and the Nelson–Aalen estimators, the two related and well-known nonparametric methods used in analyzing the survival probability and the cumulative hazard function. Then I provide a brief introduction of the life table method, initially developed and used by demographers and epidemiologists. Next, I describe a variety of testing techniques for comparing two or more group-wise survival functions. Lastly, a summary of these descriptive approaches is provided.

Survival Analysis: Models and Applications, First Edition. Xian Liu.

2.1 The Kaplan–Meier (product-limit) and Nelson–Aalen estimators

The Kaplan–Meier estimator (1958), also known as the *product-limit method*, provides a simple but effective scheme that calculates a single lifetime indicator, the survival function $S(t)$. As time t is divided into a series of intervals according to observed event or censored times, the Kaplan–Meier survival estimates are calculated by the product of a series of interval-specific conditional probabilities. This method is designed in such a simple way that the censored survival function can be easily computed by hand. The Nelson–Aalen estimator (1972), as an alternative to the Kaplan–Meier approach, calculates the cumulative hazard function using the same rationale. The application of both estimators is based on the assumption that the occurrence of censoring is independent of actual survival times.

2.1.1 Kaplan–Meier estimating procedures with or without censoring

I start the description of the Kaplan–Meier estimator with a simple example in the absence of censoring. Suppose there are ten older women who have died of breast cancer during a seven-year observation period. Using 'month' as the time scale, their survival times are ordered by rank according to the number of months elapsed from time 0 to the occurrence of the event:

Survival times in months: 5, 17, 24, 32, 40, 46, 47, 50, 59, and 74.

Given this series of survival times, the survival rate at time 0 is 1 because all ten older women are alive at the beginning of the observation. The proportion surviving to month 5 is 0.9 as nine out of those ten older women survive beyond month 5. Likewise, by the end of month 17, two women have died in total, so the proportion surviving at this time is 0.8. At month 24 and month 32, the proportions of survival are, respectively, 0.7 and 0.6. The survival rates at the following observed survival times can also be computed easily from the ratio of the number of women still alive at each survival time over value 10. While the above calculation is straightforward, the proportion surviving beyond a given month can be calculated in a different perspective. For example, the survival rate at month 17 can be estimated by the proportion of survivors at month 5 (0.9) multiplied by the proportion surviving between month 5 and month 17. At month 24, the survival probability can be calculated by the survival rate at month 17 times the proportion surviving between month 17 and month 24. Placing the previous step into the calculation, the survival rate at month 24 can be further expressed as the product of three interval-specific conditional proportions of survival. Similarly, the survival rate at month 32 can be estimated as the product of four interval-specific conditional probabilities of survival, the survival rate at month 40 the product of five conditional surviving proportions, and so forth. The survival rate at each survival time thus computed is called the Kaplan–Meier estimate. The logic involved in this estimator is that for an older woman with breast cancer who survives beyond month 40, she must survive through months 5, 17, 24, and 32 first, so that her chance of survival throughout 40 months is composed of a series of interval-specific survival rates.

Below, I take the liberty to summarize the above procedure up to month 48 (four years) in the format of a typical Kaplan–Meier table. Table 2.1 shows the procedure that the survival rate at each month is simply the product of a series of interval-specific conditional probabilities of survival. In the absence of censoring, the survival rate can be more easily obtained

Table 2.1 Kaplan–Meier survival estimates for older women with breast cancer.

Month	Calculating steps	Survival rate
0	$10/10 = 1.0$	1.0
5	$1.0 \times (9/10) = 0.9$	0.9
17	$1.0 \times (9/10) \times (8/9) = 0.9$	0.8
24	$1.0 \times (9/10) \times (8/9) \times (7/8) = 0.7$	0.7
32	$1.0 \times (9/10) \times (8/9) \times (7/8) \times (6/7) = 0.6$	0.6
40	$1.0 \times (9/10) \times (8/9) \times (7/8) \times (6/7) \times (5/6) = 0.5$	0.5
46	$1.0 \times (9/10) \times (8/9) \times (7/8) \times (6/7) \times (5/6) \times (4/5) = 0.4$	0.4
47	$1.0 \times (9/10) \times (8/9) \times (7/8) \times (6/7) \times (5/6) \times (4/5) \times (3/4) = 0.3$	0.3

Table 2.2 Kaplan–Meier survival estimates with right censoring.

Month	Calculating steps	Survival rate
0	$12/12 = 1.0$	1.00
5	$1.0 \times (11/12) = 0.92$	0.92
17	$1.0 \times (11/12) \times (10/11) = 0.83$	0.83
20^+	$1.0 \times (11/12) \times (10/11) \times (9/9) = 0.83$	0.83
24	$1.0 \times (11/12) \times (10/11) \times (9/9) \times (8/9) = 0.74$	0.74
32	$1.0 \times (11/12) \times (10/11) \times (9/9) \times (8/9) \times (7/8) = 0.65$	0.65
35^+	$0.65 \times (6/6) = 0.65$	0.65
40	$0.65 \times (6/6) \times (5/6) = 0.54$	0.54
46	$0.65 \times (6/6) \times (5/6) \times (4/5) = 0.43$	0.43
47	$0.65 \times (6/6) \times (5/6) \times (4/5) \times (3/4) = 0.32$	0.32

from the number of survivors at each observed survival time over the total number of survivors at the beginning of observation. When censoring exists, however, this ratio function does not apply very well because the survival status for a censored case is unknown. Removal of censored cases from the calculation leads to erroneous results due to the neglect of survival times for those lost to observation in the middle of a survival interval. In such situations, the Kaplan–Meier estimator has the capability to account for some types of censored data, particularly right censoring. This property is a major appeal of the Kaplan–Meier estimator, given frequent occurrences of censoring in longitudinal surveys and clinical trials.

To demonstrate how the Kaplan–Meier estimator handles right censoring, I extend the previous example by adding two older women with breast cancer who entered the study at the beginning of the investigation but are then lost to observation, one at month 20 and one at month 35. Now, the total number of older women increases to 12, with their survival times given by

Survival times in months: 5, 17, 20^+, 24, 32, 35^+, 40, 46, 47, 50, 59, and 74,

where the two censored cases are designated by the sign +. Given these survival and censored times, a revised Kaplan–Meier table is displayed in Table 2.2, which presents the proportions surviving at ten survival times after adding two censored cases. At time 5, the survival rate now increases to 0.92 (11/12) because the two censored patients are known to be alive at month 5 and are thus counted as survivors. Likewise, $S(17)$ is elevated to 0.83 after taking additional survivors into consideration. At month 20, one survivor is lost to observation, but from month 17 to month 20, none of the other survivors is deceased so $S(20)$ is still 0.83. At this time point, nine patients remain exposed to the risk of death. At month 24, another patient is deceased; therefore, with nine survivors at month 20, the proportion of survival at month 24 is computed as $(11/12) \times (10/11) \times (9/9) \times (8/9) = 0.74$. Similarly, the proportion surviving to month 32 is $(11/12) \times (10/11) \times (9/9) \times (8/9) \times (7/8) = 0.65$. At month 35, another patient is lost to observation and hence there are five patients left exposed to the risk of death and the survival rate at this time is still 0.65. Given the number of survivors at month 35, the proportions surviving to months 40, 46, and 47 are, respectively, 0.54, 0.43, and 0.32, computed by following the Kaplan–Meier estimating procedure. It is worth noting that at each observed survival time the value of the survival rate is higher than the corresponding rate without including censored cases because the survival times for the two censored patients are considered in the counting procedure.

Using the survival estimates computed in Table 2.2, I generate a plot to highlight that the Kaplan–Meier survival function follows a declining step process, using the following SAS program.

SAS Program 2.1:

```
data Kaplan_Meier;
   input Months Status@@;
datalines;

5  1 17 1 20  0 24  1 32  1 35  0 40  1 46  1 47  1 50  1
59  1  74  1
;

ods html;
ods graphics on;

proc lifetest data = Kaplan_Meier;
  time Months*Status(0);
run;

ods graphics off;
ods html close;
```

In SAS Program 2.1, I create a temporary dataset titled ‘Kaplan_Meier,’ containing only two variables: Months (survival time in months) and Status (0 = censored and 1 = not censored). Then the data of survival times and the censoring indicator STATUS are entered in order. The PROC LIFETEST procedure is used to plot the Kaplan–Meier survival function. For this simple analysis without involving other covariates, only the TIME statement is required in the PROC LIFETEST statement. For the graphic display, the ODS GRAPHICS statement is specified.

SAS Program 2.1 generates a plot of the Kaplan–Meier estimates, given in Figure 2.1, which displays the plot of the Kaplan–Meier survival estimates against the time scale,

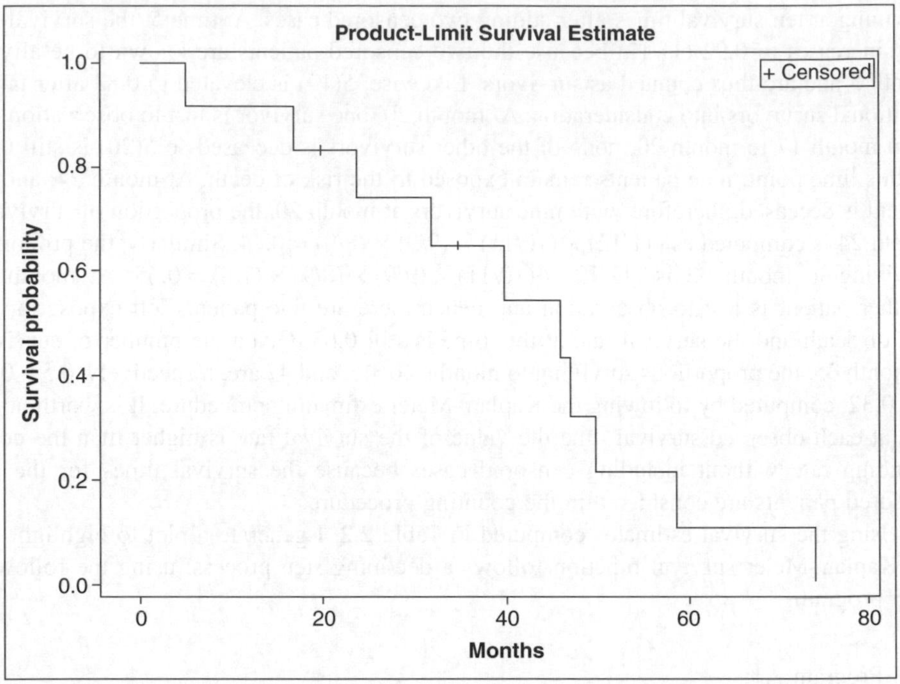

Figure 2.1 Plot of Kaplan–Meier estimates.

Months. Clearly, the Kaplan–Meier (product-limit) survival estimates follow a step function at survival times. When a death occurs, the survival curve drops vertically to a lower level of survival and then remains constant over time until another death occurs. In the plot, the symbol '+' indicates the horizontal location in months where right censoring occurs. Notice that in a standard Kaplan–Meier plot, the survival function is termed the 'survival probability,' rather than the 'survival rate' or the 'proportion surviving,' as pertaining to the large-sample approximation theory. For analytic convenience, the terms 'survival probability,' 'survival rate,' and 'proportion of survival' are interchangeable in the following text.

2.1.2 Formulation of the Kaplan–Meier and Nelson–Aalen estimators

The example given in Subsection 2.1.1 uses a very small sample of individuals, with each having a unique survival time, censored or not censored. If a large sample is used for calculating the Kaplan–Meier estimates, there may be too many lifetimes to be ranked, arranged, and computed. Additionally, in large-scale longitudinal surveys, some individuals may share the same survival times and some others may be lost to observation at exactly the same time points. In survival analysis, this shared survival time is referred to as the *tied observation time*, with observations sharing the same survival time, called the *tied cases*. In the presence of observation ties, the Kaplan–Meier estimator needs to be formulated to fit into various situations.

For a sample of n individuals, there are potentially n survival times until all experience a particular event (e.g., death). These survival times can be ordered by rank as

$$t_1 \leq t_2 \leq t_3 \leq t_4 \leq \cdots \leq t_n,$$

where t_i represents the time at which individual i experiences a particular event or right censoring ($i = 1, 2, \ldots, n$). Because at time t_i individuals with actual survival or censored times smaller than t_i have already exited, there is a specific number of survivors who remain exposed to the risk of event at t_i, denoted by n_i, where $n_1 \geq n_2 \geq \cdots \geq n_n$. As t_n here is the lifetime for the last survivor in the rank list, $n_n = 1$. If there are no observation ties, the total number of survival times is equal to the number of observations and, accordingly, survival times are ordered by

$$t_1 < t_2 < t_3 < t_4 < \cdots < t_n.$$

With the existence of tied cases at some of the survival times, however, the total number of recorded times is smaller than n.

Let d_i be the number of events at time t_i ($d_i = 1$ if there are no tied cases at t_i); then the Kaplan–Meier estimator for the probability of survival at time t is

$$\hat{S}(t) = \prod_{t_i < t} \frac{n_i - d_i}{n_i}, \tag{2.1}$$

where $\hat{S}(t)$ is the Kaplan–Meier estimate for the probability of survival at time t. As d_i can be any number including 1, Equation (2.1) takes into consideration the existence of tied observations. Although censoring is not particularly specified in this equation, its presence does not affect the validity of this formulation. If t_i is a censored survival time, for example, d_i is 0 from t_{i-1} to t_i and $n_i = n_{i-1} - 1$, so that the conditional probability of survival between t_{i-1} and t_i is 1. If t_i indicates a tied censored time with c_i being the number of censored observations tied at t_i, then $n_i = n_{i-1} - c_i$ and the conditional probability of survival between t_{i-1} and t_i is still 1.

Sometimes, specification of censored times is necessary in formalizing the survival function due to reasons of generalization. In such situations, a status indicator for a survival or a censored time, denoted by δ_{ti}, can be created where $\delta_{ti} = 0$ if t_i is a censored survival time and $\delta_{ti} = 1$ if t_i is an actual survival time. Let $\tilde{d}_i = d_i$ if $\delta_{ti} = 1$ and $\tilde{d}_i = c_i$ if $\delta_{ti} = 0$ (or $\tilde{d}_i = \min(d_i, c_i)$). Then the Kaplan–Meier estimator can be written by

$$\hat{S}(t) = \prod_{t_i < t} \left(\frac{n_i - \tilde{d}_i}{n_i} \right)^{\delta_{ti}}. \tag{2.2}$$

Clearly, when t_i is a censored survival time, $\delta_{ti} = 0$ and $\left[\left(n_i - \tilde{d}_i \right) / n_i \right] = 1$; hence the proportion surviving between t_{i-1} and t_i is 1. In contrast, when t_i is an actual survival time, $\delta_{ti} = 1$ and the term $\left[\left(n_i - \tilde{d}_i \right) / n_i \right]$ is smaller than 1, thus indicating an actual proportion of survival in the interval (t_{i-1}, t_i).

Given Equations (2.1) and (2.2), several scenarios are suggested to deal with various situations. First, if the number of events is small, the data can be arranged in the order of time without grouping and the number of censored cases in the intervening time intervals is also counted, as applied in Subsection 2.1.1. Second, if the above procedure is considered to be time consuming because of a relatively large sample size but the number of censored survival times is relatively small, some of the successive intervals only containing censored times can be combined. Lastly, when the number of events is large, some selected division points need to be specified with events and censored cases counted in corresponding intervals. For such data, a summary table may be created to display the selected time intervals, the number of events, the number of censored cases, and the probability of survival at each of the selected intervals.

From the Kaplan–Meier estimator, other lifetime functions can be readily derived given the intimate associations among various indicators described in Chapter 1. A popular application, for example, is to convert the survival function to the cumulative hazard function. Given the equation $H(t) = -\log S(t)$, the cumulative hazard function can be expressed in terms of the Kaplan–Meier survival estimate $\hat{S}(t_i)$, given by

$$\hat{H}(t) = -\log\left[\prod_{t_i<t}\left(\frac{n_i - \tilde{d}_i}{n_i}\right)^{\delta_{ti}}\right]. \tag{2.3}$$

For small x, $\log(1 + x) \approx x$. Therefore, Equation (2.3) can be further expanded:

$$\hat{H}(t) = -\sum_{t_i \le t}\delta_{t_i}\log\left(1 - \frac{\tilde{d}_i}{n_i}\right) \approx -\sum_{t_i \le t}\delta_{t_i}\left(-\frac{\tilde{d}_i}{n_i}\right) = \sum_{t_i \le t}\left(\frac{\tilde{d}_i\delta_{t_i}}{n_i}\right). \tag{2.4}$$

If censored times are not particularly specified in the formulation of the cumulative hazard function, Equation (2.4) becomes

$$\hat{H}(t) \approx \sum_{t_i \le t}\left(\frac{d_i}{n_i}\right) = \sum_{t_i \le t}[1 - \hat{s}(t_i)]. \tag{2.5}$$

Equation (2.5) is the celebrated *Nelson–Aalen estimator*, initially proposed by Nelson (1972) and later mathematically formalized and justified by Aalen (1978). Clearly, the Nelson–Aalen estimator, developed independently, is an approximation to the Kaplan–Meier estimate transformation on $H(t)$. As mentioned in Chapter 1, at a single survival time t_i, the ratio of the number of events over the number of those exposed to the risk of an event is identical to the hazard rate at t_i, and between two survival times in a step function, the hazard rates all take value 0. Consequently, the Nelson–Aalen estimator has a solid theoretical base (Aalen, 1978; Andersen *et al.*, 1993; Fleming and Harrington, 1991). In Chapter 6, I will provide a simple proof for its validity using the martingale central limit theorem.

The cumulative hazard function is frequently used to test the parametric form of the hazard function, given its intimate associations with some of the parametric distributions, as will be described in some of the later chapters. While both approaches are widely used, the Nelson–Aalen estimator on the cumulative hazard function is generally considered to behave better than the Kaplan–Meier estimator for data of small samples.

Given the mathematical association among lifetime indicators, the survival function can be expressed in terms of the Nelson–Aalen estimator, given by

$$\hat{S}(t) = \exp\left[-\hat{H}(t)\right] \approx \exp\left(-\sum_{t_i \le t}\frac{d_i}{n_i}\right), \tag{2.6}$$

or

$$\hat{S}(t) \approx \exp\left[-\sum_{t_i \le t}\left(\frac{\tilde{d}_i \delta_{ti}}{n_i}\right)\right]. \tag{2.7}$$

In the SAS software package, the Nelson–Aalen estimates of both survival probabilities and the cumulative hazard function can be made. Using the prior example of Table 2.2, here I reformat SAS Program 2.1 by adding the option 'NELSON' (or 'AALEN') in the PROC LIFETEST statement, requesting SAS to apply the Nelson–Aalen estimator, instead of the Kaplan–Meier method, for computing the probability of survival and the cumulative hazard rate at each survival time. The revised SAS program creates a temporary SAS data file named Nelson_Aalen, as displayed below.

SAS Program 2.2:

```
......

data Nelson_Aalen;
 input Months Status@@;
datalines;

5  1 17 1 20  0 24 1 32 1 35 0 40 1 46 1 47 1 50 1
59 1 74 1
;

ods html;
ods graphics on;

proc lifetest data = Nelson_Aalen NELSON;
  time Months*Status(0);
run;

ods graphics off;
ods html close;
```

SAS Program 2.2 generates a plot of the Nelson–Aalen survival estimates that is almost identical to Figure 2.1. From the output data derived from SAS Program 2.2, not presented here, the Nelson–Aalen estimates of survival probabilities are analogous to those reported in Table 2.2.

2.1.3 Variance and standard error of the survival function

When a population sample is large enough, the Kaplan–Meier estimator approximates the mean of the survival probability, asymptotically normally distributed. Given this property, the variance of this survival estimate, from the theoretical standpoint, can be well specified for assessing the dispersion of the survival probability. Nevertheless, estimation of the variance for $\hat{S}(t)$, denoted by $\hat{V}\left[\hat{S}(t)\right]$, cannot easily be formulated without further inference. The difficulty here is the ambiguity resulting from the fact that the variance estimated from a sample does not depend on all limits of an observation. In survival data, the greatest observed lifetime, denoted t^*, is often a censored time, so that $\hat{S}(t^*) > 0$ and $n_{t^*+1} = 0$.

Therefore, $\hat{S}(t)$ is undefined for $t > t^*$. When the probability of $t > t^*$ for a population is sizable, a nonparametric estimate of the variance for $S(t)$ is not highly informative. In such situations, some approximation approaches need to be applied.

A number of techniques have been developed to derive an unbiased estimator for the variance of the Kaplan–Meier survival function (Kalbfleisch and Prentice, 2002; Peto *et al.*, 1977). Originally, Kaplan and Meier (1958) used the well-known Greenwood (1926) formula to yield an estimate of the variance for $\hat{S}(t)$, and this formula remains a popular estimator in the analysis of the nonparametric survival function. Researchers prefer to use the *delta method* for the derivation of this approximation, as presented in most textbooks on survival analysis. In brief, the delta method is an approximation method involving transformations of random variables. Specifically, let X be a random variable distributed as $N(\mu, \sigma^2)$ with p.d.f. $f(x)$ and $g(X)$ be a single-valued and measurable function of X. If $g(X)$ is differentiable, its integral is the expected value of $g(X)$. Although the variance of $g(X)$ is often not directly obtainable, a linear approximation of $g(X)$ in the neighborhood of μ, through some expansion series, leads to the approximation that $V[g(X)] \approx [g'(\mu)]^2\sigma^2$. Appendix A provides a detailed description of this approximation method.

The derivation of the Greenwood formula on the Kaplan–Meier survival function takes several transformation steps. It starts with the estimation for the variance of $\log \hat{S}(t)$. Taking the log values of both sides of Equation (2.1) yields

$$\log\left[\hat{S}(t)\right] = \sum_{t_i < t} \log\left(\frac{n_i - d_i}{n_i}\right) = \sum_{t_i < t} \log[\hat{s}(t_i)], \tag{2.8}$$

where $\hat{s}(t_i)$ is the conditional probability of survival in interval (t_{i-1}, t_i). As $\hat{s}(t_i)$ can be expressed as an estimate of a proportion, its variance is

$$\hat{V}[\hat{s}(t_i)] = \frac{\hat{s}(t_i)[1 - \hat{s}(t_i)]}{n_i}. \tag{2.9}$$

Using the delta method, the variance of $\log \hat{s}(t_i)$ can be approximated from the variance of $\hat{s}(t_i)$. As the derivative of $\log(X)$ is $(1/X)$, the variance of $\log \hat{s}(t_i)$ is approximated by

$$\begin{aligned}\hat{V}[\log \hat{s}(t_i)] &\approx \left[\frac{1}{\hat{s}(t_i)}\right]^2 \left\{\frac{\hat{s}(t_i)[1 - \hat{s}(t_i)]}{n_i}\right\} \\ &\approx \frac{1 - \hat{s}(t_i)}{\hat{s}(t_i) n_i}.\end{aligned} \tag{2.10}$$

For analytic convenience, both numerator and denominator are multiplied by a common term n_i, which leads to

$$\hat{V}[\log \hat{s}(t_i)] \approx \frac{n_i[1 - \hat{s}(t_i)]}{\hat{s}(t_i)(n_i)^2}. \tag{2.11}$$

As $\hat{s}(t_i) \times n_i = (n_i - d_i)$, Equation (2.11) can be written by

$$\hat{V}[\log \hat{s}(t_i)] \approx \frac{d_i}{(n_i - d_i)n_i}. \tag{2.12}$$

Given Equation (2.12), the variance of $\log \hat{S}(t)$ can be obtained by summing up variances of all $\log \hat{s}(t_i)$ values, where $t_i \leq t$, given by

$$\hat{V}\left[\log \hat{S}(t_i)\right] \approx \sum_{t_i \leq t} \frac{d_i}{(n_i - d_i)n_i}. \tag{2.13}$$

Lastly, the variance of the survival probability $\hat{S}(t)$ can be approximated by performing a retransformation procedure using the delta method. Because the derivative of exp(X) is still exp(X), exp[log(x)] is X and hence the final equation is

$$\hat{V}\left[\hat{S}(t_i)\right] \approx \left[\hat{S}(t)\right]^2 \sum_{t_i \leq t} \frac{d_i}{(n_i - d_i)n_i}. \tag{2.14}$$

Equation (2.14) is the famous Greenwood formula, widely used in the descriptive analysis of survival data. The square root of this equation yields an estimate of the standard error for $\hat{S}(t)$. Given the Greenwood formula, once the point estimate of $S(t)$ is obtained, an approximate of its variance can be readily calculated using empirical data of d_i and n_i from a Kaplan–Meier table. Kalbfleisch and Prentice (2002) consider it valid to use a normal approximation of the distribution of $\hat{S}(t)$ with mean $S(t)$ and the variance estimate if censoring is not sizable and the sample size is large. Such validity holds whether the event time T is discrete or continuous or mixed with discrete and continuous components.

With the same rationale, the variance of the cumulative hazard rate at t can be estimated by $V\left[-\log \hat{S}(t)\right]$, using the same procedure that derives the Greenwood formula. After some algebra, the variance of the Nelson–Aalen estimator can be written by

$$\hat{V}[H(t)] \approx \sum_{t_i \leq t} \frac{d_i}{n_i^2}. \tag{2.15}$$

In SAS, the PROC LIFETEST procedure not only calculates the Kaplan–Meier survival estimates but it also computes corresponding standard errors using the square root of the Greenwood formula. SAS Program 2.1, used to generate a plot demonstrating the Kaplan–Meier estimates, also derives the probability of survival and its standard error at each survival time, as summarized in Table 2.3. The interested reader might want to practice whether his or her hand calculation agrees with the estimates reported in the table.

2.1.4 Confidence intervals and confidence bands of the survival function

Conventionally, given the estimate of the variance and a significance level α, the confidence interval of an asymptotically normally distributed estimate can be readily computed. For example, for a continuous random variable X distributed as $N(\mu, \sigma^2)$, its 95 % confidence interval with $\alpha = 0.05$ is simply given by $\bar{X} \pm 1.96\left[\hat{V}(X)\right]^{1/2}$. A serious defect, however, arises from using this conventional procedure for estimating the variance of the survival

Table 2.3 Kaplan–Meier estimates and standard errors from SAS Program 3.1.

Time (months)	Probability of survival	Survival standard error
0	1.0000	0.0000
5	0.9167	0.0798
17	0.8333	0.1076
20+	0.8333	0.1076
24	0.7407	0.1295
32	0.6481	0.1426
35+	0.6481	0.1426
40	0.5401	0.1544
46	0.4321	0.1568
47	0.3241	0.1503
50	0.2160	0.1335
59	0.1080	0.1014
74	0.0000	—

function. Whereas a standard continuous variable has range $(-\infty, \infty)$, the probability of survival ranges between 0 and 1. Given this restriction, using the standard equation can yield the value of $\hat{S}(t)$ out of its bounds, thus yielding impossible estimates. Given this concern, the confidence interval of $\hat{S}(t)$ needs to be estimated by some transformation approaches, from which the range of $\hat{S}(t)$ can be restricted.

There are a number of popular transformation functions that can be applied to derive a confidence interval of $\hat{S}(t)$ with range (0, 1). These transformation approaches include the Wilson score method, arcsine–square root transformation, logit transformation, and log–log transformation. The Wilson score method, developed by Edwin B. Wilson (1927), improves the normal approximation interval by imputing a new asymptotic variance based on a new parameter instead of the proportion itself. For the 95 % confidence, the Wilson score method derives a nearly identical interval to that derived from the normal approximation. The arcsine–square root transformation, a widely used method to compute point-wise confidence limits for the survival function, takes the arcsine of the square root of a number with the range (−1, 1). This transformation derives the variance and a confidence interval stabilizing for situations with no censoring. The logit transformation, also widely used, yields the confidence interval for the logit of $\hat{S}(t)$ first and then this logit-based interval is retransformed to the confidence limits of $\hat{S}(t)$. The reader familiar with generalized linear modeling might remember that the probability linked to a logit function takes a value between 0 and 1.

In survival analysis, the most popular transformation function for the confidence interval of $\hat{S}(t)$ is perhaps the so-called *log–log transformation*, developed by Kalbfleisch and Prentice (2002). The logic of this transformation method is that the asymptotic normal distribution of $\hat{S}(t)$ should be first transformed to a continuous function with unrestricted bounds. Specifically, they propose first to estimate the variance of the following transformed function:

$$\hat{\upsilon}(t) = \log\left[-\log \hat{S}(t)\right]. \tag{2.16}$$

Equation (2.16) specifies a well-known transformation function in survival analysis, referred to as the *log–log survival function*. As discussed in Chapter 1, $-\log S(t)$ is simply the cumulative hazard rate at time t; therefore the log–log survival function is actually the log transformation of the cumulative hazard function with a range from minus infinity to plus infinity. Given this property, the log–log survival function is also called the *log function of the cumulative hazard*.

Applying the delta method with respect to the Greenwood formula, the variance of Equation (2.16) can be derived:

$$\hat{V}[\hat{\upsilon}(t)] \approx \frac{1}{\left[\log \hat{S}(t)\right]^2} \sum_{t_i \leq t} \frac{d_i}{(n_i - d_i)n_i} \approx \frac{\hat{V}\left[\hat{S}(t)\right]}{\left[\hat{S}(t)\log \hat{S}(t)\right]}. \tag{2.17}$$

Given Equation (2.17), the confidence interval for the log–log survival function is given by

$$\log\left[-\log \hat{S}(t)\right] \pm z_{1-\alpha/2}\sqrt{\frac{\hat{V}\left[\hat{S}(t)\right]}{\left[\hat{S}(t)\log \hat{S}(t)\right]}}, \tag{2.18}$$

where $z_{1-\alpha/2}$ is the z-score for the upper $\alpha/2$ percentile of the standard normal distribution. As the log–log survival function is the log transformation of $H(t)$, the confidence interval for the survival function can be estimated by taking the exponential form of Equation (2.18) twice, which leads to

$$\left[\hat{S}(t)\right]^{1/\tilde{\theta}} \leq \left[\hat{S}(t)\right] \leq \left[\hat{S}(t)\right]^{\tilde{\theta}}, \tag{2.19}$$

where

$$\tilde{\theta} = \exp\left\{ z_{1-\alpha/2}\sqrt{\frac{\hat{V}\left[\hat{S}(t)\right]}{\left[\hat{S}(t)\log \hat{S}(t)\right]}}\right\}. \tag{2.20}$$

Equations (2.19) and (2.20) yield a confidence interval of $\hat{S}(t)$ ranging between 0 and 1. This retransformed confidence interval is considered to provide the correct coverage probability for a $(1 - \alpha)$ interval, valid even for very small samples with heavy censoring (Borgan and Liestøl, 1990). Given the nonlinearity after retransformation, however, this confidence interval is not symmetric about $\hat{S}(t)$.

As limits of an independent Kaplan–Meier survival estimate, the confidence interval of $\hat{S}(t)$ *is not associated with the entire lifetime process; rather, it only covers the true value of* $S(t)$ with probability $(1 - \alpha)$ at a single time point. Therefore, the confidence interval of the survival rate is not considered highly informative in survival analysis. For a lifetime process, it is essential statistically to combine a series of confidence intervals for the survival function, thereby constituting a $(1 - \alpha)$ confidence region for the entire survival curve. In statistics, such a confidence region is referred to as the *confidence bands*. Though closely connected with each other, the confidence bands differ conceptually and mathematically from the point-wise confidence intervals. While a point-wise confidence interval only attaches to the survival estimate at an individual time point, the confidence bands cover the entire survival curve simultaneously, with each point-wise confidence band behaving as an integral element of the whole confidence region. For this reason, confidence bands are also called *simultaneous confidence bands* or *simultaneous confidence intervals*. One of the important features in confidence bands is that if each confidence interval individually has probability (1 – α), the simultaneous coverage probability is generally less than (1 – α). Therefore, it is unacceptable to derive confidence bands by connecting the endpoints of all point-wise confidence intervals.

The derivation of confidence bands involves complex mathematical justifications and inferences. In particular, a point-wise confidence band, denoted by $\hat{S}(t) \pm \tilde{w}(t)$ with coverage probability (1 – α), satisfies the following condition for each value of t:

$$\Pr\left\{\left[\hat{S}(t) - \tilde{w}(t)\right] \leq \hat{S}(t) \leq \left[\hat{S}(t) + \tilde{w}(t)\right]\right\} = 1 - \alpha, \tag{2.21}$$

where $\tilde{w}$ is the confidence width determined by α. The lower and upper limits, $\left[\hat{S}(t) - \tilde{w}(t)\right]$ and $\left[\hat{S}(t) + \tilde{w}(t)\right]$, are sometimes denoted by $\tilde{L}$ and $\tilde{U}$, respectively.

There are two popular methods for calculating the confidence bands with respect to the Kaplan–Meier survival estimates. The first method is proposed by Hall and Wellner (1980), referred to as the *Hall–Wellner band*. The second approach, developed by Nair (1984), is called the *equal precision band*. For both methods, the confidence bands are constructed using the confidence coefficients taken from special distributions. These coefficients are provided in some textbooks and academic works (e.g., Klein and Moeschberger, 2003). Both bands can be computed by most statistical software packages including SAS (in PROC LIFETEST). Therefore, I do not include those coefficients tables in this book.

The mathematical inferences and the estimation procedures for both the Hall–Wellner and the equal precision bands are complex; for details of mathematical justifications and inferences, the interested reader is referred to Borgan and Liestøl (1990), Hall and Wellner (1980), Klein and Moeschberger (2003), and Nair (1984). Operationally, the calculation can be performed by taking the following four steps:

Step 1. Pick two time points, t_L and t_U. If the Hall–Wellner band is used, $t_L = 0$ and t_U is the event time just less than the largest observed event time; if the equal precision band is applied, t_L is just larger than the first observed event time and t_U is the same as above.

Step 2. Calculate the values of two confidence band coefficients, denoted $\acute{a}_L$ and $\acute{a}_U$, respectively, given by

$$\acute{a}_L = \frac{n\hat{V}\left[\hat{S}(t_L)\right]}{1 + n\hat{V}\left[\hat{S}(t_L)\right]} \tag{2.22}$$

and

$$\acute{a}_U = \frac{n\hat{V}\left[\hat{S}(t_U)\right]}{1 + n\hat{V}\left[\hat{S}(t_U)\right]}. \tag{2.23}$$

Step 3. Using values of $\acute{a}_L$ and $\acute{a}_U$, find the third coefficient, denoted either by $\acute{\kappa}_\alpha(\acute{a}_L, \acute{a}_U)$ for the Hall–Wellner band or by $\acute{c}_\alpha(\acute{a}_L, \acute{a}_U)$ for the equal precision band, from the tables for confidence coefficients of 100(1 – α) confidence bands.

Step 4. There are several transformation forms for the confidence bands, as for confidence intervals. With respect to the popular log–log transformation, the confidence band can be expressed as

$$\left[\hat{S}(t)\right]^{1/\tilde{\theta}} \leq \left[\hat{S}(t)\right] \leq \left[\hat{S}(t)\right]^{\tilde{\theta}}, \tag{2.24}$$

where

$$\tilde{\theta} = \exp\left\{\frac{k_\alpha(\acute{a}_L, \acute{a}_U)\left[1 + n\hat{V}\left(\hat{S}(t)\right)\right]}{\sqrt{n}\log\left[\hat{S}(t)\right]}\right\} \quad \text{for Hall–Wellner band,} \tag{2.25}$$

$$\tilde{\theta} = \exp\left\{\frac{c_\alpha(\acute{a}_L, \acute{a}_U)\sqrt{\hat{V}\left[\hat{S}(t)\right]}}{\log\left[\hat{S}(t)\right]}\right\} \quad \text{for equal precision band.} \tag{2.26}$$

In Equations (2.25) and (2.26), $\acute{\kappa}_\alpha$ or $\acute{c}_\alpha$ is the upper α fractile of the least observed upper bound. In practice, only the intervals for values of t greater than the first observed event time and smaller than the greatest observed event time need to be computed.

The two types of bands differ in several perspectives. The Hall–Wellner confidence bands are not proportional to the point-wise confidence intervals, as their derivation uses some ad hoc formulas. The equal precision method, on the other hand, yields proportional results to point-wise confidence intervals; specifically, the approach applies identical formulas to calculate confidence intervals and confidence bands, and the only difference between the two estimators is that the z-score is used to calculate confidence intervals and a different coefficient to derive confidence bands. Overall, the Hall–Wellner method provides better results than the equal precision when applying the log–log transformation, whereas the equal precision bands are more suitable when the arcsine–square root transformation is used.

To illustrate differences between confidence intervals and confidence bands for the Kaplan–Meier survival estimates, the data of older Americans described in Chapter 1 are used. In particular, I want to examine the two-year survival function among those diagnosed with cancer at baseline. In the AHEAD data, there are 39 survival times observed by the end of the 24th month, 19 actual events (those who died of cancer) and 20 censored cases. The following SAS program is constructed to estimate the survival function, confidence intervals, and confidence bands using lifetime data of those 39 individuals.

SAS Program 2.3:

```
options ls=80 ps=56 nodate number pageno=1 center;
ods select all;
ods trace off;
ods listing;
title1;
run;

data Kaplan_Meier;
 input Months Status @@;
datalines;
```

```
1 0 2 0 3 1 3 1 3 1 4 1 4 1 5 0 5 0 5 0 6 1 6 1 7 1 8 1
8 1 9 1 9 1 9 1 10 0 12 0 12 0 12 0 12 1 13 1 14 1 15 1
19 0 20 0 21 0 21 1 22 0 22 0 22 1 22 1 22 0 23 0 23 0
23 0 23 0
;

ods html;
ods graphics on;

ods select SurvivalPlot;
proc lifetest data=Kaplan_Meier OUTSURV=out1 Confband=HW Conftype=loglog
plots=survival(CB=HW);
  time Months * Status(0);
run;

proc print data=out1;
     title2 "OUTSURV data set";
     title3 "CONFBAND=all, CONFTYPE=Loglog";
run;

ods graphics off;
ods trace off;
```

In SAS Program 2.3, the input data of 39 survival times and their censoring statuses are saved in the SAS temporary dataset 'Kaplan_Meier.' The two variables, 'Months' and 'Status,' are defined previously in SAS Program 2.1. In the PROC LIFETEST statement, I ask SAS to create a temporary output dataset 'out1' containing the survival estimates and then to plot them with graphics using the ODS. To obtain the Hall–Wellner bands in the out = out1 dataset, I specify the CONFBAND = HW option (for a brief illustration, only the Hall–Wellner bands are used in this example; if both the Hall–Wellner and equal precision bands are needed, the CONFBAND = all option needs to specified). The CONFTYPE = LOGLOG option is specified to apply the log–log transformation for calculating the confidence intervals and confidence bands. Lastly, I request SAS to display a specific plot of the Hall–Wellner bands for the survival function. Other commands have been described previously.

SAS Program 2.3 derives Table 2.4, where the second column is the survival time and the third column displays whether a given survival time is an actual or a censored survival time, with 1 = censored. While the fourth column presents the Kaplan–Meier survival probabilities, the fifth and sixth columns are the lower and upper limits of the confidence interval for each survival estimate given $\alpha = 0.05$. Similarly, the last two columns demonstrate the lower and upper limits of the confidence band derived from the Hall–Wellner method. As evidenced in this table, the confidence band of each survival probability has much wider confidence limits than the corresponding confidence interval. The latter, associated independently with a single time point, seriously underestimates the true variability of the survival function. Therefore, in survival analysis, especially in clinical and epidemiological settings, the confidence bands should be regularly used for demonstrating a true confidence range of the survival function.

SAS Program 2.3 also yields a plot of the Hall–Wellner confidence bands on the Kaplan–Meier estimates, shown in Figure 2.2. The plot displays the confidence region of the survival

Table 2.4 Kaplan–Meier estimates, confidence intervals, and confidence bands.

Obs	Months	OUTSURV data aet CONFBAND=all, CONFTYPE=Loglog _CENSOR_	SURVIVAL	SDF_LCL	SDF_UCL	HW_LCL	HW_UCL
1	0	—	1.00000	1.00000	1.00000	—	—
2	1	1	1.00000	—	—	—	—
3	2	1	1.00000	—	—	—	—
4	3	0	0.91892	0.76931	0.97311	0.24868	0.99488
5	4	0	0.86486	0.70534	0.94140	0.43793	0.97480
6	5	1	0.86486	—	—	—	—
7	5	1	0.86486	—	—	—	—
8	5	1	0.86486	—	—	—	—
9	6	0	0.80522	0.63366	0.90225	0.46431	0.94066
10	7	0	0.77540	0.59982	0.88108	0.45706	0.92067
11	8	0	0.71575	0.53506	0.83624	0.42621	0.87709
12	9	0	0.62628	0.44371	0.76377	0.36158	0.80633
13	10	1	0.62628	—	—	—	—
14	12	0	0.59497	0.41254	0.73749	0.33582	0.78107
15	12	1	0.59497	—	—	—	—
16	12	1	0.59497	—	—	—	—
17	12	1	0.59497	—	—	—	—
18	13	0	0.55778	0.37391	0.70720	0.30109	0.75282
19	14	0	0.52060	0.33699	0.67587	0.26638	0.72461
20	15	0	0.48341	0.30159	0.64353	0.23199	0.69654
21	19	1	0.48341	—	—	—	—
22	20	1	0.48341	—	—	—	—
23	21	0	0.43946	0.25877	0.60648	0.18760	0.66767
24	21	1	0.43946	—	—	—	—
25	22	0	0.34181	0.17709	0.52175	0.09299	0.61559
26	22	1	—	—	—	—	—
27	22	1	—	—	—	—	—
28	22	1	—	—	—	—	—
29	23	1	—	—	—	—	—
30	23	1	—	—	—	—	—
31	23	1	—	—	—	—	—
32	23	1	—	—	—	—	—

probabilities within a two-year observation period. Notice that the Hall–Wellner confidence bands exclude the initial observed survival times because, according to Borgan and Liestøl (1990), anomalous values of the lower confidence band are often detected at the start of the survival process when the log–log or arcsine transformations are used. Consequently, displaying the Hall–Wellner bands in those local regions is not informative.

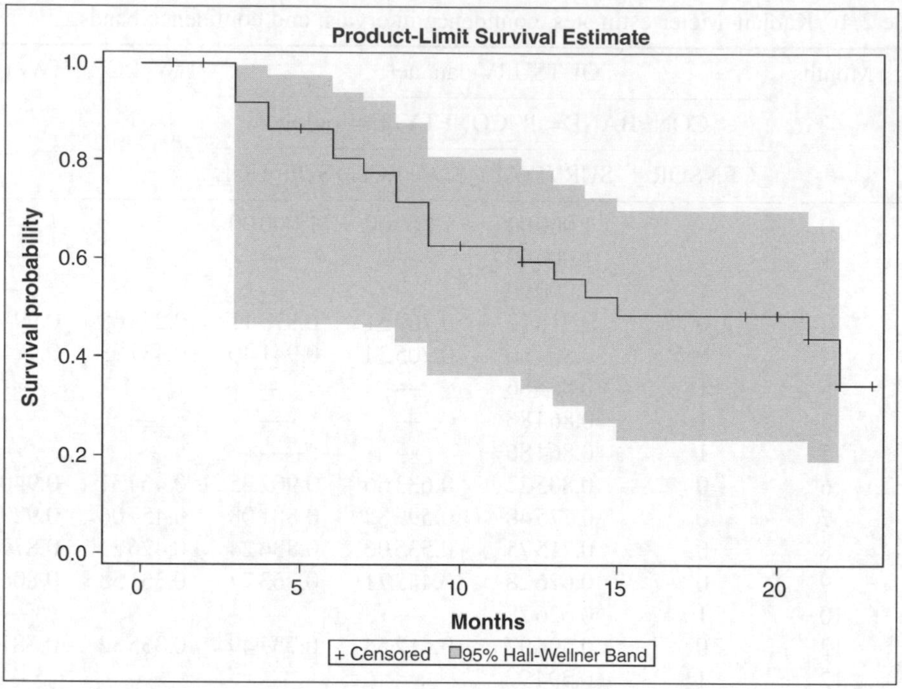

Figure 2.2 Hall–Wellner confidence bands for the probability of survival.

2.2 Life table methods

Other than the Kaplan–Meier and Nelson–Aalen estimators, a popular nonparametric approach in survival analysis is the life table method, which also has some capacity to handle right censoring. Demographers and epidemiologists have a long history of using life tables for analyzing survival data. A typical life table generates the probability of survival at a particular year of age, the life expectancy at birth, and the life expectancy remaining at an exact age, based on the hypothesis of a synthetic cohort. Separate life tables can be created for comparing mortality rates and life expectancies among individuals of different demographic and socioeconomic characteristics. Though originally designed to analyze mortality and survival, the life table method has been extended to calculate actuaries, disability-free life expectancy, geographical mobility, marital status patterns, occupational careers, and multidimensional transitions in health care (Crimmins, Hayward, and Saito, 1996; Hayward and Grady, 1990; Liu *et al.*, 1995, 1997; Rogers, 1975; Rogers, Rogers, and Belanger, 1990; Schoen, 1988; Schoen and Land, 1979; Sullivan, 1971). In a survival analysis, Gehan (1969) provides specifications of the continuous hazard function and the probability density function from discrete estimates of a life table, thereby advancing the life table method to the analysis of event times and survival processes.

In this section, I first describe Gehan's basic formulations of several continuous lifetime functions based on the theory of large-sample approximations. Next, I briefly introduce some of the advanced life table techniques, such as the multistate life table and the multidimensional Markov processes for events with frequent turnovers. Lastly, an empirical example is provided to display how to construct a life table using empirical survival data.

2.2.1 Life table indicators

Like the Kaplan–Meier estimator, a life table is created to calculate the probability of survival and its changes. In demography and epidemiology, however, the survival function in a life table is generally viewed as a function of age, rather than of time, largely due to the fact that survival data used in these fields often come from the age-specific death rates in a specific period. For analytic convenience, the probability of survival is usually multiplied by 100 000 in a conventional life table, yielding a new indicator, denoted by l_a, where the letter 'a' represents an exact age ($a = 0, 1, \ldots, \omega$), referred to as the *number of survivors on a radix*. As l_a is simply $S(a) \times 100000$, in a conventional life table $l_0 = 100000$ and $l_\omega = 0$. Using the vital registration statistics or survey data with respect to a specific period, a conventional life table is often constructed by assuming a synthetic birth cohort following current age-specific death rates (Keyfitz, 1985; Siegel and Swanson, 2004). Consequently, survival processes described in a conventional life table do not reflect actual trajectories of survival dynamics because they are derived from current mortality schedules across many population birth cohorts.

In survival analysis, the conventional life table method is extended by counting the actual number of survivors, of censored observations, and of events, from longitudinal data of event histories. Accordingly, observational time, rather than age, is used to define intervals to highlight the dynamic nature of a lifetime event. In many aspects, this modified life table method bears a tremendous resemblance to the Kaplan–Meier and Nelson–Aalen estimators, as will be seen below. To be in line with the focus of this book, therefore, many of the following specifications are based on Gehan (1969) with some minor notational modifications.

Let the survival data be grouped into $J + 1$ intervals, denoted by (t_{j-1}, t_j), where $j = 1, 2, \ldots, J + 1$, with the unit of interval j defined as $\tilde{b}_j = t_j - t_{j-1}$. By definition, $t_0 = 0$ and $t_{J+1} = \infty$, and accordingly $\tilde{b}_0 = 0$, $\tilde{b}_{J+1} = \infty$. Also, n_{j-1} is the number of individuals entering the interval (t_{j-1}, t_j) and d_j is the number of events occurring in interval j. In the absence of censoring, the difference between n_{j-1} and n_j yields the number of events in (t_{j-1}, t_j) and the ratio of the number of events over n_{j-1} generates the probability of experiencing a particular event in the interval.

In the presence of censoring, the *effective sample size* in (t_{j-1}, t_j), denoted by $\check{n}_j$, is defined and used for calculating the life table measures. Suppose c_j, the number of censored cases, falls in (t_{j-1}, t_j). The effective sample size at the start of the interval is conventionally given by

$$\check{n}_j = n_j - \frac{c_j}{2}, \tag{2.27}$$

where $(c_j/2)$ is the adjustment that only half of c_j, assumed to be evenly distributed in (t_{j-1}, t_j), should be counted in the total number of individuals exposed to the risk of the event. This adjustment is one of the key features in the life table method that counts survival times of censored cases in the estimation procedure. Accordingly, the conditional probability of experiencing the event, denoted by q_j, is estimated by

$$\hat{q}_j = \frac{d_j}{\breve{n}_j} = \frac{d_j}{n_j - \frac{c_j}{2}}, \tag{2.28}$$

where the denominator represents the unbiased amount of exposure to the risk, given the assumption of a uniform distribution of censored observations.

Given the association that $\hat{s}_j = 1 - \hat{q}_j$, the conditional probability of survival in (t_{j-1}, t_j) is

$$\hat{s}_j = 1 - \frac{d_j}{n_j - \frac{c_j}{2}}. \tag{2.29}$$

This estimate of the conditional probability is another main feature of the life table method. In the Kaplan–Meier estimator, censored survival times are counted only across intervals, as shown in Table 2.3; in the life table method, nevertheless, censored times are taken into account both across and within intervals.

The variance for the conditional probability of experiencing the event in (t_{j-1}, t_j) can be estimated by the conventional approach, given by

$$V(\hat{q}_j) = \frac{\hat{q}_j \hat{s}_j}{\breve{n}_j} = \frac{2\hat{q}_j \hat{s}_j}{2n_j - c_j}. \tag{2.30}$$

The square root of Equation (2.30) gives rise to an estimate of the standard error for $\hat{q}_j$. Notice that if n_j is small, Equation (2.30) can cause strong inconsistencies in the estimate, thereby affecting the quality of this estimator.

Given the conditional probability of the event, the survival function at the end of (t_{j-1}, t_j) is estimated as

$$\hat{S}(t_j) = \hat{S}(t_{j-1})\hat{s}_{j-1} = \prod_{j'=1}^{j} (1 - \hat{q}_{j'}). \tag{2.31}$$

As Equation (2.31) demonstrates, the life table estimator of the survival function is actually an approximation of the Kaplan–Meier method, expressed as the product of a series of interval-specific conditional probabilities of survival. When the sample size is large, the two approaches are asymptotically equivalent.

The estimation of the variance for the survival function also bears some resemblance to the estimator described in Section 2.1, given by

$$V\left[\hat{S}(t_j)\right] = \left[\hat{S}(t_j)\right]^2 \sum_{j'=1}^{j} \frac{\hat{q}_{j'}}{\hat{s}_{j'}\left(n_{j'} - \frac{c_{j'}}{2}\right)}. \tag{2.32}$$

The square root of Equation (2.32) yields an estimate for the standard error of the survival function at t_j. The reader might want to compare Equation (2.32) with the Greenwood formula (Equation (2.14)). In fact, in the absence of censoring, the variance estimate of the survival function in the life table method approximates the estimate derived from Equation (2.14).

According to Gehan (1969), the probability density function at the midpoint of (t_{j-1}, t_j), denoted by t_{mj}, can be approximated straightforwardly:

$$\hat{f}(t_{mj}) = \frac{\left[\hat{S}(t_{j-1}) - \hat{S}(t_j)\right]}{\tilde{b}_j} = \frac{\hat{S}(t_{j-1})\hat{q}_j}{\tilde{b}_j}, \tag{2.33}$$

with the variance estimator

$$\hat{V}\left[\hat{f}(t_{mj})\right] \cong \left[\hat{f}(t_{mj})\right]^2 \sum_{j'=1}^{j} \left[\frac{\hat{q}_{j'}}{\left(n_{j'} - \frac{c_{j'}}{2}\right)\hat{s}_{j'}} + \frac{\hat{s}_{j'}}{\left(n_{j'} - \frac{c_{j'}}{2}\right)\hat{q}_{j'}} \right]. \tag{2.34}$$

Obviously, the above p.d.f. estimate at the midpoint of a time interval is computed as the total probability of experiencing a particular event for the entire interval divided by the interval width $\tilde{b}_j$. The validity of Equations (2.33) and (2.34) is based on the assumption that events occurring within a time interval are evenly or linearly distributed.

Likewise, given this hypothesis, the hazard function at t_{mj} can also be estimated in the same fashion:

$$\hat{h}(t_{mj}) = \frac{2\hat{q}_j}{\tilde{b}_j(1+\hat{s}_j)} = \frac{d_j}{\tilde{b}_j\left[n_j - \frac{1}{2}(d_j + c_j)\right]}. \tag{2.35}$$

Notice that in Equation (2.35), only half of d_j, the number of events occurring in (t_{j-1}, t_j), are counted in the number of individuals exposed to the risk. As mentioned in Chapter 1, if $\tilde{b}_j$ represents a considerably wide unit of a time interval, the continuous $S(t)$ is a decreasing function within the interval, so not all n_{j-1} individuals are at risk in the entire interval. If events within the interval occur uniformly or linearly, counting half of d_j in the denominator yields a reasonable estimate of the hazard rate at the midpoint of the interval. This estimate, however, is an average, not necessarily reflecting an instantaneous rate, especially when events occur irregularly or nonlinearly. As demographers term it, Equation (2.35) essentially provides an estimate of the average hazard function (Siegel and Swanson, 2004).

Gehan (1969) also specifies an estimate for the variance of the estimated hazard rate at t_{mj}. With some notational modifications, it can be written as

$$\hat{V}\left[\hat{h}(t_{mj})\right] \cong \left[\hat{h}(t_{mj})\right]^2 \frac{1 - \left[b_j\hat{h}(t_{mj})/2\right]^2}{\left(n_j - \frac{c_j}{2}\right)\hat{q}_j}. \tag{2.36}$$

The above measures can be used when constructing a life table with the time interval as the basic unit. I would like to emphasize that the above formulas are mostly based on the theory of large-sample approximations, so the life table method is applicable only when the sample size is large enough for every time interval. If the sample size for a given interval is small (less than 20, say), the Kaplan–Meier or Nelson–Aalen estimators are preferable for an efficient nonparametric analysis of survival data. Given this restriction, the life table method is not recommended for a descriptive analysis of survival data obtained from clinical trials.

2.2.2 Multistate life tables

In survival analysis, an individual's event histories are sometimes linked to more than one single event process. At a given time, individuals may be exposed to the risks of several related events, thereby making survival processes attach to a set of competing risks. Examples of such phenomena include transitions in multiple modes of health (Crimmins, Hayward, and Saito, 1996; Land, Guralnik, and Blazer, 1994; Liu *et al.*, 1995), labor force participation (Hayward and Grady, 1990), and multidimensional transitions in health care (Liang *et al.*, 1996; Liu *et al.*, 1997). A number of demographers and statisticians have developed a series of statistical models for the description and analysis of such multidimensional processes in a life table format, generally referred to as the *multistate life table*. These models are generally associated with one or more states of origin (the state at the beginning of observation) and more than one state of destination (the state at the end of observation), which, combined, constitute a finite space for a set of stochastic and multidimensional survival processes.

To describe a multistate life table more effectively, here I provide a flow chart about transitions in functional status to aid in the interpretation of the mathematical specifications given below. Suppose that at the beginning of a time interval individuals are divided into two groups according to function status, 'functional independence' and 'functional dependence.' As observed at the origin of time, this functional status is referred to as the *state of origin*, denoted by $\tilde{i} = 1, 2$. At the end of the observation, there are three possible outcomes in terms of that individual's functional status: 'functionally independent,' 'functionally dependent,' and 'dead,' referred to as the *state of destination* and denoted by $\tilde{j} = 1, 2, 3$, respectively. Between the two functional states, 'functional independence' and 'functional dependence,' a transition can occur from either direction within the time interval, and therefore they are called the *transient states*. The third status at destination, 'dead,' is a permanently ending state, and conventionally it is called the *absorbing state*. The multidimensional transitions between these states are displayed in Figure 2.3, where $P_{\tilde{i}\tilde{j}}$ indicates a transition process from the origin state $\tilde{i}$ to the destination state $\tilde{j}$. Given the assumption

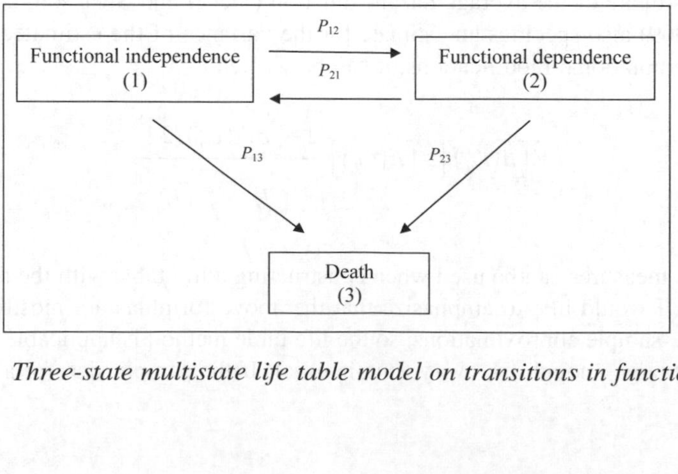

Figure 2.3 Three-state multistate life table model on transitions in functional status.

that only one transition is permitted within a specific time interval, four transition processes can be identified: from functional independence to functional dependence, from functional independence to death, from functional dependence to functional independence, and from functional dependence to death. As defined, individuals can move in and out of the transient states, as shown by the arrowed lines in Figure 2.3.

Like a conventional life table, the multistate life table estimates the probability of survival at a particular year of age, the life expectancy at birth, and the life expectancy remaining at an exact age. Each of these life table measures, however, needs to be calculated for each state of origin. Descriptively, the multistate life table is generally defined as a time-inhomogeneous and continuous-time Markov process model with finite space Ω. The state space Ω of the stochastic process has $\mathcal{K}+1$ states, where $\mathcal{K}$ is a positive integer greater than 1 (in terms of the example about transitions in functional status, $\mathcal{K}$ is 2). The $(\mathcal{K}+1)$ th state is the absorbing state. As indicated by Figure 2.3, two-way transitions are allowed between the transient states; that is, while a functionally independent person at the beginning can become functionally dependent within the time interval, an individual is permitted to recover from functional dependence within the period.

On the state space Ω, I define a stochastic process, $[\ddot{y}(t): t \geq 0]$, as seen by transition probabilities from the state of origin to the state of destination. The transition probabilities between the $\mathcal{K}+1$ states of $\ddot{y}$, assumed to be continuous, are given by

$$\tilde{\pi}_{\tilde{i}\tilde{j}}[t, \Delta t) = \Pr\left[\ddot{y}(t+\Delta t) = \tilde{j} \,\middle|\, \ddot{y}(t) = \tilde{i}\right], \tag{2.37}$$

where $\tilde{\pi}_{\tilde{i}\tilde{j}}[t, \Delta t)$ represents the probability that an individual in state $\tilde{i}$ at time t will be in state $\tilde{j}$ at time $(t + \Delta t)$. The corresponding transition force, statistically referred to as the gross flow hazard rate, is

$$h_{\tilde{i}\tilde{j}}(t) = \lim_{\Delta t \to 0} \frac{\tilde{\pi}_{\tilde{i}\tilde{j}}[t, \Delta t)}{\Delta t}, \quad \text{for } \tilde{i} \neq \tilde{j}, \tag{2.38}$$

where $h_{\tilde{i}\tilde{j}}(t)$ is the force of decrement for a transition from state $\tilde{i}$ to state $\tilde{j}$ at time t. As defined in Chapter 1, it is nonnegative but not necessarily smaller than 1.

If persistence in state $\tilde{i}$ from time t to time $(t + \Delta t)$ can be viewed as a special type of transition, its transition probability can be written by

$$\tilde{\pi}_{\tilde{i}\tilde{i}}[t, \Delta t) = 1 - \sum_{\tilde{j}=1}^{\mathcal{K}+1} \tilde{\pi}_{\tilde{i}\tilde{j}}[t, \Delta t), \quad \text{for } \tilde{j} \neq \tilde{i}. \tag{2.39}$$

The derivation of Equation (2.39) is based on the constraint that a set of transition probabilities must sum up to 1.

Likewise $h_{\tilde{i}\tilde{i}}(t)$, the force of persistence in $\tilde{i}$ at time t, is

$$h_{\tilde{i}\tilde{i}}(t) = -\lim_{\Delta t \to 0} \left[\frac{1 - \sum_{\tilde{j}=1}^{\mathcal{K}+1} \tilde{\pi}_{\tilde{i}\tilde{j}}[t, \Delta t)}{\Delta t} \right] = -\sum_{\tilde{j}=1}^{\mathcal{K}+1} h_{\tilde{i}\tilde{j}}(t), \quad \text{for } \tilde{j} \neq \tilde{i}, \tag{2.40}$$

where $h_{\tilde{i}\tilde{i}}(t)$, as a counterforce, is always nonpositive, referred to as the *force of retention* (Schoen, 1988). The transition probabilities and the forces of transition can be conveniently arranged into two $(\mathcal{K}+1)$ by $(\mathcal{K}+1)$ stochastic matrices, defined as $\Pi(t, \Delta t)$ and $\boldsymbol{h}(t)$, respectively. By definition, each row of the Π matrix sums to 1 and each row of the $\boldsymbol{h}$ matrix sums to 0.

Given $S(0) = 1$, the initial distribution of survival probability in state $\tilde{i}$, denoted by $S_{\tilde{i}}(0)$, is mathematically defined by

$$S_{\tilde{i}}(0) = \Pr\left[\ddot{y}(0) = \tilde{i}\right], \quad \text{for } \tilde{i} \in \Omega, \tag{2.41}$$

with the range (0, 1). Within the context of transitions in functional status, for example, $S_{\tilde{i}}(0)$ indicates the probability distribution of individuals in the two states of origin at time 0 given that $S_1(0) + S_2(0) = 1$. For younger populations, it is likely that no one is functionally dependent, so $S_1(0) = 1$ and $S_2(0) = 0$. Similarly, for individuals beyond a certain old age, everyone may be functionally disabled, so we have $S_1(0) = 0$ and $S_2(0) = 1$. When constructing a multistate life table, this distribution can be obtained from empirical data.

Given $S_i(0)$, the survival function at state $\tilde{i}$ can be defined as follows

$$S_{\tilde{i}}(t) = \Pr\left[\ddot{y}(t) = \tilde{i}\right] = \sum_{\tilde{k} \in \Omega} S_{\tilde{k}}(0) \tilde{\pi}_{\tilde{k}\tilde{i}}(0, t), \tag{2.42}$$

Demographers call $S_{\tilde{i}}(0)$ the radix of a multistate life table, as the sequence of $S_{\tilde{i}}(t)$ is the survival function corresponding to the Markov chain. As usually applied, $S_{\tilde{i}}(t)$ can be multiplied by a value, such as 10^6, for analytic convenience (Hoem and Jensen, 1982), thereby generating a new life table indicator, termed $l_{\tilde{i}}(t)$. In the literature of multistate life table modeling, $l_{\tilde{i}}(t)$ is referred to as the stationary population corresponding to the Markov process.

The gross flows of the stationary population are specified as the function

$$l_{\tilde{i}\tilde{j}}[t, \Delta t) = l_{\tilde{i}}(t) \tilde{\pi}_{\tilde{i}\tilde{j}}[t, \Delta t), \tag{2.43}$$

where $l_{\tilde{i}\tilde{j}}[t, \Delta t)$ represents the number of individuals in state $\tilde{i}$ at time t who are in state $\tilde{j}$ at time $(t + \Delta t)$ with respect to the stationary population. Accordingly, a $(\mathcal{K}+1)$ by $(\mathcal{K}+1)$ matrix $\boldsymbol{l}(t, \Delta t)$ can be created containing elements $l_{\tilde{i}\tilde{j}}(t, \Delta t)$, referred to as the *matrix of gross flows*.

Within the context of event times, the expected life in state $\tilde{j}$ between time t_{j-1} and time t_j spent by those in state $\tilde{i}$ at time t_{j-1} can be written as

$$\tilde{L}_{\tilde{i}\tilde{j}}(t_{j-1}, t_j) = \int_0^1 l_{\tilde{i}\tilde{j}}(t_{j-1}, u) \mathrm{d}u, \tag{2.44}$$

where the unit $(t_j - t_{j-1})$ represents a discrete interval with width $\tilde{b}_j$, often set at 1 year in demographic and epidemiologic studies. $\tilde{L}_{\tilde{i}\tilde{j}}(\cdot)$ is also called the sojourn time, representing the total person-years lived. These person-years lived at the level of gross flows can be aggregated to the level of net flows, defined by

$$\tilde{L}_{\tilde{i}}[t_{j-1}, t_j) = \sum_{\tilde{j}=1}^{\tilde{k}} \tilde{L}_{\tilde{j}\tilde{i}}[t_{j-1}, t_j) = \int_0^1 l_{\tilde{i}}[t_{j-1} + u) \mathrm{d}u, \tag{2.45}$$

where $\tilde{L}_{\tilde{i}}(t_{j-1}, t_j)$ is the person-years lived in state $\tilde{i}$ between t_{j-1} and t_j without the constraint of being in state $\tilde{i}$ at time t_{j-1}.

The above equations summarize basic specifications of a traditional multistate life table. Researchers have developed a variety of estimating algorithms to formalize these functions (Land and Schoen, 1982; Liu *et al.*, 1995; Namboodiri and Suchindran, 1987; Rogers, 1975; Schoen, 1988; Schoen and Land, 1979). Because these accounting procedures are based on varying assumptions on patterns of transitions within a discrete interval (usually one year), there are distinct differences in the results derived from those approaches as well as a general distinction between the underlying stochastic processes of a given event and accounting procedures (Hoem and Jensen, 1982). While some traditional procedures only permit a single transition within a one-year period, several refined methods relax the single-transition assumption, thereby taking into account the return of those who have left a given state at an earlier stage (Schoen, 1988).

These methods, however, may still lead to substantial bias for lifetime events with rapid turnovers because those who have returned to the state of origin may leave there again soon. The pattern of health care use, for example, typifies such rapid processes, given the frequent and intense turnovers of hospitalization and institutionalization over time. Other dynamic processes that occur rapidly over time include adolescent dating behavior, the employment experiences of marginal workers, mental disorders like depression, and the like. Indeed, the traditional accounting procedures are not capable of handling these frequent events, resulting in a characterization of life-cycle experiences at variance with the true set of the stochastic processes.

Theoretically, difficulties in estimating more intense and rapidly unfolding processes can be resolved by using shorter time intervals. If the interval unit is sufficiently short to suit the circumstances of a rapid process, it may be reasonable to assume that the rate of transition from one state to another is constant across all subintervals, thereby retaining the standard ways of estimating interval-specific transition rates. Such a strategy, however, is usually not realistic, given the scarcity of empirical data on frequent transitions. Additionally, the use of survey data from multiple random samples, which is often the case in constructing a multi-state life table, would be highly restrictive, given an insufficient sample size for each much shortened subinterval. Hence, it is necessary to adapt the conventional estimation procedures to characterize accurately the phenomena that occur intensely and rapidly over time.

For example, if use of a wide time interval is unavoidable in constructing a multistate life table, the generation of transition probabilities needs to be based on the principle of the Chapman–Kolmogorov relation (Cox and Miller, 1978), given by

$$\tilde{\pi}_{\tilde{i}\tilde{j}}^{(\check{n})} = \sum_{j=1}^{\tilde{k}} \tilde{\pi}_{\tilde{i}\tilde{j}}^{(\check{n}-1)} \tilde{\pi}_{\tilde{j}\tilde{i}}^{(I)}, \quad \check{n} = (1, 2, \ldots), \tag{2.46}$$

where $\tilde{\pi}_{\tilde{i}\tilde{j}}^{(\check{n})}$ is defined as the probability of being in state $\tilde{j}$ at time $\check{n}$ for those who are at state $\tilde{i}$ at time 0, termed the *n-step transition probability*. Similarly, $\tilde{\pi}_{\tilde{i}\tilde{j}}^{(\check{n}-1)}$ is an $(\check{n}-1)$-step transition probability and $\tilde{\pi}_{\tilde{i}\tilde{j}}^{(I)}$ is a one-step transition probability. This Markov process equation indicates that, in the presence of repeated transitions within a time interval, the $\check{n}$-step transition probability is virtually the outcome of a series of one-step transition probabilities within an interval represented by $\check{n}$ steps. Other multistate life table indicators need to be adapted as well, according to repeated flows of transitions.

The mathematical algorithms of a multistate life table for events with rapid processes are complex, so I do not describe the detailed procedures further in this text. The interested reader is referred to Liu *et al*. (1997).

2.2.3 Illustration: Life table estimates for older Americans

In this subsection, I provide an empirical example to demonstrate how to construct a life table using the SAS code. Empirical data come from a random sample of older Americans diagnosed with lung cancer. Event time is measured as the number of months elapsed from the time of diagnosis to the time of death or the time of censoring. Given the information of actual survival and censored times, I first create a dataset containing the number of events and the number of censored cases in each month for a total of 12 months. Below is the SAS program for this study.

SAS Program 2.4:

```
title 'survival of older persons diagnosed with lung cancer';

data Life_Table;
  keep Freq Months Censored;
  retain Months -.5;
  input fail withdraw @@;
  Months + 1;
  Censored = 0;
  Freq = fail;
  output;
  Censored = 1;
  Freq = withdraw;
  output;
  datalines;

16 0 22 5 19 3 20 4 27 2 20 11 21 32 38 59 40 61
24 33 18 19 23 36
;
.........
```

In this program, I create three variables for the construction of the life table: Months (defined earlier), Censored (1 = censored, 0 = not censored), and Freq (the frequency variable). From the above program, two types of observations are created for each time interval, one indicating the event observations and the other the censored observations. As displayed, input data are the frequencies of events and censored cases in each month.

The next step is to specify the ODS GRAPHICS ON statement for generating graphics of the survival and hazard curves and invoke the PROC LIFETEST again to calculate various life table estimates. As a result, the remainder of SAS Program 2.4 is given below.

SAS Program 2.4 (continued):

```
.........
ods graphics on;

proc lifetest data = Life_Table method = lt intervals = (0 to 11 by 1)
              plots = (s, ls, lls, h, p);
```

```
   time Months * Censored(1);
   freq Freq;
run;

ods graphics off;
```

In SAS Program 2.4 (continued), I ask SAS to compute the life table survival estimates by specifying METHOD = LT. The INTERVALS = (0 to 11 by 1) option specifies that estimates for 12 intervals (0 to 11) are computed. The PLOTS = (s, ls, lls, h, p) option requests SAS to display graphs of the life table survival function estimate, negative log of the estimate (the cumulative hazard function), log of the negative log of the estimate (the log–log survival function), estimated density function at the midpoint of each interval, and estimated hazard function.

As a result of SAS Program 2.4, SAS constructs a life table containing the requested survival function estimates and the standard errors (each function is described in Subsection 2.2.1) and five requested lifetime graphs. While the life table thus produced includes a large amount of data, I only display a portion of the estimates in this text, as summarized in Table 2.5. The table shows that among the older persons diagnosed with lung cancer, the survival probability throughout the first month is 0.97 with a standard error of 0.01. As time progresses, the probability of survival declines initially and then accelerates in later stages of the observation period. The five-month probability of survival is about 0.86 (*SE* = 0.01). In the 10th month, the survival rate is slightly higher than 0.5, suggesting that about half of those older persons are expected to survive throughout 10 months. By the end of the 12th month, the chance of survival is only 0.34 with a standard error of 0.03. This twelve-month survival rate indicates that for older persons diagnosed with lung cancer, only about 35 % are expected to survive beyond a one-year period.

SAS Program 2.4 also produces many other survival estimates, such as the conditional probability of failure, the median residual lifetime, the probability density function, the

Table 2.5 Life table survival estimates for patients with lung cancer.

Interval (t_{i-1}, t_i)	Number failed	Number censored	Effective sample size	Survival function	Standard error of survival
0–1	16	0	553.0	1.0000	0.0000
1–2	22	5	534.5	0.9711	0.0071
2–3	19	3	508.5	0.9311	0.0108
3–4	20	4	486.0	0.8963	0.0130
4–5	27	2	463.0	0.8594	0.0149
5–6	20	11	429.5	0.8093	0.0168
6–7	21	32	388.0	0.7716	0.0180
7–8	38	59	321.5	0.7299	0.0192
8–9	40	61	223.5	0.6436	0.0214
9–10	24	33	136.5	0.5284	0.0241
10–11	18	19	86.5	0.4355	0.0263
11–12	23	36	41.0	0.3449	0.0282

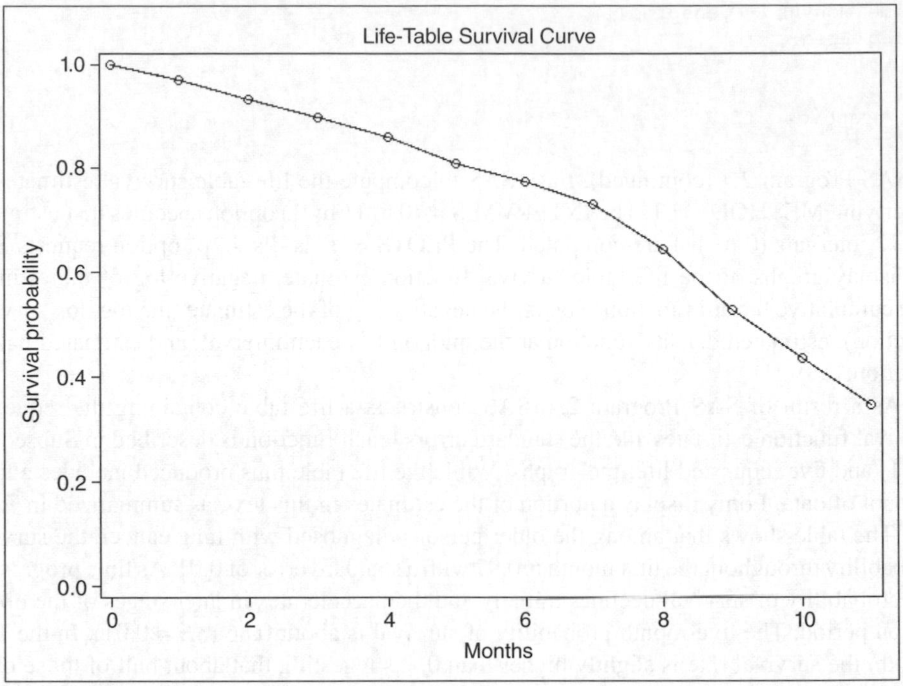

Figure 2.4 Life-table survival function for older persons with lung cancer.

hazard rate, and the standard error of each of these life table measures. The interested reader might want to rerun SAS Program 2.4 for viewing more results.

As mentioned above, five graphs are produced from SAS Program 2.4. Here, I select for display the graphs of the survival function and the cumulative hazard function, the two lifetime functions I consider to be most important for the description of survival processes for a population. First, Figure 2.4 displays the plot of the life table survival function estimate. It is interesting to note that in the first seven months or so, the survival function declines linearly; nevertheless, from that time point forward the probability of survival drops more sharply, highlighting the increased mortality acceleration in later months of the observation interval.

The next plot, Figure 2.5, displays the negative log of the survival estimates, the cumulative hazard function, and an accelerated cumulative hazard function over time. As will be discussed in Chapter 3, if the plot of the negative log of the survival function versus survival time approximates a straight line, the hazard function is constant, thereby highlighting an exponential distribution of survival times. If it is not, as shown by the above curve, the hazard function does not tend to be constant within this twelve-month period.

2.3 Group comparison of survival functions

The Kaplan–Meier estimator can be applied to compare survival functions by adding certain stratification factors. The stratification factors often selected include treatments in clinical

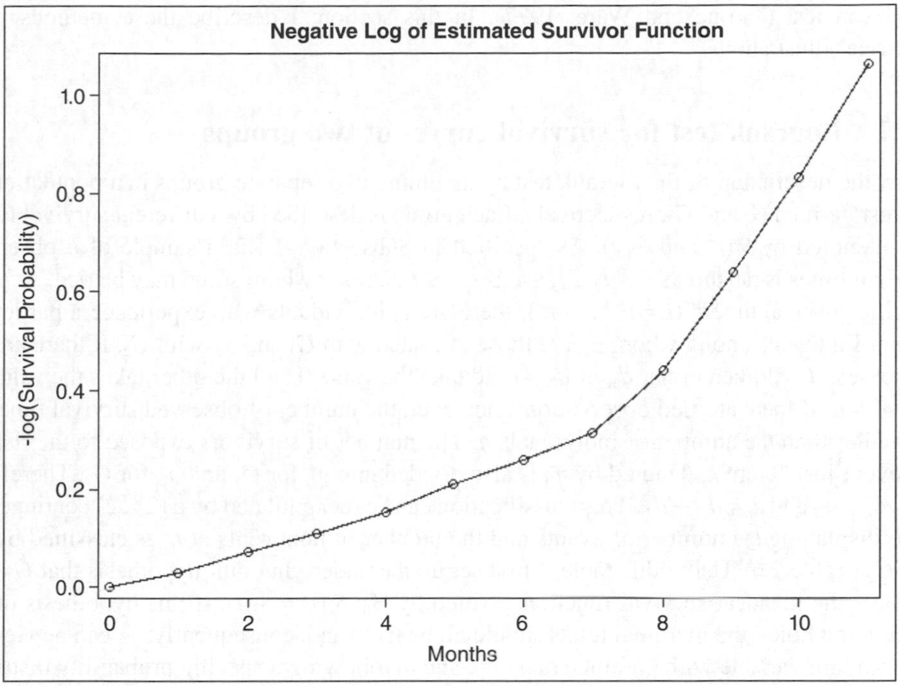

Figure 2.5 Negative log of the estimated survival function (the cumulative Hazard function) for older persons diagnosed with lung cancer.

trials and such sociodemographic variables as age group, gender, ethnicity, and marital status. In comparing the survival functions between two or more groups, an observed difference can be either the outcome of an actual disparity or a reflection of the sampling error. Therefore, it is essential to perform significance tests for determining whether an observed difference is true.

Significance tests on survival curves of different population groups generally begin with a null hypothesis, denoted by H_0, assuming no statistically significant difference. A significance level α, the predetermined critical value in a probability distribution, is regularly used to help determine whether to accept or reject the H_0 hypothesis. In particular, if the p-value of an observed difference is less than or equal to α, the difference is considered statistically significant, thereby resulting in the rejection of the underlying null hypothesis. If the p-value is greater than α, the null hypothesis is probably true and a group difference in the survival function may occur merely by chance.

Statisticians use various probability functions for hypothesis testing, the normal and the chi-squared distributions being the most widely applied. In survival analysis, there are a number of methods that can be used to test group differences in the survival function statistically. These techniques include, but are not limited to, the Mantel–Haenszel logrank test (Mantel and Haenszel, 1959), the Peto and Peto logrank test (Peto and Peto, 1972), the Gehan generalized Wilcoxon rank sum test (Gehan, 1967), the Peto and Peto and Prentice generalized Wilcoxon test (Peto and Peto, 1972; Prentice, 1978), and the Tarone and Ware modified

Wilcoxon test (Tarone and Ware, 1977). In this section, I describe these methods with empirical illustrations.

2.3.1 Logrank test for survival curves of two groups

I start the description of the logrank test by assuming two separate groups in a population of interest, termed G_1 and G_2, respectively. Each group is described by a different survival function, denoted by $S_1(t)$ and $S_2(t)$. As specified in Subsection 2.1.2, a sample of n observed survival times is ranked as $t_1 \leq t_2 \leq t_3 \leq t_4 \leq \cdots \leq t_n$, among whom some may be tied. At each specific survival time t_i ($i = 1, \ldots, n'$), there are d_i individuals who experience a particular event of interest, among whom d_{1i} are those affiliated with G_1 and d_{2i} with G_2. If there are no tied cases, $d_i = 1$, then either d_{1i} or d_{2i} would take the value 0 and the other takes the value 1, and $n' = n$. If there are tied observations, however, the number of observed survival times n' is smaller than the number of individuals n. The number of survivors exposed to the risk of the event just before t_i, denoted by n_i, is also divided into n_{1i} for G_1 and n_{2i} for G_2. Therefore, $n_i = n_{1i} + n_{2i}$ and $d_i = d_{1i} + d_{2i}$. This classification can be recapitulated by a (2×2) contingency table displaying the number of events and the number of nonevents at t_i, as classified by G_1 and G_2 (Table 2.6). Using this table, I first set up the underlying null hypothesis that G_1 and G_2 have the identical survival function, written by H_0: $S_1(t) = S_2(t)$. If this hypothesis of no association holds, the marginal totals should all be fixed and, consequently, d_{1i} can be viewed as a random variable with parameters n_i, n_{1i}, and d_i following a specific probability distribution called *hypergeometric distribution* (Peto and Peto, 1972). A detailed description of the hypergeometric distribution is provided in Chapter 3 (Section 3.7).

Briefly, the hypergeometric probability of having d_{1i} in n_{1i}, given the fixed values of n_i, n_{1i}, and d_i, can be written by

$$\Pr\left(\tilde{Y}_{1i} = d_{1i}\right) = \frac{\binom{d_i}{d_{1i}}\binom{n_i - d_i}{n_{1i} - d_{1i}}}{\binom{n_i}{n_{1i}}}, \tag{2.47}$$

where $\tilde{Y}_{1i}$ is the random variable for d_{1i}. Specification of each binomial coefficient in Equation (2.47) is described in Section 3.7.

The hypergeometric random variable d_{1i}, given n_i, n_{1i}, and d_i, is well defined, with the expected value

Table 2.6 Number of events and of nonevents at t_i in two groups.

Group	Event		Total
	Yes	No	
G_1	d_{1i}	$n_{1i} - d_{1i}$	n_{1i}
G_2	d_{2i}	$n_{2i} - d_{2i}$	n_{2i}
Total	d_i	$n_i - d_i$	n_i

$$\mathrm{E}(d_{1i}; n_i, n_{1i}, d_i) = \frac{d_i n_{1i}}{n_i} \tag{2.48}$$

and variance

$$V(d_{1i}; n_i, n_{1i}, d_i) = \frac{d_i(n_i - d_i)n_{1i}n_{2i}}{n_i^2(n_i - 1)}. \tag{2.49}$$

As will be further discussed in Chapter 3, the interpretation of Equation (2.48) is straightforward: if the variable d_{1i} is random, its expected value is simply the proportion of n_i selected to n_{1i}, then multiplied by the total number of events d_i. In other words, if the null hypothesis holds, d_i should be proportionally allocated into G_1 and G_2. Therefore, from the variability of the observed d_{1i}, the null hypothesis on the association between survival and group can be statistically tested given a value of α.

Mantel and Haenszel (1959) propose to sum the differences between d_{1i} and $\mathrm{E}(d_{1i})$ for all observed survival times, given by

$$\breve{D} = \sum_{i=1}^{n'} [d_{1i} - \mathrm{E}(d_{1i})], \tag{2.50}$$

where $\breve{D}$ is the sum of differences between the observed and the expected values of d_{1i} over all the observed survival times. Likewise, the variance of $\breve{D}$ is the sum of the variances of d_{1i} over the total number of survival times:

$$V(\breve{D}) = \sum_{i=1}^{n'} V(d_{1i}). \tag{2.51}$$

As $\breve{D}$ tends to be normally distributed with increasing sample size, its standardized form has mean zero and variance 1, written by

$$\frac{\breve{D}}{\sqrt{\mathrm{var}(\breve{D})}} \sim N(0,1).$$

Therefore, a z-score can be derived for testing the independence of survival and group, with the test statistic defined as

$$z = \frac{\sum_{i=1}^{n'} [d_{1i} - \mathrm{E}(d_{1i})]}{\sqrt{\sum_{i=1}^{n'} \mathrm{var}(d_{1i})}}. \tag{2.52}$$

Given the standard procedure for the z-test, significance testing on the null hypothesis can be performed: if the z-score is smaller than z_α, the null hypothesis that H_0: $S_1(t) = S_2(t)$ should be accepted with the conclusion that survival and group are independent. If $z \le z_\alpha$, on the other hand, the H_0 hypothesis should be rejected, implying that G_1 and G_2 are probably subject to two different survival processes.

When the total number of observed events is large, a more plausible statistic for testing the difference in two group-specific survival functions is to convert the standard normal to the chi-square distribution. Statistically, the square of a standard normal random variable has a chi-squared distribution, so a robust and efficient test statistic based on the chi-square distribution, generally denoted by Q, is

$$Q_{\text{logrank}} = \frac{\sum_{i=1}^{n'} [d_{1i} - \mathrm{E}(d_{11})]^2}{\sum_{i=1}^{n'} \mathrm{var}(d_{1i})} \sim \chi^2(1), \tag{2.53}$$

where $\chi^2(1)$ indicates the chi-square distribution with one degree of freedom for two groups. If the Q score is greater than or equal to the score associated with α, the p-value is lower than or equal to α and thus the null hypothesis is to be rejected. If the p-value is lower than α, then the difference in the two survival functions is probably due to sampling error, so H_0 is accepted. Generally, the p-values generated from both z-score and Q-score are identical when the sample size is large.

Peto and Peto (1972) and Prentice (1978) mathematically formalize the logrank test developed by Mantel and Haenszel (1959). This formalization includes the derivation of logrank scores for survival data with right censoring, starting with the specification of a real-valued random variable $\tilde{Y}$ with c.d.f. $F(t)$ and survival curve $S(t) = 1 - F(t)$. Suppose that $S_k(t_i, \theta_i)$ is a survival function parameterized by θ_i, where $\theta_i = \theta_{1i}$ for G_1 and $\theta_i = \theta_{2i}$ for G_2, and $k = 1, 2$. Here, the test on the independence of survival and group can be performed in terms of the parameter θ with the null hypothesis H_0: $\theta_{1i} = \theta_{2i} = \theta_i$. The parameter θ_i can be linked to a parametric distribution and estimated from a specific parametric likelihood function, denoted by $\hat{\theta}_i$. By such specifications, the logrank test can be expressed in terms of ordered residuals relative to a parametric distribution (Andersen *et al.*, 1982; Prentice, 1978).

Given a continuous survival function, the hazard rate for $G_k(k = 1, 2)$ at t_i, given $\hat{\theta}_i$, is given by

$$\hat{h}_k(t_i, \hat{\theta}_i) = -\frac{\mathrm{d}\log \hat{S}_k(t_i, \hat{\theta}_i)}{\mathrm{d}t_i}. \tag{2.54}$$

Therefore, the cumulative hazard rate for $G_k(k = 1, 2)$ at t_i, given $\hat{\theta}_i$, is

$$\hat{H}_k(t_i, \hat{\theta}_i) = -\log \hat{S}_k(t_i, \hat{\theta}_i), \tag{2.55}$$

where the function S_k is known and continuous.

In the presence of censoring and without ties, let $\upsilon_{1i} = 0$ if d_{1i} is right censored; otherwise $\upsilon_{1i} = 1$. Assuming θ_0 is a fixed form of θ_i for all t values, the fixed overall parameter θ_0, under the null hypothesis, can be estimated by

$$\hat{\theta} = \frac{\sum d_{1i}}{\sum -\log S(\upsilon_{1i})}. \tag{2.56}$$

As $S(\upsilon_{1i})$ is relative to the occurrence of a single event, the denominator in Equation (2.56) is the expected number of total events from t_0 to survival time t_i in G_1. Alternatively, Equation (2.56) can be mathematically expressed as

$$\hat{\theta} = \frac{\sum_{i=1}^{n_i'} \frac{d_{1i}}{n_{1i}}}{\int_0^{n_i'} h_1(u)\,\mathrm{d}u}. \tag{2.57}$$

Therefore, the estimate of θ_0 can be expressed as the Nelson–Aalen estimate over the cumulative hazard function from a continuous distribution.

Given the null hypothesis and letting

$$e_{1i} = -\theta_0 \log S(\upsilon_{1i}), \tag{2.58}$$

Peto and Peto (1972) specify the following equations:

$$\mathrm{E}(e_{1i}) = \mathrm{E}\left[-\log S^{\theta_0}(\upsilon_{1i})\right] = \mathrm{E}(d_{1i}) = \mathrm{var}(d_{1i} - e_{1i}), \tag{2.59}$$

which is regardless of the fixed censoring point of $\tilde{Y}_{1i}$.

Let $O_{ki} = d_{ki}$ and $E_{ki} = e_{ki}$ ($i = 1, \ldots, n'$; $k = 1, 2$) in a traditional fashion. Under the null hypothesis, $\mathrm{E}(O_{ki} - E_{ki}) = 0$ and $\mathrm{var}(O_{ki} - E_{ki}) = \mathrm{E}(E_{ki})$. As a result, a test statistic can be expressed by

$$Q_{\mathrm{logrank}} \approx \sum_k \sum_i \frac{(O_{ki} - E_{ki})^2}{\mathrm{var}(O_{ki} - E_{ki})} \sim \chi^2(1). \tag{2.60}$$

Equation (2.60) agrees with Equation (2.53) using a different expression. According to Equation (2.59), Equation (2.60) further reduces to

$$Q_{\mathrm{logrank}} \approx \sum_k \sum_i \frac{(O_{ki} - E_{ki})^2}{\hat{E}_{ki}} \sim \chi^2(1). \tag{2.61}$$

Equation (2.61) indicates that the Mantel–Haenszel statistic is basically an approximate to the familiar Pearson chi-square test for equality of two groups. The term 'logrank test' actually comes from Peto and Peto's inference, in which the method uses the log transformation of the survival function to test a series of ranked survival times. In the absence of censoring, as Andersen *et al.* comment (Andersen et al., 1993, p. 349), the logrank test generates test scores approximately linearly related to the log rank of the observations ordered from the largest to the smallest (the so-called Savage test).

2.3.2 The Wilcoxon rank sum test on survival curves of two groups

The original Wilcoxon two-sample rank sum test (Wilcoxon, 1945) is perhaps the most popular nonparametric testing technique for two population groups. Traditionally, this test has been widely used as an alternative to the paired t-test when the assumption of normality cannot be satisfied. In particular, the Wilcoxon method is applied to the ordinal or continuous response variables with the null hypothesis that the distribution of a given variable is the same for two population groups. The test is based on the calculation of a statistic, generally called U, whose distribution under the null hypothesis is known.

Gehan (1967) and Breslow (1970) extend the Wilcoxon rank sum test to the context of survival analysis. Before describing the extended approach handling right censoring, I review the Wilcoxon rank sum test for uncensored data for familiarizing the reader with this type of test. Suppose n_1 and n_2 individuals are allocated randomly into G_1 and G_2, with $n_1 + n_2 = n$. Then the observations are rank ordered by group:

$$(n_{11}, n_{12}, \ldots, n_{1n_1}) \text{ and } (n_{21}, n_{22}, \ldots, n_{2n_2}).$$

All the observations are then arranged into a single ranked series, regardless of which group they belong to, given by

$$\{n_{(1)} < n_{(2)} < \cdots < n_{(n_1+n_2)}\}.$$

The ranks for observations in G_1 are added up:

$$R_1 = \sum_{i'=1}^{n_1} R_{1i'}, \tag{2.62}$$

where $R_{1i'}$ is the rank of $n_{1i'}$ in $n_{(i)}$, where $i' = 1, \ldots, n_1$). R_2 can be obtained by adding ranks of $n_{2i''}$ in $n_{(i)}$, where $i'' = 1, \ldots, n_2$.

Given that the ranked observations are survival times that follow cumulative distribution functions $F_1(n_1)$ and $F_2(n_2)$, I specify the null hypothesis that H_0: $F_1(t) = F_2(t)$. The Wilcoxon rank sum test is based on the calculation of the statistic U, whose distribution under the null hypothesis is known, written by

$$\frac{R_1 - E(R_1)}{\sqrt{\text{var}(R_1)}} \sim N(0,1), \tag{2.63}$$

where

$$\text{E}(R_1) = \frac{n_2(n_1 + n_2 + 1)}{2} \tag{2.64}$$

and

$$\text{var}(R_1) = \frac{n_1 n_2 (n_1 + n_2 + 1)}{12}. \tag{2.65}$$

The U score can be tested according to the distribution specified in Equation (2.63). Specifically, for testing the null hypothesis the following counting process is specified:

$$U(n_{1i'}, n_{2i''}) = U_{i'i''} = \begin{cases} +1 & \text{if } n_{1i'} > n_{2i''}, \\ 0 & \text{if } n_{1i'} = n_{2i''}, \text{ where } i' = 1, \ldots, n_1 \text{ and } i'' = 1, \ldots, n_2. \\ -1 & \text{if } n_{1i'} < n_{2i''}, \end{cases} \tag{2.66}$$

The total U score is defined by

$$U = \sum_{i',i''} U_{i'i''}. \tag{2.67}$$

As defined by Equation (2.67), U is the cumulative number of observations in G_2 whose rank is definitely less than $n_{1i'}$ minus the number of observations in G_2 whose rank is definitely greater than $n_{1i'}$. Therefore, if the null hypothesis is true, the value of the U-score should be zero.

From the above equations, a close relationship between U and R_1 can be identified, given by

$$R_1 = \frac{n_1(n_1 + n_2 + 1) + U}{2}. \tag{2.68}$$

As a result, U can be expressed in terms of R_1:

$$U = 2R_1 - n_1(n_1 + n_2 + 1). \tag{2.69}$$

Gehan's approach (1965) adapts Equation (2.67) to survival processes in the presence of right censoring. Let $t_{i'}$ and $t_{i''}$ be actual survival times and $t_{i'}^{+}$ and $t_{i''}^{+}$ censored times for G_1 and G_2, respectively. Then, Gehan redefines the $U_{i'i''}$ score as

$$U_{i'i''}^{\text{Gehan}} = \begin{cases} +1 & \text{if } t_{i'} > t_{i''} \text{ or } t_{i'}^{+} \geq t_{i''}, \\ 0 & \text{if } t_{i'} = t_{i''} \text{ or } \left(t_{i'}^{+}, t_{i''}^{+}\right) \text{ or } t_{i'}^{+} < t_{i''} \text{ or } t_{i''}^{+} < t_{i'}, \\ -1 & \text{if } t_{i'} < t_{i''} \text{ or } t_{i'} \leq t_{i''}^{+}. \end{cases} \tag{2.70}$$

In Gehan's approach, whether a censored observation is counted as 1, 0, or −1 depends on the timing of censoring as compared to survival times of the other group. If censoring occurs to a member of G_1 but the censored time is greater than or equal to the actual survival time for a given member of G_2, the rank of the actual survival time for the member of G_1 is greater than the actual survival time for the member of G_2. Consequently, the score should be 1. In contrast, if the actual survival time for the member of G_1 is less than or equal to the censored time for the member of G_2, the rank of the survival time for the member of G_1 is definitely less than the actual survival time for the member of G_2. Then the value −1 should be assigned. If censoring occurs to an individual in one group before an event takes place for a matched member in the other group, a comparison of their ranks is difficult, so the score is simply 0.

A summary statistic for observation i' ($i' = 1, \ldots, n_1$), denoted by $W_{i'}$, is defined by

$$W_{i'} = \sum_{i''=1}^{n_2} U_{i'i''}^{\text{Gehan}}. \tag{2.71}$$

Equation (2.71) indicates that for an individual of G_1 with event time i', $W_{i'}$ is the number of observations in G_2 whose lifetimes are definitely less than $t_{i'}$ minus the number whose survival times are definitely greater than $t_{i'}$, taking into account the occurrence of right censoring. If survival is truly independent of group, survival times should be randomly distributed; then the expected value of $W_{i'}$ is 0. Given this rationale, the Gehan statistic, denoted by W, is

$$W = \sum_{i'=1}^{n_1} W_{i'} = \sum_{i'} \sum_{i''} U_{i'i''}^{\text{Gehan}}, \tag{2.72}$$

where the sum is over all n_1-versus-n_2 comparisons.

If the null hypothesis holds, the statistic W has the properties

$$\mathrm{E}(W) = 0, \tag{2.73}$$

$$\mathrm{var}(W) = \frac{n_1 n_2}{(n_1 + n_2)(n_1 + n_2 - 1)} \sum_{i'=1}^{n_1} W_{i'}^2. \tag{2.74}$$

Finally, the null hypothesis that $S_1(t) = S_2(t)$ can be tested by the Q test, given by

$$Q_{\text{Wilcoxon}} = \frac{[W - E(W)]^2}{\mathrm{var}(W)} \sim \chi^2(1). \tag{2.75}$$

Therefore, given the value of α, the equality of survival curves between G_1 and G_2 can be statistically tested by the p-value of the above chi-square distributed statistic. This method is the so-called *generalized Wilcoxon test* in survival analysis. From Equation (2.75), the reader might notice its striking similarity to the logrank test.

As the number of individuals exposed to the risk of a particular event decreases with the rank of survival times, the generalized Wilcoxon rank sum test implicitly uses the number of exposures just before a survival time as weight for the derivation of the statistic. This implied feature is the major difference between the generalized Wilcoxon test and the logrank test. As more weights are given to differences in the survival function at smaller t values, Tarone and Ware (1977) suggest the use of the square root of n_i as the weight to perform the generalized Wilcoxon test, so that a more balanced Q statistic can be derived.

Peto and Peto (1972) and Prentice (1978) advocate a different scoring method in the presence of censoring, using the Kaplan–Meier survival estimates. Here, the status indicator is used for a survival or a censored time, defined as $\delta_{ti'}$, where $\delta_{ti'} = 0$ if $t_{i'}$ is a censored survival time and $\delta_{ti'} = 1$ if $t_{i'}$ is an actual survival time. Then the $W_{i'}$ is redefined as

$$W_{i'} = \begin{cases} \hat{S}(t_{i'+1}) + \hat{S}(t_{i'-1}) - 1 & \text{if } \delta_{ti'} = 1, \\ \hat{S}(t_{i'+1}) - 1 & \text{if } \delta_{ti'} = 0. \end{cases} \tag{2.76}$$

Accordingly, the overall test score, W, is redefined as the sum of the scores generated by performing Equation (2.76) for G_1. In the presence of tied cases, this test score is reformulated by

$$W = \sum_{i'=1}^{n_1} W_{i'} d_{i'}. \tag{2.77}$$

The Peto and Peto (1972) and Prentice (1978) generalization of the Wilcoxon test is considered to be preferable to Gehan's approach because their generalized scores are consistent for an exact observation in the presence of right censoring. In Gehan's method, scores at particular survival times vary according to the pattern of censoring imposed on the observations, so that differences in the pattern of censoring between G_1 and G_2 can somewhat affect the quality of a test (Andersen *et al.*, 1993; Peto and Peto, 1972).

In general, compared to the logrank test, the generalized Wilcoxon rank sum test is sensitive to early differences between two survival curves, given the assignment of weight to each observation. Tarone and Ware (1977) argue that these two popular approaches can be unified by a general counting system in which they differ only in the choice of weight. This characterization enables statisticians to develop generalized procedures with choices of weight, as described in Subsection 2.3.3.

2.3.3 Comparison of survival functions for more than two groups

In empirical analyses, researchers often need to compare survival processes among more than two population groups. In biomedical studies, for example, there are frequently more than two treatments or testing groups in clinical trials. In survey data analysis, scientists are often interested in whether or not the occurrence of a particular event differs among several socioeconomic and demographic groups for gaining important information with policy implications. Given survival data allocated into more than two population groups, the theoretical question is whether any of those population subgroups differs from any others in the survival function.

Technically, tests on survival curves of more than two groups are simply the extension of the two-sample perspectives described above. Suppose there are K different groups, where $K > 2$, denoted by $G_1, G_2, \ldots, G_K$, respectively. In the presence of right censoring, the survival data from group k ($k = 1, \ldots, K$) is

$$(t_{k1}, \delta_{k1}), (t_{k2}, \delta_{k2}), \ldots, (t_{kn_k}, \delta_{kn_k}),$$

where δ_{ki} is the censoring status indicator defined earlier. In this survival data structure, at each survival time t_i ($i = 1, \ldots, n'$) the sample n_i is allocated into K groups, given by $n_{1i}, n_{2i}, \ldots, n_{Ki}$. Likewise, d_i is divided into $d_{1i}, d_{2i}, \ldots, d_{Ki}$, where d_{ki} is defined as the number of individuals in G_k who experience a particular event of interest at survival time t_i. Therefore, $n_i = n_{1i} + n_{2i} + \cdots + n_{Ki}$ and $d_i = d_{1i} + d_{2i} + \cdots + d_{Ki}$. If there are no tied observations, one of the d_{ki} takes the value 1 and the others take the value 0. This classification can be illustrated by a ($K \times 2$) contingency table displaying the number of events and the number of nonevents at t_i, as classified by K groups (Table 2.7). Using this table, the null hypothesis to be tested is that all K groups are subject to an identical survival function, written by H_0: $S_1(t) = S_2(t) = \cdots = S_K(t)$. This null hypothesis is to be rejected if one of the $S_k(t)$ values deviates significantly from any of the others. A $\chi^2(K - 1)$ test can be performed by comparing the observed and the expected values of events, by extending the methods described in Subsections 2.3.1 and 2.3.2.

With K groups involved in a comparison, a matrix expression of mathematical equations is more convenient. Let $\boldsymbol{O}_i = [d_{1i}, \ldots, d_{(K-1)i}]$ be a vector for the observed number of events in group 1 to group ($K - 1$) at event time t_i. Given a series of numbers of exposure, denoted $n_{1i}, n_{2i}, \ldots, n_{Ki}$, the distribution of counts in $\boldsymbol{O}_i$ is assumed to follow a multivariate hypergeometric function, conditional on both the row and the column totals (a detailed description of the hypergeometric distribution is provided in Chapter 3). This multivariate hypergeometric distribution, under the null hypothesis, is associated with a mean vector

Table 2.7 Number of events and of exposures at t_i in $\boldsymbol{K}$ groups.

Group	Event		Total
	Yes	No	
G_1	d_{1i}	$n_{1i} - d_{1i}$	n_{1i}
G_2	d_{2i}	$n_{2i} - d_{2i}$	n_{2i}
—			
G_K	d_{Ki}	$n_{Ki} - d_{Ki}$	n_{Ki}
Total	d_i	$n_i - d_i$	n_i

$$\mathbf{E}_i = \left[\frac{d_i n_{1i}}{n_i}, \frac{d_i n_{2i}}{n_i}, \frac{d_i n_{(K-1)i}}{n_i}\right]' \tag{2.78}$$

and a variance–covariance matrix

$$\boldsymbol{V}_i = \begin{bmatrix} v_{11i} & v_{12i} & \cdots & v_{1(K-1)i} \\ & v_{22i} & \cdots & v_{2(K-1)i} \\ & & \ddots & \\ & & & v_{(K-1)(K-1)i} \end{bmatrix}. \tag{2.79}$$

In the standard logrank test, the kth diagonal element in $\boldsymbol{V}_i$ is defined as

$$v_{kki} = \frac{n_{ki}(n_i - n_{ki})d_i(n_i - d_i)}{n^2(n_i - 1)} \tag{2.80}$$

and the $k\iota$th off-diagonal element is

$$v_{k\iota i} = \frac{n_{ki}n_{\iota i}d_i(n_i - d_i)}{n^2(n_i - 1)}, \tag{2.81}$$

where $k \neq \iota$.

With $(K - 1)$ degrees of freedom, the Q score for the logrank test of the $(K \times 1)$ table can be written as

$$Q_{\text{logrank}} = (\boldsymbol{O} - \mathbf{E})'\boldsymbol{V}^{-1}(\boldsymbol{O} - \mathbf{E}) \sim \chi^2(K-1), \tag{2.82}$$

where

$$\boldsymbol{O} = \sum_{i=1}^{n'} \boldsymbol{O}_i, \quad \mathbf{E} = \sum_{i=1}^{n'} \mathbf{E}_i, \quad \text{and} \quad \boldsymbol{V} = \sum_{i=1}^{n'} \boldsymbol{V}_i.$$

It is recognizable that the procedures of comparing survival curves for more than two groups, as formulated by Equations (2.78) through (2.82), are simply the expansion of the logrank test on two groups described in Subsection 2.3.1. The logrank test, however, does not consider group weight in calculating the test statistic. This procedure may not cause serious bias when comparing two population samples, given relatively similar numbers of individuals. In comparing more than two survival curves, however, this problem can be serious because the number of individuals is usually unevenly allocated. Using weights can reduce sensitivity to early or late departures in testing the relationship among multiple samples (Klein and Moeschberger, 2003). As a result, some other techniques in this area, like the generalized Wilcoxon sum rank test and its modified version, may be used as alternatives.

As indicated earlier, some scientists (Klein and Moeschberger, 2003; Tarone and Ware, 1977) suggest that the logrank test and the modified Wilcoxon rank sum statistic can be specified in a way that they differ only in the choice of weight. This clarification results in the standardization of various techniques for comparing survival data of different population groups. Specifically, this unification is conducted by defining a weight function $w_k(t)$, given the property that $w_k(t) = 0$ whenever n_{ki} is 0.

Let $t_1 \le t_2 \le t_3 \le t_4 \le \cdots \le t_n$ be the distinct survival times in a combined sample and $w(t_i)$ be a positive weight function at event time t_i. Then the rank test statistic for comparing survival functions of K groups have the form of a K-dimensioned vector $\ddot{\boldsymbol{\upsilon}} = (\ddot{\upsilon}_1, \ddot{\upsilon}_2, \ldots, \ddot{\upsilon}_K)'$ with $\ddot{\upsilon}_k$ $(k = 1, 2, \ldots, K)$,given by

$$\ddot{\upsilon}_k = \sum_{i=1}^{n'} w(t_i)\left(d_{ki} - \frac{n_{ki}d_i}{n_i}\right). \tag{2.83}$$

The estimated variance–covariance matrix of $\ddot{\boldsymbol{\upsilon}}$, $\boldsymbol{V} = (V_{k\iota})$, is defined as

$$V_{k\iota} = \sum_{i=1}^{n'} w^2(t_i)\left[\frac{(n_i n_{\iota i}\delta_{k\iota} - n_{ki}n_{\iota i})d_i(n_i - d_i)}{n^2(n_i - 1)}\right], \tag{2.84}$$

where $\delta_{k\iota}$ is 1 if $k = \iota$ and 0 otherwise. The term $\ddot{\upsilon}_k$ $(k = 1, 2, \ldots, K)$ is a weighted sum of observed minus expected numbers of events under the null hypothesis of identical survival curves. Given the standardization, the overall test statistic, denoted by Q_{standard}, is generally written as a multivariate sandwich equation $\ddot{\boldsymbol{\upsilon}}'\boldsymbol{V}^{-1}\ddot{\boldsymbol{\upsilon}}$. To spread it out with consideration of weights, the equation is

$$Q_{\text{standard}} = \left[\sum_{i=1}^{n'} \boldsymbol{w}_i(\boldsymbol{O}_i - \mathbf{E}_i)\right]' [\boldsymbol{w}_i \boldsymbol{V}_i \boldsymbol{w}_i]^{-1} \left[\sum_{i=1}^{n'} \boldsymbol{w}_i(\boldsymbol{O}_i - \mathbf{E}_i)\right] \sim \chi^2(K-1) \tag{2.85}$$

where $\boldsymbol{w}_{\text{i}} = \text{diag}(w_{\text{i}})$ for a $(K - 1)$ by $(K - 1)$ diagonal matrix.

Equation (2.85) is used as a generalized formula for testing survival curves of K groups, in which several models of this sort are reflected with differences only in the choice of weight. As a standardized expression, Equation (2.85) can also be applied to a two-group comparison as a special case with $K = 2$.

Given a unified specification, differences in various methods can be evaluated by examining the specification of weight for each testing method. The logrank test is based on the comparison between the observed and the expected numbers of events at each event time regardless of the distribution of n, so that $\boldsymbol{w}_{\text{i}}$ is an identity matrix over all event times for this test. Gehan's Wilcoxon rank sum test takes into account the distribution of sample size across all t_i values and, therefore, in this test $\boldsymbol{w}_{\text{i}} = \text{diag}(n_{\text{i}})$. Tarone and Ware (1977) suggest, as mentioned previously, that more weight should be assigned to later differences between the observed and the expected numbers of events, so that, in this method, $\boldsymbol{w}_{\text{i}} = \text{diag}(n_{\text{i}})^{1/2}$. In the Peto–Peto Wilcoxon test, on the other hand, the Kaplan–Meier estimate for the pooled sample, $\hat{S}(t)$, is used as the weight. Based on the survival function of a pooled sample, instead of survival times and censoring distributions, the Peto–Peto weight specification is believed to have the capacity of generating more reliable results when censoring patterns differ over individual samples (Prentice and Marek, 1979).

Prentice (1978) and Andersen *et al.* (1982) propose a method to modify the weight used by the Peto–Peto method. They contend that in the Peto–Peto test, the Kaplan–Meier estimator for $S(t)$ should be replaced by the following estimator:

$$\bar{S}(t) = \prod_{t_i \le t} \left(1 - \frac{d_i}{n_i + 1}\right). \tag{2.86}$$

According to Prentice (1978) and Andersen *et al.* (1982), Equation (2.86) provides a consistent estimator of $S(t)$ under mild conditions on censoring. The test with such a weight is called the *modified Peto–Peto test*. When n is large, however, the modified Peto–Peto test generates very close or even identical results to those derived from the test originally proposed by Peto and Peto (1972).

There are some other tests on survival curves of different population groups dealing with other lifetime situations, such as the stratified and logrank tests for trend. For those additional testing techniques, the interested reader can refer to Collett (2003), Lawless (2003), and Klein and Moeschberger (2003).

2.3.4 Illustration: Comparison of survival curves between married and unmarried persons

To display how to perform various statistical tests on differences in the survival function between two or more population groups, I provide an empirical example about marital status and the probability of survival among older Americans. In particular, I want to estimate the five-year survival function among currently married and currently not married persons separately, and then assess whether or not the two survival curves differ significantly. In the survival data of older Americans, there is a variable called ‘Married,’ with 1 = ‘currently married’ and 0 = else, used for stratifying the survival data. The null hypothesis is that the survival curve for the individuals who are ‘currently married’ does not differ distinctively from the survival curve among the ‘currently not married,’ written by H_0: $(S_1(t) = S_2(t)$. I propose to use the above-mentioned five methods to test this hypothesis.

The SAS program for performing the five tests largely assembles SAS Program 2.1, with the addition of the variable ‘Married’ in the PROC LIFETEST statement as the stratification factor, shown below.

SAS Program 2.5:

```
...........

proc format;
  value Rx 1 = 'Married' 0 = 'Not married';

.........
```

```
ODS graphics on;

proc lifetest data = new plots = survival(atrisk = 0 to 60 by 10);
  time Months * Status(0);
  strata married / test = all;
run;

ODS graphics off;
```

Compared to SAS Program 2.1, this program adds the stratification factor 'Married,' a PROC FORMAT statement that specifies values of that factor, and a STRATA option in the PROC LIFETEST statement. The PLOTS = survival option requests SAS to plot the survival curves and the 'ATRISK =' option specifies the time points at which the numbers exposed to the risk of death are displayed. In the STRATA statement, the TEST = all option specifies that all the nonparametric test scores are calculated.

SAS Program 2.5 yields a large quantity of output data. Therefore, I select to display the basic descriptive information and the results of the five tests in the following table.

SAS Program Output 2.1:

The LIFETEST Procedure

Summary of the Number of Censored and Uncensored Values

Stratum	married	Total	Failed	Censored	Percent Censored
1	Married	1090	181	909	83.39
2	Not married	892	218	674	75.56
Total		1982	399	1583	79.87

Rank Statistics

married	Log-Rank	Wilcoxon	Tarone	Peto	Modified Peto	Fleming
Married	-43.348	-76900	-1820	-39.368	-39.345	-39.556
Not married	43.348	76900	1820	39.368	39.345	39.556

Test of Equality over Strata

Test	Chi-Square	DF	Pr > Chi-Square
Log-Rank	19.2336	1	<.0001
Wilcoxon	19.1857	1	<.0001
Tarone	19.1951	1	<.0001
Peto	19.6290	1	<.0001
Modified Peto	19.6285	1	<.0001

The first part of SAS Program Output 2.1 presents the distribution of the total sample, of the number of events, and of the number of censored observations, classified by marital status. Of 1982 individuals, 1090 are currently married and 892 currently not married. There are 399 persons who are deceased by the end of the 60th month, among whom 181 are currently married and 218 are currently not married. Additionally, 1583 older persons are right censored: 909 'currently married' and 674 'currently not married.'

The second section of the output table displays the test scores, varying over different methods as anticipated. The final section demonstrates the test results on the five methods described previously. Those tests generate very close chi-square statistics assuming a $\chi^2(1)$ distribution, especially those generated from the Peto–Peto and the modified Peto–Peto tests. With a negligible difference (19.6290 versus 19.6285), the modified Peto–Peto test is not shown to improve the original estimate significantly in this example. Each of the test scores attaches to a *p*-value, all smaller than 0.0001. Given the consistency of the test scores and the corresponding *p*-values, it can be concluded that the null hypothesis should be rejected; that is, the survival curve for currently married persons differs significantly from the survival curve among their unmarried counterparts.

In SAS Program 2.5, the PLOT = SURVIIVAL option requests SAS to produce two survival curves, one for currently married and one for currently not married. The graph in Figure 2.6 is the resulting plot, where the survival curves for the two groups, currently married and currently not married, are displayed, along with the number of older persons

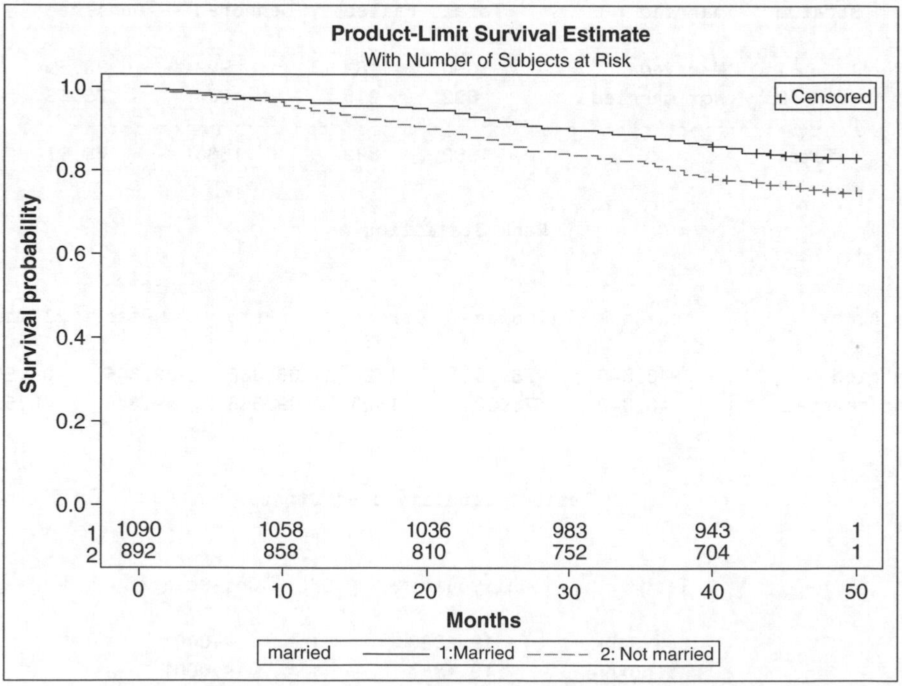

Figure 2.6 Plot of survival curves for currently married and currently not married persons.

exposed to the risk of death at month 0, 10, 20, 30, 40, and 50. The dominance of the survival curve among currently married older persons is obvious as the probability of survival declines at a much slower pace than does the curve among the 'currently not married.' The two survival curves start to separate after month 0, then the separation widens consistently over time. According to the results of the five tests, the separation between the two survival curves is statistically significant, demonstrating that older Americans who are currently married are expected to live longer than those currently not married.

2.4 Summary

This chapter describes some widely used descriptive approaches in survival analysis. Both the Kaplan–Meier and Nelson–Aalen estimators are described extensively, including the derivation of variances, confidence intervals, and confidence bands for the survival function. As most lifetime indicators are intimately associated, the Kaplan–Meier and Nelson–Aalen estimators can be applied to estimate other lifetime measures, given relevant formulas described in Chapter 1. Additionally, I provide a brief introduction about the life table method. While a life table accounts for survival times of censored observations both across and within fixed intervals, in many aspects the life table estimates approximate those generated from the Kaplan–Meier and the Nelson–Aalen approaches. One distinct advantage of using the Kaplan–Meier and Nelson–Aalen estimators over the life table method is the flexibility of using data with a small sample size, which is perhaps the reason why the life table method is rarely applied in biomedical studies.

In this chapter, I also describe several popular methods for testing survival functions of two or more population groups statistically, including the logrank test, Gehan's generalized Wilcoxon rank sum test, the Peto–Peto logrank and Wilcoxon methods, and the Tarone and Ware modified test. All these methods can be articulated by a unified formula in which they differ only in the choice of weight. This characterization facilitates the development of computer software procedures that program all those methods within an integrated estimating process, as exemplified by the programmed options in SAS PROC LIFETEST. While all these techniques often generate very close and even identical testing results, the logrank and Gehan's generalized Wilcoxon rank sum tests are the most widely used approaches to compare two or more group-specific survival curves.

As a stratification factor can be causally associated with some other explanatory factors, there are potentially conflicting possibilities for a bivariate relationship between a single covariate and survival outcomes. Methodologically, one of the potential possibilities is a spurious association, defined as a mathematical relationship in which two factors have no actual causal connection but look correlated due to the existence of one or more 'lurking' or confounding variables. A good example is found in a study of the relationship between education and smoking behavior among older Taiwanese (Liu, Hermalin, and Chuang, 1998). In the traditional Chinese culture, the majority of older Taiwanese women are illiterates, but, at the same time, they are less likely to smoke cigarettes and more likely to survive than older men. Consequently, a descriptive analysis displays a strong positive association between education and smoking cigarettes among older Taiwanese, a phenomenon contrary to what is expected. This observed association is obviously spurious because most lowly educated Taiwanese women do not smoke, thereby confounding the actual association between education and smoking behavior. After the lurking variable 'gender' is controlled, the association between education and smoking behavior among older Taiwanese becomes significantly negative. Therefore, caution must apply when performing the descriptive approaches described in this chapter. These methods only have the capability to provide tentative results in survival analysis. There are some exceptions in this regard, including some of the clinical trials in which the potential confounding effects are taken into account in the process of randomization.

3

Some popular survival distribution functions

The distribution of event time T often follows some distinct patterns. These recognizable survival shapes have enabled statisticians and mathematicians to develop a variety of parametric models for describing survival processes. Empirically, parametric survival models have been widely employed, particularly in the field of industrial reliability analyses, when a known family of distributions can be identified and validated to reflect the history of a dynamic event.

In this chapter, I describe several popular families of parametric time distributions, including the exponential, Weibull, gamma, lognormal, log-logistic, and Gompertz and other Gompertz-type distributions. These parametric distributional functions have been used frequently in the fields of biostatistics, epidemiology, biology, gerontology, demography, sociology, and biomedicine. Serving as fundamentals for understanding more complicated survival models described in later chapters, the mathematical specifications, interpretations, and properties of these parametric models are extensively described and discussed. Some other families of lifetime distributions are also briefly summarized. Likelihood functions of some of these parametric distributions are described in Chapter 4, where covariates are introduced into those parametric models. Additionally, I include the hypergeometric distribution in this chapter, a discrete function widely applied in the analysis of lottery and gambling patterns. In survival analysis, this distribution is used to perform the popular logrank test on survival differences between two or more population subgroups, as discussed in Chapter 2.

3.1 Exponential survival distribution

Among the families of the parametric time distributions, the exponential distribution is the simplest function because its specification is based on a single parameter. Let λ be a constant rate of change; the survival function at time t with the exponential distribution is given by

$$S(t; \lambda) = \mathrm{e}^{-\lambda t}, \tag{3.1}$$

Survival Analysis: Models and Applications, First Edition. Xian Liu.

where λ is the constant rate of change throughout the interval $(0, \infty)$. Given Equation (3.1), the hazard rate in the exponential distribution can be written as

$$h(t;\lambda) = -\frac{1}{S(t;\lambda)}\frac{\mathrm{d}S(t;\lambda)}{\mathrm{d}t} = -\frac{\frac{\mathrm{d}}{\mathrm{d}t}\mathrm{e}^{-\lambda t}}{\mathrm{e}^{-\lambda t}} = \frac{\mu \mathrm{e}^{-\lambda t}}{\mathrm{e}^{-\lambda t}} = \lambda. \tag{3.2}$$

Consequently, the underlying property of the exponential distribution is the specification of a constant hazard rate, given by

$$h(t; T \sim \exp) \equiv \lambda. \tag{3.3}$$

The exponential cumulative hazard function, denoted by $H(t; \lambda)$, can be easily derived from Equation (3.3):

$$H(t;\lambda) = -\log S(t;\lambda) = -\log\{\exp[-(\lambda t)]\} = \lambda t. \tag{3.4}$$

Equation (3.4) shows that when the hazard rate is constant, the cumulative hazard rate is simply the product of the rate and time.

From Equation (3.1), the p.d.f. of the exponential distribution can also be readily specified:

$$f(t;\lambda) = h(t;\lambda)S(t;\lambda) = \lambda \mathrm{e}^{-\lambda t}, \quad t = 0, 1, \ldots, \infty. \tag{3.5}$$

Similarly, the c.d.f. at time t can be written as

$$F(t;\lambda) = 1 - S(t;\lambda) = 1 - \mathrm{e}^{-\lambda t}. \tag{3.6}$$

As the constant rate determines the scale of a hazard function, λ is often referred to as the scale parameter.

Taking natural log values on both sides of Equation (3.1) yields

$$\log S(t;\lambda) = -\lambda t. \tag{3.7}$$

Clearly, the log survival function is linearly associated with time t. Hence, a graph of $\log S(t; \lambda)$ versus t yields a straight line in the exponential distribution of T. This feature of the exponential distribution is often used for a graphical check of exponentiality with empirical data, which will be discussed further in Chapter 4.

To demonstrate patterns of lifetime processes with different values of λ, I display six p.d.f. and six c.d.f. curves with $\lambda = 0.5$, $\lambda = 1.0$, $\lambda = 1.5$, $\lambda = 2.0$, $\lambda = 2.5$, and $\lambda = 3.0$, respectively. Below is an SAS program to derive a graph presenting these six p.d.f. curves, with t ranging from 0 to 10.

SAS Program 3.1:

```
options ls=80 ps=58 nodate pageno=1 number center;
ods select all;
```

```
ods trace off;
ods listing;
title1;
run;

data Exponential_pdf;
    do e_scale = 0.5 to 3.0 by 0.5;
    do t = 0.1 to 10 by .1;
    exponential_pdf=PDF('EXPONENTIAL',t,e_scale);
    output;
    end;
    end;
run;

goptions targetdevice=winprtc reset=global gunit=pct border cback=white
        colors=(black red blue)
        ftitle=swissxb ftext=swissxb htitle=2 htext=1.5;

proc gplot data=Exponential_pdf;
    plot exponential_pdf * t = e_scale;
    symbol1 c=black  i=splines  l=1  v=plus;
    symbol2 c=red    i=splines  l=2  v=diamond;
    symbol3 c=blue   i=splines  l=3  v=square;
    symbol4 c=green  i=splines  l=4  v=circle;
    symbol5 c=magenta i=splines  l=5  v=triangle;
    symbol6 c=brown  i=splines  l=6  v=star;
    title1 "Figure 3.1 Exponential pdf varying parm";
    run;
quit;
```

SAS Program 3.1 produces a p.d.f. graph (Figure 3.1) linked to a series of λ values by using the p.d.f. function in the DATA statement and the PROC GPLOT procedure. Figure 3.1 demonstrates that a constant hazard rate is linked with a decreasing function of p.d.f. because $S(t)$ decreases over t.

If the 'PDF' option in SAS Program 3.1 is replaced with 'CDF,' with the title and some other statements revised accordingly, then the graph of the c.d.f. function is produced (Figure 3.2). The c.d.f. plot shows that given a smaller value of λ, the c.d.f. function of the exponential distribution tends to be more rectangularized.

Because in the exponential time distribution the hazard rate is constant, the expected life is simply the reciprocal of λ. Given $S(0) = F(\infty) = 1$, we have

$$1 = \int_0^{\infty} f(t)\mathrm{d}t = \int_0^{\infty} h(t)S(t)\mathrm{d}t. \tag{3.8}$$

In the construct of the exponential distribution, Equation (3.8) can be extended to

$$1 = \int_0^{\infty} h(t;\lambda)\mathrm{e}^{-\lambda t}\,\mathrm{d}t = \lambda\int_0^{\infty} \mathrm{e}^{-\lambda t}\,\mathrm{d}t = \lambda \mathrm{E}(T_0). \tag{3.9}$$

Consequently, the expected lifetime is defined as

$$\mathrm{E}(T_0;\lambda) = \frac{1}{\lambda} = \lambda^{-1}, \tag{3.10}$$

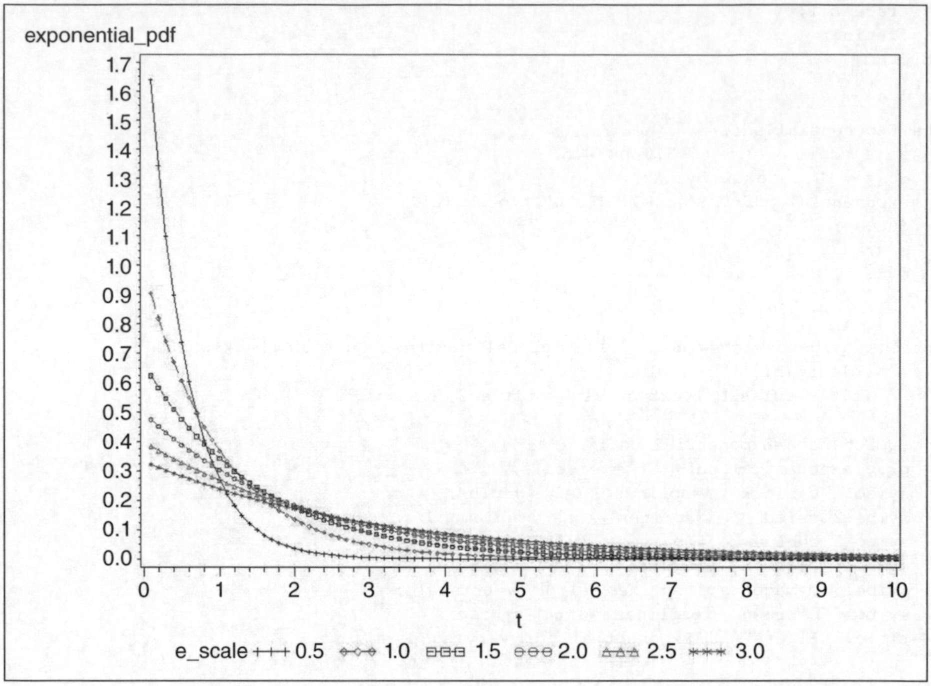

Figure 3.1 Exponential p.d.f. varying parm (parameter).

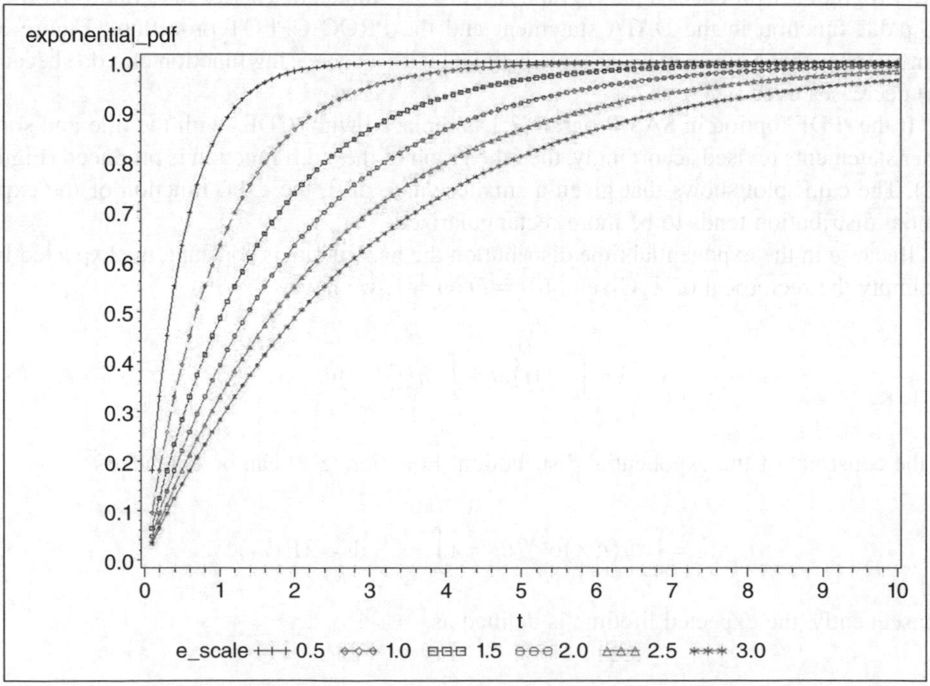

Figure 3.2 Exponential c.d.f. function.

with variance of T

$$\operatorname{var}(T; \lambda) = \frac{1}{\lambda^2}. \tag{3.11}$$

Because $E(T_0; \lambda)$ is the expected duration of life, λ^{-1} is sometimes regarded as a rate parameter of the exponential distribution. Some researchers use this scale rate to reparameterize the exponential distribution for analytic convenience in certain situations. For example, let $\tilde{\gamma} = \lambda^{-1}$; then the p.d.f. of lifetime T can be rewritten as

$$f(t; \tilde{\gamma}) = \frac{e^{-t/\tilde{\gamma}}}{\tilde{\gamma}}, \quad t = 0, 1, \ldots, \infty. \tag{3.12}$$

Equation (3.12) can be defined as a one-parameter extreme value function. Given the definition of the scale parameter $\tilde{\gamma}$, the expected value of event time T and its variance can be rewritten by $\tilde{\gamma}$ and $\tilde{\gamma}^2$, respectively. The two scale parameters λ and $\tilde{\gamma}$ take the same value if and only if $\lambda = 1$, referred to as the standard exponential distribution.

The median value of the exponential survival function, denoted by t_m, can be obtained from λ or $\tilde{\gamma}$. The condition that $S(t_m) = 0.5$ leads to the following equation:

$$S(t_m) = 0.5 = e^{-\lambda t_m}, \tag{3.13}$$

which can be converted to

$$t_m = \frac{1}{\lambda}\log(2) = \tilde{\gamma} \times \log(2). \tag{3.14}$$

Given that λ is independent of t, another important property of the exponential distribution is the so-called *memorylessness*. This property is mathcmatically defined as

$$\Pr[T \in (t, t+1) | T \geq t] = \Pr[T \in (t+1, t+2) | T \geq t+1] \quad \text{for all } t \geq 0. \tag{3.15}$$

As λ is constant at all times, the expected life is also memoryless of t. This property suggests that at any time and whatever the past survival experience, the expected time remaining in the lifetime process is unchanged, given an exponential distribution of T.

In reality, the lifetime process rarely follows an exponential distribution featured by a constant hazard rate, so its usability is somewhat limited. Mortality, incidence of disease, marriage disruption, health status transitions, unemployment, drug use recidivism, and other popular topics in survival analysis all seem highly associated with time or age. Nevertheless, some special lifetime events may be considered roughly to follow the exponential distribution, in which occurrences of events are not distinctly associated with time. Car accidents within a territorial domain, for example, tend to have a stable rate over time if environmental factors remain unchanged. The chance of breaking a plate seems not a function of time, so the probability of its occurrence is more or less constant over time. For those events, the expected life remaining can be readily estimated by taking the reciprocal of the observed failure rate. Given a recently reported rate of car accidents, for example, I am able to calculate the expected months elapsed until the next car accident occurs to anyone residing in the same area. From the rate of breaking a plate, I can estimate in how many years a new set of plates should be purchased. What is interesting is that if none of my plates is broken in five years, the expected years remaining for not breaking another plate is the same as five years ago because the process of breaking a plate is memoryless.

As event occurrences within a short period are sometimes relatively stable, some scientists have used the exponential distribution to model survival processes within a limited time interval. In population studies, the death rate, incidence rate of a specific disease, or rate of resolution from disability are often assumed to be constant within a single age range. This characteristic has enabled some demographers to estimate a series of age-specific hazard rates by using the exponential survival model. Crimmins, Hayward, and Saito (1996), for example, use the exponential function to calculate a variety of rates for construction of active life tables among older Americans.

3.2 The Weibull distribution and extreme value theory

Among all families of parametric time distributions, the Weibull model is perhaps the most widely applied parametric function in survival analysis due to its simplicity and flexibility. Additionally, the Weibull function can be formulated by two approaches: the proportional hazard rate model and the accelerated time failure process.

3.2.1 Basic specifications of the Weibull distribution

The Weibull probability distribution of event time T, a continuous function, is featured by the use of two parameters – a scale parameter λ and a shape parameter $\tilde{p}$. With two parameters functioning simultaneously, the Weibull distribution, compared with the exponential distribution, provides a parametric model with additional flexibility. The notation $T \sim \text{Weib}(\lambda, \tilde{p})$ is generally used to denote that the event time T has a Weibull distribution with parameters λ and $\tilde{p}$.

Specifically, the survival function with the Weibull distribution is given by

$$S(t; \lambda, \tilde{p}) = \exp\left[-(\lambda t)^{\tilde{p}}\right]. \tag{3.16}$$

Given the intimate associations among various lifetime measures, the hazard function in the Weibull distribution can be readily derived from Equation (3.16):

$$h(t; \lambda, \tilde{p}) = -\frac{\frac{\mathrm{d}}{\mathrm{d}t}\mathrm{e}^{-(\lambda t)^{\tilde{p}}}}{\mathrm{e}^{-(\lambda t)^{\tilde{p}}}} = \frac{\lambda \tilde{p} t^{\tilde{p}-1}\exp\left[-(\lambda t)^{\tilde{p}}\right]}{\exp\left[-(\lambda t)^{\tilde{p}}\right]} = \lambda \tilde{p}(\lambda t)^{\tilde{p}-1}. \tag{3.17}$$

Given Equation (1.8), the cumulative hazard function $H(t; \lambda, \tilde{p})$ can be written as

$$H(t; \lambda, \tilde{p}) = -\log S(t; \lambda, \tilde{p}) = -\log\left\{\exp\left[-(\lambda t)^{\tilde{p}}\right]\right\} = (\lambda t)^{\tilde{p}}. \tag{3.18}$$

Taking natural log values on both sides of Equation (3.18) gives rise to

$$\log[-\log S(t;\lambda,\tilde{p})] = \log\lambda + \tilde{p}\log t. \tag{3.19}$$

It is clear that given the relationship specified in Equation (3.19), a plot of log $H(t; \lambda, \tilde{p})$ versus log t should display a straight line with slope $\tilde{p}$ if data come from a Weibull distribution. Statisticians and demographers take advantage of this relationship to assess whether empirical survival data follow a Weibull distribution, as will be displayed in Chapter 4.

Specifications of $S(t)$ and $h(t)$ lead to the following equation for the Weibull p.d.f. function:

$$f(t;\lambda,\tilde{p}) = h(t)S(t) = \lambda\tilde{p}(\lambda t)^{\tilde{p}-1}\exp\left[-(\lambda t)^{\tilde{p}}\right]. \tag{3.20}$$

Likewise, the c.d.f. at time t is derived by

$$F(t;\lambda,\tilde{p}) = 1 - S(t;\lambda,\tilde{p}) = 1 - \exp\left[-(\lambda t)^{\tilde{p}}\right]. \tag{3.21}$$

From Equation (3.21), the reader can easily identify that, when $\tilde{p} = 1$, the Weibull survival function reduces to the exponential survival probability and other Weibull lifetime functions would accordingly become the indicators following the exponential distribution. Therefore, the exponential time distribution is a special case of the Weibull function given $\tilde{p} = 1$. It is also identifiable that when $\tilde{p} > 1$, the hazard rate increases in a nonlinear fashion over t; when $\tilde{p} < 1$, the hazard rate decreases in a nonlinear form with t. Therefore, when the value of $\tilde{p}$ is given and $\tilde{p} \neq 1$, the hazard rate is either monotonically increasing or monotonically decreasing over a life course. Given this feature, one of the fundamental properties for the Weibull distribution is *monotonicity*.

Some statisticians and economists prefer to use the reciprocal of λ as the scale factor for analytic convenience. Given $\lambda^* = 1/\lambda$, the hazard function can be reexpressed as

$$h(t;\lambda^*,\tilde{p}) = \frac{\tilde{p}}{\lambda^*}\left(\frac{t}{\lambda^*}\right)^{\tilde{p}-1}. \tag{3.22}$$

Other Weibull functions can be also reparameterized by replacing λ with λ^*. One advantage of using λ^* as the scale parameter is that more complex Weibull properties, such as moments, the mean and variance of T, and the skewness, can be more conveniently formulated.

To demonstrate the impact the Weibull shape parameter poses on the Weibull distribution, below I display six hazard rate and six p.d.f. functions, given six values of $\tilde{p}$: 0.5, 1.0, 1.5, 2.0, 2.5, and 3.0. When deriving those curves, the value of λ is fixed at 1.0 and t ranges from 0 to 10. The following SAS program is written for the derivation of a graph displaying six hazard rate curves.

SAS Program 3.2:

```
options ls=80 ps=58 nodate pageno=1 number center;
ods select all;
ods trace off;
ods listing;
```

```
title1;
run;

data Weibull_hazard;
    w_scale = 1;
    do w_shape = 0.25 to 1.5 by 0.25;
    do t = 0.1 to 10 by .1;
    Weibull_hazard = (w_shape*w_scale) * (w_scale*t)**(w_shape - 1) ;
    output;
       end;
    end;
run;

goptions targetdevice=winprtc reset=global gunit=pct border cback=white
    colors=(black red blue) ftitle=swissxb ftext=swissxb htitle=2 htext=1.5;

proc gplot data=Weibull_hazard;
    plot Weibull_hazard * t = w_shape;
    symbol1 c=black     i=splines  l=1  v=plus;
    symbol2 c=red         i=splines  l=2  v=diamond;
    symbol3 c=blue       i=splines  l=3  v=square;
    symbol4 c=green     i=splines  l=4  v=circle;
    symbol5 c=magenta  i=splines  l=5  v=triangle;
    symbol6 c=brown     i=splines  l=6  v=star;
    title1 "Figure 3.3. Weibull hazard function";
    run;
quit;
```

The SAS software package does not specify the hazard function in the DATA step. Therefore, the equation of the hazard function needs to be written manually in the program. SAS Program 3.2 yields the plot of the hazard function in Figure 3.3, which displays $h(t)$ as monotonically decreasing over time for w_shape < 1, monotonically increasing for w_shape > 1, and constant for w_shape = 1 (the exponential function). It also indicates that $h(t)$ is highly sensitive to the change in the shape parameter and can take a value greater than 1. Therefore, theoretically defining the continuous hazard function as the conditional probability is inappropriate in this specific example.

The p.d.f. function can be derived by replacing the hazard equation in Program 3.2 with the 'PDF' function. With specification of a new title, a graph of the p.d.f. function with six values of p is displayed in Figure 3.4.

The reader might be interested in comparing the plots of the hazard and the p.d.f. functions. As it is a standardized measure relative to the survival rate and is highly sensitive to the change in the shape parameter, the hazard rate is a preferable lifetime indicator for displaying the relative risk of a particular event in survival analysis. Notice also that the change in the value of λ, not displayed here, modifies the scale on the t axis, but not on the basic shape.

The derivation of the expected survival time in the Weibull distribution, denoted by $E[T_0; T \sim \text{Weib}(\lambda, \tilde{p})]$ or $E(T; \lambda, \tilde{p})$, is mathematically complex. After some algebra, the expected survival time and its variance $V(T)$ can be calculated by the following two equations:

$$E(T; \lambda, \tilde{p}) = \lambda^{-1}\Gamma\left(1+\frac{1}{\tilde{p}}\right), \tag{3.23}$$

$$V(T; \lambda, \tilde{p}) = \frac{1}{\lambda^2}\left\{\Gamma\left(1+\frac{2}{\tilde{p}}\right)-\left[\Gamma\left(1+\frac{1}{\tilde{p}}\right)\right]^2\right\}, \tag{3.24}$$

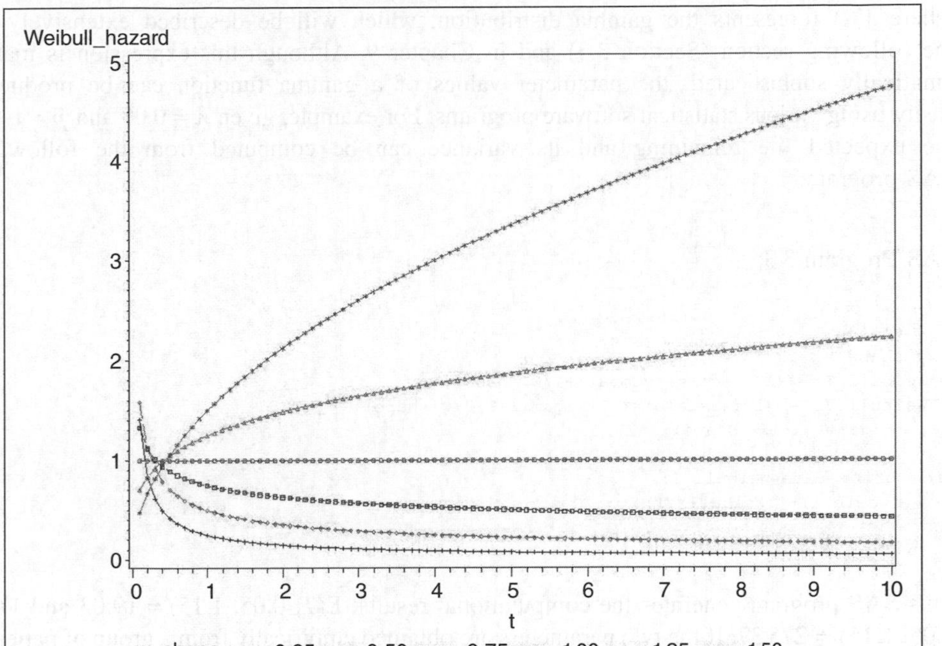

Figure 3.3 Weibull hazard function.

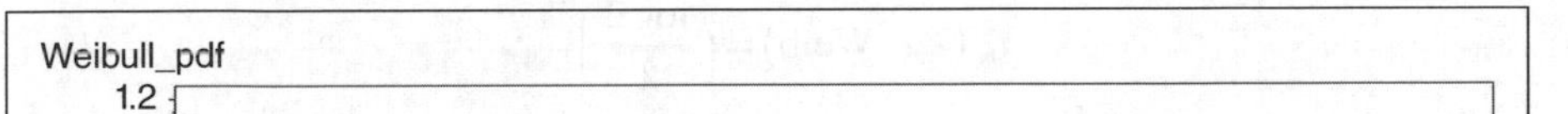

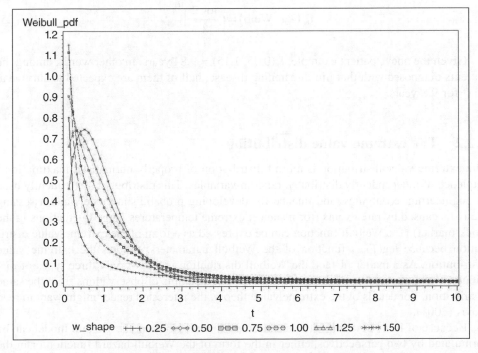

Figure 3.4 Weibull p.d.f. varying shape parm.

where Γ(.) represents the gamma distribution, which will be described extensively in the following section (Section 3.3) and in Chapter 9. Although this expression is mathematically sophisticated, the parameter values of a gamma function can be produced easily using various statistical software programs. For example, given $\lambda = 0.01$ and $\tilde{p} = 1.15$, the expected life remaining and its variance can be computed from the following SAS program.

SAS Program 3.3:

```
data Weibull_T;
   w_scale = 0.05;
   w_shape = 1.15;
   Weibull_T = (1/w_scale)*gamma(1+1/w_shape);
   Weibull_VT = (1/(w_scale)**2)*((gamma(1+2/w_shape))
     - (gamma(1+1/w_shape))**2);

proc print data=Weibull_T;
   var Weibull_T Weibull_VT;
run;
```

This SAS program generates the computational results: E(T; 0.05, 1.15) = 19.03 and V(T; 0.05, 1.15) = 275.37. If the two parameters are obtained empirically from a group of patients diagnosed with a life-threatening disease, then the estimated mean survival time for those patients is about 19 years, with the variance of survival times being 275.4 years.

The median survival time of a Weibull distribution is also well defined, given by

$$t_m(T \sim \text{Weib}) = \left(\frac{\log 2}{\lambda}\right)^{1/\tilde{p}}. \tag{3.25}$$

Given the above patient example, t_m(0.05, 1.15) = 9.84 years. In other words, among the patients diagnosed with that life-threatening disease, half of them are expected to survive at least for 9.8 years.

3.2.2 The extreme value distribution

The extreme value distribution is a limit distribution of properly normalized maxima for a sequence of independently distributed random variables. This distribution is frequently used in engineering, economics, and finance for developing probabilistic models and assessing the risks caused by rare events (for instance, extreme temperatures, large fluctuations in the stock market). The Weibull function can be expressed as a form of the extreme value distribution because log(T), a function of the Weibull parameters, follows the extreme value distribution. As a matter of fact, the Weibull distribution is one of only three types of distributions that model the maximum or minimum of a sample of observations from the same distribution. For details of the extreme value theory, the interested reader might want to read Coles (2001).

Because of its association with the extreme value distribution, the Weibull model can be formulated by two perspectives, either in the form of the Weibull hazard function or in the form of the extreme value distribution of log(T). Many statisticians consider it more convenient to use the extreme value distribution for the formalization of the Weibull parameters, given its high flexibility and generalizability. The two sets of model parameters, hazard or extreme value, are interrelated. For this reason, in many computer software packages, including SAS, the Weibull survival and probability density functions are specified in terms of the extreme value distribution, and, accordingly, $S(t; \lambda, \tilde{p})$ and $f(t; \lambda, \tilde{p})$ are defined as inverse functions (SAS, 2009, Volume 3).

Let $Y = \log(T)$, $p^* = 1/\tilde{p}$, and $\tilde{u} = \log(\lambda^*) = -\log(\lambda)$. The survival and the p.d.f. functions can be written in the form of the extreme value distribution, given by

$$S(t) = \exp\left[-\exp\left(\frac{y-\tilde{u}}{p^*}\right)\right], \quad -\infty < y < \infty$$

$$f(t) = (p^*)^{-1}\exp\left[\frac{y-\tilde{u}}{p^*} - \exp\left(\frac{y-\tilde{u}}{p^*}\right)\right]. \quad -\infty < y < \infty$$

Given the parameters of the extreme value distribution, the Weibull parameters can be calculated given the expressions $\tilde{p} = 1/p^*$ and $\lambda = \exp(-\tilde{u})$. Frequently, applied statisticians use the Weibull distribution in situations dealing with the minimum of random variables, whereas the extreme value distribution is applied as an approximation to model the maxima. Although they are not directly estimated in most computer software packages, the Weibull parameters can be easily obtained from the parameter estimates derived from the extreme value model. In some of the later chapters, I will further discuss the Weibull model and its likelihood function, and, accordingly, the issue of parameter conversion between the Weibull and the extreme value distributions will be repeatedly encountered in the text that follows.

The Weibull distribution is probably the most popular and most widely applied parametric model in survival analysis. Its high applicability largely resides in the flexibility and monotonicity of the distribution. In health research, for example, human mortality and morbidity generally follow an increasing pattern after the age of 10, which can be adequately described by the Weibull distribution. In gerontological studies, the Weibull model is considered the most appropriate perspective to describe survival processes among older persons within a limited time interval, as it correctly reflects the monotonic trend of old-age mortality (Liu, 2000). In Chapter 4, I will further describe how to estimate parameters based on the Weibull and the extreme value distributions using the maximum likelihood estimator, which accounts for censored observations and the effects of covariates.

3.3 Gamma distribution

In Section 3.2, I briefly described the gamma distribution as a two-parameter family of continuous probability distributions. It has a scale parameter λ (some statisticians specify the reciprocal of λ as the scale parameter) and a shape parameter $\tilde{k}$, where $\tilde{k} > 0$ and $\lambda > 0$. The gamma function, generally denoted by $\Gamma(\tilde{k})$, is mathematically defined as

$$\Gamma(\tilde{k}) = \int_0^\infty t^{\tilde{k}-1} e^{-t}\, dt. \tag{3.26}$$

After some algebra, the p.d.f. of the gamma distribution, generally written as $f[t; T \sim \Gamma(\lambda, \tilde{k})]$, is given by

$$f\left[t; T \sim \Gamma(\lambda, \tilde{k})\right] = \frac{\lambda(\lambda t)^{\tilde{k}-1} e^{-\lambda t}}{\Gamma(\tilde{k})}, \quad t > 0. \tag{3.27}$$

From Equation (3.26), a series of $\Gamma(\tilde{k})$ may be calculated such that $\Gamma(1) = 1$, $\Gamma(2) = 1$, $\Gamma(3) = 2$, $\Gamma(4) = 6$, $\Gamma(5) = 24$, and so on. Consequently, for any positive integer $\tilde{k}$ the density function of the gamma distribution can be rewritten by

$$f\left[t; T \sim \Gamma(\lambda, \tilde{k})\right] = \frac{\lambda(\lambda t)^{\tilde{k}-1} e^{-\lambda t}}{(\tilde{k}-1)!}, \quad t > 0. \tag{3.28}$$

It can be identified that when $\tilde{k} = 1$, the gamma density function reduces to the exponential density function, so the exponential distribution is also a special case of the gamma distribution.

When $\lambda = 1$, Equation (3.27) reduces to the one-parameter gamma distribution, also referred to as the standard gamma distribution of T, written as

$$f\left[t; T \sim \Gamma(\tilde{k})\right] = \frac{t^{\tilde{k}-1} e^{-t}}{\Gamma(\tilde{k})}, \quad t > 0, \tag{3.29}$$

with its c.d.f. defined as

$$F\left[t; T \sim \Gamma(\tilde{k})\right] = \int_0^t \frac{t^{\tilde{k}-1} e^{-u}}{\Gamma(\tilde{k})} du, \quad t > 0. \tag{3.30}$$

Equation (3.30) is called the *incomplete gamma function*. Specifications of the survival and hazard functions for the gamma distribution are based on this incomplete function. The survival function, denoted by $S[t; T \sim \Gamma(\tilde{k})]$, is given by

$$S\left[t; T \sim \Gamma(\tilde{k})\right] = 1 - F\left[t; T \sim \Gamma(\tilde{k})\right]. \tag{3.31}$$

Similarly, the gamma distributed hazard function can be expressed as

$$h\left[t; T \sim \Gamma(\tilde{k})\right] = \frac{f\left[t; T \sim \Gamma(\tilde{k})\right]}{S\left[t; T \sim \Gamma(\tilde{k})\right]} = \frac{\lambda(\lambda t)^{\tilde{k}-1} e^{-\lambda t}}{\Gamma(\tilde{k})\{1 - F\left[t; T \sim (\tilde{k})\right]\}}. \tag{3.32}$$

In order to understand the properties of the gamma distribution graphically, I illustrate six p.d.f. and six hazard rate functions of the standard gamma distribution. With λ fixed as

1.0, the six values of $\tilde{k}$ are, respectively, 0.5, 1.5, 2.5, 3.5, 4.5, and 5.5. An SAS program is presented below for the derivation of a graph displaying six p.d.f. curves of the gamma distribution.

SAS Program 3.4:

```
options ls=80 ps=58 nodate pageno=1 number center;
ods select all;
ods trace off;
ods listing;
title1;
run;

data Gamma_pdf;
    g_scale = 1;
    do g_shape = 0.5 to 5.5 by 1.0;
    do t = 0.1 to 10 by .1;
    Gamma_pdf=PDF('GAMMA',t,g_shape,g_scale);
    output;
         end;
    end;
run;

goptions targetdevice=winprtc reset=global gunit=pct border cback=white
       colors=(black red blue)
       ftitle=swissxb ftext=swissxb htitle=2 htext=1.5;

proc gplot data=Gamma_pdf;
    plot Gamma_pdf * t = g_shape;
    symbol1 c=black   i=splines  l=1  v=plus;
    symbol2 c=red     i=splines  l=2  v=diamond;
    symbol3 c=blue    i=splines  l=3  v=square;
    symbol4 c=green   i=splines  l=4  v=circle;
    symbol5 c=magenta i=splines  l=5  v=triangle;
    symbol6 c=brown   i=splines  l=6  v=star;
    title1 "Figure 3.5. Gamma pdf varying shape parm";
    run;
quit;
```

SAS Program 3.4 generates the plot shown in Figure 3.5, which displays the gamma p.d.f. curves associated with each of the values selected for k. Generally, the smaller the value of k, the more skewed the p.d.f. function looks. When the value of $\tilde{k}$ is lower than 1, the p.d.f. is a monotonically decreasing function over t; when $\tilde{k}$ is large, on the other hand, the gamma p.d.f. approximates a normal distribution. Therefore, the gamma distribution is a very flexible function for the description of various lifetime events, given the variety of shapes associated with different values of the gamma parameters. Such flexibility in modeling empirical survival data will be discussed further in Chapters 4 and 9.

The gamma hazard function can be derived by revising the DATA statement in SAS code, given in the following program.

SAS Program 3.5:

```
......

Data Gamma_hazard;
    g_scale = 1;
```

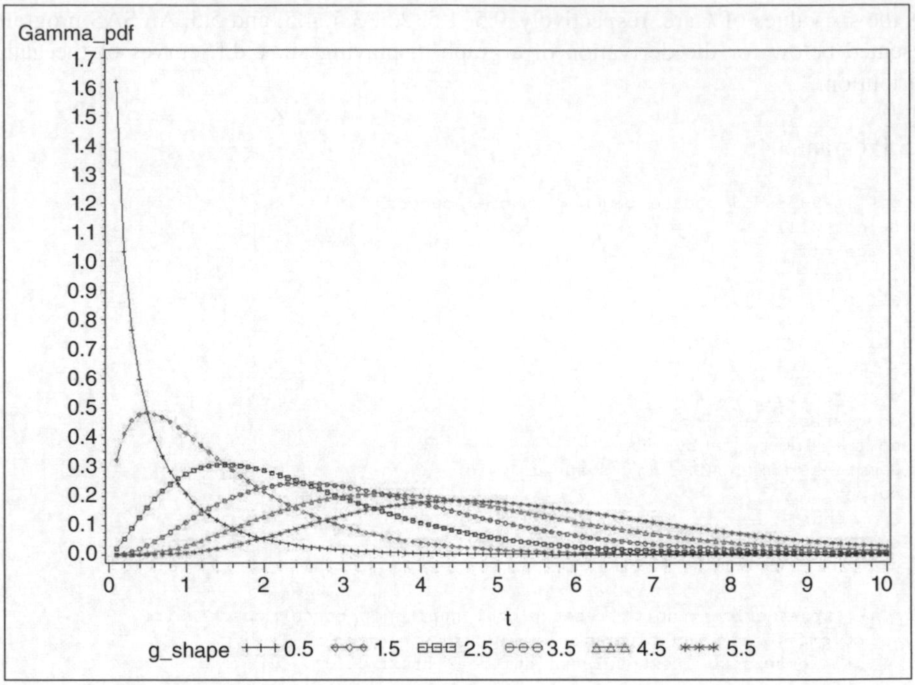

Figure 3.5 Gamma p.d.f. varying shape parm.

```
    do g_shape = 0.5 to 5.5 by 1.0;
    do t = 0.1 to 10 by .1;
          Gamma_pdf = PDF('GAMMA',t,g_shape,g_scale);
          Gamma_cdf = CDF('GAMMA',t,g_shape,g_scale);
          Gamma_survival = 1 - Gamma_cdf;
          Gamma_hazard =   Gamma_pdf / Gamma_survival;
    output;
       end;
    end;
run;
......
```

Given the above revisions, the PROC GPLOT procedure generates a series of Gamma_hazard curves along with time t, shown in Figure 3.6. The figure suggests that when $\tilde{k} < 1$, the hazard rate is a monotonically decreasing function; when $\tilde{k} > 1$, $h(t)$ is monotonically increasing over time. When $\tilde{k} = 1$, not shown in the plot, the hazard rate is constant throughout all times following the exponential distribution.

The expected lifetime and the variance of the gamma distribution are well defined. After much algebra, $E[T; T \sim \Gamma(\lambda, \tilde{k})]$ and $V[T; T \sim \Gamma(\lambda, \tilde{k})]$ are written as

$$E[T; T \sim \Gamma(\lambda, \tilde{k})] = \frac{\tilde{k}}{\lambda}, \tag{3.33}$$

$$V[T; T \sim \Gamma(\lambda, \tilde{k})] = \frac{\tilde{k}}{\lambda^2}. \tag{3.34}$$

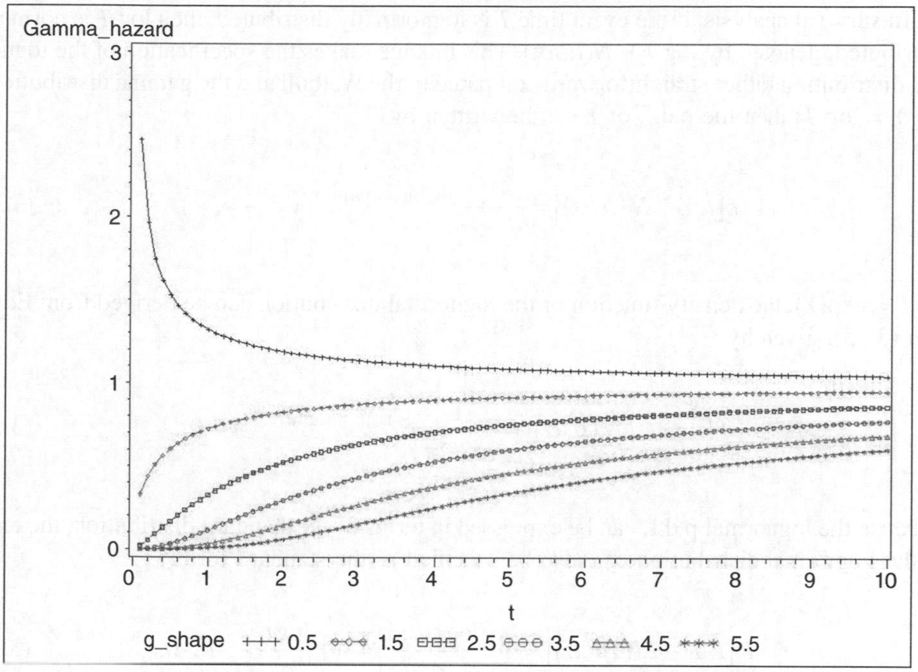

Figure 3.6 Gamma hazard rate function.

For analytic convenience, λ and $\tilde{k}$ are often assumed to take the same value in empirical studies, thereby reducing the gamma distribution to a one-parameter function. As a result, the expected value of T reduces to 1 with $V(T) = 1/\lambda = 1/\tilde{k}$.

The gamma distribution is useful for modeling survival processes that do not fit into a symmetrical distribution, although it is not as popular as the Weibull, lognormal, and log-logistic functions. Given its flexibility on the shape description, the gamma density function can be used to derive a wide variety of skewed distributions. In studies of human mortality, the probability distribution of health is often found to be severely skewed because of the strong 'selection of the fittest' effect in survival processes. Consequently, in biological studies the gamma distribution is frequently used to model lifetime events with unobserved heterogeneity (Manton and Stallard, 1979; Vaupel, Manton, and Stallard, 1979; Wild, 1983; Yashin and Iachine, 1995), as will be described extensively in some of the later chapters.

3.4 Lognormal distribution

The lognormal distribution is another popular parametric function widely used in survival analysis. Its high applicability lies in the fundamental property that the logarithm of a lognormal distribution is normally distributed with mean μ and variance σ^2, thus fitting ideally to the tradition of generalized linear modeling. In mathematical literature, the lognormal distribution is denoted by $T \sim LN(\mu, \sigma^2)$.

In survival analysis, if the event time T is lognormally distributed, then log T is normally distributed, denoted by $\log T \sim N(\mu, \sigma^2)$. This linkage makes the specification of the lognormal distribution rather straightforward compared to the Weibull and the gamma distributions. Let $Y = \log T$; then the p.d.f. of Y can be written by

$$f[t; Y \sim N(\mu, \sigma)] = \frac{1}{\sqrt{2\pi}\sigma} \mathrm{e}^{-1/2[(y-\mu)/\sigma]^2}, \quad y \in (-\infty, \infty). \tag{3.35}$$

As $T = \exp(Y)$, the density function of the lognormal distribution can be derived from Equation (3.35), given by

$$f[t; T \sim LN(\mu, \sigma)] = \frac{1}{t\sigma\sqrt{2\pi}} \mathrm{e}^{-1/2[(\log t-\mu)/\sigma]^2}, \quad t > 0. \tag{3.36}$$

Because the lognormal p.d.f. can be expressed in terms of the standard distribution, the c.d.f. of the lognormal distribution can also be specified as the standard form:

$$F[t; T \sim LN(\mu, \sigma)] = \Phi\left(\frac{\log t - \mu}{\sigma}\right) = \Phi\left(\frac{\log t}{\sigma}\right), \quad t > 0, \tag{3.37}$$

where $\Phi(\cdot)$ represents the cumulative normal distribution function, also referred to as the probit function. The survival function is

$$S[t; T \sim LN(\mu, \sigma)] = 1 - \Phi\left(\frac{\log t}{\sigma}\right). \tag{3.38}$$

Likewise, the hazard function is given by

$$h[t; T \sim LN(\mu, \sigma)] = \frac{f[t; T \sim LN(\mu, \sigma)]}{\Phi[t; T \sim LN(\mu, \sigma)]} = \frac{\frac{1}{t\sigma}\varphi\left(\frac{\log t}{\sigma}\right)}{\Phi\left(\frac{-\log t}{\sigma}\right)}, \tag{3.39}$$

where $\varphi(\cdot)$ is the probability density function of the normal distribution. Therefore, the cumulative hazard function can be readily derived, written as

$$H[t; T \sim LN(\mu, \sigma)] = -\log S[t; T \sim LN(\mu, \sigma)] = -\log\left[1 - \Phi\left(\frac{\log t}{\sigma}\right)\right]. \tag{3.40}$$

Using the above lognormal equations and adapting the SAS code programmed for the previously described parametric distributions, various lognormal distribution functions can

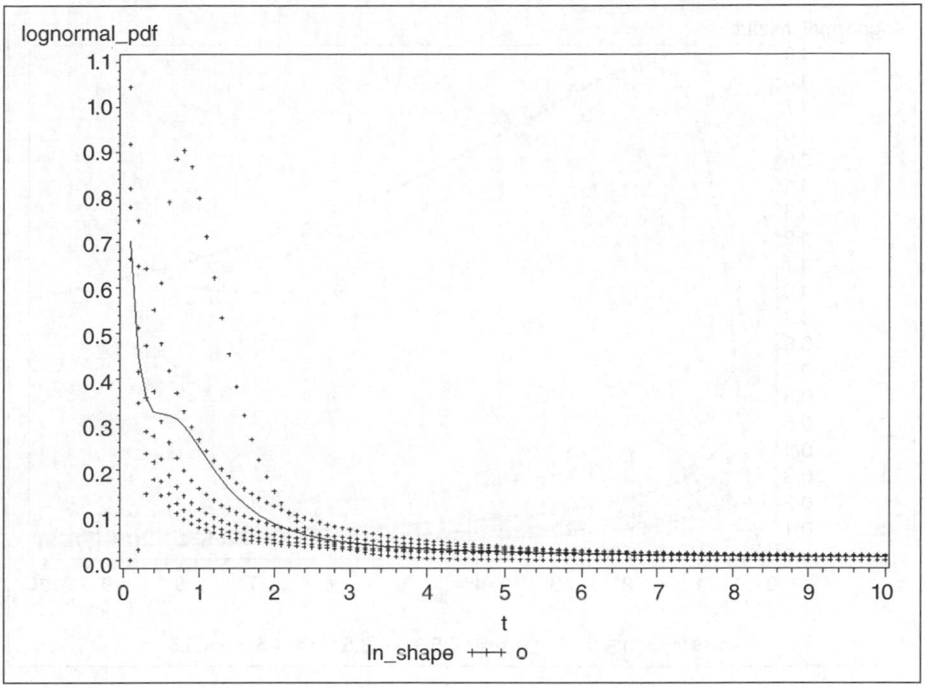

Figure 3.7 Lognormal p.d.f. varying shape parm.

be derived. Specifically, let $\mu = 0$; I select six values of σ to display six curves of the lognormal p.d.f. and six lognormal hazard functions. The six values of σ are, respectively, 0.5, 1.5, 2.5, 3.5, 4.5, and 5.5. The plot demonstrating the p.d.f. is shown in Figure 3.7 (the SAS programs for the lognormal distribution are not particularly presented because they are simply the modified versions of the programs previously described). Figure 3.7 shows that the p.d.f. of the lognormal distribution is a positively skewed function. As a higher σ results in greater skewness, σ is defined as the shape parameter of the lognormal distribution.

The next plot displays the lognormal hazard functions associated with different values of σ. Figure 3.8 displays the general pattern of the lognormal hazard function. The hazard rate at time 0 has the value 0, increases to a maximum somewhere in the t axis, then decreases consistently, and finally approaches 0 as t tends to infinity. When the value of the scale parameter σ is smaller than 0, the lognormal function describes a lifetime pattern that increases over time initially and then decreases.

Notice that μ and σ^2 in the above equations are not the mean and variance of T. Neither can we take $\exp(\mu)$ as the mean of T or $\exp(\sigma^2)$ as the variance of T because the transformation from one function to another reflects the transformation of the entire distribution, rather than of an expected value. Because the lognormal distribution of T is skewed, $E[T; T \sim LN(\mu, \sigma)] \neq \mu$ and $V[T; T \sim LN(\mu, \sigma)] \neq \sigma^2$.

When the event time T is a lognormally distributed random variable, its expected value, variance, and median are mathematically defined by

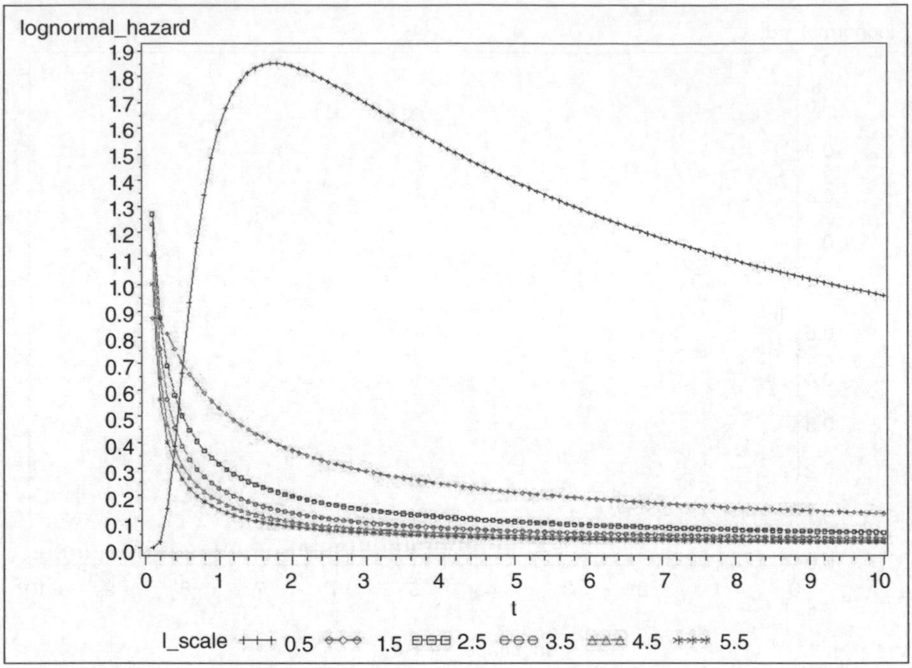

Figure 3.8 Lognormal hazard rate function.

$$\mathrm{E}[T; T \sim LN(\mu, \sigma)] = \exp\left(\mu + \frac{\sigma^2}{2}\right) = \exp\left(\frac{\sigma^2}{2}\right), \tag{3.41}$$

$$\begin{aligned} V[T; T \sim LN(\mu, \sigma)] &= \exp(2\mu)\{\exp[2\sigma^2 - \exp(\sigma^2)]\} \\ &= \exp[2\sigma^2 - \exp(\sigma^2)], \end{aligned} \tag{3.42}$$

$$t_m[T \sim LN(\mu, \sigma)] = \exp(\mu) = 1. \tag{3.43}$$

The positive skewness of the lognormal distribution implies that the median, $t_m[T; T \sim LN(\mu, \sigma)]$, lies below $\mathrm{E}[T; T \sim LN(\mu, \sigma)]$, with equality holding if and only if $\sigma^2 = 0$. Therefore, the lognormal mean of T is always greater than 1 unless the variance is 0. It should also be remembered that the lognormal function is a positively skewed distribution.

The lognormal distribution is frequently used as the multiplicative product of independent random variables, observed or unobserved. It can be used as a retransformed error term from normally distributed random errors in generalized linear modeling. Those regression techniques will be described and discussed extensively in Chapters 8 and 9.

3.5 Log-logistic distribution

The lognormal distribution is widely used to describe events whose rate increases initially and decreases consistently afterwards. This distribution, however, works well only in the absence of censoring. When there are considerable censored observations in survival data, the log-logistic distribution provides an appropriate option to describe a lifetime event that can be captured by the lognormal function. Generally, the shape of the log-logistic distribution is analogous to the lognormal distribution but with heavier tails. Another important feature of the log-logistic distribution is that it has a closed form for the cumulative distribution, the survival, and the hazard functions, unlike those of the lognormal model, thereby serving as a preferable distributional form to model a lifetime event that changes direction.

Mathematically, the log-logistic distribution of T is the antilogarithm of the familiar logistic distribution, as its name readily suggests. Given this, the logarithm of event time T follows a logistic distribution if T is distributed as log-logistic. Therefore, like the case of the Weibull model and the extreme value distribution, the log-logistic function can be approached from two perspectives.

Let $Y = \log T$. The density function of Y is defined as the familiar logistic distribution, given by

$$f(y) = \frac{\widehat{b}^{-1}\exp\left[(y-\tilde{u})/\widehat{b}\right]}{\left\{1+\exp\left[(y-\tilde{u})/\widehat{b}\right]\right\}^2}, \quad y \in (-\infty, \infty), \tag{3.44}$$

where $\tilde{u}$ and $\widehat{b}$ are parameters for the logistic function of Y, written as $Y \sim Logist(\tilde{u}, \widehat{b})$. Let $\lambda = \exp(\tilde{u})$ and $\widehat{p} = \widehat{b}^{-1}$. The antilogarithm of Equation (3.44) yields the density function of T:

$$f(t) = \frac{(\widehat{p}/\lambda)(t/\lambda)^{\widehat{p}-1}}{\left[1+(t/\lambda)^{\widehat{p}}\right]^2}, \quad t > 0, \tag{3.45}$$

where λ and $\widehat{p}$ are parameters of the log-logistic distribution, generally expressed as $T \sim LLogist(\lambda, \widehat{p})$. The c.d.f. of T is then given by

$$F[t; T \sim LLogist(\lambda, \widehat{p})] = \frac{1}{1+(t/\lambda)^{-\widehat{p}}}. \tag{3.46}$$

The survival and hazard rate functions of T can then be readily derived given their intimate associations with the p.d.f. and c.d.f. of T:

$$S[t; T \sim LLogist(\lambda, \widehat{p})] = 1 - F[t; T \sim LLogist(\lambda, \widehat{p})] = \left[1+(t/\lambda)^{\widehat{p}}\right]^{-1}, \tag{3.47}$$

$$h[t; T \sim LLogist(\lambda, \widehat{p})] = \frac{f[t; T \sim LLogist(\lambda, \widehat{p})]}{S[t; T \sim LLogist(\lambda, \widehat{p})]} = \frac{(\widehat{p}/\lambda)(t/\lambda)^{\widehat{p}-1}}{1+(t/\lambda)^{\widehat{p}}}. \tag{3.48}$$

As performed previously, I create two graphs of the log-logistic distributions, the p.d.f. and the hazard functions. Specifically, I let $\lambda = 1$ and give six values of $\widehat{p}$: 0.5, 1.5, 2.5, 3.5, 4.5, and 5.5. The SAS program is similar to the preceding examples except for

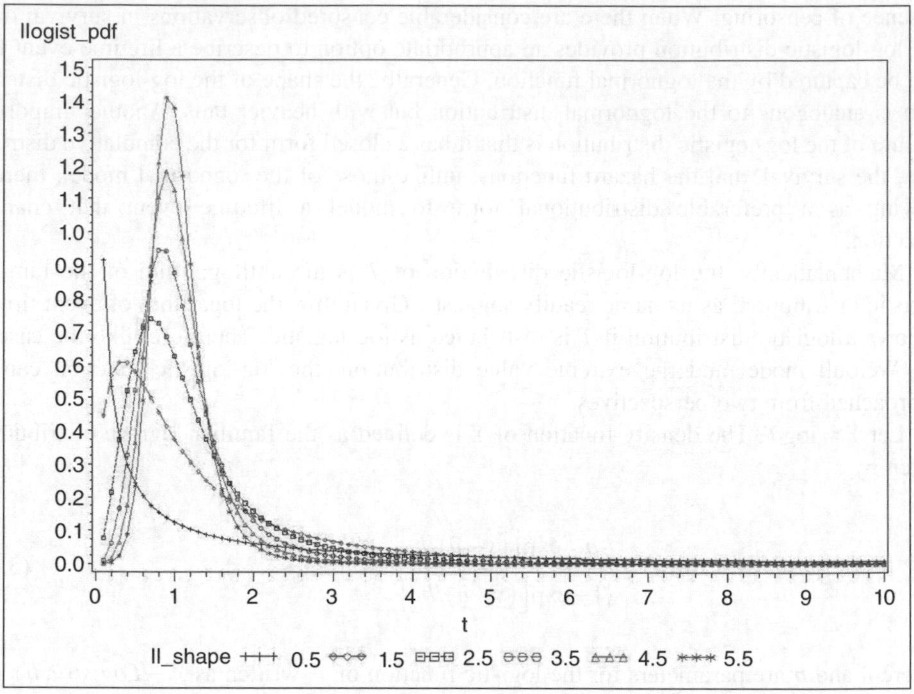

Figure 3.9 Log-logistic p.d.f. varying shape parm.

the concrete equation and function specifications and is therefore not presented. Using the input data, equations, and the relevant SAS code, the plot demonstrating six p.d.f. curves is shown first.

Figure 3.9 looks similar to the corresponding graph for the lognormal distribution in Figure 3.7. The next plot demonstrates six corresponding hazard functions given the log-logistic distribution. The similarities and differences between Figures 3.10 and 3.8 are both striking. From Figure 3.10, several important features regarding the log-logistic distribution can be summarized and discussed. First, unlike the popular Weibull model, the log-logistic distribution describes a nonmonotonic hazard function. Second, when $\hat{p} \leq 1$, the hazard rate decreases over t monotonically; when $\hat{p} > 1$, the hazard function increases initially and then decreases consistently over t, with the shape being unimodal. Third, as mentioned earlier, the cumulative distribution function of the log-logistic distribution, which can be written by $F[t; T \sim LLogist(\lambda, \hat{p})]$, can be expressed in a closed form; therefore this parametric function is useful to analyze data with censoring. There are some other features which, linked to the capability of allowing for group differences, will be discussed in Chapter 4.

After much algebra, the expected T, the variance, and the median in the log-logistic distribution are mathematically defined by

$$E[T; T \sim LLogist(\lambda, \hat{p})] = \frac{\lambda(\pi/\hat{p})}{\sin(\pi/\hat{p})}, \quad \text{for } \hat{p} > 1, \tag{3.49}$$

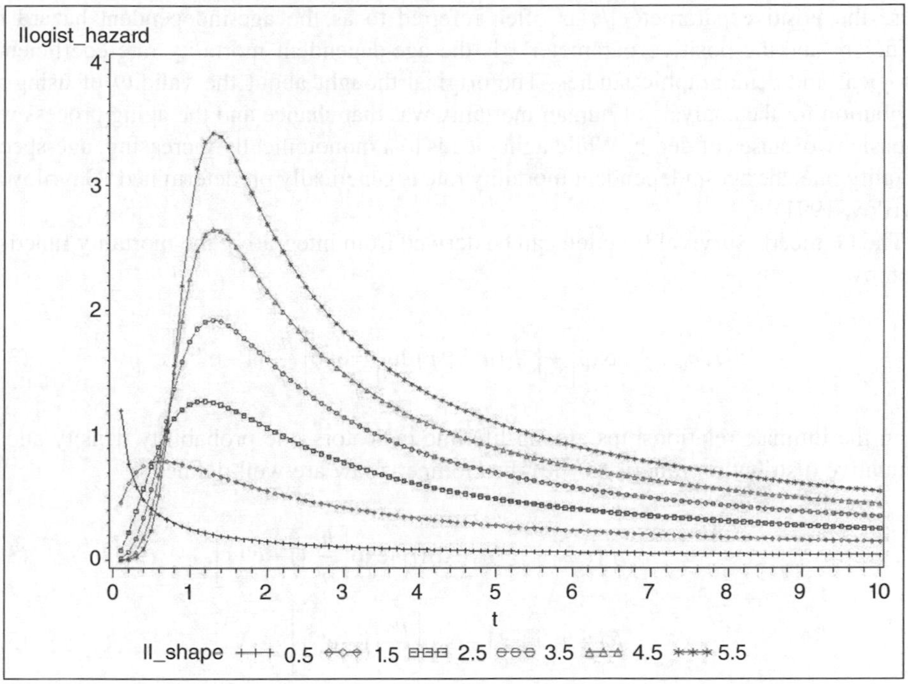

Figure 3.10 Log-logistic hazard rate function.

$$V[T; T \sim LLogist(\lambda, \tilde{p})] = \frac{\lambda^2}{\frac{2(\pi/\tilde{p})}{\sin 2(\pi/\tilde{p})} - \frac{(\pi/\tilde{p})^2}{\sin^2(\pi/\tilde{p})}}, \quad \text{for } \tilde{p} > 2, \tag{3.50}$$

$$t_m[T \sim LLogist(\lambda, \tilde{p})] = \lambda. \tag{3.51}$$

Mathematical inferences for the above three equations and other properties of the log-logistic distribution involve complex algebra, and therefore they are not further elaborated in this text. In Chapter 4, I will describe the log-logistic distribution and its statistical inference when model covariates are included.

3.6 Gompertz distribution and Gompertz-type hazard models

Of various survival functions, the Gompertz (1820, 1825) law has perhaps been the most widely used quantitative description of human mortality and survival by mathematical biologists and demographers. This mathematical function illustrates an exponential mortality schedule, particularly over the range 40–80 years (Eakin and Witten, 1995; Finch, Pike, and Witten, 1990; Hirsch, Liu, and Witten, 2000; Liu and Witten, 1995; Riggs, 1990). The classical Gompertzian mortality function is simply given by

$$h(t; h_0, r) = h_0 e^{rt}, \tag{3.52}$$

where the positive parameter h_0 is often referred to as the age-independent hazard rate coefficient and the positive parameter r is the age-dependent mortality rate coefficient in biological and demographic studies. The original thought about the validity of using this distribution for the analysis of human mortality was that chance and the aging process were the basic two causes of death. While aging leads to a monotonically increasing, age-specific mortality rate, the age-independent mortality rate is genetically predetermined (Gavrilov and Gavrilov, 1991).

The Gompertz survival function can be derived from integrating the mortality functions, given by

$$S(t; h_0, r) = \exp\left[-\int_0^t h(u; h_0, r)\,\mathrm{d}u\right] = \exp\left[\frac{h_0}{r}\left(1 - \mathrm{e}^{rt}\right)\right]. \tag{3.53}$$

Given the intimate relationships among lifetime indicators, the probability density and the cumulative distribution functions with the Gompertz law are well defined:

$$f(t; h_0, r) = h_0 \exp(rt) \exp\left[\frac{h_0}{r}\left(1 - \mathrm{e}^{rt}\right)\right], \tag{3.54}$$

$$F(t; h_0, r) = 1 - \exp\left[\frac{h_0}{r}\left(1 - \mathrm{e}^{rt}\right)\right]. \tag{3.55}$$

First, I illustrate a graph of six Gompertz hazard functions, with the value of h_0 fixed at 0.05 and six selected values of r, which are 0.05, 0.075, 0.10, 0.0125, 0.0150, and 0.175. The SAS program for this step is not presented, given the similarities to the previous programs. The resulting plot is shown in Figure 3.11.

Equation (3.52) and Figure 3.11, both analytically and graphically, demonstrate that the Gompertz hazard function follows an exponential form; that is, not only does the hazard rate increase over t, but the rate of change in the hazard rate also increases over time. Therefore, the Gompertzian hazard rate is never concave. Notice that here the term 'exponential' refers to the hazard function, whereas in the exponential distribution the exponential form is associated with the survival function.

Some scientists have used the log transformation of Equation (3.52) to display a transformed linear function, given by

$$\log h(t; h_0, r) = \log h_0 + rt. \tag{3.56}$$

With the same input data, the subsequent plot displays the log-linear result given by Equation (3.56) (Figure 3.12). Clearly, the log transformation of the hazard function given a Gompertz distribution is linearly associated with time. Because of this feature, it is common in demographic research to calculate the logarithms of age-specific death rates as an important population measure and plot such mortality transforms against age (Horiuchi and Coale, 1990).

More recently, there has been increasing skepticism about the validity of the Gompertz model as an accurate portrayal of human mortality. Some empirical studies demonstrate that, at advanced ages, the rate of increase over time slows down and, as a result, the trajectory of mortality falls off from a convex Gompertz curve (Carey *et al.*, 1992; Vaupel, Manton,

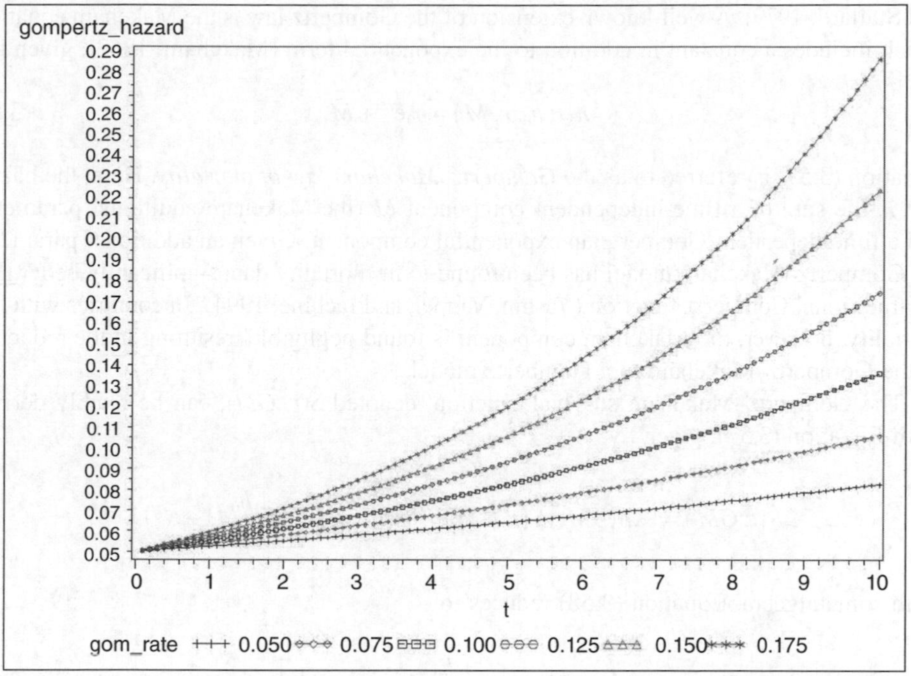

Figure 3.11 Gompertz hazard rate function.

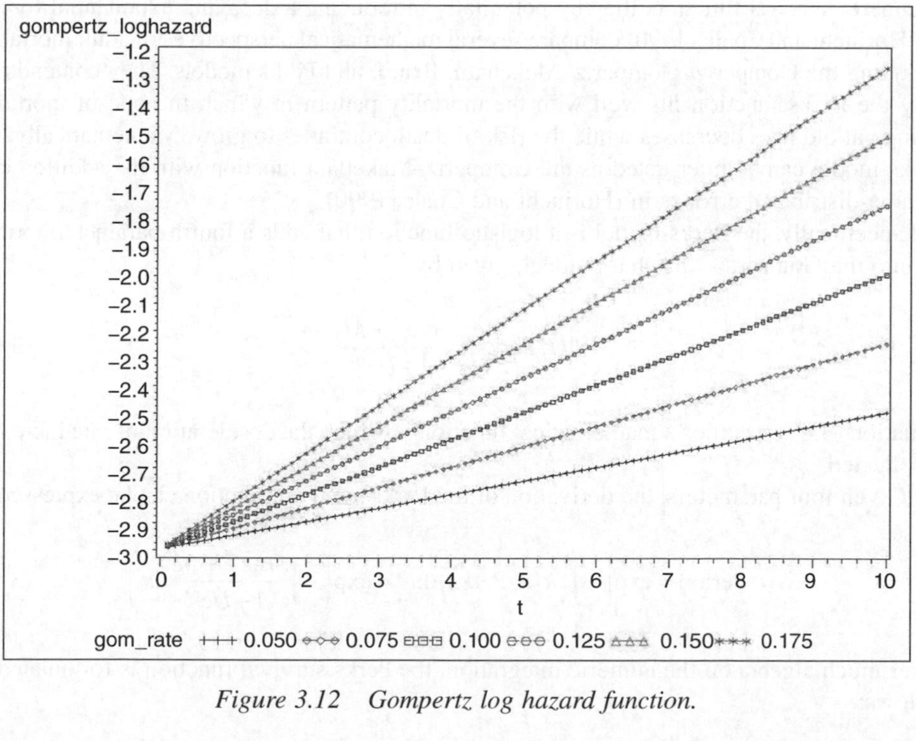

Figure 3.12 Gompertz log hazard function.

and Stallard, 1979). A well-known extension of the Gompertz law is the Makeham equation, which includes a constant in addition to the exponential term (Makeham, 1867), given by

$$h\left(t; h_0, r, \tilde{M}\right) = h_0 \mathrm{e}^{rt} + \tilde{M}. \tag{3.57}$$

Equation (3.57) is referred to as the *Gompertz–Makeham law of mortality*. Here, the hazard rate is the sum of a time-independent component $\tilde{M}$ (the Makeham additional parameter) and a time-dependent Gompertzian exponential component. Given an additional parameter, the Gompertz–Makeham model has been found to fit mortality data significantly better than the traditional Gompertz function (Yashin, Vaupel, and Iachine, 1994). In countries with low mortality, however, the Makeham component is found negligible, resulting in the reduction of the Gompertz–Makeham to a Gompertz model.

The Gompertz–Makeham survival function, denoted $S(t;\ GM)$, can be readily derived from Equation (3.57), given by

$$S(t; GM) = \exp\left(-\tilde{M}t\right) S(t; h_0, r) = \exp\left(-\tilde{M}t\right) \exp\left[\frac{h_0}{r}\left(1 - \mathrm{e}^{rt}\right)\right]. \tag{3.58}$$

With some algebra, Equation (3.58) reduces to

$$S(t; GM) = \exp\left[\frac{h_0}{r}\left(1 - \mathrm{e}^{rt}\right) - \tilde{M}t\right]. \tag{3.59}$$

Therefore, the addition of the Makeham constant adds a multiplicative effect to the original Gompertz survival function, thereby potentially introducing a decaying exponential force.

Horiuchi and Coale (1990) compare several mathematical perspectives of adult mortality, including the Gompertz, Gompertz–Makeham, Beard, and Perks models. They contend that only the Perks function fits well with the mortality pattern in which the rate of mortality change at old ages decreases while the risk of death continues to grow. Mathematically, the Perks model can be interpreted as the Gompertz–Makeham function with the addition of a gamma-distributed error term (Horiuchi and Coale, 1990).

Specifically, the Perks model is a logistic function that adds a fourth parameter, termed $\breve{U}$, into the Gompertz–Makeham model, given by

$$h(t; \text{Perks}) = \frac{h_0 \mathrm{e}^{rt} + \tilde{M}}{1 + \breve{U}\mathrm{e}^{rt}}. \tag{3.60}$$

Equation (3.60) specifies a mathematical function in which the deceleration of rate increases is reflected.

Given four parameters, the derivation of the Perks survival function can be expressed as

$$S(t; \text{Perks}) = \exp\left[-\int_0^t h(u; \text{Perks})\,\mathrm{d}u\right] = \exp\left(-\int_0^t \frac{h_0 \mathrm{e}^{ru} + \tilde{M}}{1 + \breve{U}\mathrm{e}^{ru}}\,\mathrm{d}u\right). \tag{3.61}$$

After much algebra on the numeric integration, the Perks survival function is formulated as follows:

$$S(t;\,\text{Perks}) = \exp\left\{-\left[\left(\tilde{M}+\frac{h_0}{\breve{U}}\right)t - \frac{h_0}{\breve{U}r}\log\left(\breve{U}+e^{-rt}\right)+\frac{\tilde{M}}{r}\log\left(1+\breve{U}e^{rt}\right)\right.\right. \tag{3.62}$$
$$\left.\left. -\frac{1}{r}\left(\tilde{M}-\frac{h_0}{\breve{U}}\right)\log\left(1+\breve{U}\right)\right]\right\}.$$

To highlight differences in the predicted hazard rates generated from the Gompertz, the Gompertz–Makeham, and the Perks models, respectively, I use the 1973–1977 death registration data of Swedish women aged from 55 to 95 years to create a plot displaying the hazard functions generated from the three approaches. The parameter estimates for each model are presented in Horiuchi and Coale (1990, p. 259). The methods about how to derive such parameters from empirical data are described in Chapter 9. The following SAS program constructs this plot with known parameter estimates.

SAS Program 3.6:

```
* Calculating hazard rates from Gompertz, Makeham, and Perks models *;

options ls=80 ps=58 nodate;
ods select all;
ods trace off;
ods listing;
title1;
run;

data Gompertz_Makeham_Perks;
  do group = 1 to 3;
  do t = 55 to 105 by 0.1;
  if group = 1 then hazard = 0.00399*exp(0.11180*(t-55));
  if group = 2 then hazard = 0.00073 + (0.00355*exp(0.11545*(t-55)));
  if group = 3 then hazard = (0.0023*exp(0.13876*(t-55)))/(1 + 0.00367*exp(0.13876*(t-55)));
  output;
  end;
  end;
run;

proc format;
  value group_fmt 1 = 'Gompertz'
                  2 = 'Makeham'
                  3 = 'Perks';
run;

goptions targetdevice=winprtc reset=global gunit=pct border cback=white
      colors=(black red blue)
      ftitle=swissxb ftext=swissxb htitle=2 htext=1.5;

proc gplot data=Gompertz_Makeham_Perks;
  format group group_fmt.;
  plot hazard * t = group;
    symbol1 c=black  i=splines  l=1  v=plus;
    symbol2 c=red    i=splines  l=2  v=diamond;
    symbol3 c=blue   i=splines  l=3  v=square;
    title1 "Figure 3.13. Hazard rate functions for Gompertz, Makeham and Perks models";
    run;
quit;
```

SAS program 3.6 produces a plot displaying the hazard functions derived from the three parametric distributions. I extend the age range from 55–100 to 55–105 for displaying mortality patterns for centenarians. In the calculating equations, the time t is given by $(t - 55)$ because the parameters are derived in an age range starting with 55, so that, when calculating a series of hazard rates, $h(0)$ actually indicates the hazard rate at age 55. The outcome of SAS Program 3.6 is given in the graph in Figure 3.13, where three mortality functions from age 55 to age 105 are compared. It is interesting to note that prior to age 85, the three hazard curves almost coincide with each other. After age 90 or so, the Perks function separates distinctly from the other two hazard schedules. From the shapes of the three hazard curves, some basic differences in the three models can be identified. Whereas both the Gompertz and the Gompertz–Makeham distributions display an exponential function over age, the Perks function predicts a trend of mortality deceleration in later life. Compared to the observed data, not shown in the plot, the Perks model reflects the closest set of the hazard rates at ages older than 85 years, therefore displaying its high applicability in modeling mortality at advanced ages. By contrast, the Gompertz and the Gompertz–Makeham models are not sensitive at all to the observed mortality deceleration and thus fit poorly to the empirical data beyond age 85.

Notice that among the parametric models delineated in this chapter, the Weibull distribution, monotonic and flexible, also has the capability to describe mortality deceleration at older ages.

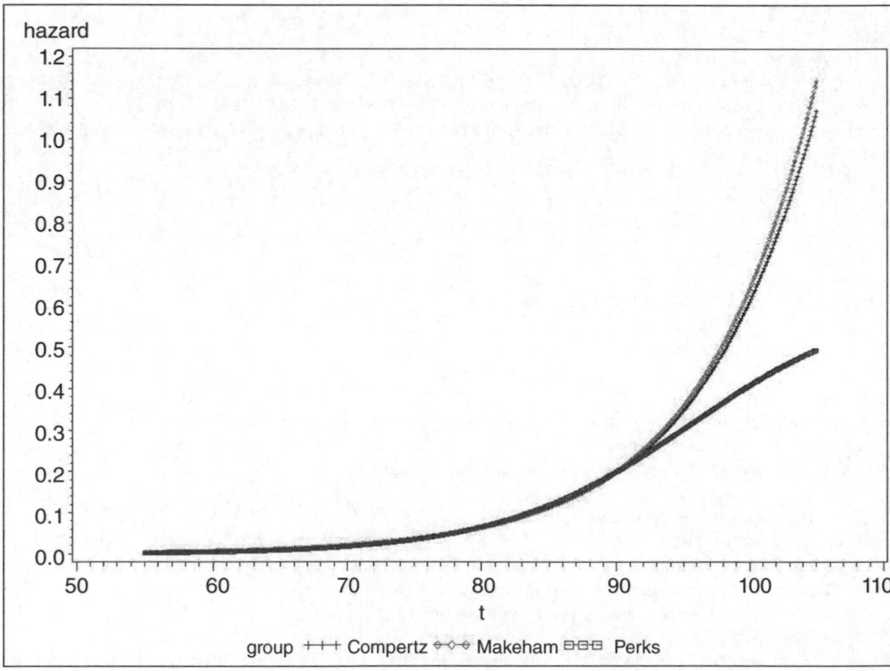

Figure 3.13 Hazard rate functions for Gompertz, Makeham, and Perks models.

3.7 Hypergeometric distribution

The hypergeometric distribution is a discrete probability function describing the number of 'successes' in a sequence of n draws without replacement from a finite population. Though not originally related to lifetime processes, the hypergeometric distribution is used in survival analysis for formalizing the logrank test on survival curves of two or more population subgroups, as briefly presented in Chapter 2 (Mantel and Haenszel, 1959; Peto and Peto, 1972). This distribution, specifically, is associated with the following two conditions: (i) a sample of n is randomly selected without replacement from a population of N individuals and (ii) in the population, D items are classified as 'successes' and $(N - D)$ items as 'failures.' The specification of these two conditions highlights the conceptual difference between the hypergeometric and the binomial distributions. Whereas a binomial experiment, also called the Bernoulli trials, requires a constant probability on every trial, in the hypergeometric distribution the probability of a success changes on every trial given selection without replacement.

To describe the hypergeometric distribution, first I define a random variable $\tilde{Y}$ that follows the hypergeometric probability function with parameters N, D, and n. This random variable is used to specify the probability of getting d successes and $(n - d)$ failures in n items, which can be expressed in the form of a combination:

$$\Pr\left(\tilde{Y}=d\right)=\frac{\begin{array}{c}(\text{number of ways getting } d \text{ successes})\\ \times(\text{number of way getting } n-d \text{ failures})\end{array}}{(\text{total number of ways selecting } n \text{ items from } N)}.$$

In the above equation, three counting processes are specified. In terms of the denominator, there are N ways to select the first item, $N - 1$ ways to select the second item, . . . , and $N - n$ ways to select the nth item. Consequently, using the binomial coefficient, the total number of ways to select n items from N can be mathematically expressed as

$$\text{Total number of ways selecting } n \text{ items from } N=\frac{N!}{n!(N-n)!}. \tag{3.63}$$

In the tradition of the binomial distribution, Equation (3.63) can be more conveniently written by

$$\text{Total number of ways selecting } n \text{ items from } N=\binom{N}{n}. \tag{3.64}$$

Likewise, the two terms in the numerator can be expressed by

$$\text{Total number of ways of getting } d \text{ successes}=\binom{D}{d}, \tag{3.65}$$

$$\text{Total number getting } n-d \text{ failures}=\binom{N-D}{n-d}. \tag{3.66}$$

Given Equations (3.64) through (3.66), the probability of getting d successes in n items is mathematically defined as

$$\Pr\left(\tilde{Y}=d\right)=\frac{\binom{D}{d}\binom{N-D}{n-d}}{\binom{N}{n}}, \tag{3.67}$$

where the binomial coefficient is defined as the coefficient in the polynomial expansion.

Equation (3.67) is referred to as the *hypergeometric distribution formula*, from which the hypergeometric probability, given values of d, N, n, and D, can be readily computed. The expected value of the hypergeometric distribution and its variance are well defined, given by

$$E\left(\tilde{Y};N,n,D\right)=\frac{nD}{N} \tag{3.68}$$

and

$$V\left(\tilde{Y};N,n,D\right)=\frac{nD(N-d)(N-n)}{N^2(N-1)}. \tag{3.69}$$

As indicated in Chapter 2, Equation (3.68) is straightforward for interpretation: given the randomness of selection, the expected value of the random variable $\tilde{Y}$ is simply the proportion of the total number N selected to the sample n multiplied by the total number of 'successes' in the population N; that is, in the hypergeometric distribution n is expected to be proportionally allocated to be d or $(n - d)$.

Below, I provide a simple example to demonstrate how to calculate the hypergeometric probability given values of N, n, and D. Suppose that we have a population of 50 older persons ($N = 50$), among whom 10 have a given chronic disease ($D = 10$). Drawing 5 persons randomly from those 50 individuals ($n = 5$), I want to know the probability of getting two persons diagnosed with that chronic disease in the sample, given a hypergoemetric distribution. Placing these numbers in Equation (3.67) leads to

$$\Pr(d=2;50,5,10)=\frac{\binom{10}{2}\binom{50-10}{5-2}}{\binom{50}{5}}=\frac{\dfrac{10!}{2!(10-2)!}\,\dfrac{40!}{3!(40-3)!}}{\dfrac{50!}{5!(50-5)!}}$$

$$=\frac{\dfrac{10\times 9}{2}\,\dfrac{40\times 39\times 38}{6}}{\dfrac{50\times 49\times 48\times 47\times 46}{5\times 4\times 3\times 2}}=\frac{45\times 9880}{2\,118\,760}=0.2098.$$

Therefore, the probability of getting two persons diagnosed with the chronic disease in a sample of 5 is 0.2098.

Similarly, the expected value and variance for the number of individuals with that chronic disease are given by

$$E(\tilde{Y}; 50, 5, 10) = \frac{5 \times 10}{50} = 1,$$

$$V(\tilde{Y}; 50, 5, 10) = \frac{5 \times 10(50-10)(50-5)}{50^2(50-1)} = \frac{88\,000}{122\,500} = 0.7184.$$

Therefore, I am expected to get 1 person diagnosed with the chronic disease in a sample of 5, with variance 0.7184. The reader might want to do some additional exercises about the hypergeometric distribution by using different sets of values.

3.8 Other distributions

There are some other lifetime distributions occasionally used in survival analysis. Researchers sometimes encounter phenomena that follow an extremely unbalanced distribution, where the probability of a population that is related to a low level of some characteristics is very high and then it decreases steadily as the level increases. The Pareto distribution can be used to describe profiles of such a type of event. This distribution is originally developed and applied by economists to describe the allocation of wealth among individuals; more recently, it is extended to describe many other situations in which the distribution of 'high' to 'low' is found. Mathematically, the Pareto distribution of a random variable X is associated with two parameters: one is a positive value representing the minimum possible value of X and the other, also positive, is called the Pareto index by economists. The p.d.f. and other related functions of the Pareto distribution are all well defined. In survival analysis, the Pareto function can be applied to model survival processes among AIDS patients or the mortality decline over age in the population aged 10 years or younger.

In natural and physical sciences, the inverse Gaussian distribution is sometimes applied to analyze positively skewed survival data. It has also been used to analyze fluctuations in the stock market. Mathematically, the inverse Gaussian distribution is a family of a continuous time process with a drift parameter and a dispersion parameter, where the drift parameter is mathematically defined as the mean of the distribution. When the drift parameter is 1, the inverse Gaussian distribution reduces to the Wald distribution, a popular distributional function in general statistics. With properties analogous to those of the lognormal distribution, this distribution is nonmonotonic, initially increasing and then decreasing over time, and eventually approaching a constant value as the lifetime becomes infinite. From empirical data, it is easy to estimate the two parameters of the inverse Gaussian distribution. This unique functional form can be used to model a wide range of distributions, from a highly skewed, given a smaller value of the dispersion parameter, to an almost normal distribution, where the dispersion parameter tends to infinity. The name 'inverse Gaussian distribution' may cause some confusion because there is no general sampling rule or transformational procedure by which the inverse Gaussian variable can be generated from a normal distribution (Chhikara and Folks, 1989). The interested reader wishing to learn more about the inverse Gaussian distribution is referred to Chhikara and Folks (1989).

3.9 Summary

In this chapter, some basic parametric distributions are described and summarized. In addition, a number of plots are generated to help the reader understand better the underlying properties and features of various parametric distributions. In Chapter 4, I will continue to describe some of the parametric models, such as the exponential, the Weibull, and log-logistic functions, as associated with covariates, statistical inferences for derivation of parameter estimates, and techniques about hypothesis testing. Therefore, it is essential for the reader to get a solid foundation in order to understand more complicated models, likelihood functions, and the detailed estimating procedures. For example, the Weibull model has been widely used in both biomedical and observational studies, but it is often expressed as a function of the extreme value distribution, and therefore the Weibull parameters are often derived from those estimated for an extreme value distribution model. Given this transformation, the conversion of the Weibull and the extreme value parameters, as detailed in Section 3.2, is worth paying special attention to.

4

Parametric regression models of survival analysis

In some sense, regression modeling is the hallmark of the modern survival analysis, especially in behavioral science. As indicated in Chapter 2, descriptive approaches do not possess the capability to test causal effects because some 'lurking' covariates can significantly confound the true association between two factors under examination. Regression modeling provides a powerful methodology to test theoretical hypotheses about causality and compare effects across population groups, given its capacity to adjust for the influences of potential confounders. In survival analysis, regression models are used for analyzing the causal linkage between an outcome lifetime variable (such as the hazard rate, the event time, or the survival function) and one or more independent variables, with one or more variables serving as controls. As the specification of independent and control variables involves prior knowledge and theoretical hypotheses, construction of a lifetime regression model needs to be guided by existing theories, previous findings, and specific research questions. Therefore, regression modeling, both generally and with specific regard to survival analysis, is a theory-based methodology, not just an amalgamation of mathematical rules, statistical procedures, and algebraic manipulations.

In this chapter, I describe parametric regression modeling on survival data, which generally points to statistical techniques combining a known parametric distribution of survival times with multivariate regression modeling procedures. In particular, I first portray general specifications and statistical inferences of parametric regression modeling. Then, several widely used parametric regression models, such as the exponential, the Weibull, and the log-logistic regression models, are illustrated with empirical examples. Some other parametric regression models are also briefly described. Special attention is paid to the Weibull regression model, given its widespread applicability in survival analysis and high flexibility in describing empirical lifetime data. Lastly, I summarize the chapter with a comparison of several key parametric regression models.

Survival Analysis: Models and Applications, First Edition. Xian Liu.

4.1 General specifications and inferences of parametric regression models

Like constructing other types of regression models, parametric regression modeling in survival analysis starts with the specification of parameters. First, for illustrative convenience, I specify a causal model involving a number of factors, including one or more independent variables and one or more control variables, and a dependent lifetime variable. Statistically, both the independent and the control variables are regarded as covariates in a multivariate regression model. According to a specific theoretical framework, the covariates, denoted by $\boldsymbol{x}$, a $1 \times M$ vector containing elements $(x_1, x_2, \ldots)'$, are those causally associated with the dependent lifetime outcomes. The dependent variable is the event time T, which may be censored. In parametric regression perspectives, this dependent variable is assumed to follow a known probability distribution whose parameters may depend on $\boldsymbol{x}$. The effect of covariates on the parameters can be modeled either using the survival time or the hazard rate at time t as a function of a parameter vector $\boldsymbol{\theta}$. Empirically, $\boldsymbol{x}$ may contain explanatory variables (independent and control) and some theoretically relevant interactions predictive of the survival time or of the hazard rate, such as medical treatment, severity of a given medical condition, and the interaction between those two variables in a typical biomedical study. The elements in $\boldsymbol{x}$ are sometimes called the *exogenous variables* as their causes are not generated within a regression model.

There are two popular perspectives in terms of parametric regression modeling. The first perspective is the parametric hazard rate model in which covariates impact the hazard function. In this class of parametric regression modeling, the proportional hazard rate model, in which the effects of covariates are assumed to be multiplicative, is most common. The second class uses the log transformation of event times as the outcome measure, often assumed to be linearly associated with covariates. In this section, I describe general specifications of these two approaches and the associated likelihood functions in the presence of right censoring.

4.1.1 Specifications of parametric regression models on the hazard function

In terms of parametric regression models on the hazard function, each observation under investigation is assumed to be subject to an instantaneous hazard rate, $h(t)$, of experiencing a particular event, where $t = 0, 1, \ldots, \infty$. Because the hazard rate is always nonnegative, the effects of covariates are generally specified as a multiplicative term $\exp(\boldsymbol{x}'\boldsymbol{\beta})$, where $\boldsymbol{\beta}$ represents a vector of regression coefficients to be estimated. Consequently, the hazard rate model on the causal relationships between covariates and lifetime processes is written by

$$h(t|\boldsymbol{x}) = h_0(t)\exp(\boldsymbol{x}'\boldsymbol{\beta}) \tag{4.1}$$

where $h_0(t)$ denotes a known baseline hazard function for continuous time T and $\boldsymbol{\beta}$ provides a set of the effects of covariates on the hazard rate, with the same length as $\boldsymbol{x}$. As can be seen from Equation (4.1), the effects of $\boldsymbol{x}$ on the hazard rate are multiplicative, or proportional, so that the predicted value of $h(t)$, given $\boldsymbol{x}$, denoted by $\hat{h}(t|\boldsymbol{x})$, can be restricted in the range $(0, \infty)$. Nonmultiplicativity of the effects of given covariates, if it exists, can be captured by specification of one or more interaction terms, contained in $\boldsymbol{x}$. Given this specification, the class of parametric regression models represented by Equation (4.1) is generally referred to as the *proportional hazard rate model*. In this survival perspective, all individuals are assumed to follow a univariate hazard function, with individual heterogeneity primarily reflected in the proportional scale change for a stratification of distinct population subgroups; that is, any two individuals have hazard rates that are constant multiples of one another (Lawless, 2003). The concept of *proportionality* in this context, nevertheless, points more to a statistical perspective than to a substantive linkage. With specification of interaction terms for some covariates, for example, the effects of those variables are no longer proportional or multiplicative. The issue of nonproportionality will be discussed further in later chapters.

The term $h_0(t)$ in Equation (4.1) represents a parametric baseline hazard function within the context of parametric regression modeling, attaching to a particular probability distribution of event time T. For example, if the baseline hazard rate is constant throughout an observation interval, we have $h_0(t) \equiv \lambda$, which leads to an *exponential regression model*, given by

$$h(t, \boldsymbol{x}; T \sim Exp) = \lambda \exp(\boldsymbol{x}'\boldsymbol{\beta}). \tag{4.2}$$

Equation (4.2) shows that the exponential regression model on the hazard rate is simply the product of a constant baseline hazard rate and a multiplicative term representing the effect of the covariate vector $\boldsymbol{x}$.

Similarly, when the observed hazard function varies monotonically over time, the Weibull regression model may be applied, given by

$$h(t, \boldsymbol{x}; T \sim \text{Weib}) = \lambda \tilde{p}(\lambda t)^{\tilde{p}-1} \exp(\boldsymbol{x}'\boldsymbol{\beta}), \tag{4.3}$$

where the definitions of λ and $\tilde{p}$ are described in Chapter 3 (Section 3.2). Equation (4.3) displays the Weibull regression mode as the Weibull distributional function, represented by Equation (3.17), multiplied by the effect term $\exp(\boldsymbol{x}'\boldsymbol{\beta})$.

Given its intimate association with the hazard function, the survival function for T given $\boldsymbol{x}$ can be readily derived from Equation (4.1):

$$\begin{aligned} S(t; \boldsymbol{x}) &= \exp\left[-\int_0^t h_0(u)du \exp(\boldsymbol{x}'\boldsymbol{\beta})\right] \\ &= \exp\left[-\exp(\boldsymbol{x}'\boldsymbol{\beta})\int_0^t h_0(u)du\right] \\ &= \exp[-\exp(\boldsymbol{x}'\boldsymbol{\beta}) H_0(t)], \end{aligned} \tag{4.4}$$

where $H_0(t)$ is defined as the continuous cumulative baseline hazard function at time t.

After some algebra, Equation (4.4) can be converted to the following formation:

$$\begin{aligned} S(t; \boldsymbol{x}) &= \{\exp[-H_0(t)]\}^{\exp(\boldsymbol{x}'\boldsymbol{\beta})} \\ &= [S_0(t)]^{\exp(\boldsymbol{x}'\boldsymbol{\beta})}, \end{aligned} \tag{4.5}$$

where $S_0(t)$ is the baseline survival function, mathematically defined as

$$S_0(t) = \exp\left[-\int_0^t h_0(u)\,\mathrm{d}u\right]$$
$$= \exp[-H_0(t)].$$

Equation (4.5) demonstrates that the survival function at t given $\boldsymbol{x}$ can be expressed as the baseline survival function $S_0(t)$ raised to the power of the multiplicative effects of covariates on the hazard function.

Given Equations (4.1) and (4.5), the probability density function of T given $\boldsymbol{x}$ is

$$f(t;\boldsymbol{x}) = h_0(t)\exp(\boldsymbol{x}'\boldsymbol{\beta})\exp\left[-\exp(\boldsymbol{x}'\boldsymbol{\beta})\int_0^t h_0(u)\,\mathrm{d}u\right]. \tag{4.6}$$

Parametric regression models on the hazard rate can be conveniently expressed in terms of a generalized linear regression function. Taking log values on both sides of Equation (4.1) yields

$$\log[h(t|\boldsymbol{x})] = \log[h_0(t)] + \boldsymbol{x}'\boldsymbol{\beta}$$
$$= \alpha^* + \boldsymbol{x}'\boldsymbol{\beta}, \tag{4.7}$$

where α^* is the logarithm of the baseline hazard function, serving as the intercept in this transformed linear regression function.

Equation (4.7) reflects some distinct similarities between the hazard rate model and other types of generalized linear regression models, such as the logistic regression. Without specification of an explicit baseline hazard function, however, Equation (4.7) does not display a direct link between $\boldsymbol{x}$ and event time T. Additionally, the model does not conveniently include a term representing random disturbances as do other generalized linear models. Empirically, specification of an error term in Equation (4.7) may raise some prediction problems because the hazard rate is not observable. These limitations can be well addressed by using another family of parametric regression models that regresses the logarithm of the event time over covariates, as described below.

4.1.2 Specifications of accelerated failure time regression models

As indicated earlier, parametric regression models in survival analysis can be created on log time over covariates, from which a different set of parameters needs to be specified. Suppose that $Y = \log T$ is linearly associated with the covariate vector $\boldsymbol{x}$. Then

$$Y = \mu^* + \boldsymbol{x}'\boldsymbol{\beta}^* + \tilde{\sigma}\varepsilon, \tag{4.8}$$

where $\boldsymbol{\beta}^*$ is a vector of regression coefficients on Y or $\log T$, μ^* is referred to as the intercept parameter, and the parameter $\tilde{\sigma}$ is an unknown scale parameter. The term ε represents random errors that follow a particular parametric distribution of T with survival function S, cumulative distribution function F, and probability density function f. Compared to Equation (4.7), Equation (4.8) looks more like a standard generalized linear regression model, thereby producing tremendous appeal for statisticians. With the location term ($\boldsymbol{x}'\boldsymbol{\beta}^*$) and scale parameter

$\tilde{\sigma}$, the baseline parametric distribution of survival times can be conveniently modeled by a term of additive random disturbances ($\log T_0$).

Using the equation $\log T \geq \log t$, the survival function, conditional on $\boldsymbol{x}$, can be expressed in the form of an extreme value distribution, as discussed in Chapter 3. Given Equation (4.8), the survival function for the ith individual is

$$\begin{aligned} S_i(t) &= \mathrm{P}\left[\left(\mu^* + \boldsymbol{x}_i'\boldsymbol{\beta}^* + \tilde{\sigma}\varepsilon_i\right) \geq \log t\right] \\ &= \mathrm{P}\left(\varepsilon_i \geq \frac{\log t - \mu^* - \boldsymbol{x}_i'\boldsymbol{\beta}^*}{\tilde{\sigma}}\right). \end{aligned} \tag{4.9}$$

Let ε_i be a component of the error vector $\boldsymbol{\varepsilon}$, $S(t) = \Pr(\varepsilon_i \geq t)$, $F(t) = \Pr(\varepsilon_i < t)$, and $f(t) = \mathrm{d}F(t)/\mathrm{d}t$. Because the term $\boldsymbol{x}'\boldsymbol{\beta}^*$ is independent of the disturbance parameter ε_i, the survival function $S(t)$ with respect to $\log T$ can be modeled by specifying a random component and a fixed component, given by

$$S(t|\boldsymbol{x}) = S_0\left(\frac{\log t - \mu^* - \boldsymbol{x}'\boldsymbol{\beta}^*}{\tilde{\sigma}}\right), \quad -\infty < \log t < \infty, \tag{4.10}$$

where S_0, independent of $\boldsymbol{x}$, is the survival function of the distribution of ε and $\boldsymbol{x}'\boldsymbol{\beta}^*$ defines the location of T, referred to as an *accelerated factor*.

As $H(t) = -\log S(t)$, the cumulative hazard function can be expressed in terms of Equation (4.10):

$$\begin{aligned} H(t|\boldsymbol{x}) &= -\log S_0\left(\frac{\log t - \mu^* - \boldsymbol{x}'\boldsymbol{\beta}^*}{\tilde{\sigma}}\right) \\ &= H_0\left(\frac{\log t - \mu^* - \boldsymbol{x}'\boldsymbol{\beta}^*}{\tilde{\sigma}}\right), \quad -\infty < \log t < \infty. \end{aligned} \tag{4.11}$$

where H_0 is the cumulative hazard function of $\boldsymbol{\varepsilon}$.

Similarly, by differentiating Equation (4.11), the corresponding hazard function is

$$h(t|\boldsymbol{x}) = \frac{1}{\tilde{\sigma}t} h_0\left(\frac{\log t - \mu^* - \boldsymbol{x}'\boldsymbol{\beta}^*}{\tilde{\sigma}}\right), \quad -\infty < \log t < \infty. \tag{4.12}$$

where h_0 is the baseline hazard function for the distribution of ε_i, also independent of $\boldsymbol{x}$.

Given its simplicity and flexibility, the above log-linear model, as represented by Equation (4.10), can be applied to formulate a large number of families of parametric distributions in survival analysis, including the exponential, the Weibull, the extreme value, the normal, the logistic, the lognormal, and the gamma distributions. In contrast, the parametric proportional hazard perspective only applies to few parametric distributions. A selected distribution of ε_i defines the formation of the intercept, scale, and shape parameters, in turn deriving the survival, the hazard, and the density functions, as will be described extensively in the following sections.

As defined, if $Y = \log T$ follows an extreme value distribution, T has an *accelerated failure time distribution* (Lawless, 2003; Meeker and Escobar, 1998). As the effect of covariate vector $\boldsymbol{x}$ on T changes the location, but not the shape, of a distribution of T, the parametric regression models that can be formulated by Equation (4.10) are generally referred to as *accelerated failure time (AFT) regression models* or *log-location-scale regression models* (in much of the following text, I call them simply the AFT regression models). One added advantage of using the specification of the AFT regression is that it covers a wide range of the survival time distribution, given the range of $\log T$ $(-\infty, \infty)$.

Using the above description, the AFT regression perspective can also be formulated with respect to the random variable T, rather than to $\log T$, for convenience of specifying a likelihood function. As Equation (4.8) is a log-linear model, exponentiation of both sides of this equation leads to

$$\begin{aligned} T &= \exp(\mu^* + \boldsymbol{x}'\boldsymbol{\beta}^*)\exp(\sigma\varepsilon) \\ &= \exp(\mu^* + \boldsymbol{x}'\boldsymbol{\beta}^*)\tilde{E}, \end{aligned} \tag{4.13}$$

where $\tilde{E} = \exp(\sigma\boldsymbol{\varepsilon}) > 0$ has the hazard function $h_0(\tilde{e})$ and is independent of $\boldsymbol{\beta}^*$. Because $\exp(\boldsymbol{x}'\boldsymbol{\beta}^*)$ is positive valued, T is restricted in the range $(0, \infty)$. Given the equation $T \geq t$, the survival function for the ith individual can be mathematically expressed by

$$S_i(t) = \mathrm{P}(T_i \geq t) = \mathrm{P}\left[\exp(\mu^* + \boldsymbol{x}'\boldsymbol{\beta}^* + \tilde{\sigma}\varepsilon_i) \geq t\right]. \tag{4.14}$$

As the term $\boldsymbol{x}'\boldsymbol{\beta}^*$ is independent of the disturbance parameter, the survival function $S(t)$ can be written by two separate components:

$$S_i(t) = S_0\left[t\exp(\boldsymbol{x}'\boldsymbol{\beta}^*)\right], \tag{4.15}$$

where S_0 is a fully specified survival function, defined as

$$S_0(t) = \mathrm{P}\left[\exp(\mu^* + \tilde{\sigma}\varepsilon) \geq t\right].$$

The hazard function for T can be readily derived from Equation (4.15), given its intimate relationship with the survival function:

$$h(t|\boldsymbol{x}) = h_0\left[t\exp(-\boldsymbol{x}'\boldsymbol{\beta}^*)\right]\exp(-\boldsymbol{x}'\boldsymbol{\beta}^*). \tag{4.16}$$

From Equation (4.16), the survival function can be respecified in terms of the AFT hazard function:

$$\begin{aligned} S(t|\boldsymbol{x}) &= \exp\left\{-\int_0^t h_0\left[u\exp(-\boldsymbol{x}'\boldsymbol{\beta}^*)\right]\exp(-\boldsymbol{x}'\boldsymbol{\beta}^*)\,\mathrm{d}u\right\} \\ &= \exp\left\{-H_0\left[t\exp(-\boldsymbol{x}'\boldsymbol{\beta}^*)\right]\right\}. \end{aligned} \tag{4.17}$$

Given Equations (4.16) and (4.17), the density function in the formation of such an AFT perspective is defined as

$$f(t; \boldsymbol{x}) = h_0\left[t\exp(-\boldsymbol{x}'\boldsymbol{\beta}^*)\right]\exp(-\boldsymbol{x}'\boldsymbol{\beta}^*)\exp\left\{-H_0\left[t\exp(-\boldsymbol{x}'\boldsymbol{\beta}^*)\right]\right\}. \tag{4.18}$$

In the AFT regression models, the effect of covariates determines the time scale in such a way that if $\exp(\boldsymbol{x}'\boldsymbol{\beta}^*) > 1$, the effect of the covariate vector $\boldsymbol{x}$ is to decelerate the survival process, and if $\exp(\boldsymbol{x}'\boldsymbol{\beta}^*) < 1$, the effect is to accelerate it (Lawless, 2003). Obviously, such multiplicative effects of covariates on survival times take the opposite direction to those on the hazard function – $\exp(\boldsymbol{x}'\boldsymbol{\beta})$ – unless two corresponding coefficients are both 0. Statistically, the two sets of regression coefficients are intimately associated and mutually convertible if a parametric distribution of T can be formulated by both the proportional hazard and the AFT perspectives.

While the parametric hazard rate and the AFT models represent two different parametric families, two parametric functions can be expressed in terms of both perspectives – the exponential and the Weibull distributions. In the Weibull regression model, for example, the two sets of regression coefficients, $\boldsymbol{\beta}$ and $\boldsymbol{\beta}^*$, reflect two parameter sets under the same parametric distribution of T; therefore, one set of parameters can be readily converted to the other. As a special case of the Weibull regression model, the exponential regression model has the same feature. These issues will be extensively discussed in the following two sections.

4.1.3 Inferences of parametric regression models and likelihood functions

Statistical inference of parametric regression models is performed to specify likelihood functions for the estimation of the parameter vector $\boldsymbol{\theta}$ in the presence of censoring. Specifically, a likelihood function with survival data describes the probability of a set of parameter values given observed lifetime outcomes. As generally applied in generalized linear regression, it is more convenient to generate parameter estimates by maximizing a log-likelihood function than by maximizing a likelihood function itself, given its relative simplicity. The unique aspect of statistical inference in survival analysis is the way of handling censoring. For analytic convenience, censoring is usually assumed to be random; that is, conditional on model parameters, censored times are assumed to be independent of each other and of actual survival times. If this assumption holds, censoring is noninformative, so that unbiased parameter estimates can be derived.

For considering right censoring in a likelihood function of parametric regression modeling, I first review some general conditions and random processes described in Chapter 1. Specifically, for each individual in a random sample and with the definition of a parameter vector $\boldsymbol{\theta}$, survival processes can be described by three random variables $(t_i, \delta_i, \boldsymbol{x}_i)$. The random variable of time t_i is defined as

$$t_i = \min(T_i, C_i) \tag{4.19}$$

and δ_i is given by

$$\begin{cases} \delta_i = 0 \text{ if } T_i > t_i, \\ \delta_i = 1 \text{ if } T_i = t_i. \end{cases} \tag{4.20}$$

The random variables contained in the covariate vector $\boldsymbol{x}$ are specified earlier.

Given these random variables, a likelihood function with respect to the parameter vector $\boldsymbol{\theta}$ for a random sample of n individuals can be readily specified:

$$L(\boldsymbol{\theta}) = \prod_{i=1}^{n} L_i(\theta)$$

$$= \prod_{i=1}^{n} f(t_i; \boldsymbol{\theta}, \boldsymbol{x}_i)^{\delta_i} S(t_i; \boldsymbol{\theta}, \boldsymbol{x}_i)^{1-\delta_i}. \tag{4.21}$$

As defined, the likelihood function $L(\boldsymbol{\theta})$ is the probability of a set of parameter values given n observed lifetime outcomes. When $\delta_i = 1$, $L_i(\boldsymbol{\theta})$ is the probability density function for the occurrence of a particular event as the second term in the second equation is 1. Likewise, when $\delta_i = 0$, $L_i(\boldsymbol{\theta})$ is the survival function for a censored time as the first term is 1. In either case, individual i's survival time, actual or censored, is accounted for in the likelihood.

The above likelihood function can be expanded in terms of a parametric regression model on the hazard rate characterized with a baseline hazard function and a vector of regression coefficients $\boldsymbol{\beta}$ including the intercept parameter. Suppose that the survival data with random variables $(t_i, \delta_i, \boldsymbol{x}_i)$ come from a parametric hazard rate regression with parameter vector $\boldsymbol{\theta}$. Then the likelihood function can be written as

$$L(\boldsymbol{\theta}) = \prod_{i=1}^{n} [h_0(t)\exp(\boldsymbol{x}_i'\boldsymbol{\beta})]^{\delta_i} \exp\left[-\int_0^t h_0(u)\exp(\boldsymbol{x}_i'\boldsymbol{\beta})\mathrm{d}u\right]. \tag{4.22}$$

With the hazard and the survival functions explicitly expressed in Equation (4.22), a third function, the p.d.f. of T, is implicitly reflected therein because, when $\delta_i = 1$, the product of the first and second terms on the right of the equation gives rise to the density function.

Taking log values on both sides of Equation (4.22), a log-likelihood function is

$$\log L(\boldsymbol{\theta}) = \sum_{i=1}^{n} \left\{\delta_i \log[h_0(t)\exp(\boldsymbol{x}_i'\boldsymbol{\beta})] - \int_0^t [h_0(u)\exp(\boldsymbol{x}_i'\boldsymbol{\beta})]\mathrm{d}u\right\}$$

$$= \sum_{i=1}^{n} \left\{\delta_i [\log h_0(t) + (\boldsymbol{x}_i'\boldsymbol{\beta})] - \int_0^t h_0(u)\mathrm{d}u \exp(\boldsymbol{x}_i'\boldsymbol{\beta})\right\}. \tag{4.23}$$

Clearly, the log-likelihood function is computationally simpler than the likelihood function itself because products become sums and exponents transform to coefficients. Thus, it is easier to maximize this log-likelihood function with respect to the unknown parameter vector $\boldsymbol{\theta}$, which may contain some specific functional factors as well as regression coefficients, given a specific baseline distributional function. The generalization of a maximum likelihood estimator for $\boldsymbol{\theta}$ in the hazard rate regression model will be described in next subsection.

The likelihood function can be also constructed in terms of the AFT regression perspective. In the presence of right censoring, the likelihood function of an AFT regression model, given Equations (4.17) and (4.18), is

$$L(\theta) = \prod_{i=1}^{n} \{h_0(t)[t\exp(-\boldsymbol{x}_i'\boldsymbol{\beta}^*)]\exp(-\boldsymbol{x}'\boldsymbol{\beta}^*)\}^{\delta_i} \exp\{-H_0[t\exp(-\boldsymbol{x}'\boldsymbol{\beta}^*)]\}, \tag{4.24}$$

where the parameter vector $\boldsymbol{\theta}$ now contains different components from those on the hazard function.

The log-likelihood function of an AFT regression model can be derived by taking log values of both sides of Equation (4.24), given by

$$\log L(\boldsymbol{\theta}) = \sum_{i=1}^{n} \left\langle \delta_i \log\left\{h_0(t)\left[t\exp(-\boldsymbol{x}_i'\boldsymbol{\beta}^*)\right]\exp(-\boldsymbol{x}'\boldsymbol{\beta}^*)\right\} - H_0\left[t\exp(-\boldsymbol{x}'\boldsymbol{\beta}^*)\right]\right\rangle$$
$$= \sum_{i=1}^{n} \left\{\delta_i\left[\log h_0(t) + \log t - (\boldsymbol{x}_i'\boldsymbol{\beta})^2\right] - H_0\left[t\exp(-\boldsymbol{x}'\boldsymbol{\beta}^*)\right]\right\}. \tag{4.25}$$

Maximization of Equation (4.25) with respect to $\boldsymbol{\theta}$ yields the maximum likelihood (ML) estimates of the parameters contained in $\boldsymbol{\theta}$ in the AFT perspective.

4.1.4 Procedures of maximization and hypothesis testing on ML estimates

There are standard procedures to maximize a likelihood function with respect to the parameter vector $\boldsymbol{\theta}$, thereby generating robust, efficient, and consistent parameter estimates. Specifically, the process starts with the construction of a score statistic vector, denoted by $\tilde{U}_i(\boldsymbol{\theta})$ for individual i and mathematically defined as the first partial derivatives of the log-likelihood function with respect to $\boldsymbol{\theta}$, given by

$$\tilde{U}_i(\boldsymbol{\theta}) = \frac{\partial}{\partial \boldsymbol{\theta}} \log L_i(\boldsymbol{\theta}) = \left[\frac{\partial}{\partial \theta_m} \log L_i(\boldsymbol{\theta})\right]_{M\times 1}, \tag{4.26}$$

where M is the dimension of $\boldsymbol{\theta}$ and θ_m is the mth component in $\boldsymbol{\theta}$ ($m = 1, \ldots, M$). This generalized likelihood function can apply to either Equation (4.23) or Equation (4.25) given different components in $\boldsymbol{\theta}$. The minus second derivatives of the log-likelihood function yields the estimator of variances and covariances for $\tilde{U}_i(\boldsymbol{\theta})$:

$$\tilde{V}_i(\boldsymbol{\theta}) = -\left(\mathrm{E}\frac{\partial^2 \log L_i}{\partial \theta_m \theta_{m'}}\right)_{M\times M}. \tag{4.27}$$

With right censoring assumed to be noninformative, the central limit theorem applies to the generation of the following total score statistic:

$$\tilde{U}(\boldsymbol{\theta}) = \sum_{i=1}^{n} \tilde{U}_i(\boldsymbol{\theta}). \tag{4.28}$$

Statistically, $\tilde{U}(\boldsymbol{\theta})$ is asymptotically normal, given the large-sample approximation to the joint distribution of parameters, with mean 0 and variance–covariance matrix

$$\tilde{V}(\boldsymbol{\theta}) = \sum_{i=1}^{n} \tilde{V}_i(\boldsymbol{\theta}).$$

Consequently, the parameter vector $\boldsymbol{\theta}$ can be estimated efficiently by solving the equation

$$\tilde{U}(\boldsymbol{\theta}) = \frac{\partial}{\partial \boldsymbol{\theta}} \log L(\boldsymbol{\theta}) = \mathbf{0}. \tag{4.29}$$

The above procedure is the formalization of a typical maximum likelihood estimator (MLE). The vector containing MLE parameter estimates are generally referred to as $\hat{\boldsymbol{\theta}}$. For a large sample, $\hat{\boldsymbol{\theta}}$ is the unique solution of $\tilde{U}(\boldsymbol{\theta}) = \mathbf{0}$, so that $\hat{\boldsymbol{\theta}}$ is consistent for $\boldsymbol{\theta}$ and distributed as multivariate normal, given by

$$\hat{\boldsymbol{\theta}} \sim N\left[\mathbf{0}, \tilde{V}(\boldsymbol{\theta})^{-1}\right]. \tag{4.30}$$

This asymptotic distribution facilitates testing of hypotheses on $\boldsymbol{\theta}$. Specifically, the above maximum likelihood estimator is based on the observed Fisher information matrix, denoted by $\boldsymbol{I}(\hat{\boldsymbol{\theta}})$, given by

$$\boldsymbol{I}(\hat{\boldsymbol{\theta}}) = -\left(\frac{\partial^2 \log L(\hat{\boldsymbol{\theta}})}{\partial \hat{\theta}_m \hat{\theta}_{m'}}\right)_{M \times M}. \tag{4.31}$$

As can be easily recognized, $\tilde{V}(\boldsymbol{\theta})$, formulated in Equation (4.27), contains the expected values of $\boldsymbol{I}(\hat{\boldsymbol{\theta}})$.

As the replacement of $\tilde{V}(\boldsymbol{\theta})$ with $\boldsymbol{I}(\hat{\boldsymbol{\theta}})$ does not affect the asymptotic distributions of $\tilde{U}(\boldsymbol{\theta})$, the term

$$\tilde{U}'(\hat{\boldsymbol{\theta}}) \boldsymbol{I}(\hat{\boldsymbol{\theta}})^{-1} \tilde{U}(\hat{\boldsymbol{\theta}}) \tag{4.32}$$

is distributed asymptotically as $\chi^2_{(M)}$, so that the hypotheses about $\boldsymbol{\theta}$ can be statistically tested given a value of α, the degree of freedom, and the null hypothesis $H_0: \hat{\boldsymbol{\theta}} = \boldsymbol{\theta}$ or simply $\hat{\boldsymbol{\theta}} = \mathbf{0}$. This test statistic on $\hat{\boldsymbol{\theta}}$ is the well-known score test.

The inverse of the observed information matrix yields the estimators of the variances and covariances for parameter estimates. For the parametric hazard regression model, for example, the variance–covariance matrix for the estimates of $\boldsymbol{\beta}$ can be written as

$$\boldsymbol{\Sigma}(\hat{\boldsymbol{\beta}}) = \boldsymbol{I}(\hat{\boldsymbol{\beta}})^{-1}. \tag{4.33}$$

The standard errors of $\boldsymbol{\beta}$ can be estimated by taking the square roots of the diagonal elements contained in $\boldsymbol{\Sigma}(\hat{\boldsymbol{\beta}})$.

As $\hat{\boldsymbol{\theta}}$ is asymptotically $N_M[\boldsymbol{\theta}, \boldsymbol{I}(\theta)^{-1}]$, $\sqrt{n}(\hat{\boldsymbol{\theta}} - \boldsymbol{\theta})$ is asymptotically $N_M[\mathbf{0}, n\boldsymbol{I}(\theta)^{-1}]$. Consequently, hypothesis testing on $\hat{\boldsymbol{\theta}}$ can also be performed by another test statistic for $H_0: \hat{\boldsymbol{\theta}} = \boldsymbol{\theta}$:

$$(\hat{\boldsymbol{\theta}} - \boldsymbol{\theta})' \boldsymbol{I}(\hat{\boldsymbol{\theta}})(\hat{\boldsymbol{\theta}} - \boldsymbol{\theta}), \tag{4.34}$$

which is also distributed as $\chi^2_{(M)}$. Specifically, $\boldsymbol{I}(\hat{\boldsymbol{\theta}})/n$ is an asymptotically consistent estimator for $\boldsymbol{I}(\boldsymbol{\theta})/n$. This test statistic, referred to as the Wald statistic, can be used to test a subtest of parameters, as will be introduced in Chapter 5.

The third main test for null hypotheses of parameter estimates in $\hat{\boldsymbol{\theta}}$ uses the likelihood ratio test. The likelihood ratio with respect to $\boldsymbol{\theta}$ is

$$LR(\boldsymbol{\theta}) = \frac{L(\boldsymbol{\theta})}{L(\hat{\boldsymbol{\theta}})}, \tag{4.35}$$

where $L(\boldsymbol{\theta})$ is the likelihood function for the model without one or more parameters, whereas $L(\hat{\boldsymbol{\theta}})$ is the likelihood function containing all parameters.

In the likelihood ratio test, the null hypothesis about $\boldsymbol{\theta}$ can be set either as H_0: $\boldsymbol{\theta} = \hat{\boldsymbol{\theta}}$ for all components in $\hat{\boldsymbol{\theta}}$ or as H_0: $\theta_m = \hat{\theta}_m$ for a single component in $\boldsymbol{\theta}$. Under such a null hypothesis, the likelihood ratio statistic, written by

$$\Lambda = 2\log L(\hat{\boldsymbol{\theta}}) - 2\log L(\boldsymbol{\theta}), \tag{4.36}$$

is asymptotically distributed as $\chi^2_{(M)}$. Consequently, statistical testing can be performed with larger values of Λ associated with smaller p-values, thereby providing more evidence against H_0. More specifically, if Λ is associated with a p-value smaller than α, the null hypothesis about $\hat{\boldsymbol{\theta}}$ should be rejected. When the likelihood ratio test is performed on all components in $\hat{\boldsymbol{\theta}}$, the likelihood ratio test displays the model fit statistic with empirical data. This test can also be conducted for one or more components in $\boldsymbol{\theta}$, but the parameters need to be partitioned for reparametrization (Kalbfleisch and Prentice, 2002; Lawless, 2003).

There are several modifications of the −2 log-likelihood statistic, such as Akaike's information criterion (*AIC*), the Bayesian information criterion (*BIC*), and the corrected version of the *AIC* (*AICC*). As they usually generate very close fit statistics as the likelihood ratio test, especially in large samples, I do not describe these modified statistics further in this text.

4.2 Exponential regression models

If survival data arise from an exponential distribution, the hazard rate is constant throughout all values of t, as specified by Equation (4.2). At the same time, the exponential regression can be approached by another family of parametric regression modeling that regresses the log survival time over covariates. An important feature of the exponential regression is that the estimated regression coefficients derived from the hazard rate and the AFT models have identical absolute values but with opposite signs, and also they share exactly the same standard errors. This section describes statistical inferences of the exponential regression model in terms of both the proportional hazard and the accelerated failure time functions. An empirical example is provided for practical illustration.

4.2.1 Exponential regression model on the hazard function

Equation (4.2) specifies the hazard rate as the product of a constant baseline hazard rate λ and the multiplicative effect term $\exp(\boldsymbol{x}'\boldsymbol{\beta})$. To further simplify this exponential regression equation, statisticians often view $\log \lambda$ as a special coefficient and place it into the regression coefficient vector $\boldsymbol{\beta}$. As a result, the first element of $\boldsymbol{x}$ contains value 1 and the first element of $\boldsymbol{\beta}$ contains value $\log \lambda$. Then Equation (4.2) can be simplified by

$$h(t, \boldsymbol{x}; T \sim Exp) = \exp(\boldsymbol{x}'\boldsymbol{\beta}). \tag{4.37}$$

When all components of $\boldsymbol{x}$ except the first element are 0, $h(t, \boldsymbol{x}; T \sim Exp) = \lambda$, given $\exp(\log \lambda) = \lambda$, thereby giving rise to the baseline hazard rate. Likewise, if all covariates are centered at sample means, the constant baseline hazard rate is the expected hazard for the population a given sample represents.

Equation (4.37) derives the following survival function given the exponential distribution of event time T:

$$S(t, \boldsymbol{x}; T \sim Exp) = \exp[-t \exp(\boldsymbol{x}'\boldsymbol{\beta})]. \tag{4.38}$$

Given specifications of the hazard and the survival functions, the density function of T, conditional on $\boldsymbol{x}$, is

$$f(t, \boldsymbol{x}; T \sim Exp) = \exp(\boldsymbol{x}'\boldsymbol{\beta})\exp[-t \exp(\boldsymbol{x}'\boldsymbol{\beta})]. \tag{4.39}$$

With the assumption of noninformative censoring, the likelihood function of the exponential regression model with respect to $\boldsymbol{\beta}$ is written as

$$L(\boldsymbol{\beta}) = \prod_{i=1}^{n} \{\exp(\boldsymbol{x}'\boldsymbol{\beta})\exp[-t \exp(\boldsymbol{x}'\boldsymbol{\beta})]\}^{\delta_i} \{\exp[-t \exp(\boldsymbol{x}'\boldsymbol{\beta})]\}^{1-\delta_i}. \tag{4.40}$$

After some algebra, Equation (4.40) reduces to

$$L(\boldsymbol{\beta}) = \prod_{i=1}^{n} \exp(\delta_i \boldsymbol{x}_i'\boldsymbol{\beta})\exp[-t_i \exp(\boldsymbol{x}_i'\boldsymbol{\beta})]. \tag{4.41}$$

Then, the log-likelihood function with respect to $\boldsymbol{\beta}$ is

$$\log L(\boldsymbol{\beta}) = \sum_{i=1}^{n} \delta_i \boldsymbol{x}_i \boldsymbol{\beta} - \sum_{i=1}^{n} t_i \exp(\boldsymbol{x}_i'\boldsymbol{\beta}). \tag{4.42}$$

Maximization of Equation (4.42) with respect to $\boldsymbol{\beta}$ yields the MLE estimates in the exponential regression model on the hazard rate. In particular, the score statistic vector $\tilde{\boldsymbol{U}}_i(\boldsymbol{\beta})$ within the construct of exponential regression modeling contains components

$$\tilde{U}_m(\boldsymbol{\beta}) = \frac{\partial \log L(\boldsymbol{\beta})}{\partial \beta_m} = \sum x_{mi} [\delta_i - t_i \exp(\boldsymbol{x}_i'\boldsymbol{\beta})], \quad m = 1, \ldots, M. \tag{4.43}$$

The Fisher information matrix of the second partial derivatives of the log likelihood function with respect to $\boldsymbol{\beta}$ is

$$I(\hat{\boldsymbol{\beta}}) = -\left[\frac{\partial^2 \log L(\boldsymbol{\beta})}{\partial \beta_m \partial \beta_{m'}}\right]_{M \times M} = \sum x_{mi} x_{m'i} t_i \exp(\boldsymbol{x}_i' \boldsymbol{\beta}). \tag{4.44}$$

In empirical research, the observed information matrix is generally used to yield asymptotic results given the large-sample approximation theory and the central limit theorem. As indicated earlier, its inverse is regularly applied as the approximated variance–covariance matrix of parameter estimates. The standard error estimates are the square roots of the diagonal elements in the inverse of the observed information matrix. As commonly known in the estimation of a regression model, high correlation between two covariates may yield ill effects on the quality of ML parameter estimates. Therefore, if the covariate vector $\boldsymbol{x}$ contains one or more interaction terms, the covariates used for constructing those interactions need to be rescaled to be centered at their sample means or at some specific values for reducing numeric instability and collinearity.

As demonstrated by Equation (4.37), given the covariate effect term $\exp(\boldsymbol{x}'\boldsymbol{\beta})$, any two individuals are subject to hazard rates that are multiplicative or proportional to one another throughout all t values. This feature can be extended to the condition that the ratio of two hazard rates associated with two successive integer values of a covariate can be expressed in terms of $\exp(b_m)$. Let b_0 be the intercept ($\log \lambda$) and b_m be the regression coefficient of covariate x_m, both contained in the coefficient vector $\boldsymbol{\beta}$. Also let two successive integer values of x_m be x_{m0} and $x_{m0} + 1$. If all other covariates are scaled to 0, the ratio of the hazard rates for $x_m = x_{m0}$ and $x_m = x_{m0} + 1$, denoted by $HR(x_{m0}, x_{m0} + 1)$, is given by

$$\begin{aligned} HR(x_{m0}, x_{m0}+1) &= \frac{\lambda \exp[b_0 + b_m(x_{m0}+1)]}{\lambda \exp(b_0 + b_m x_{m0})} \\ &= \exp[(x_{m0} + 1 - x_{m0}) b_m] \\ &= \exp(b_m). \end{aligned} \tag{4.45}$$

Given this simple inference, the term $\exp(b_m)$ is referred to as *the hazard ratio of covariate m*, with the abbreviated term HR. This definition holds for all proportional hazard regression models, including the Weibull regression model and the semi-parametric regression model described in later chapters. Exponentiation of elements in the coefficient vector $\boldsymbol{\beta}$ thus yields a hazard ratio vector. Such a relative risk holds when other covariates take nonzero values because the additional terms would appear in both the numerator and the denominator in Equation (4.45) and thereby can cancel out.

For proportional hazard rate models, an individual hazard ratio displays the multiplicative effect on the hazard rate with a 1-unit change in a given covariate. If the covariate is a dichotomous variable, the hazard ratio has an intuitive meaning of relative risk. For example, the hazard ratio for gender (1 = female, 0 = male) shows the proportion of the hazard rate for women as relative to the hazard rate for men, other variables being equal. In the case of a continuous covariate, the hazard ratio presents the increased risk ($HR > 1$) or the decreased risk ($HR < 1$) of experiencing a particular event with a 1-unit increase in the value of a given covariate.

Computing $100 \times [\exp(b_m) - 1]$ yields the percentage change in the hazard rate with a 1-unit change in covariate x_m. Consider the gender example: if the hazard ratio is 0.75, the value of $100 \times (0.75 - 1) = -25$, indicating a 25 % reduction in the hazard rate for women as compared to the hazard rate for men, other variables remaining constant.

4.2.2 Exponential accelerated failure time regression model

As indicated in Chapter 2, the exponential distribution can be modeled as an accelerated failure time function. Let $Y = \log T$ and $\tilde{\gamma} = \lambda^{-1}$. Then Equation (4.2) can be written in a linear form as

$$Y = \mathbf{x}'\boldsymbol{\beta}^* + \varepsilon_{\text{exp}}, \tag{4.46}$$

where ε_{exp} can be viewed as a special case of the extreme value distribution with the scale parameter equaling 1 (the extreme value distribution is briefly described in Chapter 3 and will be discussed further in Section 4.3). The term $\log\tilde{\gamma}$ is included in $\boldsymbol{\beta}^*$ as an intercept parameter. Exponentiation of both sides of this equation leads to the following AFT model:

$$\begin{aligned} T &= \exp(\mathbf{x}'\boldsymbol{\beta}^*)\exp(\varepsilon_{\text{exp}}) \\ &= \exp(\mathbf{x}'\boldsymbol{\beta}^*)\tilde{E}_{\text{exp}}, \end{aligned} \tag{4.47}$$

where $\tilde{E}$ follows an exponential distribution, as defined. Given the above specifications, the survival function is

$$S(t; \mathbf{x}, \boldsymbol{\beta}^*) = \exp[-\exp(y - \mathbf{x}'\boldsymbol{\beta}^*)], \tag{4.48}$$

where $y = \log(t)$. Accordingly, the density function can be expressed in terms of the extreme value distribution, given by

$$f(t; \mathbf{x}, \boldsymbol{\beta}^*) = \exp[(y - \mathbf{x}'\boldsymbol{\beta}^*) - \exp(y - \mathbf{x}'\boldsymbol{\beta}^*)]. \tag{4.49}$$

Given the density and the survival functions, the likelihood function with respect to $\boldsymbol{\beta}^*$ is

$$L(\boldsymbol{\beta}^*) = \prod_{i=1}^{n} \{\exp[(y - \mathbf{x}'\boldsymbol{\beta}^*) - \exp(y - \mathbf{x}'\boldsymbol{\beta}^*)]\}^{\delta_i} \{\exp[-\exp(y - \mathbf{x}'\boldsymbol{\beta}^*)]\}^{1-\delta_i}. \tag{4.50}$$

The log-likelihood function is

$$\log L(\boldsymbol{\beta}^*) = \sum_{i=1}^{n} \delta_i (y - \mathbf{x}'\boldsymbol{\beta}^*) - \exp(y - \mathbf{x}'\boldsymbol{\beta}^*). \tag{4.51}$$

According to the procedures described earlier, maximizing the above log-likelihood function with respect to $\boldsymbol{\beta}^*$ yields the MLE estimates of $\tilde{\gamma}$ and the regression coefficients.

The second partial derivative of this function, for a single component, is defined as

$$\frac{\partial^2 L(\boldsymbol{\beta}^*)}{\partial \beta_m \beta_{m'}} = -\sum_{i=1}^{n} x_{mi} x_{m'i} \exp(y - \mathbf{x}'\boldsymbol{\beta}^*). \tag{4.52}$$

The variance–covariance matrix of $\boldsymbol{\beta}^*$ can be derived from the inverse of the observed information matrix $\boldsymbol{I}\left(\hat{\boldsymbol{\beta}}^*\right)$, from which the null hypothesis can be statistically tested, as described in Subsection 4.1.3.

In the exponential accelerated failure time model, the hazard rate given $\boldsymbol{x}$ is regarded as the inverse function of Equation (4.48), given by

$$h(t; \boldsymbol{x}, \boldsymbol{\beta}^*) = \exp(-\boldsymbol{x}'\boldsymbol{\beta}^*), \tag{4.53}$$

where $\log \tilde{\gamma}$ is the first element in $\boldsymbol{\beta}^*$. A comparison between Equations (4.53) and (4.37) demonstrates that as $[\exp(-\boldsymbol{x}'\boldsymbol{\beta}^*)]$ is equivalent to $\exp(\boldsymbol{x}'\boldsymbol{\beta})$, $\boldsymbol{\beta}^* = -\boldsymbol{\beta}$. Additionally, the standard errors of the hazard and AFT parameter estimates are equal. Therefore, the estimation of either the hazard rate or the AFT perspective yields both sets of parameter estimates through some straightforward transformation.

As $\exp(\boldsymbol{x}'\boldsymbol{\beta}^*)$ represents a vector of multiplicative effects on T, the individual term $\exp(b_m^*)$ indicates the ratio of survival times for $x_m = x_{m0}$ and $x_m = x_{m0} + 1$, referred to as the *time ratio of covariate m* or TR. Consequently, exponentiation of the elements in the coefficient vector $\boldsymbol{\beta}^*$ yields a time ratio vector. An individual time ratio displays the multiplicative effect on T with a 1-unit change in a given covariate. Suppose that covariate x_m is a dichotomous variable representing gender with 1 = female and 0 = male. Then the time ratio displays the proportion of survival time for women as relative to the survival time for men, other variables being equal. In the case of a continuous covariate, the time ratio presents whether the survival time for the occurrence of a particular event increases ($TR > 1$) or decreases ($TR < 1$) with a 1-unit change in the value of a covariate of interest. Like the hazard ratio, interpreting a time ratio is much like interpreting an odds ratio for a logistic regression model. The term $100[\exp(b_j^*) - 1]$ represents the percentage change in the event time with a 1-unit change in covariate x_m, other covariates being fixed. As $\boldsymbol{\beta}^*$ and $\boldsymbol{\beta}$ take opposite signs, the time ratio and the corresponding hazard ratio bear opposite directions as deviating from unity.

Given the estimates of $\boldsymbol{\beta}^*$, the exponential survival function can be approximated given values of $\boldsymbol{x}$. Some other functions, intimately related to the distribution of T, are also obtainable, either from $\boldsymbol{\beta}^*$ or from $\boldsymbol{\beta}$. For example, according to Equation (3.14), the estimated median time to the occurrence of a particular event is

$$t_m(\boldsymbol{x}, \boldsymbol{\beta}) = \frac{\log 2}{\exp(\boldsymbol{x}'\boldsymbol{\beta})} = \exp(\boldsymbol{x}'\boldsymbol{\beta}^*)\log 2. \tag{4.54}$$

Likewise, the estimated pth percentile of the survival time distribution, given $\boldsymbol{x}$, can be estimated by replacing the value of $\log 2$ with $\log 1/(1 - p)$:

$$t_p(\boldsymbol{x}, \boldsymbol{\beta}) = \frac{\log\left(\frac{1}{1-p}\right)}{\exp(\boldsymbol{x}'\boldsymbol{\beta})} = \exp(\boldsymbol{x}'\boldsymbol{\beta}^*)\log\left(\frac{1}{1-p}\right). \tag{4.55}$$

Therefore, with the estimates of $\boldsymbol{\beta}$ available, the median and various percentiles of survival time can be estimated by placing values of $\boldsymbol{x}$ into either of the above two equations.

4.2.3 Illustration: Exponential regression model on marital status and survival among older Americans

In Section 2.3.4, I provide an empirical example about marital status and the probability of survival among older Americans. Although the survival curve for currently married persons is found to differ significantly from the curve among the currently not married, this relationship can be confounded by some 'lurking' covariates. In the present illustration, I reexamine this association by considering two potential confounders – age and educational attainment. I consider these two covariates because each of them is often observed to be causally associated with both marital status and mortality, and thus may potentially yield some confounding effects.

In the analysis, marital status is a dichotomous variable with 1 = 'currently married' and 0 = else, named 'Married.' An individual's age is the actual years of age and educational attainment, an approximate proxy for socioeconomic status, is measured as the total number of years in school, assuming the influence of education on mortality to be a continuous process (Liu, Hermalin and Chuang, 1998). Both control variables are measured at the AHEAD baseline survey and are then rescaled to be centered at the sample means for convenience of analysis. The two centered control variables are termed, respectively, 'Age_mean' and 'Educ_mean.' My goal is to assess whether the significant difference in the probability of survival between currently married and currently not married persons holds after adjusting for the confounding effects of age and educational attainment. For illustrating how to apply the exponential regression model, I estimate a one-year survival function, assuming the baseline hazard rate to be constant within this relatively short observation interval.

In the SAS system, the PROC LIFEREG procedure is used to fit parametric regression models. This procedure is entirely based on the AFT perspective; as a result, it does not directly model the hazard rate and does not produce the corresponding hazard ratio. In the exponential regression perspective, however, parameter estimates on log(survival time) can be readily converted to the parameter estimates on the log(hazard) and the hazard ratios by using the SAS ODS procedure.

Below is the SAS program for the estimation of the exponential regression model on marital status and survival.

SAS Program 4.1:

```
options ps=56;
libname pclib 'C:\<the location that contains the dataset "chapter4_data>;;
options _last_=pclib.chapter4_data;

proc format;
  value Rx 1 = 'Married' 0 = 'Not married';

data new;
  set pclib.chapter4_data;
  format Married Rx.;

......

Censor = 1;
  if death = 0 then Censor = 1;
```

```
proc SQL;
  create table new as
  select *, age-mean(age) as age_mean,
  educ-mean(educ) as educ_mean
  from new;
quit;

* Compute estimates of the exponential regression model *;
ods graphics on ;
ods output Parameterestimates = Exponential_AFT;
proc lifereg data=new outest=Exponential_outest;
  class married;
  model  duration*Censor(1)  =  married  age_mean  educ_mean  /  dist  =  Exponential;
  output out = new1 cdf = prob;
run;
ods graphics off;
ods output close;

* Compute and print correspoing PH estimates and HR *;
data Exponential_AFT;
  if _N_ = 1 then set Exponential_outest;
  set Exponential_AFT;
  PH_beta = -1*estimate;
  AFT_beta = estimate;
  HR = exp(PH_beta);
  option nolabel;

proc print data = Exponential_AFT;
  id Parameter;
  var AFT_beta PH_beta HR;
  format PH_beta 8.5 HR 5.3;
  title1 "LIFEREG/Exponential on duration";
  title2 "ParameterEstimate dataset e/PH_beta & HR computed manually";
  title4 "PH_beta = -1*AFT_beta";
  title6 "HR = exp(PH_beta)";
run;

proc sgplot data = new1;
  scatter x = duration y = prob / group = married;
  discretelegend;
  title1 "Figure 4.1. Cumulative distribution function: Exponential";
run;
```

In SAS Program 4.1, a temporary SAS data file 'New' is created from the dataset chapter4_data. The dichotomous variable Censor is constructed, with 1 = censored and 0 = not censored. The SAS PROC SQL procedure creates two centered covariates as controls – Age_mean and Educ_mean – which are then saved into the temporary SAS data file for further analysis.

In the SAS LIFEREG procedure, I first ask SAS to estimate the regression coefficients of covariates on log(duration), with parameter estimates saved in the temporary SAS output file Exponential_AFT. In this step, the CLASS statement specifies the variable 'Married' as a classification variable. The MODEL statement specifies three covariates, with the distribution specified as exponential. The OUTPUT statement creates the output dataset New1. Given the option 'cdf = Prob,' the temporary dataset New1 contains the variable Prob created to yield the cumulative distribution function at the observed responses.

The following part converts the saved log time coefficients (AFT_beta) into log hazard coefficients (PH_beta) and hazard ratios (HR). Then I request SAS to print three sets of parameter estimates: regression coefficients on log(duration), regression coefficients on log(hazards), and hazard ratios. For exponential regression models, the conversion from AFT parameter estimates to the HR estimates is conducted simply by changing the sign of each parameter estimate. Because both sets of parameter estimates, AFT and PH, share the same standard errors, conversion of standard errors is unnecessary.

Lastly, the PROC SGPLOT procedure produces a graph of the cumulative distribution values versus the variable Duration. Some of the analytic results from SAS Program 4.1 are presented below.

SAS Program Output 4.1:

```
                    The LIFEREG Procedure

                      Model Information

          Data Set                              WORK.NEW
          Dependent Variable               Log(duration)
          Censoring Variable                      censor
          Censoring Value(s)                           1
          Number of Observations                    2000
          Noncensored Values                          56
          Right Censored Values                     1944
          Left Censored Values                         0
          Interval Censored Values                     0
          Number of Parameters                         4
          Name of Distribution               Exponential
          Log Likelihood                    -301.3722192


           Number of Observations Read          2000
           Number of Observations Used          2000

                        Fit Statistics

       -2 Log Likelihood                        602.744
       AIC (smaller is better)                  610.744
       AICC (smaller is better)                 610.764
       BIC (smaller is better)                  633.148

          Analysis of Maximum Likelihood Parameter Estimates

                            Standard   95% Confidence     Chi-
Parameter        DF Estimate   Error       Limits        Square Pr > ChiSq

Intercept         1   5.8817  0.1768   5.5351   6.2283 1106.15     <.0001
married        0  1   0.4064  0.2912  -0.1644   0.9772    1.95     0.1629
married        1  0   0.0000   .        .        .        .         .
age_mean          1  -0.0605  0.0215  -0.1027  -0.0184    7.93     0.0049
educ_mean         1   0.0268  0.0371  -0.0458   0.0994    0.52     0.4698
Scale             0   1.0000  0.0000   1.0000   1.0000
Weibull Shape     0   1.0000  0.0000   1.0000   1.0000

                LIFEREG/Exponential on duration
       ParameterEstimate dataset e/PH_beta & HR computed manually

                    PH_beta = -1*AFT_beta

                      HR = exp(PH_beta)

         Parameter        AFT_beta      PH_beta       HR

         Intercept         5.88173     -5.88173    0.003
         married           0.40642     -0.40642    0.666
         married           0.00000      0.00000    1.000
         age_mean         -0.06052      0.06052    1.062
         educ_mean         0.02679     -0.02679    0.974
         Scale             1.00000     -1.00000    0.368
         Weibull Shape     1.00000     -1.00000    0.368
```

In SAS Program Output 4.1, the model information and a statistic of model fitness are presented first. There are 56 uncensored (deaths) and 1944 right-censored observations, given a fairly short observation interval. As all covariates are measured at baseline and the vital status for each individual is known, all censored observations are of Type I right censoring. The log-likelihood for this exponential regression model is −301.3722, and this statistic is often used for comparing the goodness of fit among multiple models, as will be described in Chapter 8. The section of fit statistics displays four indicators of model fitness, with the −2 log-likelihood statistic described earlier. In summary, values of these four statistics are close, generating the same conclusion about model fitting for this analysis.

The table of ML parameter estimates demonstrates the LIFEREG estimates on log(duration) derived from the maximum likelihood procedure. The intercept, 5.8817 ($SE = 0.1768$), is statistically significant at $\alpha = 0.05$. Within a fairly short observation period of 12 months, however, currently married persons do not display a significantly different survival function from the curve among currently not married after adjusting for the effects of age and educational attainment. Because the variable 'Married' is dichotomous with one degree of freedom, the parameter estimate is given only for currently not married persons (in PROC LIFEREG, the group with the greatest value is treated as the reference). Consequently, the intercept provides an estimate for a currently married older person with an average age and an average educational attainment. For the two control variables, age is negatively associated with survival time, statistically significant ($\chi^2 = 7.93$; $p = 0.0049$). Educational attainment, on the other hand, is positively linked to survival time, which is not statistically significant ($\chi^2 = 0.52$; $p = 0.4698$).

The last table in SAS Program Output 4.1 presents the three sets of parameter estimates – AFT_beta, PH_beta, and HR. In the exponential regression model, as mentioned above and can be seen from the table, the PH_beta of a given covariate is simply the AFT_beta value times −1. The hazard ratio of each covariate (HR) is presented to highlight the multiplicative effect on the mortality of older Americans within a one-year time interval. For example, a one-year increase in age would increase the hazard rate by 6 % ($HR = 1.06$), other variables being equal.

Figure 4.1 displays the cumulative distribution function contained in the output dataset New1 for currently married and currently not married older persons. Two c.d.f.'s are shown without demonstrating a clear pattern of mortality differences. As 'month' is used as the time scale, there are substantial tied observations, especially in later months. This lack of association between marital status and survival might be due to the short observation interval, during which the impact of married life on the probability of survival cannot be captured. For a longer observation interval, on the other hand, the selection of the exponential regression model is obviously not appropriate because the hazard rate, especially among older persons, increases over time.

Another possibility for this lack of association is misspecification of the baseline distributional function of T. Although hazard rates within a one-year period are often considered to be relatively stable, this assumption might not be entirely appropriate for older persons. A graphical check on the distribution of the hazard rate can provide some implications concerning whether or not the exponential distribution is a good fit for the present analysis. Given this reason, I plot a graph of negative log survival versus time for the entire sample, using the Kaplan–Meier survival estimates. The plot should display a straight line if the survival data within a one-year interval arise from an exponential distribution, as indicated in Chapter 3. The SAS program for plotting this curve is given below.

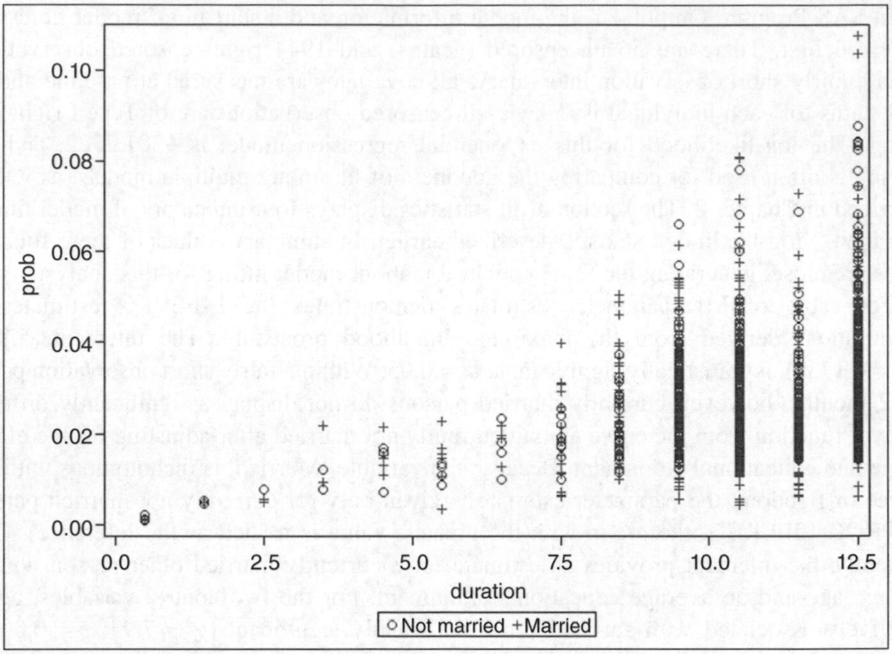

Figure 4.1 Cumulative distribution function: exponential.

SAS Program 4.2:

```
......
Status = 1;
if death=0 or time > 12 then Status = 0;

ods html;
ods graphics on;

ods select NegLogSurvivalPlot;
lifetest data = new OUTSURV = out1 plots = logsurv;
 time duration * Status(0);
run;

proc print data=out1;
    title1 "Figure 4.2.3-2. Log S(t) versus t";
run;

ods graphics off;
ods trace off;
```

In SAS Program 4.2, I replace the variable Censor with the variable Status (1 = event, 0 = censored) for executing the PROC LIFETEST procedure, constructing a negative log $\hat{S}(t)$ versus t plot using the Kaplan–Meier survival estimates. The ODS Graphics is enabled by specifying the ODS GRAPHICS ON statement with the ODS select name as NegLogSur-

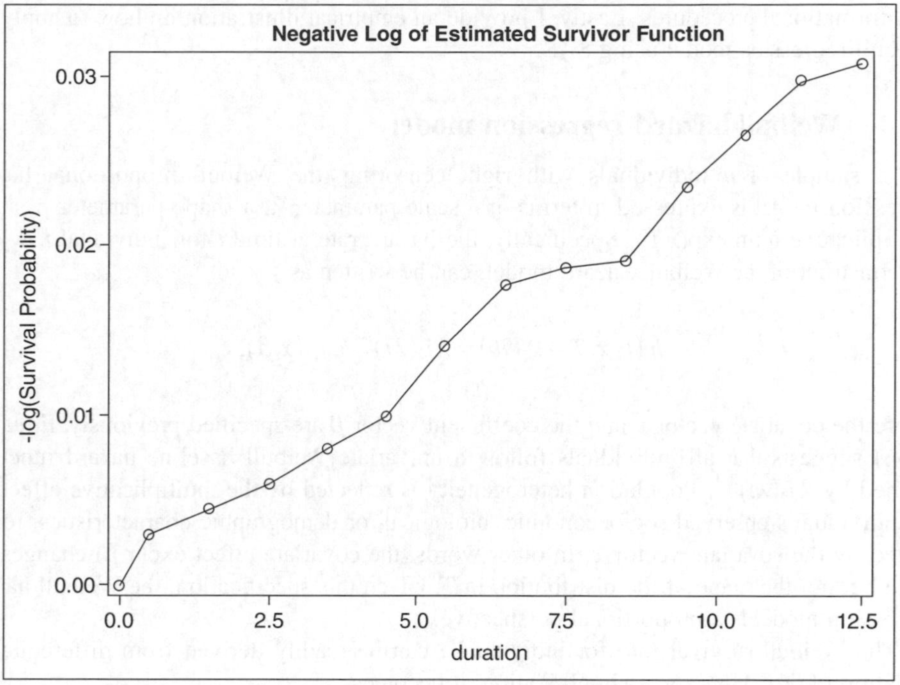

Figure 4.2 Plot of negative log survival versus time.

vivalPlot. In the PROC LIFETEST statement, the option PLOTS = LOGSURV asks SAS to construct the graph of negative $\log \hat{S}(t)$ versus t. SAS Program 4.2 yields the plot in Figure 4.2, where the negative log $S(t)$ versus t displays a roughly straight line, though with substantial variations, thus suggesting that the use of the exponential distributional function for a one-year observation interval is probably not unreasonable among older Americans. It must be emphasized that this graphical check cannot be used to make a final decision on an underlying distribution of survival data. More plausible checking methods will be discussed in Chapters 5 and 6.

4.3 Weibull regression models

Like exponential regression models, the Weibull regression can be approached in terms of two lifetime functions. As a result, the Weibull parameters can be estimated either by the Weibull proportional hazard or by the accelerated failure time model. Given the underlying distributional function of T, one set of parameter estimates can be easily converted to the other through some transformational procedures.

This section first describes the basic specifications and inferences of both the proportional hazard and the AFT regression models. Then I specify the intimate associations between the Weibull proportional hazard and AFT parameters, with a detailed description of the transformational procedures. Lastly, I provide an empirical illustration on how to apply the Weibull regression model using SAS.

4.3.1 Weibull hazard regression model

For a sample of n individuals with right censoring, the Weibull proportional hazard regression model is expressed in terms of a scale parameter λ, a shape parameter $\tilde{p}$, and a multiplicative term $\exp(\boldsymbol{x}'\boldsymbol{\beta})$. Specifically, the hazard rate at time t for individual i, within the construct of the Weibull hazard model, can be written as

$$h_i(t, \boldsymbol{x}; T \sim Weib) = \lambda\tilde{p}(\lambda t)^{\tilde{p}-1}\exp(\boldsymbol{x}_i'\boldsymbol{\beta}), \tag{4.56}$$

where the covariate vector $\boldsymbol{x}$ and the coefficient vector $\boldsymbol{\beta}$ are specified previously. Equation (4.56) suggests that all individuals follow a univariate Weibull baseline hazard function, defined by $\lambda\tilde{p}(\lambda t)^{\tilde{p}-1}$. Population heterogeneity is reflected by the multiplicative effects of an individual's observed socioeconomic, biological, or demographic characteristics, represented by the covariate vector $\boldsymbol{x}$. In other words, the covariate effect $\exp(\boldsymbol{x}'\boldsymbol{\beta})$ changes the scale but not the shape of the distribution in T. Given this specification, the Weibull hazard regression model is a proportional perspective.

The Weibull survival rate for individual i can be readily derived from differentiating Equation (4.56). After some simplification, it becomes

$$S_i(t, \boldsymbol{x}; T \sim Weib) = \exp\left[-\exp(\boldsymbol{x}_i'\boldsymbol{\beta})\lambda t^{\tilde{p}}\right]. \tag{4.57}$$

By definition, the density function of T in the Weibull distribution can be expressed by the product of the Weibull hazard function and the survival function. Consequently, the likelihood function of n observations is

$$L(\lambda, \tilde{p}, \boldsymbol{x}) = \prod_{i=1}^{n}\left[\lambda\tilde{p}(\lambda t)^{\tilde{p}-1}\exp(\boldsymbol{x}_i'\boldsymbol{\beta})\right]^{\delta_i}\exp\left[-\exp(\boldsymbol{x}_i'\boldsymbol{\beta})\lambda t^{\tilde{p}}\right]. \tag{4.58}$$

In Equation (4.58), if $\delta_i = 1$, $L_i(\lambda, \tilde{p}, \boldsymbol{x})$ is the density function for a particular event, given the product of the two terms on the right of equation; when $\delta_i = 0$, $L_i(\lambda, \tilde{p}, \boldsymbol{x})$ is the survival function for a censored survival time as the first term on the right of the equation is 1.

Taking log values on both sides of Equation (4.58), the log-likelihood function is

$$\log L(\lambda, \tilde{p}, \boldsymbol{x}) = \sum_{i=1}^{n}\Big\{\delta_i\left[\log\lambda + \log\tilde{p} + (\tilde{p}-1)\log(\lambda t) + \boldsymbol{x}_i'\boldsymbol{\beta}\right] - \left[\exp(\boldsymbol{x}_i'\boldsymbol{\beta})(\lambda t)^{\tilde{p}}\right]\Big\}. \tag{4.59}$$

After some algebra, Equation (4.59) can be simplified, removing a term that does not involve unknown parameters, given by

$$\log L(\lambda, \tilde{p}, \boldsymbol{x}) = \sum_{i=1}^{n} \{\delta_i [\log(\lambda \tilde{p}) + \tilde{p} \log t_i + \boldsymbol{x}_i' \boldsymbol{\beta}] - \lambda \exp(\boldsymbol{x}_i' \boldsymbol{\beta}) t^{\tilde{p}}\}. \tag{4.60}$$

Maximizing Equation (4.60) requires that this log-likelihood function be differentiated with respect to model parameters λ, $\tilde{p}$, and $\boldsymbol{\beta}$. I do not, however, elaborate on the concrete estimating procedures for the proportional hazard parameters because in most statistical software packages the more flexible AFT function is used to generate the standard parametric parameters from which the proportional hazard parameter estimates can be obtained by some simple transformations.

Once the maximum likelihood estimates of parameters λ, $\tilde{p}$, and $\boldsymbol{\beta}$ are derived, the hazard, survival, and other related functions can be approximated, given values of selected values of $\boldsymbol{x}$. Whereas the hazard and survival functions can be estimated by applying Equations (4.56) and (4.57), the estimated median survival time, given $\boldsymbol{x}$, is

$$\hat{t}_m\left(\hat{\lambda}, \hat{\tilde{p}}, \boldsymbol{x}\right) = \left[\frac{\log 2}{\hat{\lambda} \exp\left(\boldsymbol{x}'\hat{\boldsymbol{\beta}}\right)}\right]^{1/\hat{\tilde{p}}}. \tag{4.61}$$

Equation (4.61) is simply the extension of Equation (3.25), with the addition of an effect term. Similarly, the estimated pth percentile of the survival time distribution, conditional on $\boldsymbol{x}$, can be estimated by replacing the value of $\log 2$ with $\log 1/(1-p)$:

$$\hat{t}_p\left(\hat{\lambda}, \hat{\tilde{p}}, \boldsymbol{x}\right) = \left[\frac{\log\left(\frac{1}{1-p}\right)}{\hat{\lambda} \exp\left(\boldsymbol{x}'\hat{\boldsymbol{\beta}}\right)}\right]^{1/\hat{\tilde{p}}}. \tag{4.62}$$

In the above equation, the reader might want to be aware of the difference between $\tilde{p}$, the Weibull shape parameter, and p, the probability value in a time distribution.

As the Weibull hazard regression model is a proportional function, the term $\exp(b_m)$ reflects the hazard ratio of covariate x_m, highlighting the proportional change in the hazard rate with a 1-unit increase in x_m, other covariates being unchanged.

4.3.2 Weibull accelerated failure time regression model

The Weibull function is often formulated in the form of the extreme value distribution because $\log(T)$, which can be expressed as a function of the Weibull parameters, follows the extreme value distribution. More important, if $\log T$ has an extreme value distribution, the survival time T follows an accelerated failure time distribution that can be applied to many families of parametric distributions, as described in Section 4.1. Given this flexibility, the Weibull regression model can be more conveniently specified and estimated within the structure of the AFT regression perspective.

Let $Y = \log(T)$ and $p^* = 1/\tilde{p}$ be the scale parameter. Replacing $\log t$ and $\tilde{\sigma}$ in Equation (4.9) with y and p^*, the Weibull survival function of T can be written as an AFT regression model:

$$S(t; \boldsymbol{x}, \boldsymbol{\beta}^*, p^*) = \exp\left[-\exp\left(\frac{y - \boldsymbol{x}'\boldsymbol{\beta}^*}{p^*}\right)\right], \quad -\infty < y < \infty. \tag{4.63}$$

Notice that Equation (4.63) is a simplified expression. As indicated in Subsection 4.1.2, the coefficient vector $\boldsymbol{\beta}^*$ includes an intercept parameter μ^*. While intimately related to the Weibull hazard rate parameter λ, the parameter μ^* will be further specified and discussed in Subsection 4.3.3.

In view of the fact that $S(t)$ can be expressed in terms of an accelerated failure time function, the Weibull hazard function can be formulated as an inverse in terms of the AFT regression model, given by

$$h(t; \boldsymbol{x}, \boldsymbol{\beta}^*, p^*) = (p^*)^{-1} \exp\left(\frac{y - \boldsymbol{x}'\boldsymbol{\beta}^*}{p^*}\right), \quad -\infty < y < \infty. \tag{4.64}$$

The value of p^* determines the shape of the Weibull hazard function. If $p^* = 1$, the Weibull AFT model reduces to the exponential AFT regression model and, consequently, the hazard function is constant (or we can say the exponential AFT regression model is a special case of the Weibull AFT regression model with $p^* = 1$). When $p^* > 1$, the hazard rate decreases over time. When $0.5 < p^* < 1$, the hazard increases at a decreasing rate, with its shape being concave. When $0 < p^* < 0.5$, the hazard rate increases with an increasing rate, and its shape is convex. Lastly, when $p^* = 0.5$, the hazard rate is constantly increasing.

With the Weibull survival and hazard functions defined as the AFT inverse functions, the AFT density function in the Weibull regression model can be easily written within the formation of an AFT regression:

$$\begin{aligned} f(t; \boldsymbol{x}, \boldsymbol{\beta}^*, p^*) &= \exp\left[-\exp\left(\frac{y - \boldsymbol{x}'\boldsymbol{\beta}^*}{p^*}\right)\right](p^*)^{-1} \exp\left(\frac{y - \boldsymbol{x}'\boldsymbol{\beta}^*}{p^*}\right) \\ &= (p^*)^{-1} \exp\left[\frac{y - \boldsymbol{x}'\boldsymbol{\beta}^*}{p^*} - \exp\left(\frac{y - \boldsymbol{x}'\boldsymbol{\beta}^*}{p^*}\right)\right], \quad -\infty < y < \infty. \end{aligned} \tag{4.65}$$

As can be seen from Equation (4.65), the Weibull AFT regression model is simply an extension of the exponential AFT regression model with the addition of a scale parameter p^*. The reader might want to compare Equations (4.63) and (4.65) with Equations (4.48) and (4.49) for such associations.

After some simplification, the likelihood function with respect to $\boldsymbol{\beta}^*$ for the Weibull AFT regression model is

$$L(\boldsymbol{\beta}^*, p^*) = \prod_{i=1}^{n} \left[(p^*)^{-1} \exp\left(\frac{y - \boldsymbol{x}'\boldsymbol{\beta}^*}{p^*}\right)\right]^{\delta_i} \exp\left[-\exp\left(\frac{y - \boldsymbol{x}'\boldsymbol{\beta}^*}{p^*}\right)\right]. \tag{4.66}$$

According to Equation (4.66), the likelihood refers to either a density function when $\delta_i = 1$, or the probability of survival when $\delta_i = 0$, so survival times for both events and censored cases are accounted for.

The log-likelihood function with respect to Equation (4.66) is

$$\log L(\boldsymbol{\beta}^*, p^*) = \sum_{i=1}^{n} \left\{ \delta_i \left[(-\log p^*) + \left(\frac{y - \boldsymbol{x}'\boldsymbol{\beta}^*}{p^*} \right) \right] \right\} - \exp\left(\frac{y - \boldsymbol{x}'\boldsymbol{\beta}^*}{p^*} \right). \quad (4.67)$$

Maximizing this log-likelihood function with respect to $\boldsymbol{\beta}^*$ and p^* yields the MLE estimates of the Weibull AFT model parameters. Here, as the estimating procedures are standard, described extensively in Section 4.1, I do not elaborate on the detailed inference. Given the above specifications in the AFT formulation, used by most major statistical software packages like SAS, the survival, density, and hazard functions in the Weibull proportional hazard model are regularly considered to be the inverse functions of the AFT parameters. As a result, given the Weibull AFT parameter estimates, the parameter estimates of the Weibull proportional hazard models can be obtained by transforming the AFT parameters, as presented in Subsection 4.3.3.

4.3.3 Conversion of Weibull proportional hazard and AFT parameters

As indicated in Chapter 3, the Weibull AFT parameters can be expressed as transforms of the Weibull hazard model parameters, and it is also true for vice versa. A comparison between Equations (4.56) and (4.64) or between (4.57) and (4.63) can help the reader better to understand the mathematical associations between the two sets of Weibull parameters.

Let $Y = \log(T)$, $p^* = 1/\tilde{p}$. Then the parameters in the Weibull proportional hazard regression model can be expressed in terms of the Weibull AFT parameters, given by

$$\lambda = \exp\left(-\frac{\mu^*}{p^*} \right), \quad (4.68)$$

$$\beta_m = -\frac{\beta_m^*}{p^*}, \quad (4.69)$$

where μ^* is the intercept parameter, defined in Subsection 4.1.2, with its value being the first element in the coefficient vector $\boldsymbol{\beta}^*$.

Similarly, the Weibull AFT parameters can be formulated with respect to the Weibull proportional hazard model parameters:

$$\mu^* = -\frac{\log \lambda}{\tilde{p}}, \quad (4.70)$$

$$\beta_m^* = -\frac{\beta_m}{\tilde{p}}. \quad (4.71)$$

While the conversion of the Weibull parameters is straightforward, transformation of the standard errors from one perspective to the other is more complex. Because the Weibull parameters, either the AFT or the proportional hazard, follow an asymptotic multivariate normal distribution, the transformation of a covariance matrix is regularly considered within an integrated multivariate framework. The delta method, described in Appendix A, is generally applied to approximate the variance and covariance transforms, viewing the original and the transformed variances and covariances as two random matrices.

I start with the Weibull AFT regression model. Suppose that $\boldsymbol{\theta}_1$ is a random vector of the Weibull AFT parameters $\left(\hat{\boldsymbol{\theta}}_1 = \hat{\theta}_{11}, \ldots, \hat{\theta}_{1M}\right)'$ with mean μ and variance matrix $\hat{V}\left(\hat{\boldsymbol{\theta}}_1\right)$, and $\hat{\boldsymbol{\theta}}_2 = g\left(\hat{\boldsymbol{\theta}}_1\right)$ is a transform of $\hat{\boldsymbol{\theta}}_1$ where g is the link function specified by Equations (4.68) and (4.69). From the Taylor series expansion,

$$\hat{\boldsymbol{\theta}}_2 = g\left(\hat{\boldsymbol{\theta}}_1\right) = g(\boldsymbol{\mu}) + \left[\frac{\partial g(\boldsymbol{\theta}_1)}{\partial \boldsymbol{\theta}_1}\middle| \boldsymbol{\theta}_1 = \boldsymbol{\mu}\right]'(\boldsymbol{\theta}_1 - \boldsymbol{\mu}) + \mathrm{O}\left(\|\boldsymbol{\theta}_1 - \boldsymbol{\mu}\|^2\right), \tag{4.72}$$

where $\left(\|\boldsymbol{\theta}_1 - \boldsymbol{\mu}\|^2\right)$ is of a higher order. A first-order Taylor series expansion of $g\left(\hat{\boldsymbol{\theta}}_1\right)$ gives rise to an approximation of mean

$$\mathrm{E}\left[g\left(\hat{\boldsymbol{\theta}}_1\right)\right] \approx g(\boldsymbol{\mu}) \tag{4.73}$$

and the variance–covariance matrix $\hat{V}\left(\hat{\boldsymbol{\theta}}_2\right)$:

$$V\left[g\left(\hat{\boldsymbol{\theta}}_1\right)\right] \approx \left[\frac{\partial g(\boldsymbol{\theta}_1)}{\partial \boldsymbol{\theta}_1}\middle| \boldsymbol{\theta}_1 = \boldsymbol{\mu}\right]' V_{\hat{\theta}_1} \left[\frac{\partial g(\boldsymbol{\theta}_1)}{\partial \boldsymbol{\theta}_1}\middle| \boldsymbol{\theta}_1 = \boldsymbol{\mu}\right]. \tag{4.74}$$

Because $g\left(\hat{\boldsymbol{\theta}}_1\right)$ in the Weibull regression is a smooth nonlinear function of the $\hat{\boldsymbol{\theta}}_1$ values, $g\left(\hat{\boldsymbol{\theta}}_1\right)$ can be approximated by a linear function of $\hat{\boldsymbol{\theta}}_1$, in the region with a nonnegligible likelihood. Consequently, the variance–covariance matrix $\hat{V}\left(\hat{\boldsymbol{\theta}}_2\right)$ can be formulated in the following linear form (Meeker and Escobar, 1998):

$$\begin{aligned} V\left[g\left(\hat{\boldsymbol{\theta}}_1\right)\right] \approx & \sum_{m=1}^{M} \left[\frac{\partial g(\boldsymbol{\theta}_1)}{\partial \theta_{1m}}\right]^2 V\left(\hat{\boldsymbol{\theta}}_1\right) \\ & + \sum_{m=1}^{M} \sum_{\substack{m'=1 \\ m' \neq m}}^{M} \left[\frac{\partial g(\boldsymbol{\theta}_1)}{\partial \theta_{1m}}\right]\left[\frac{\partial g(\boldsymbol{\theta}_1)}{\partial \theta_{1m'}}\right] \mathrm{cov}(\theta_{1m}, \theta_{1m'}). \end{aligned} \tag{4.75}$$

The second component on the right of Equation (4.75) can be omitted if the elements in $\hat{\boldsymbol{\theta}}_1$ are uncorrelated.

Klein and Moeschberger (2003) expand Equation (4.75) by creating an example for times to death from laryngeal cancer. For convenience of further analysis and simplification, some of the transformational equations are displayed below, with certain notational modifications:

$$\begin{aligned} \mathrm{cov}\left(\hat{\beta}_m, \hat{\beta}_{m'}\right) \approx & \frac{\mathrm{cov}\left(\hat{\beta}_m^*, \hat{\beta}_{m'}^*\right)}{\left(\hat{p}^*\right)^2} - \frac{\hat{\beta}_m^* \,\mathrm{cov}\left(\hat{\beta}_{m'}^*, \hat{p}^*\right)}{\left(\hat{p}^*\right)^3} - \frac{\hat{\beta}_{m'}^* \,\mathrm{cov}\left(\hat{\beta}_{m}^*, \hat{p}^*\right)}{\left(\hat{p}^*\right)^3} \\ & + \frac{\hat{\beta}_{m'}^* \hat{\beta}_m^* V\left(\hat{p}^*\right)}{\left(\hat{p}^*\right)^4}, \quad m, m' = 1, \ldots, M; \end{aligned} \tag{4.76}$$

$$V(\hat{\lambda}) \approx \exp\left(-2\frac{\hat{\mu}^*}{\hat{p}^*}\right)\left[\frac{V(\hat{\mu}^*)}{(\hat{p}^*)^2} - 2\frac{\hat{\mu}^* \operatorname{cov}(\hat{\mu}^*, \hat{p}^*)}{(\hat{p}^*)^3} + \frac{(\hat{\mu}^*)^2 V(\hat{p}^*)}{(\hat{p}^*)^4}\right]; \tag{4.77}$$

$$V(\tilde{p}) \approx \frac{V(\hat{p}^*)}{(\hat{p}^*)^4}; \tag{4.78}$$

$$\operatorname{cov}(\hat{\beta}_m, \hat{\lambda}) \approx \exp\left(-\frac{\hat{\mu}^*}{\hat{p}^*}\right)\left[\frac{\operatorname{cov}(\hat{\beta}^*_m, \hat{\mu}^*)}{(\hat{p}^*)^2} - \frac{\hat{\beta}^*_j \operatorname{cov}(\hat{\beta}^*_m, \hat{p}^*)}{(\hat{p}^*)^3} - \frac{\hat{\mu}^* \operatorname{cov}(\hat{\mu}^*, \hat{p}^*)}{(\hat{p}^*)^3} + \frac{\hat{\beta}^*_m \hat{\mu}^* V(\hat{p}^*)}{(\hat{p}^*)^4}\right], \quad m = 1, \ldots, M; \tag{4.79}$$

$$\operatorname{cov}(\hat{\beta}_m, \tilde{p}) \approx \frac{\operatorname{cov}(\hat{\beta}^*_m, \hat{p}^*)}{(\hat{p}^*)^3} - \frac{\hat{\beta}^*_m V(\hat{p}^*)}{(\hat{p}^*)^4}, \quad m = 1, \ldots, M; \tag{4.80}$$

$$\operatorname{cov}(\hat{\lambda}, \tilde{p}) \approx \exp\left(-\frac{\hat{\mu}^*}{\hat{p}^*}\right)\left[\frac{\operatorname{cov}(\hat{\mu}^*, \hat{p}^*)}{(\hat{p}^*)^3} - \frac{\hat{\mu}^* V(\hat{p}^*)}{(\hat{p}^*)^4}\right]. \tag{4.81}$$

The square roots of the transformed variances for the Weibull proportional hazard parameters yield the estimated standard errors, in turn deriving corresponding confidence intervals for the transforms. Based on the above expanded equations, Klein and Moeschberger (2003) transform the standard errors of the Weibull AFT coefficients to the standard errors of the proportional hazard coefficients using the data of patients with cancer of the larynx. The results are presented in Tables 12.1 and 12.2 of their book.

With more parameters specified, the expansion of Equation (4.75) to transform variances and covariances becomes much more tedious and cumbersome. Allison (2010) discusses the characteristics of the Weibull hazard function for different values of the scale p^* and presents related graphs (Figure 2.3, p. 21). He notes that test results of the null hypothesis on $\log T$ coefficients also serve as the results of the null hypothesis on log hazard coefficients. This is a reasonable proposition because the baseline distribution of $\log T$ and $\log h(t)$ are actually two transformed profiles of the Weibull baseline distribution of T. As a result, corresponding estimates in $\hat{\boldsymbol{\theta}}_1$ and $\hat{\boldsymbol{\theta}}_2$ should be subject to the same p-values with identical Wald statistics. This association suggests that test results from the Weibull AFT regression model can be borrowed to perform the significance test on the estimated regression coefficients in the Weibull hazard rate regression models, without performing the transformation of the AFT variance–covariance matrix for the proportional hazard parameter estimates.

Given this intimate association, standard errors of the estimated regression coefficients and the scale parameter contained in $\hat{\boldsymbol{\theta}}_2$ can be approximated by using a much simpler approach. Here, I first demonstrate the transformation of the standard error for a single estimated regression coefficient $\hat{\beta}^*_m$. Suppose that the two regression coefficients, $\hat{\beta}^*_m$ and $\hat{\beta}_m$, have exactly the same p-value associated with a common Wald statistic distributed as χ^2.

Given the large-sample approximate normal distribution of the ML estimator, it is reasonable to establish the following equation of approximation:

$$\frac{\beta_m^*}{SE(\beta_m^*)} \approx \frac{-\beta_m}{SE(\beta_m)}. \tag{4.82}$$

Multiplying both the denominator and numerator on the right side of Equation (4.82) with the scale parameter p^* yields

$$\frac{\beta_m^*}{SE(\beta_m^*)} \approx \frac{-\beta_m(p^*)}{SE(\beta_m)(p^*)}. \tag{4.83}$$

Because $-\beta_j p^* = \beta_j^*$, we have

$$SE(\beta_m) \approx \frac{SE(\beta_m^*)}{p^*}. \tag{4.84}$$

Therefore, the standard error of $\hat{\beta}_m$ can be approximated from the standard error of $\hat{\beta}_m^*$ over the scale parameter p^*. Standard errors of other hazard regression coefficients can be estimated using the same approach. Consequently, the tedious computation of the delta method can be avoided.

Using the same logic, the standard error of $\tilde{p}$, the shape parameter for the Weibull proportional hazard model, is

$$SE(\tilde{p}) \approx \frac{SE(p^*)}{(p^*)^2}. \tag{4.85}$$

The interested reader might want to practice how Equation (4.85) is derived. Notice that squaring Equation (4.85) gives rise to Equation (4.78) about $V(\tilde{p})$ derived from the delta method.

To highlight the applicability of the above simplified calculations, I transform the standard errors of the Weibull AFT coefficients presented in Table 12.1 of Klein and Moeschberger's (2003) book to the standard errors of the Weibull proportional hazard coefficients, using Equations (4.84) and (4.85). Table 4.1 displays the original AFT parameter estimates and their standard errors, the transformed proportional hazard coefficients, the transformed standard errors of the proportional hazard parameters from Klein and Moeschberger's calculation (KM SE), and the transformed standard errors from Equations (4.84) and (4.85).

The transformed standard errors of the PH regression coefficients and the scale parameter from the simple approach are almost identical to those calculated from the delta method. I do not report the transformed standard error estimate of the intercept parameter because the application of Equation (4.84) yields the transformed standard error of $\log\hat{\lambda}$ (β_0) rather than the standard error for the scale parameter $\hat{\lambda}$ itself. Therefore, while the standard error of the

Table 4.1 Parameter estimates of Weibull AFT regression and the PH transforms.

Variable	Parameter estimate	Standard error	PH parameter estimate	KM SE for transforms	SE from new equations
Scale	0.88	0.11	1.13	0.14	0.14
Z_1	–0.15	0.41	0.17	0.46	0.47
Z_2	–0.59	0.32	0.66	0.36	0.36
Z_3	–1.54	0.36	1.75	0.42	0.41
Z_4	–0.02	0.01	0.02	0.01	0.01

model intercept is less important, the standard error of $\hat{\lambda}$ can be obtained by using the delta method.

Such a transformation, from the Weibull AFT variance–covariance matrix to the corresponding matrix for the proportional hazard parameter estimates, can also be performed by applying the bootstrap approximation method. Specifically, bootstrap sampling is used to simulate the repeated sampling process in a large number of bootstrap samples for computing the needed standard errors or confidence intervals of certain estimators, thereby reducing the dependence on large-sample approximation. The number of bootstrap samples is generally recommended as between 2000 and 5000. Theoretically, the bootstrapping method derives a range of an estimator, rather than a one-on-one transform, because each procedure can derive a unique set of parameter estimates. Additionally, the bootstrap approximation does not account for covariance between parameters and thus may introduce some specification problems. Therefore, this approach is a second-choice alternative when the large-sample approximation is valid and the likelihood-based methods are not too demanding computationally. This approximation method is standard, not specifically designed for survival analysis. Therefore, I do not describe the detailed procedures of bootstrap further in this text. The interested reader can read Efron and Tibshirani (1993) for more details.

I would like to make a recommendation that if the estimation of confidence intervals is not needed, the researcher might want to use the *p*-values of the AFT parameter estimates directly for the significant test on the Weibull proportional hazard parameters, thus saving the energy of performing further computations.

4.3.4 Illustration: A Weibull regression model on marital status and survival among older Americans

In Subsection 4.3.3, I examined the association between marital status and the probability of survival among older Americans for a twelve-month observation, adjusting for the confounding effects of age and educational attainment. The results did not display a significant effect of current marriage on the one-year mortality of older Americans. This lack of association, as indicated earlier, might be due to a relatively short observation interval, during which the impact of married life on the probability of survival cannot be captured.

In the present illustration, I revisit this topic by extending the observation period from 12 to 48 months (four years). The underlying null hypothesis is that currently married older persons do not have a better chance of survival than do those not currently married within a much lengthened observation period. With an extended observation interval, I specify a Weibull distribution of survival time to model the baseline survival function among older Americans. As previously specified, marital status is a dichotomous variable: 1 = 'currently married' and 0 = else, with the variable name given as 'Married.' Age and educational attainment are used as the control variables, and their centered measures, 'Age_mean' and 'Educ_mean,' are applied in the regression analysis.

As the hazard rate, especially among older persons, tends to increase over time, the use of the Weibull regression model is theoretically reasonable because of its monotonic property. As mentioned in Chapter 3, if the survival data arise from a Weibull distribution, the plot of $\log\left[-\log\hat{S}(t)\right]$ versus $\log(t)$ should display a roughly linear line. Given this feature, I first plot such a graph before starting the formal regression analysis, using the Kaplan–Meier survival estimates. The SAS program for plotting this curve is given below.

SAS Program 4.3:

```
......
ods graphics on;

ods select LogNegLogSurvivalPlot;
proc lifetest data = new OUTSURV = out1 plots = loglogs;
 time Months * Status(0);
run;
```

In SAS Program 4.3, I use the variable Status (1 = event, 0 = censored) again for executing the PROC LIFETEST procedure to construct a log negative $\log\hat{S}(t)$ versus log t plot using the Kaplan–Meier survival estimates. The ODS Graphics is enabled by specifying the ODS GRAPHICS ON statement with the ODS select name switching to LogNegLogSurvivalPlot. In the PROC LIFETEST statement, the option PLOTS = LOGLOGS tells SAS to construct a graph of the log negative $\log\hat{S}(t)$ function versus $\log t$ from the survival data of older Americans. SAS Program 4.3 yields the plot in Figure 4.3.

The plot of the $\log\left[-\log\hat{S}(t)\right]$ versus log (months) displays an approximately straight curve, thereby indicating the use of the Weibull regression in the present illustration to be reasonable. Nevertheless, plotting the graph of a linear relationship between a transformed survival function and a transformed time function is a tentative, rough approach for a functional check; it cannot be used to make a final decision regarding whether or not a given parametric regression fits the survival data, as also indicated in Section 4.2.

Next, the PROC LIFEREG procedure is used to fit the Weibull regression model on the survival data of older Americans. In the SAS system, the PROC LIFEREG procedure is based on the AFT perspective, so that it does not directly estimate hazard rate parameters. The Weibull parameter estimates on log(hazards), however, can be obtained from the estimates on the log(survival time) by using the SAS ODS procedure. Below is the SAS program for the estimation of the Weibull regression parameters on marital status and survival for a four-year period.

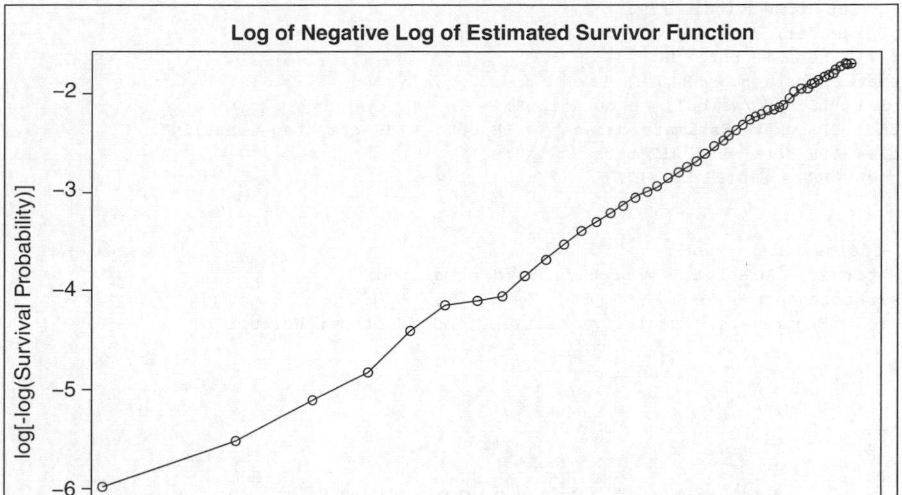

Figure 4.3 Plot of log negative log survival versus log time.

SAS Program 4.4:

......

```
* Compute xbeta estimates of the Weibull accelerated failure time model *;
ods graphics on ;
ods output Parameterestimates = Weibull_AFT;
proc lifereg data=new outest=Weibull_outest;
  class married;
  model duration*Censor(1) = married age_mean educ_mean / dist = Weibull;
  output out = new1 cdf = prob;
run;
ods graphics off;
ods output close;

* Compute and print corresponding PH estimates and HR *;
data Weibull_AFT;
  if _N_=1 then set Weibull_outest(keep= _SCALE_);
  set Weibull_AFT;
  string = upcase(trim(Parameter));
  if (string ne 'SCALE') & (string ne 'WEIBULL SHAPE')
  then PH_beta = -1*estimate/_SCALE_;
  else if PH_beta = .;
  AFT_beta = estimate;
  HR = exp(PH_beta);
  drop _SCALE_;
options nolabel;
```

```
proc print data=Weibull_AFT;
  id Parameter;
  var AFT_beta PH_beta HR;
  format PH_beta 8.5 HR 5.3;
  title1 "LIFEREG/Weibull on duration";
  title2 "ParameterEstimate dataset w/PH_beta & HR computed manually";
  title4 "PH_beta = -1*AFT_beta/Scale";
  title6 "HR = exp(PH_beta)";
run;

proc sgplot data = new1;
  scatter x = duration y = prob / group = married;
  discretelegend;
  title1 "Figure 4.4. Cumulative distribution function: Weibull";
run;
```

SAS Program 4.4 is a revised version of SAS Program 4.1, given the adjustment of the code for fitting a Weibull regression model. Therefore, the earlier part of the program is not presented. Briefly, in the omitted part a temporary SAS data file 'New' is created from the dataset chapter4_data. The survival time variable 'duration' is now specified in terms of a 48-month observation period. Accordingly, the dichotomous variable 'Censor,' 1 = censored and 0 = not censored, is redefined to conform to a 48-month observation window, with the Type I right censoring fixed at the end of the 48-month interval. The construction of the two centered control variables, Age_mean and Educ_mean, is saved into the temporary SAS data file 'New' for the Weibull regression analysis.

In SAS Program 4.4, I first ask SAS to estimate the regression coefficients of covariates on log(duration), with parameter estimates saved in the temporary SAS output file Weibull_AFT. The MODEL statement specifies three covariates, with the time distribution specified as Weibull. In SAS, the DIST = WEIBULL option can be omitted because the LIFEREG procedure fits the default Type 1 extreme-value distribution by using log(duration) as the response, equivalent to fitting the Weibull AFT regression model. The OUTPUT statement creates the output dataset New1.

The next section converts the saved Weibull log time coefficients (AFT_beta) into the Weibull log hazard coefficients (PH_beta) and the Weibull hazard ratios (HR), given the formulas in Subsection 4.3.3. Compared to SAS Program 4.1, an additional parameter SCALE is now displayed in the transformation procedure. Next, I request SAS to print three sets of parameter estimates – the regression coefficients on log(duration), the regression coefficients on log(hazards), and the hazard ratios. The test results of the null hypothesis on log time coefficients also serve as the results of the null hypothesis on log hazard coefficients because the two sets of the Weibull parameter estimates share the same p-values. As a result, in the present illustration I borrow test results from the Weibull AFT regression models to perform the significance tests on the regression coefficients in the Weibull hazard rate regression model. If needed, calculation of the standard errors for proportional hazard coefficients can be easily programmed in SAS.

Lastly, the PROC SGPLOT procedure is used to produce a plot of the cumulative distribution values versus the variable Duration. Some of the analytic results from SAS Program 4.4 are presented below.

SAS Program Output 4.2:

```
                        The LIFEREG Procedure

                          Model Information

              Data Set                                WORK.NEW
              Dependent Variable                 Log(duration)
              Censoring Variable                        censor
              Censoring Value(s)                             1
              Number of Observations                      2000
              Noncensored Values                           332
              Right Censored Values                       1668
              Left Censored Values                           0
              Interval Censored Values                       0
              Number of Parameters                           5
              Name of Distribution                     Weibull
              Log Likelihood                       -1132.63769

                           Fit Statistics

          -2 Log Likelihood                         2265.275
          AIC (smaller is better)                   2275.275
          AICC (smaller is better)                  2275.305
          BIC (smaller is better)                   2303.280

              Analysis of Maximum Likelihood Parameter Estimates

                                   Standard   95% Confidence     Chi-
Parameter            DF Estimate     Error        Limits       Square Pr > ChiSq

Intercept             1   5.3314    0.1071   5.1215   5.5414 2477.89     <.0001
married    Married    1  -0.0547    0.0946  -0.2401   0.1307    0.33     0.5631
married    Not married 0  0.0000         .        .        .       .          .
age_mean              1  -0.0588    0.0076  -0.0737  -0.0439   60.13     <.0001
educ_mean             1   0.0163    0.0121  -0.0074   0.0400    1.82     0.1773
Scale                 1   0.7944    0.0425   0.7154   0.8822
Weibull Shape         1   1.2588    0.0673   1.1336   1.3978

                     PH_beta = -1*AFT_beta/Scale

                          HR = exp(PH_beta)

              Parameter        AFT_beta     PH_beta      HR

              Intercept         5.33143    -6.71104   0.001
              married          -0.05470     0.06886   1.071
              married           0.00000     0.00000   1.000
              age_mean         -0.05879     0.07401   1.077
              educ_mean         0.01631    -0.02054   0.980
              Scale             0.79443           .       .
              Weibull Shape     1.25877           .       .
```

In SAS Program Output 4.2, the class level information and a statistic of model fitness are presented first. There are 332 uncensored observations (deaths) and 1668 right-censored observations, giving a much extended observation interval. As mentioned in the previous example, all censored observations are of Type I right censoring. The log likelihood for this Weibull regression model is −1132.6377. The section of fit statistics displays four indicators of model fitness, with the −2 log-likelihood statistic probably being the mostly widely used. In summary, values of these four statistics are close, generating the same conclusion about model fitting for this analysis.

The table Analysis of Maximum Likelihood Parameter Estimates displays the LIFEREG estimates on log(duration) given the Weibull distribution, derived from the maximum likelihood procedure. The intercept, 5.3314 ($SE = 0.1071$), is very strongly statistically significant. With a much extended observation period, however, currently married older persons are still not shown to have a significantly higher survival probability than the currently not married, after adjusting for the effects of age and education ($\beta_1 = 0.0547$, $p = 0.5631$). Therefore, it is likely that the bivariate association between marital status and survival, shown in Chapter 2 and statistically significant, is spurious. For the two control variables, age is negatively and statistically significantly associated with survival time ($\beta_2 = -0.0588$, $p < 0.0001$). Educational attainment is positively linked to survival time, but this effect is not statistically significant ($\beta_3 = 0.0163$, $p = 0.1773$). Here, the AFT coefficients estimated for the Weibull regression model are similar to those for the exponential regression within a shortened observation interval. The Weibull shape parameter $\tilde{p}$ is simply the reciprocal of the AFT parameter estimate p^* ($1/0.7944 = 1.2588$). The value of $\tilde{p}$, greater than 1, exhibits a monotonically increasing hazard function within the 48-month interval, as expected. This shape parameter estimate can be easily tested by $(\tilde{p} - 1.0)/SE$, which is statistically significant ($0.2588/0.0673 = 3.8455$, $p < 0.01$).

The last section in SAS Program Output 4.2 presents the three sets of the Weibull parameter estimates – AFT_beta, PH_beta, and HR. The hazard ratio of each covariate (HR) is presented to highlight the multiplicative effects of covariates on the mortality of older Americans within a four-year time interval. For example, a one-year increase in age would increase the hazard rate by about 8 % ($HR = 1.077$), other variables being equal. This effect, again, displays tremendous similarity to the hazard ratio in the exponential regression model.

The plot in Figure 4.4 displays the cumulative distribution function, contained in the output dataset New1, for currently married and currently not married older persons. Two cumulative distribution functions from the Weibull regression model are displayed, one for currently married older persons (o) and one for those currently not married (+). Even with an extended observation period, the plot does not demonstrate a clear pattern of the relationship between marital status and the cumulative probability of death. This lack of association, after controlling for the two 'lurking' variables, might be due to the fact that the probability of survival and marital status are both affected by age and education, so that the bivariate association between current marriage and survival, statistically significant, is spurious without a true causal relationship. A competing explanation is that the extension of the observation period to four years is still not long enough to capture the impact of current marriage on the mortality of older Americans. In any case, this illustration of multivariate regression analysis highlights the importance of performing regression modeling for testing a hypothesis on the causal linkage between two factors in a survival analysis.

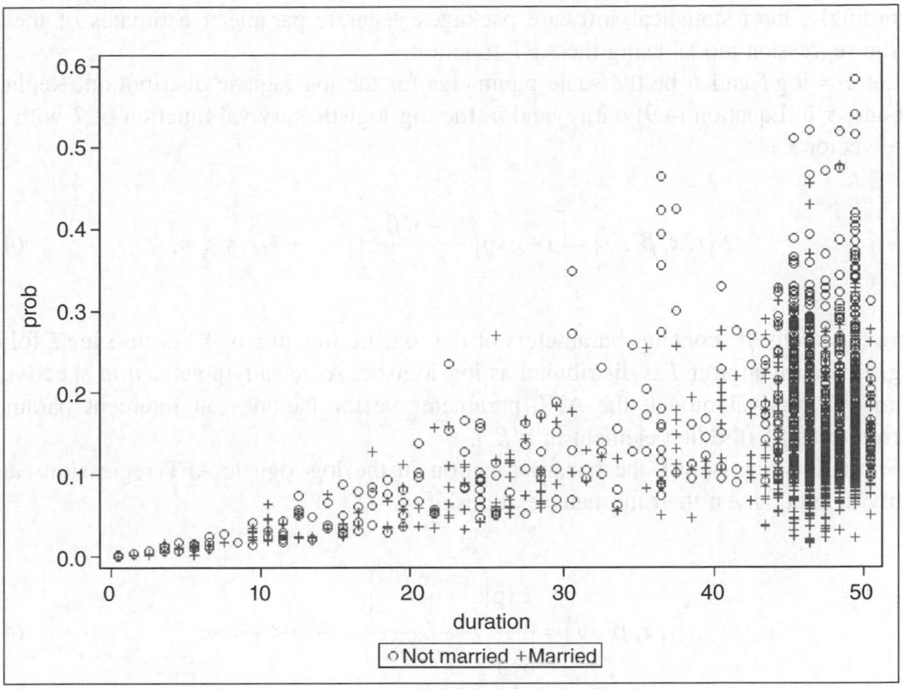

Figure 4.4 Cumulative distribution function: Weibull.

4.4 Log-logistic regression models

The Weibull proportional hazard rate model is popular in biomedical and demographic studies because it is easy to understand and the distribution agrees with most schedules of human mortality and morbidity. This regression model, however, has limitations under certain circumstances. The Weibull distribution is monotonic, so cannot be used to describe lifetime events in which the hazard rate changes direction. For example, human mortality decreases over age before reaching age 10, and then it increases steadily until all cohort members die out. Obviously, it is inappropriate to use the Weibull function to describe this long-standing process. As indicated in Chapter 3, there are several parametric lifetime functions that describe events whose rate changes direction over the life course. Lognormal and log-logistic functions are perhaps the most popular perspectives in this regard. When there are considerable censored observations in empirical data, the log-logistic distribution is believed to provide more accurate parameter estimates than the lognormal model, thereby serving as a preferable distributional function to model survival data with heavy censoring.

This section describes the log-logistic regression model and its statistical inference. In line with the previous two sections, an empirical illustration is provided to show how to apply this parametric regression model in empirical research.

4.4.1 Specifications of the log-logistic AFT regression model

The log-logistic regression model is formally specified as an accelerated failure time function because it can be conveniently expressed in the formation of Equations (4.8) and (4.9).

Accordingly, most statistical software packages generate parameter estimates of the log-logistic regression model using the AFT function.

Let $Y = \log T$ and $\hat{b}$ be the scale parameter for the log-logistic distribution. Replacing $\log t$ and $\tilde{\sigma}$ in Equation (4.9) with y and $\hat{b}$, the log-logistic survival function of T with covariate vector $\boldsymbol{x}$ is

$$S\left(t; \boldsymbol{x}, \boldsymbol{\beta}^*, \hat{b}\right) = \left[1 + \exp\left(\frac{y - \boldsymbol{x}'\boldsymbol{\beta}^*}{\hat{b}}\right)\right]^{-1}, \quad -\infty < y < \infty, \tag{4.86}$$

where the vector $\boldsymbol{\beta}^*$ contains parameters of the logistic function of Y because $\log T$ follows a logistic distribution if T is distributed as log-logistic. As usually practiced in specifying a parametric survival model, the AFT parameter vector includes an intercept parameter, referred to as μ^* (the first element in $\boldsymbol{x}'\boldsymbol{\beta}^*$).

From Equation (4.86), the hazard function in the log-logistic AFT regression can be readily defined, given their intimate relationship:

$$h\left(t; \boldsymbol{x}, \boldsymbol{\beta}^*, \hat{b}\right) = \frac{\exp\left(\frac{y - \boldsymbol{x}'\boldsymbol{\beta}^*}{\hat{b}}\right)}{\hat{b}\left(1 + \frac{y - \boldsymbol{x}'\boldsymbol{\beta}^*}{\hat{b}}\right)}, \quad -\infty < y < \infty. \tag{4.87}$$

With the AFT survival and the hazard functions specified, the density function of T in the log-logistic accelerated failure time regression model is

$$f\left(t; \boldsymbol{x}, \boldsymbol{\beta}^*, \hat{b}\right) = \frac{\exp\left(\frac{y - \boldsymbol{x}'\boldsymbol{\beta}^*}{\hat{b}}\right)}{\hat{b}\left[1 + \frac{y - \boldsymbol{x}'\boldsymbol{\beta}^*}{\hat{b}}\right]\left[1 + \exp\left(\frac{y - \boldsymbol{x}'\boldsymbol{\beta}^*}{\hat{b}}\right)\right]}, \quad -\infty < y < \infty. \tag{4.88}$$

Given the above three basic log-logistic AFT regression functions, the likelihood function for a sample of n individuals is given by

$$L\left(\boldsymbol{x}, \boldsymbol{\beta}^*, \hat{b}\right) = \prod_{i=1}^{n} \left\{\frac{\exp\left(\frac{y - \boldsymbol{x}'\boldsymbol{\beta}^*}{\hat{b}}\right)}{\hat{b}\left(1 + \frac{y - \boldsymbol{x}'\boldsymbol{\beta}^*}{\hat{b}}\right)}\right\}^{\delta_i} \left[1 + \exp\left(\frac{y - \boldsymbol{x}'\boldsymbol{\beta}^*}{\hat{b}}\right)\right]^{-1}, \quad -\infty < y < \infty. \tag{4.89}$$

Clearly, the contribution of an event time to the likelihood is the density because when $\delta_i = 1$, the product of the hazard rate and the probability of survival defines a density function. If the observation is censored, $\delta_i = 0$, so the likelihood is the probability of survival.

The corresponding log-likelihood function can then be readily specified:

$$\log L\left(\boldsymbol{x},\boldsymbol{\beta}^*,\widehat{b}\right)=\sum_{i=1}^{n}\delta_i\left\{-\log\widehat{b}+\left(\frac{y-\boldsymbol{x}'\boldsymbol{\beta}^*}{\widehat{b}}\right)-2\log\left[1+\exp\left(\frac{y-\boldsymbol{x}'\boldsymbol{\beta}^*}{\widehat{b}}\right)\right]\right\}$$
$$-(1-\delta_i)\log\left[1+\exp\left(\frac{y-\boldsymbol{x}'\boldsymbol{\beta}^*}{\widehat{b}}\right)\right]. \tag{4.90}$$

Analogous to inferences for other parametric regression models, maximizing the above log-likelihood function with respect to the model parameters yields the MLE estimates of the log-logistic AFT regression model. The inverse of the observed information matrix generates the variance–covariance matrix of the log-logistic parameter estimates. As the estimating procedures follow the standard algorithms, as described extensively in Section 4.1, I do not elaborate the concrete equations for the derivation of parameter estimates in the log-logistic AFT regression model.

4.4.2 Retransformation of AFT parameters to untransformed log-logistic parameters

The AFT regression modeling is widely applied for the derivation of parameter estimates due to its flexibility and convenience. The log-logistic regression model is no exception. Some statisticians, however, consider it more convenient to interpret analytic results using the original, or untransformed, log-logistic parameters on survival time per se. This stance highlights the importance of converting thc log-logistic AFT function into the untransformed log-logistic distribution, given parameter estimates obtained from the AFT perspective.

For retransformation of the log-logistic AFT parameters to the original log-logistic parameters on survival times, first I specify the log-logistic parameters on T in terms of the AFT parameters on $\log T$, given by

$$\lambda=\exp\left(-\frac{\mu^*}{\widehat{b}}\right), \tag{4.91}$$

$$\beta_j=-\frac{\beta_j^*}{\widehat{b}}, \tag{4.92}$$

$$\widehat{p}=\frac{1}{\widehat{b}}, \tag{4.93}$$

where μ^* is the intercept parameter, the first element in the coefficient vector $\boldsymbol{\beta}^*$. In form, these log-logistic transforms are much like those specified for the Weibull proportional hazard transforms although the log-logistic function cannot be expressed as a proportional hazard function. As a result, the transformation procedures described in Subsection 4.3.3 can be well applied for the log-logistic regression.

Given the specification of the above untransformed log-logistic regression parameters, the survival function given $\boldsymbol{x}$ can be written in the form of the untransformed log-logistic perspective, given by

$$S(t; \boldsymbol{x}, \boldsymbol{\beta}, \lambda, \tilde{p}) = \left[1+\lambda \exp(\boldsymbol{x}'\boldsymbol{\beta})t^{\tilde{p}}\right]^{-1}. \tag{4.94}$$

The reader might want to compare Equation (4.94) with Equation (4.86) for a better understanding of the implications of such a transformation. Given a univariate log-logistic distribution of T, the two sets of parameters just reflect two profiles of the same distributional function, thus being intimately associated. In other words, the parameters on $\log T$ can be easily transformed into the parameters on T.

Given such an intimate relationship, the log-logistic hazard rate can be written as a function of the untransformed parameters on event time T:

$$h(t; \boldsymbol{x}, \boldsymbol{\beta}, \lambda, \tilde{p}) = \frac{\lambda \tilde{p} \exp(\boldsymbol{x}'\boldsymbol{\beta})t^{\tilde{p}-1}}{1+\lambda \exp(\boldsymbol{x}'\boldsymbol{\beta})t^{\tilde{p}}}. \tag{4.95}$$

Equation (4.95) derives exactly the same hazard rate as that from Equation (4.84), using a different expression for the formation with a new set of parameters.

As can be expressed by the product of the survival and the hazard functions, the p.d.f. of the original log-logistic regression on T is

$$f(t; \boldsymbol{x}, \boldsymbol{\beta}, \lambda, \tilde{p}) = \frac{\lambda \tilde{p} \exp(\boldsymbol{x}'\boldsymbol{\beta})t^{\tilde{p}-1}}{\left[1+\lambda \exp(\boldsymbol{x}'\boldsymbol{\beta})t^{\tilde{p}}\right]^2}. \tag{4.96}$$

Given the above specifications, the log-logistic regression model on T can be articulated by retransforming the AFT parameter estimates.

The variance–covariance matrix of parameter estimates λ, $\boldsymbol{\beta}$, and $\tilde{p}$ can be approximated by applying the delta method, with the procedure described in Subsection 4.3.3. As displayed in 4.3.3, however, standard errors of the untransformed parameter estimates, except for μ^*, can be approximated by using a much simpler approach based on the large-sample approximate normal distribution of the ML estimators (see Equations (4.84) and (4.85)). If the value of the standard error is not of particular concern, the significance test on $\boldsymbol{\beta}$ and $\tilde{p}$ can be performed by borrowing the test results on $\boldsymbol{\beta}^*$ and $\tilde{b}$, particularly since the two sets of regression coefficients share the same p-values.

Unlike the case in the Weibull regression model, the term $\exp(\boldsymbol{x}'\boldsymbol{\beta})$ in the log-logistic regression cannot be viewed as the proportional effects on the lifetime outcome. This effect vector, however, can be understood as representing odds ratios on the probability of survival at time t. According to the specification of the logistic regression model, the odds of the survival rate at t, given $\boldsymbol{x}$, is

$$\text{Odds}\left[S(t; \boldsymbol{x}, \boldsymbol{\beta}, \lambda, \tilde{p})\right] = \frac{S(t; \boldsymbol{x}, \boldsymbol{\beta}, \lambda, \tilde{p})}{1-S(t; \boldsymbol{x}, \boldsymbol{\beta}, \lambda, \tilde{p})} = \frac{\left[1+\lambda \exp(\boldsymbol{x}'\boldsymbol{\beta})t^{\tilde{p}}\right]^{-1}}{\left[\lambda \exp(\boldsymbol{x}'\boldsymbol{\beta})t^{\tilde{p}}\right]^{-1}}. \tag{4.97}$$

Given $[\exp(\boldsymbol{x}'\boldsymbol{\beta})]^{-1} = \exp(-\boldsymbol{x}'\boldsymbol{\beta})$, Equation (4.97) can be rewritten as

$$\text{Odds}\left[S(t; \boldsymbol{x}, \boldsymbol{\beta}, \lambda, \tilde{p})\right] = \exp(-\boldsymbol{x}'\boldsymbol{\beta})\frac{\left[1+\lambda t^{\tilde{p}}\right]^{-1}}{\left[\lambda t^{\tilde{p}}\right]^{-1}} = \exp(-\boldsymbol{x}'\boldsymbol{\beta})\frac{S(t|\boldsymbol{x}=0)}{1-S(t|\boldsymbol{x}=0)}. \tag{4.98}$$

Conceivably, a single effect term $\exp(-b_m)$ indicates the change in the individual odds of surviving with a 1-unit increase in covariate x_m, other variables being equal. This interpretation highlights the fact that the term $\exp(-\boldsymbol{x}'\boldsymbol{\beta})$ is odds proportional to the probability of survival. Given a special link to the logistic distribution, the log-logistic survival function is the only parametric survival model that possesses both the proportional odds and the AFT representations (Klein and Moeschberger, 2003).

4.4.3 Illustration: The log-logistic regression model on marital status and survival among the oldest old Americans

In Subsection 4.3.4, I reexamined the association between marital status and the probability of survival among older Americans for a 48-month observation, adjusting for the confounding effects of age and educational attainment. The results did not confirm current marriage to have a statistically significant impact on the four-year survival rate of older persons. The use of the Weibull regression model is considered to be theoretically sound because the death rate generally monotonically increases among older persons. Some scientists contend, however, that the population hazard rate is the average risk among surviving individuals who are physically selected from the 'survival of the fittest' process (Hougaard, 1995; Liu *et al.*, 2010; Vaupel, Manton, and Stallard, 1979). Empirically, the observed hazard function for a population or a population subgroup is often found to rise exponentially at younger and middle age, and then the rate of increase will be leveled-off or even decline at some oldest ages. This phenomenon is thought to be because selection eliminates less fit individuals from a given population as its age increases. Its mortality rate increases less rapidly with age than it would otherwise be because the surviving members of the population are the ones who are most fit.

In the present illustration, I analyze the association between marital status and survival among older persons aged 85 or over, generally termed the oldest old. Given such an old population, I assume a log-logistic distribution of survival time, seeking to capture the possible nonmonotonic process among those oldest old. Using this parametric regression model, the shape parameter of the log-logistic regression model displays whether the hazard rate is monotonic over time. The Weibull regression model, though highly flexible in general situations, does not have the capability to capture the possible directional change over time in the hazard rate.

As previously specified, marital status is a dichotomous variable: 1 = 'currently married' and 0 = else, with the variable name given as 'Married.' Specification of age and educational attainment remains the same, and their centered measures, 'Age_mean' and 'Educ_mean,' are used in the regression analysis as control variables. The following SAS program estimates the log-logistic regression model on marital status and survival among the oldest old Americans within a 4-year observation period.

SAS Program 4.5:

```
......

* Compute xbeta estimates of the log-logistic accelerated failure time model *;
ods graphics on ;
ods output Parameterestimates = Llogistic_AFT;
```

```
proc lifereg data=new outest=Llogistic_outest; where age ge 85;
  class married;
  model duration*Censor(1) = married age_mean educ_mean / dist = Llogistic;
  output out = new1 cdf = prob;
run;
ods graphics off;
ods output close;

* Compute and print corresponding untransformed estimates and OR *;
data Llogistic_AFT;
  if _N_=1 then set Llogistic_outest(keep=_SCALE_);
  set Llogistic_AFT;
  string = upcase(trim(Parameter));
  if (string ne 'SCALE') & (string ne 'Llogistic SHAPE')
  then UT_beta = -1*estimate/_SCALE_;
  else if UT_beta = .;
  AFT_beta = estimate;
  OR = exp(-UT_beta);
  P = 1 / _SCALE_;
  drop _SCALE_;
options nolabel;

proc print data=Llogistic_AFT;
  id Parameter;
  var AFT_beta UT_beta OR P;
  format UT_beta 8.5 OR 5.3;
  title1 "LIFEREG/Llogistic on duration";
  title2 "ParameterEstimate dataset ll/UT_beta & OR computed manually";
  title4 "UT_beta = -1*AFT_beta/Scale";
  title6 "OR = exp(-UT_beta)";
run;
```

SAS Program 4.5 bears tremendous resemblance to SAS Program 4.4, with some code adjustments for fitting the log-logistic regression. In the early part of the program, not presented, the procedures of constructing temporary SAS data files ('NEW,' 'NEW1') and specifying various variables are exactly the same as in SAS Program 4.4.

In the SAS LIFEREG procedure, I first ask SAS to estimate the parameters on log(duration), with parameter estimates saved in the temporary SAS output file Llogistic_AFT. The 'WHERE AGE GE 85' option informs SAS that only the oldest old persons are analyzed. The CLASS and MODEL statements also remain the same except for the specification of the DIST = LLOGISTIC option. The OUTPUT statement is identical to SAS Program 4.4, which creates the output dataset New1 containing the variable Prob to display the cumulative distribution function at observed responses.

The next section converts the saved log-logistic log time coefficients (AFT_beta) to the log-logistic untransformed time coefficients (UT_beta) and odds ratios (OR), using the formulas described in Subsection 4.4.2. Notice, compared to SAS Program 4.4, that the parameter estimation of OR takes the opposite direction, as deviated from 1, to the corresponding hazard ratios in the Weibull model because the proportional odds in the log-logistic regression reflect multiplicative changes in the probability of survival, rather than in the hazard rate. Next, I request SAS to print three sets of parameter estimates – the regression coefficients on log(duration), the regression coefficients on time duration itself, and the odds ratios on the probability of survival. As mentioned previously, test results of the null hypothesis on log time coefficients also serve as the results of the null hypothesis testing on time coefficients.

The main body of the analytic results from SAS Program 4.5 is presented in the following output table.

SAS Program Output 4.3:

```
                        The LIFEREG Procedure

                          Model Information

              Data Set                          WORK.NEW
              Dependent Variable           Log(duration)
              Censoring Variable                  censor
              Censoring Value(s)                       1
              Number of Observations                 193
              Noncensored Values                      66
              Right Censored Values                  127
              Left Censored Values                     0
              Interval Censored Values                 0
              Number of Parameters                     5
              Name of Distribution              LLogistic
              Log Likelihood                -161.9482104


                            Fit Statistics

           -2 Log Likelihood                     323.896
           AIC (smaller is better)               333.896
           AICC (smaller is better)              334.217
           BIC (smaller is better)               350.210


           Analysis of Maximum Likelihood Parameter Estimates

                                  Standard   95% Confidence     Chi-
Parameter            DF Estimate     Error       Limits       Square Pr > ChiSq

Intercept             1   4.5877    0.3415   3.9183   5.2571  180.46     <.0001
married   Married     1  -0.2498    0.1828  -0.6081   0.1086    1.87     0.1719
married   Not married 0   0.0000     .        .        .        .         .
age_mean              1  -0.0242    0.0256  -0.0744   0.0259    0.90     0.3440
educ_mean             1   0.0022    0.0214  -0.0398   0.0441    0.01     0.9192
Scale                 1   0.5344    0.0611   0.4271   0.6687

                    UT_beta = -1*AFT_beta/Scale

                        OR = exp(-UT_beta)

        Parameter     AFT_beta      UT_beta       OR        P

        Intercept      4.58770     -8.58444     5348     1.87118
        married       -0.24977      0.46736    0.627     1.87118
        married        0.00000      0.00000    1.000     1.87118
        age_mean      -0.02422      0.04533    0.956     1.87118
        educ_mean      0.00217     -0.00406    1.004     1.87118
        Scale          0.53442       .          .        1.87118
```

In SAS Program Output 4.3, there are 193 oldest old persons in the survival data, among whom are 66 uncensored (deaths) and 127 right censored. As indicated earlier, all censored observations are of Type I right censoring. The log-likelihood for this log-logistic AFT regression model is −161.9482, yielding the–2 log-likelihood statistic at 323.896.

The table Analysis of Maximum Likelihood Parameter Estimates displays the LIFEREG log-logistic parameter estimates on log(duration), derived from the maximum likelihood procedure. The intercept, 4.5877 (*SE* = 0.3414), is statistically significant. None of the three regression coefficients is statistically significant, perhaps because, at the oldest ages, all differentials in the probability of survival have vanished thanks to the 'selection of the fittest' effect. The log-logistic untransformed shape parameter $\widehat{p}$ is simply the reciprocal of the AFT parameter estimate $\widehat{b}$ (1/0.5344 = 1.8712), presented at the last column of the last section. The value of $\widehat{p}$, greater than 1, indicates a nonmonotonic hazard function; namely, among the oldest old Americans, the hazard rate tends to increase initially and then decrease as time progresses. This untransformed shape parameter estimate on survival time can be easily tested by $(\widehat{p}-1.0)/SE$, analogous to the formula for the Weibull proportional hazard shape parameter. Obviously, this shape parameter estimate is statistically significant, reflecting the existence of a selection effect among the oldest old Americans (the selection issues will be discussed extensively in Chapter 9).

The last section also presents the three sets of the log-logistic parameter estimates – AFT_beta, UT_beta, and OR. The odds ratio (OR), or proportional odds (PO), of each covariate is displayed to highlight the multiplicative effect on the odds of survival among the oldest old Americans. For example, a one-year increase in age would lower the individual odds of survival by 4.4 % (*HR* = 0.956), other covariates being equal.

Although the value of $\widehat{p}$, greater than 1, suggests a nonmonotonic trend in the hazard rate, it may be interesting to examine whether the hazard schedules of the two marital status groups really change direction within a four-year observation period. Accordingly, below I use the SAS PROC GPLOT procedure to generate two hazard rate curves for the oldest old, one for currently married and one for currently not married. Equation (4.95) is applied, using the parameter estimates on survival time because they are more interpretable. In estimating these hazard curves, the values of control variables are fixed at sample means, so that the functions for those currently married and those currently not married can be compared effectively without being confounded. Because age and educational attainment are both centered at their sample means, their XBETA values need not be considered in calculating the predicted hazard rates. The SAS program for this plot is provided as follows.

SAS Program 4.6:

```
* Calculating hazard rates for log-logistic regression model *;

options ls=80 ps=58 nodate;
ods select all;
ods trace off;
ods listing;
title1;
run;

data Llogistic;
  do group = 1 to 2;
  do t = 1 to 50 by 0.1;
```

```
  if group = 1 then hazard = (0.00019 * 1.87118 * exp(0.46736) * (t**0.87118))
       / (1 + 0.00019 * exp(0.46736)  * (t**1.87118));
  if group = 2 then hazard =  (0.00019 * 1.87118 * exp(0)  * (t**0.87118))
       / (1 + 0.00019 * exp(0)  * (t**1.87118));
  output;
  end;
  end;
run;

proc format;
  value group_fmt 1 = 'Not currently married'
             2 = 'Currently married'
run;

goptions targetdevice=winprtc reset=global gunit=pct border cback=white
        colors=(black red blue)
        ftitle=swissxb ftext=swissxb htitle=2 htext=1.5;

proc gplot data = Llogistic;
  format group group_fmt.;
  plot hazard * t = group;
    symbol1 c=black  i=splines l=1 v=plus;
    symbol2 c=red     i=splines l=2 v=diamond;
    title1 "Figure 4.6. Hazard functions for currently married and currently not
married persons";
    run;
quit;
```

SAS Program 4.6 produces two hazard functions for currently married and currently not married older persons, respectively. The value of λ, $\exp(-4.58770/0.53442) = 0.00019$, is derived from Equation (4.91). The resulting plot is displayed in Figure 4.5, which demonstrates that within the four-year observation period, the hazard rates for currently married and currently not married oldest old increase consistently, but the rate of increase is decreasing (the second derivative of the hazard function is negative). Therefore, the value of $\widehat{p}$ greater than 1 simply represents a long-term nonmonotonic trend in the mortality of the oldest old; it does not describe an actual nonmonotonic process within a limited observation period. Therefore, these two log-logistic curves can also be described by using the Weibull regression model regardless of the value of $\widehat{p}$.

It is also interesting to note that the oldest old Americans who are currently married have higher mortality rates than do their counterparts who are currently not married, although this effect is not statistically significant. The emergence of this pattern among the oldest old is perhaps related to changes in the distribution of an individual 'frailty' due to the selection effect. This issue will be further discussed in Chapter 9.

A competing possibility for the absence of a significant association between marital status and the mortality of oldest old Americans comes from the fact that a four-year observation period is still not stretched out enough to capture the dynamics of the effect. In Chapter 5, I will analyze this issue by specifying a much longer observation interval using the Cox proportional model.

4.5 Other parametric regression models

As can be summarized from previous sections, each of the exponential, the Weibull, and the log-logistic regression models has its unique characteristics and practicability in survival

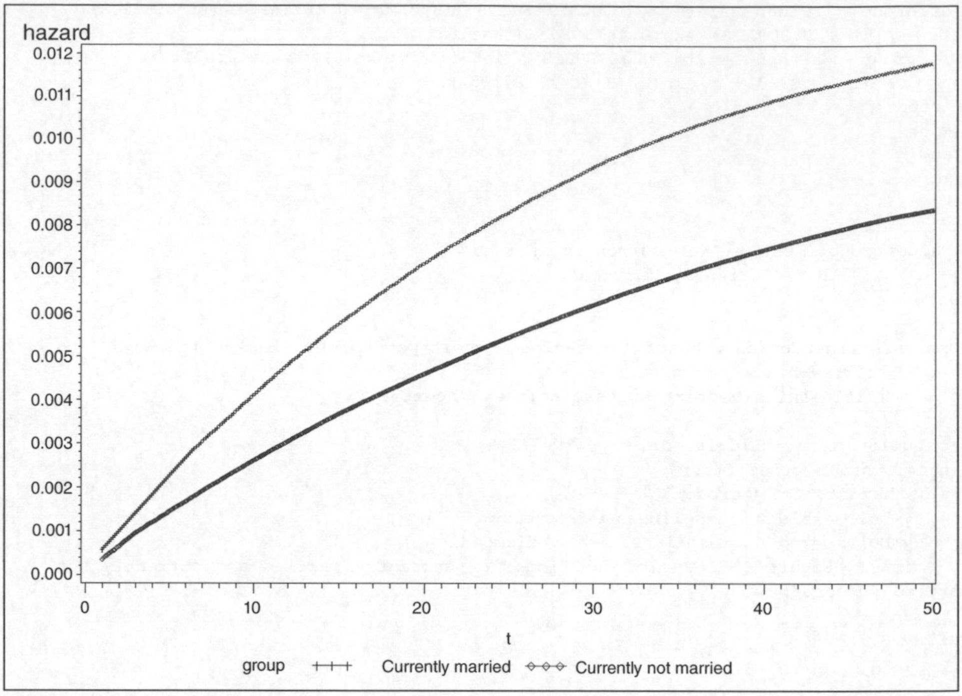

Figure 4.5 Hazard functions for currently married and currently not married persons.

analysis. The exponential regression model describes the survival data with a constant baseline hazard rate, whereas the Weibull regression model provides a flexible perspective to portray the hazard function, which is monotonically increasing or decreasing over time. Unlike the above two parametric models, the log-logistic regression model simulates nonmonotonic processes of the relative risk on the hazard rate that increase initially and then consistently decrease in the later stage of a life course.

There are some other regression models that have also seen tremendous applications in survival analysis, each corresponding to a specific pattern of survival processes. In this section, I briefly introduce two additional parametric models: the lognormal and the gamma regression models.

4.5.1 The lognormal regression model

As mentioned in Chapter 3, the lognormal distribution is another popular parametric function for the description of a nonmonotonic process in the hazard function. Its wide applicability is based on its simplicity because the logarithm of a lognormal distribution is normally distributed with mean μ and variance σ^2. Given the lognormal distribution, the AFT survival function, given covariate vector $\boldsymbol{x}$ and parameter vector $\boldsymbol{\beta}^*$, can be modeled by

$$S\left(t; \boldsymbol{x}, \boldsymbol{\beta}^*, \breve{b}\right) = 1 - \Phi\left(\frac{y - \boldsymbol{x}'\boldsymbol{\beta}^*}{\breve{b}}\right), \quad -\infty < y < \infty, \tag{4.99}$$

where $\Phi(\cdot)$ indicates the standard normal cumulative distribution function (the probit function), $\breve{b}$ is the scale parameter for the lognormal distribution, and the coefficient vector $\boldsymbol{\beta}^*$ includes an intercept parameter μ^*. The probability density function of the lognormal regression model is

$$f\left(t; \boldsymbol{x}, \boldsymbol{\beta}^*, \breve{b}\right) = \frac{1}{\sqrt{2\pi\sigma}} \exp\left[-\frac{1}{2}\left(\frac{y - \boldsymbol{x}'\boldsymbol{\beta}^*}{\breve{b}}\right)^2\right], \quad -\infty < y < \infty. \tag{4.100}$$

With the survival and density functions specified, the hazard function can be readily formulated as the ratio of $f\left(t; \boldsymbol{x}, \boldsymbol{\beta}^*, \breve{b}\right)$ over $S\left(t; \boldsymbol{x}, \boldsymbol{\beta}^*, \breve{b}\right)$. It then follows that the log-likelihood function can be written for the derivation of lognormal parameter estimates by using the standard estimating procedures described in Section 4.1.

Though simpler in formulation than the log-logistic regression model, the lognormal regression model does not behave well in the presence of heavy censoring. Accordingly, this model can be applied to describe nonmonotonic hazards only when the survival data do not contain many censored observations.

4.5.2 Gamma distributed regression models

The gamma distribution is often used as a part of a regression model in survival analysis. In particular, the gamma model has been applied for reflecting a skewed distribution of random errors when the assumption of normality on individual disturbances cannot be satisfied. As described in Chapter 3, the density function of a gamma distribution is

$$f(t) = \frac{\lambda(\lambda t)^{\tilde{k}-1} \mathrm{e}^{-\lambda t}}{\Gamma\left(\tilde{k}\right)}, \quad t > 0. \tag{4.101}$$

where $\tilde{k}$ is the shape parameter and λ is the scale parameter. The mean and variance of survival time T for the gamma distribution are

$$\mathrm{E}[T; T \sim \Gamma(\lambda, \tilde{k})] = \frac{\tilde{k}}{\lambda}, \tag{4.102}$$

$$V[T; T \sim \Gamma(\lambda, \tilde{k})] = \frac{\tilde{k}}{\lambda^2}. \tag{4.103}$$

When the gamma distribution is used to address skewed disturbances, the hazard rate model with an arbitrarily assigned error term can be written as

$$\mathrm{E}\left[h\left(t, \boldsymbol{x}, \tilde{k}, \lambda\right)\right] = \frac{h_0(t)\exp(\boldsymbol{x}'\boldsymbol{\beta})\tilde{k}}{\lambda} = h_0(t)\exp\left[\boldsymbol{x}'\boldsymbol{\beta} + \log\left(\frac{\tilde{k}}{\lambda}\right)\right]. \tag{4.104}$$

Given the flexibility of the gamma distribution, the above specification has been applied in modeling bivariate survival times and individual frailty (Vaupel, Manton, and Stallard, 1979; Wild, 1983; Yashin and Iachine, 1995). For convenience of analysis, researchers often impose the conditions that $\lambda = \tilde{k}$ and $\sigma^2 = 1/\tilde{k} = 1/\lambda$. Without these conditions, the estimation of a gamma distributed regression model becomes tedious and cumbersome due to the addition of more model parameters. In Chapter 9, I will describe the use of the gamma model as a statistical means to account for selection bias in survival data with dependence.

With the specification of one more parameter, the gamma distribution is extended to the *generalized gamma model*. This extended gamma distribution is sometimes used to test the efficiency of the exponential, the Weibull, and lognormal regression models because this distribution contains those parametric functions as special cases. Given three parameters, the hazard function can take a variety of shapes, thus possessing the capability to model some complicated lifetime events. When a parametric regression model involves a large number of covariates, however, the use of the generalized gamma function can cause overparameterization and overfitting of survival data, thereby making the model statistically inefficient.

4.6 Parametric regression models with interval censoring

The above descriptions of parametric regression models are based on the assumption that all censored observations are right censored. In reality, the exact timing for the occurrence of a particular event is often not observed, and instead the information available to the researcher is only a time interval (t_{i-1}, t_i) during which an event occurs. In clinical trials and most observational surveys of a panel design, all event times are recorded in terms of specific time intervals, rather than of exact time points, thus suggesting interval censoring. When a time interval is small, T_i can be approximated by taking the midpoint of a particular interval, as mentioned in Chapter 1. When the interval is large, however, regular inference of survival processes may overlook some important information, in turn leading to some bias in parameter estimates.

This section describes valid inferences to tackle the issue of interval censoring in the regression analysis. An empirical illustration is then provided to demonstrate how to perform such analysis using SAS. The inference for left censoring bears some resemblance to that of interval censoring, but it is not particularly displayed in this text.

4.6.1 Inference of parametric regression models with interval censoring

Inference of parametric regression models with interval censoring is generally based on the assumption that the time span of a censored interval is independent of the underlying exact failure time. Given this assumption, the estimating approach for interval censoring is simply the combination of the standard procedures on right-censored survival data and the basic likelihood function for interval censoring, provided in Chapter 1.

For a random sample of n individuals with independent interval censoring, the event time for the ith individual is denoted by $T_i \in \left(\overline{l}_i, \overline{r}_i\right]$, where $i = 1, 2, \ldots n$, and $\overline{l}$ and $\overline{r}$ indicate left and right endpoints of a particular time interval in which the event occurs. Suppose $\overline{l}_i < \overline{r}_i$ for all $i = 1, \ldots, n$ ($\overline{l}_i$ may be 0 and $\overline{r}_i$ may be ∞), and $\overline{L}_i < \overline{R}_i$ are the observed left and right endpoints for the interval censored T_i. It follows that the likelihood of experiencing a particular event for the ith individual is

$$L_i(\boldsymbol{\theta}) = F(\bar{R}_i; \boldsymbol{\theta}) - F(\bar{L}_i; \boldsymbol{\theta}), \tag{4.105}$$

where $F(t;\, \boldsymbol{\theta})$ is the cumulative distribution function for the event time given $\boldsymbol{\theta}$.

Assuming a continuous parametric function for the distribution of F, the likelihood function with respect to $\boldsymbol{\theta}$ for a sample of n individuals can be conveniently written as an AFT function:

$$\begin{aligned} L(\boldsymbol{\theta}) &= \prod_{i=1}^{n} [F(\tilde{u}_i) - F(\tilde{v}_i)] \\ &= \prod_{i=1}^{n} [S(\tilde{v}_i) - S(\tilde{u}_i)], \end{aligned} \tag{4.106}$$

where $S(t;\, \boldsymbol{\theta})$ is the parametric survival function and $\tilde{u}_i$ and $\tilde{v}_i$ are defined by

$$\tilde{u}_i = \frac{\log \bar{R}_i - \mu^* - \boldsymbol{x}_i'\boldsymbol{\beta}}{\tilde{\sigma}},$$

$$\tilde{v}_i = \frac{\log \bar{L}_i - \mu^* - \boldsymbol{x}_i'\boldsymbol{\beta}}{\tilde{\sigma}}.$$

Equation (4.106) shows that each observation contributes two pieces of information to the likelihood, $S(\bar{L}_i, \boldsymbol{\theta}_i)$ and $S(\bar{R}_i, \boldsymbol{\theta}_i)$, which follow the same distributional function. As defined, when both $\bar{L}_i$ and $\bar{R}_i$ are observed and $\bar{L}_i < \bar{R}_i$, the observation is interval censored; when both $\bar{L}_i$ and $\bar{R}_i$ are observed but $\bar{L}_i = \bar{R}_i$, $L_i(\boldsymbol{\theta})$ is the density function of T_i. Likewise, if $\bar{L}_i$ is observed but $\bar{R}_i$ is not, the observation is right censored.

Taking log values on both sides of Equation (4.106) yields the log likelihood function of independent interval censored data:

$$\log L(\boldsymbol{\theta}) = \sum_{i=1}^{n} \log[S(\tilde{v}_j) - S(\tilde{u}_j)]. \tag{4.107}$$

With interval censoring assumed to be random, the total score statistic is

$$\frac{\partial}{\partial \boldsymbol{\theta}} \log L(\boldsymbol{\theta}) = \sum_{i=1}^{n} \frac{\partial [S(\bar{L}_i, \boldsymbol{\theta}) - S(\bar{R}_i, \boldsymbol{\theta})] / \partial \boldsymbol{\theta}}{S(\bar{L}_i, \boldsymbol{\theta}) - S(\bar{R}_i, \boldsymbol{\theta})}. \tag{4.108}$$

As a standard procedure, the maximum likelihood estimates of $\boldsymbol{\theta}$ can be obtained by the solution of $\partial \log L(\boldsymbol{\theta}) / \partial \boldsymbol{\theta} = \boldsymbol{0}$. The information matrix for interval-censored survival data can be obtained by applying the term $-\partial^2 \log L(\boldsymbol{\theta}) / \partial \boldsymbol{\theta} \partial \boldsymbol{\theta}'$, with its inverse yielding the approximates of the variances and covariances for parameter estimates with interval censoring. In the SAS system, interval censoring can be handled by applying the PROC LIFEREG procedure, as shown in the following illustration.

4.6.2 Illustration: A parametric survival model with independent interval censoring

In Subsection 4.3.4, I provided an empirical example of the Weibull regression model on marital status and the probability of survival among older Americans, using 'month' as the time scale. Strictly speaking, this specification of event time can cover up some information of variability in survival times because the measure 'month' in fact records the midpoint of a time interval. For example, a duration of 10.5 months actually represents all event times ranging from 10.00 months to 10.99 months.

In the present illustration, I revise SAS Program 4.4 by fitting a Weibull regression model that particularly specifies interval censored survival times. My intention is to examine whether the previous model of right censoring is subject to significant bias on the Weibull parameter estimates. Other parts of this revised Weibull regression model, including specification of covariates, remain the same as described in Section 4.3.

Specifically, I first create two time variables, time1 and time2, specifying the lower and upper endpoints of a given censoring interval, respectively. As mentioned earlier, if both values of time1 and time2 for an individual are observed and the lower value (time1) is less than the upper value (time2), the observation is interval censored. If the upper value is missing, the lower endpoint serves as the right-censored value. If the lower value is greater than the upper value or both values are missing, the observation is not used in the estimation. (Left-censored observations, not covered by this illustration, can be indicated by the condition that if the lower value is missing, the upper value is used as the left-censored value.) The following SAS program constructs the two time variables. Using these two endpoints, the Weibull regression model is respecified with interval censored data.

SAS Program 4.7:

```
......
if death = 0 then time1 = duration + 1;
  else time1 = duration;

if death = 0 then time2 = .;
  else time2 = duration + 1;
......

proc lifereg data=new outest=Weibull_outest;
  class married;
  model (time1, time2) = married age_mean educ_mean / dist = Weibull;
  output out = new1;
run;
......
```

Other parts of the SAS code, designated by dots, are exactly the same as those in SAS Program 4.4.

In SAS Program 4.7, the variables time1 and time2 are created (the variable 'duration' is now an integer, rather than a midpoint), with time1 specified as the lower and time2 as the upper endpoints of a censoring interval. Nonmissing values of both time1 and time2 indicate the occurrence of a death within the interval (time1, time2); therefore, SAS treats the observation as interval censored. If time1 is not missing but time2 is missing, the observation is viewed as right censored, with time1 moving forward by one unit (duration + 1) as the right-censored survival time. Compared to SAS Program 4.4, the only difference in the PROC LIFEREG procedure is the specification of two endpoints in the MODEL statement. Specifically, replacing the 'MODEL DURATION*CENSOR(1) =' statement in SAS Program 4.4, two endpoint variables are now specified in a parenthesis after the word MODEL, with the first being the lower value and the second being the upper value.

SAS Program 4.7 yields the following SAS output.

SAS Program Output 4.4:

```
                          The LIFEREG Procedure

                            Model Information

            Data Set                                    WORK.NEW
            Dependent Variable                        Log(time1)
            Dependent Variable                        Log(time2)
            Number of Observations                          2000
            Noncensored Values                                 0
            Right Censored Values                           1668
            Left Censored Values                               0
            Interval Censored Values                         332
            Number of Parameters                               5
            Name of Distribution                         Weibull
            Log Likelihood                          -2139.390037


                              Fit Statistics

           -2 Log Likelihood                      4278.780
           AIC (smaller is better)                4288.780
           AICC (smaller is better)               4288.810
           BIC (smaller is better)                4316.785


              Analysis of Maximum Likelihood Parameter Estimates

                               Standard   95% Confidence     Chi-
Parameter            DF Estimate   Error      Limits        Square Pr > ChiSq

Intercept             1   5.3371  0.1069   5.1276  5.5466 2493.00   <.0001
married   Married     1  -0.0547  0.0943  -0.2397  0.1302    0.34   0.5618
married   Not married 0   0.0000   .        .       .        .       .
age_mean              1  -0.0587  0.0076  -0.0736 -0.0439   60.29   <.0001
educ_mean             1   0.0163  0.0121  -0.0074  0.0399    1.82   0.1771
Scale                 1   0.7923  0.0424   0.7134  0.8800
Weibull Shape         1   1.2621  0.0676   1.1364  1.4017

                      PH_beta = -1*AFT_beta/Scale

                           HR = exp(PH_beta)

            Parameter         AFT_beta      PH_beta       HR

            Intercept          5.33707     -6.73602    0.001
            married           -0.05473      0.06908    1.072
            married            0.00000      0.00000    1.000
            age_mean          -0.05874      0.07414    1.077
            educ_mean          0.01628     -0.02054    0.980
            Scale              0.79232       .          .
            Weibull Shape      1.26212       .          .
```

The log-likelihood value for the Weibull regression model with interval censoring is −2139.39, compared to −1132.638 estimated for the Weibull model of right censoring (see SAS Program Output 4.2). Accordingly, the −2 log-likelihood statistic, following a chi-square distribution, is 4278.78 for the interval-censored survival model, compared to 2265.275 in the right-censored model. The increase in the value of this statistic is not surprising because, in estimating the interval-censored parameters, each observation contributes two pieces of information to the total likelihood. Similar to the previous model, values of all four model fit statistics are very close, thereby generating the same conclusion on model fitness.

With respect to the maximum likelihood parameter estimates, the PROC LIFEREG procedure on the interval-censored data yields almost identical results to those obtained from the Weibull regression model with right censoring. The intercept, 5.3371 ($SE = 0.1069$), differs very slightly from 5.3314 ($SE = 0.1071$) estimated for the previous Weibull model. Additionally, the two Weibull regression models, right or interval censored, generate an equal regression coefficient of marital status ($\beta_1 = -0.0547$), with only a tiny difference in the standard error (0.0943 versus 0.0946). The regression coefficients of age and educational attainment are almost the same, with identical values of standard errors. Given such similarities, the corresponding proportional hazard coefficients and the hazard ratios are very close to those reported in SAS Program Output 4.2. The Weibull scale and shape parameters are also similar between the two Weibull regression models.

The above comparison provides very strong evidence that when a time interval for event occurrences is not uncommonly wide, the use of the midpoint as the substitute for an exact event time is appropriate and statistically efficient.

4.7 Summary

This chapter describes general inferences of parametric regression modeling and a number of specific parametric regression models that are widely used in survival analysis. Parametric regression models can be approached by two perspectives, the proportional hazard rate model and the accelerated failure time regression model. Each of those two approaches has its own strengths and limitations. In such scientific disciplines as medicine, biology, epidemiology, and sociology, researchers are inclined to analyze variability in the hazard rate as a function of model covariates because the hazard model describes the relative risk of an event occurrence in a direct, straightforward fashion. Therefore, the proportional hazard regression model becomes the most applied approach in those fields. On the other hand, statisticians prefer to apply the accelerated failure time perspective for specifying and estimating various parametric survival models, given its functional flexibility and statistical applicability for a large number of families of parametric distributions. Fortunately, for the parametric regression models that can be expressed in terms of both perspectives, one set of parameter estimates can be readily converted to the other set through mathematical transformations, including conversion of standard errors and confidence intervals.

Of various parametric regression models, the exponential, the Weibull, and the log-logistic functions are perhaps the most widely applied regression models in survival analysis. The exponential regression model is used to describe survival processes characterized by a constant baseline hazard rate. The Weibull regression model, on the other hand, portrays a hazard rate function that monotonically increases or decreases over time. Because many survival processes follow a monotone pattern, the flexible Weibull regression perspective boasts widespread applications in a variety of disciplines, ranging from medicine to sociology, epidemiology, engineering, and so forth. Unlike the above two parametric perspectives, the log-logistic regression model delineates nonmonotonic risk processes, with the hazard rate increasing initially and then consistently decreasing in the late stage of a life course.

If a particular probability distribution of survival data can be identified and validated, statistical inference based on a parametric regression perspective is considered more efficient and more precise than those derived from survival models in the absence of an explicit distributional function (Collett, 2003), particularly for survival data with a small sample size (Holt and Prentice, 1974). Given such statistical strengths, parametric regression modeling is popular in some disciplines where a true distributional function of survival times can be easily identified (e.g., industrial reliability analysis, mathematical biological studies). In other disciplines, however, ascertaining a parametric distribution is not a simple undertaking. The major concern is the selection effect inherent in survival processes. Because frailer individuals tend to die sooner, the estimation of individual mortality risks, aging progression, and mortality differentials among various population subgroups can be biased by some unobservable characteristics. Consequently, a particular observed parametric pattern of survival can be just an artifact shaped by successive exits of frailer subjects. Such uncertainty has gradually made parametric regression modeling a much less applied technique than the semi-parametric regression model.

5

The Cox proportional hazard regression model and advances

As indicated in Chapter 4, a common criticism of using a parametric regression model to analyze survival data is the difficulty in ascertaining the validity of an underlying parametric distribution in survival times. With the selection effect operating throughout the life course, a parametric distribution may not necessarily reflect the true individual trajectories of survival processes; therefore, parameter estimates, derived from a regression model associated with a misspecified distribution of lifetimes, can be biased. Additionally, many researchers are more interested in the effects of covariates on the risk of an event occurrence than in the shape of a specific failure time distribution. While the proportional hazard model is highly welcomed in many applied disciplines, the application of parametric regression models is sometimes inconvenient because only the exponential and the Weibull functions can be formulated as a proportional hazard model. Given these concerns, it is highly useful to create a regression model that yields valid estimates of covariate effects on the hazard function while avoiding the specification of an underlying distributional function. Technically, developing such a regression model is not unrealistic. If all individuals are subject to a common baseline distribution of survival and differences in the hazard rate can be primarily reflected through the multiplicative effect of covariates, the underlying distribution of survival times becomes a constant and thus can potentially cancel out from a specific likelihood function. In the year 1972, David Cox masterfully developed a proportional hazard model, which derives robust, consistent, and efficient estimates of covariate effects using the proportional hazards assumption while leaving the baseline hazard rate unspecified (Cox, 1972). Since then, the *Cox proportional hazard model*, often simply referred to as the *Cox model*, has become the most widely applied regression perspective in survival analysis. Technically, the Cox model uses the maximum likelihood algorithm for a partial likelihood function, with the estimating approach referred to as a *partial likelihood*.

In this chapter, I first describe basic specifications of the Cox model and the detailed procedures of a partial likelihood. Next, the statistical techniques handling tied observations

Survival Analysis: Models and Applications, First Edition. Xian Liu.

in estimating the Cox model are delineated, followed by a section portraying how to estimate a survival function from the hazard rate estimates of the Cox model without specifying an underlying hazard function. Some other advances of the proportional hazard model are also introduced in the chapter, such as the hazard model with time-dependent covariates, the stratified proportional hazard model, and the management of left truncated survival data. Additionally, in Section 5.7, I describe several coding schemes for specifying qualitative factors and the statistical inference of local tests in the Cox model. In each section except 5.1, I illustrate an empirical example with one or two SAS programs. Lastly, I summarize the chapter with comments on the Cox model and its refinements.

5.1 The Cox semi-parametric hazard model

In this section, I describe the basic specifications of the Cox proportional hazard model, the partial likelihood, and the estimating procedures in the presence of right censoring.

5.1.1 Basic specifications of the Cox proportional hazard model

I start the description of the Cox model with the general specification of the proportional hazard rate model given in Subsection 4.1.1. Each observation under investigation is assumed to be subject to an instantaneous hazard rate, $h(t)$, of experiencing a particular event, where $t = 0, 1, \ldots, \infty$. Analogous to the parametric proportional hazard model, the effect of covariates in the Cox model is specified by a multiplicative term $\exp(\boldsymbol{x}'\boldsymbol{\beta})$, given the nonnegative nature of the hazard function. The basic equation of the Cox model is exactly the same as Equation (4.1), given by

$$h(t|\boldsymbol{x}) = h_0(t)\exp(\boldsymbol{x}'\boldsymbol{\beta}). \tag{5.1}$$

Though identical in form, the detailed specification of Equation (5.1) differs from Equation (4.1). In the Cox model, the term $h_0(t)$ represents an arbitrary and unspecified baseline hazard function for continuous time T, whereas in the parametric perspective it represents a specific distributional function. The coefficient vector $\boldsymbol{\beta}$ provides a set of covariate effects on the hazard rate, with the same length as $\boldsymbol{x}$. The effects of $\boldsymbol{x}$ on the hazard rate are assumed to be multiplicative, so that the predicted value of $h(t)$ given $\boldsymbol{x}$, denoted by $\hat{h}(t|\boldsymbol{x})$, varies in the range $(0, \infty)$. Exponentiation of a specific regression coefficient generates the hazard ratio (HR) of covariate x_m.

Suppose covariate x_m is a dichotomous variable with $x_{m1} = 1$ and $x_{m0} = 0$. Let other covariates all take the value 0; the hazard ratio of covariate x_m is

$$\begin{aligned} HR_m &= \frac{h_0(t)\exp\left(x_{m1}\hat{\beta}_m\right)}{h_0(t)\exp\left(x_{m0}\hat{\beta}_m\right)} \\ &= \exp\left[\left(x_{m1} - x_{m0}\right)\hat{\beta}_m\right] \\ &= \exp\left(\hat{\beta}_m\right), \end{aligned} \tag{5.2}$$

where $\hat{\beta}_m$ is the estimate of the regression coefficient for covariate x_m. This definition of relative risk, independent of $h_0(t)$, holds when other covariates are not zero because additional terms appearing in both the numerator and the denominator would cancel out in Equation (5.2). This specification can be readily extended to the case of a continuous covariate.

Independent of the unspecified baseline hazard function, the hazard ratio provides an uncomplicated indicator to measure the effect of a given covariate on the hazard rate. If a specific covariate is a dichotomous variable, the hazard ratio displays an intuitive meaning of the relative risk, as also discussed in Chapter 4. For example, if the regression coefficient of cancer (1 = yes, 0 = no) on mortality is 1.60, the hazard ratio is exp(1.60) = 4.95, suggesting that those with cancer are about 5 times as likely to die as those without cancer, other covariates being equal. For a continuous covariate, the hazard ratio displays the extent to which the risk increases ($HR > 1$) or decreases ($HR < 1$) with a 1-unit increase in the value of that covariate.

Broadly, the hazard ratio can also be calculated to reflect the proportional change in the hazard rate with a $\dot{w}$-unit increase in x_m, given by

$$\begin{aligned} HR_{\dot{w}} &= \frac{\exp\left[\left(x_{m0}+\dot{w}\right)\hat{\beta}_m\right]}{\exp\left(x_{m0}\hat{\beta}_m\right)} \\ &= \exp\left[\left(x_{m0}+\dot{w}-x_{m0}\right)\hat{\beta}_m\right] \\ &= \exp\left(\dot{w}\hat{\beta}_m\right) \\ &= \exp\left(\hat{\beta}_m\right)^{\dot{w}}. \end{aligned} \tag{5.3}$$

In the above equation, the measure $\exp\left(\dot{w}\hat{\beta}_m\right)$ is referred to as the $\dot{w}$-unit hazard ratio, reflecting the multiplicative change in the hazard rate with a $\dot{w}$-unit increase in covariate x_m. This multiunit hazard ratio is useful for displaying the effect of a continuous or an interval covariate with a small metric unit. For example, a 1-unit hazard ratio of age may not be meaningful enough to reflect the true influence because age has a very small unit given a range of (0, ω). Under such circumstances, the measure $\exp\left(10\times\hat{\beta}_{\text{age}}\right)$ is a more appropriate choice for displaying the impact an individual's age has on the relative risk to the occurrence of a particular event.

In empirical studies, some researchers prefer to use the equation $\{100 \times [\exp(b_m) - 1]\}$, which gives rise to the percentage change in the hazard rate with a 1-unit change in covariate x_m. Consider the cancer example: if the hazard ratio is 5 for cancer patients, the value of $[100 \times (5 - 1)]$ is 400, in turn indicating a 400 % increase in the mortality rate for those diagnosed with cancer as compared to those not diagnosed.

In the Cox model, all individuals are assumed to follow an unspecified nuisance function $h_0(t)$, and therefore population heterogeneity is primarily reflected in proportional scale changes as a function of $\exp(\boldsymbol{x}'\boldsymbol{\beta})$. I want to emphasize again, however, that the concept of *proportionality* here addresses a statistical perception, and the specification of an interaction term or the addition of an arbitrarily assigned random effect can easily spoil the proportionality hypothesis.

Given the specification of the hazard function, the survival probability, given $\boldsymbol{x}$, can be developed in the same fashion as Equation (4.5):

$$S(t;\boldsymbol{x}) = [S_0(t)]^{\exp(\boldsymbol{x}'\boldsymbol{\beta})}, \tag{5.4}$$

where $S_0(t)$ is the baseline survival function, defined as

$$S_0(t) = \exp\left[-\int_0^t h_0(u)\,du\right]$$
$$= \exp[-H_0(t)].$$

In the Cox model, the baseline survival function is unspecified because $h_0(t)$ is an unspecified nuisance function. Practically, the baseline survival function can be understood as the survival function when all covariates are scaled 0, as can be easily deduced from Equation (5.4). Therefore, the substantive meaning of $S_0(t)$ is related to how covariates are created. If covariates are rescaled to be centered at sample means, for example, the baseline survival function indicates a mean survival function for the population that an underlying random sample represents, or the survival probability for an 'average' individual in that population.

Equation (5.4) also shows that the survival function at t, given covariate vector $\boldsymbol{x}$, is simply the baseline survival function $S_0(t)$ raised to the power of the multiplicative effects of covariates on the hazard function. Therefore, with an estimate of the underlying survival function $S_0(t)$, the survival probability for each individual can be estimated given the values of covariates and the estimated regression coefficients $\hat{\boldsymbol{\beta}}$. While not explicitly specified in Equation (5.4), the $S_0(t)$ estimate can be obtained from some other lifetime indicators, thus generating estimates of the complete survival function. The implications of Equation (5.4) will be discussed further in Section 5.3.

Given Equations (5.1) and (5.4), the density function of T given $\boldsymbol{x}$ is

$$f(t;\boldsymbol{x}) = h_0(t)\exp(\boldsymbol{x}'\boldsymbol{\beta})\exp\left[-\exp(\boldsymbol{x}'\boldsymbol{\beta})\int_0^t h_0(u)\,du\right]. \tag{5.5}$$

Equation (5.5) indicates that, in the Cox model, the density function is not explicitly specified either, because $h_0(t)$ is unspecified.

The Cox model can be conveniently expressed in terms of a log-linear model, with covariates assumed to be linearly associated with the log $h(t)$ function. Taking log values on both sides of Equation (5.1) yields

$$\log[h(t|\boldsymbol{x})] = \log[h_0(t)] + \boldsymbol{x}'\boldsymbol{\beta}$$
$$= i^* + \boldsymbol{x}'\boldsymbol{\beta}, \tag{5.6}$$

where i^* is the log of the baseline hazard function in the proportional hazard model. While explicitly specified as the intercept factor in the parametric hazard regression model, this log transformed baseline hazard function is unspecified in the Cox model because $h_0(t)$ is unspecified. Hence, the Cox model is a log-linear regression model without specifying an intercept. As the above specifications differ from both the nonparametric and the parametric perspectives, the Cox model is also called the *semi-parametric regression model*.

As summarized, the Cox model is a simplified perspective of parametric regression modeling described in Chapter 4. The development of the partial likelihood function, presented below, facilitates the validity and reliability of the simplification.

5.1.2 Partial likelihood

The estimation of the original Cox proportional hazard model starts with ordering a random sample of n individuals according to the rank of survival times, assuming no observation ties, given by

$$t_1 < t_2 < t_3 < t_4 \cdots < t_n.$$

Rather than specifying a full likelihood function for Equation (5.1), Cox (1972) considers the conditional probability that an individual experiences a particular event at time t_i ($i = 1, 2, \ldots, n$) given that he or she is one of $\mathcal{r}$ individuals at risk to the event at t_i (those with $T \geq t_i$). Let $\mathcal{R}(t_i)$ be the risk set, consisting of all individuals not experiencing the event and uncensored just prior to t_i. In a discrete interval (t_i, $t_i + \Delta$), the conditional probability that individual i experiences the event given the risk set $\mathcal{R}(t_i)$ can be written by

$$\frac{\mathrm{P}[\text{individual } i \text{ with covariates } \boldsymbol{x}_i \text{ experiences event in time interval} (t_i, t_i + \Delta)]}{\sum_{l \in \mathcal{R}(t_i)} \mathrm{P}[\text{invidual } l \text{ experiences event in } (t_i, t_i + \Delta)]}. \tag{5.7}$$

Because the baseline hazard has an arbitrary form in the Cox model, intervals between successive survival times do not provide information on the multiplicative effects of covariates on the hazard function. Let t be a continuous function. Then the conditional probability transforms to a continuous hazard function, as specified in Chapter 1. Hence, given $\Delta \to 0$, Equation (5.7) becomes

$$\frac{\text{hazard rate at } t_i \text{ for individual } i \text{ with covariates } \boldsymbol{x}_i}{\sum_{l \in \mathcal{R}(t_i)} \text{hazard rate at } t_i \text{ for individual } l}. \tag{5.8}$$

As both the numerator and the denominator are represented by the hazard function given $\Delta \to 0$, Equation (5.8) maintains the characterization of the conditional probability that an individual experiences an event at time t_i given $\mathcal{r}$ individuals who are exposed to the risk at t_i. This specification agrees with the Nelson–Aalen estimator described in Chapter 2.

Equation (5.8) can be written in the form of a regression model with a parameter vector $\boldsymbol{\beta}$, written by

$$\begin{aligned} \frac{h(t_i; \boldsymbol{x}_i)}{\sum_{l \in \mathcal{R}(t_i)} h(t_i; \boldsymbol{x}_l)} &= \frac{h_0(t_i)\exp(\boldsymbol{x}_i'\boldsymbol{\beta})}{\sum_{l \in \mathcal{R}(t_i)} h_0(t_i)\exp(\boldsymbol{x}_l'\boldsymbol{\beta})} \\ &= \frac{\exp(\boldsymbol{x}_i'\boldsymbol{\beta})}{\sum_{l \in \mathcal{R}(t_i)} \exp(\boldsymbol{x}_l'\boldsymbol{\beta})}. \end{aligned} \tag{5.9}$$

In the above formulation, the baseline hazard function appears in both the numerator and the denominator of the equation, so that it can cancel out in the final equality. Essentially, the second equation in (5.9) still denotes the conditional probability that an individual experiences a particular event at time t_i given all the individuals exposed to that risk at t_i. With the common terms eliminated, it provides an incomplete hazard function without specifying the distribution of h_0.

The joint likelihood for $\boldsymbol{\beta}$, the only parameters to be estimated in the Cox model, is simply specified as the product of Equation (5.9) over all t_i values, given by

$$L_p(\boldsymbol{\beta}) = \prod_{i=1}^{n} \left[\frac{\exp(\boldsymbol{x}_i'\boldsymbol{\beta})}{\sum_{l \in \mathcal{R}(t_i)} \exp(\boldsymbol{x}_l'\boldsymbol{\beta})} \right]^{\delta_i}, \tag{5.10}$$

where $L_p(\cdot)$ represents an incomplete likelihood function and δ_i is the censoring indicator such that $\delta_i = 1$ if t_i is an event time and $\delta_i = 0$ if t_i is a censored time. As defined, the partial likelihood function $L_p(\boldsymbol{\beta})$ is the probability of a set of regression coefficient values given n observed lifetime outcomes, actual or censored survival times. When $\delta_i = 1$, $L_{pi}(\boldsymbol{\beta})$ is the conditional probability of an event occurrence given the risk set $\mathcal{R}(t_i)$. As no information about h_0 contributes to it, the above incomplete likelihood function is generally referred to as the *partial likelihood function* in survival analysis.

As $L_{pi}(\boldsymbol{\beta})$ is simply 1 when $\delta_i = 0$, the product of the conditional probabilities for all right-censored observations are also 1, thus suggesting that the conditional probabilities over all right-censored cases do not make any contribution to the partial likelihood. Consequently, these censored cases can be unaccounted for in the partial likelihood equation without influencing the total partial likelihood. Therefore, it is statistically tenable to simplify Equation (5.10) by only multiplying the conditional probabilities over all events:

$$L_p(\boldsymbol{\beta}) = \prod_{i=1}^{d} \frac{\exp(\boldsymbol{x}_i'\boldsymbol{\beta})}{\sum_{l \in \mathcal{R}(t_i)} \exp(\boldsymbol{x}_l'\boldsymbol{\beta})}, \tag{5.11}$$

where d is the total number of events, ordered by rank. Equation (5.11) reflects the fact that each actual event, or failure, contributes a factor to the above simplified likelihood function while the conditional probabilities of censored observations do not play a role in partial likelihood. This equation is the standard partial likelihood function originally created by Cox. Notice that this simplification does not mean that all censored observations are excluded because, at each t_i, the risk set $\mathcal{R}(t_i)$ includes all observations censored at times later than t_i.

Taking log values on both sides of Equation (5.11), a log partial likelihood function is

$$\log L_p(\boldsymbol{\beta}) = \sum_{i=1}^{d} \left\{ \boldsymbol{x}_i'\boldsymbol{\beta} - \sum_{i=1}^{d} \log \left[\sum_{l \in \mathcal{R}(t_i)} \exp(\boldsymbol{x}_l'\boldsymbol{\beta}) \right] \right\}. \tag{5.12}$$

Like maximization of a complete likelihood function in parametric regression modeling, the above log partial likelihood function can be mathematically maximized with respect to the unknown parameter vector $\boldsymbol{\beta}$ that contains the regression coefficients of covariates without an intercept factor. As the partial likelihood depends on the ordering of actual survival times, hazard rates are unrelated to survival times and intervals between events. This characteristic indicates that the baseline hazard distribution is inherent in the ordering of survival times without a known shape. As the partial likelihoods are based on the number of events, rather than on the total number of individuals in a random sample, the application of the Cox model requires a considerably larger sample for estimating model parameters than does parametric regression modeling, especially in analyzing events that do not frequently occur.

5.1.3 Procedures of maximization and hypothesis testing on partial likelihood

Maximization of the partial likelihood function is performed with respect to the parameter vector $\boldsymbol{\beta}$ by using the standard procedures described in Chapter 4. As generally applied, the process starts with the construction of a score statistic vector, denoted by $\tilde{\boldsymbol{U}}_i(\boldsymbol{\beta})$ and mathematically defined as the first partial derivatives of the log partial likelihood function with respect to $\boldsymbol{\beta}$. The total score statistic for the mth covariate ($m = 1, \ldots, M$) is

$$\tilde{U}(\beta_m) = \frac{\partial}{\partial \beta_m} \log L_p(\boldsymbol{\beta}) = \sum_{i=1}^{d} \left[x_{im} - \frac{\sum_{l \in \mathcal{R}(t_i)} x_{lm} \exp(\boldsymbol{x}_l' \boldsymbol{\beta})}{\sum_{l \in \mathcal{R}(t_i)} \exp(\boldsymbol{x}_l' \boldsymbol{\beta})} \right]$$

$$= \sum_{i=1}^{d} \{ x_{im} - \mathrm{E}[x_m | \mathcal{R}(t_i)] \}, \tag{5.13}$$

where

$$\mathrm{E}[x_m | \mathcal{R}(t_i)] = \frac{\sum_{l \in \mathcal{R}(t_i)} x_{lm} \exp(\boldsymbol{x}_l' \boldsymbol{\beta})}{\sum_{l \in \mathcal{R}(t_i)} \exp(\boldsymbol{x}_l' \boldsymbol{\beta})}.$$

It is worth noting that the score statistic can be conveniently simplified as a permutation test based on residuals computed for the regression on covariates, rather than on the regression coefficients themselves, as also indicated in Chapter 4. In modern survival analysis, the score statistic plays an extremely important role in developing advanced techniques on the hazard model residuals and the asymptotic variance estimators for analyzing clustered survival data, as will be described extensively in some of the later chapters.

Following the standard maximum likelihood estimating procedures, the coefficient vector $\boldsymbol{\beta}$ in the partial likelihood function can be estimated by solving the equation

$$\tilde{\boldsymbol{U}}(\boldsymbol{\beta}) = \frac{\partial}{\partial} \log L_p(\boldsymbol{\beta}) = \boldsymbol{0}, \tag{5.14}$$

where

$$\tilde{\boldsymbol{U}}(\boldsymbol{\beta}) = (\partial \log L_p / \partial \beta_1, \ldots, \partial \log L_p / \partial \beta_M)'.$$

The above generalization is a typical maximum likelihood estimator (MLE). Hence, statistically the partial likelihood estimator is essentially no different from the standard maximum likelihood perspective, the only difference being that maximization is performed on a partial rather than a complete function.

As indicated in Chapter 4, for a large sample, $\hat{\boldsymbol{\beta}}$ is the unique solution of $\tilde{\boldsymbol{U}}(\boldsymbol{\beta}) = \mathbf{0}$, so that $\hat{\boldsymbol{\beta}}$ is consistent for $\boldsymbol{\beta}$ and distributed as multivariate normal, which, conventionally, can be expressed as

$$\hat{\boldsymbol{\beta}} \sim N\left[\boldsymbol{\beta}, \tilde{V}(\boldsymbol{\beta})^{-1}\right]. \tag{5.15}$$

Operationally, the estimation of $\boldsymbol{\beta}$ is generally performed through an iterative scheme, with $\hat{\boldsymbol{\beta}}^0 = \mathbf{0}$ as the initial step, using the Newton–Raphson method. The series of $\hat{\boldsymbol{\beta}}$ in the iterative scheme is generally denoted by $\hat{\boldsymbol{\beta}}^{\tilde{j}}$ ($\tilde{j} = 1, 2, \ldots$). The iterative scheme terminates when $\hat{\boldsymbol{\beta}}^{\tilde{j}+1}$ is sufficiently close to $\hat{\boldsymbol{\beta}}^{\tilde{j}}$. Consequently, the maximum likelihood estimate of $\boldsymbol{\beta}$ can be operationally defined as $\hat{\boldsymbol{\beta}} = \hat{\boldsymbol{\beta}}^{\tilde{j}+1}$.

Like estimating a parametric regression model, the asymptotic normal distribution of $\hat{\boldsymbol{\beta}}$ facilitates hypothesis testing on $\boldsymbol{\beta}$. In particular, the variance estimator of $\boldsymbol{\beta}$ is based on an $M \times M$ observed information matrix (M is the number of covariates), denoted by $\boldsymbol{I}\left(\hat{\boldsymbol{\beta}}\right)$ and mathematically defined as

$$\boldsymbol{I}\left(\hat{\boldsymbol{\beta}}\right) = -\left(\frac{\partial^2 \log L\left(\hat{\boldsymbol{\beta}}\right)}{\partial \hat{\boldsymbol{\beta}}^2}\right)_{M \times M}, \tag{5.16}$$

with the (m, m')th element specified as

$$\begin{aligned} I_{mm'}(\boldsymbol{\beta}) = {} & \sum_{i=1}^{d} \{\mathrm{E}[x_{im} x_{im'} | \mathcal{R}(t_i)]\} \\ & - \sum_{i=1}^{d} \{\mathrm{E}[x_{im} | \mathcal{R}(t_i)] E[x_{im'} | \mathcal{R}(t_i)]\}, \end{aligned} \tag{5.17}$$

where

$$\mathrm{E}[x_{im} x_{im'} | \mathcal{R}(t_i)] = \frac{\sum_{l \in \mathcal{R}(t_i)} x_{lm} x_{lm'} \exp(\boldsymbol{x}_l' \boldsymbol{\beta})}{\sum_{l \in \mathcal{R}(t_i)} \exp(\boldsymbol{x}_l' \boldsymbol{\beta})}.$$

If Equation (5.16) is correctly assumed, then $\sqrt{n}\left(\hat{\boldsymbol{\beta}} - \boldsymbol{\beta}\right)$ converges to an M-dimensional normal vector with mean 0 and a covariance matrix $\boldsymbol{\Sigma}\left(\hat{\boldsymbol{\beta}}\right)$ that can be consistently estimated by

$$\boldsymbol{\Sigma}\left(\hat{\boldsymbol{\beta}}\right) = \boldsymbol{I}\left(\hat{\boldsymbol{\beta}}\right)^{-1}. \tag{5.18}$$

Therefore, the variance estimator of $\boldsymbol{\beta}$ for the Cox model is simply the inverse of the Fisher observed information matrix.

In form, Equation (5.18) is exactly the same as Equation (4.33), with both estimators following the standard procedures of maximization. The standard errors of $\boldsymbol{\beta}$ can be obtained by taking the square roots of the diagonal elements in $\boldsymbol{\Sigma}(\hat{\boldsymbol{\beta}})$. Similarly, the squared z-score, the ratio of each component in $\hat{\boldsymbol{\beta}}$ over its standard error, follows a chi-square distribution with one degree of freedom under the null hypothesis that $\hat{\boldsymbol{\beta}} = \mathbf{0}$. The information matrix evaluated at this null hypothesis is defined as $\boldsymbol{I}(\mathbf{0})$. The corresponding vector of scores, denoted by $\tilde{\boldsymbol{U}}(\mathbf{0})$, tends to be distributed as multivariate normal with mean 0 and a covariance matrix $\boldsymbol{I}(\mathbf{0})^{-1}$ for large samples. As a result, the score test statistic on $\hat{\boldsymbol{\beta}} = \mathbf{0}$ is

$$\boldsymbol{U}(\mathbf{0})' \boldsymbol{I}(\mathbf{0})^{-1} \boldsymbol{U}(\mathbf{0}), \tag{5.19}$$

which is distributed asymptotically as chi-square with M degrees of freedom under the null hypothesis. If there are no tied survival times, this score test in the Cox model is identical to the logrank test (Klein and Moeschberger, 2003; Lawless, 2003).

Given the same null hypothesis, $\hat{\boldsymbol{\beta}}$ is asymptotically normally distributed with mean 0 and the covariance matrix $\boldsymbol{I}(\hat{\boldsymbol{\beta}})^{-1}$ given the large sample approximation theory and the central-limit theorem. Accordingly, the Wald test statistic is defined by

$$\hat{\boldsymbol{\beta}}' \boldsymbol{I}(\hat{\boldsymbol{\beta}})^{-1} \hat{\boldsymbol{\beta}}, \tag{5.20}$$

which is also distributed asymptotically as chi-square with M degrees of freedom under the null hypothesis. Based on the maximum likelihood estimation procedures, specifications of both the score and the Wald test statistics have a tremendous resemblance to those for parametric hazard models. The Wald test statistic can be used to test a subtest of the estimated regression coefficients in $\hat{\boldsymbol{\beta}}$, which will be described in Section 5.7.

Also analogous to parametric regression modeling, hypothesis testing of $\hat{\boldsymbol{\beta}}$ in the Cox model can be performed by using the partial likelihood ratio test. For example, the partial likelihood ratio with respect to all elements in $\hat{\boldsymbol{\beta}}$ is defined as

$$LR(\boldsymbol{\beta}) = \frac{L_p(\mathbf{0})}{L_p(\hat{\boldsymbol{\beta}})}, \tag{5.21}$$

where $L_p(\mathbf{0})$ is the partial likelihood function for the model without covariates (termed the empty model) and $L_p(\hat{\boldsymbol{\beta}})$ is the partial likelihood function containing all covariates.

The null hypothesis about $\boldsymbol{\beta}$ can be written as H_0: $\hat{\boldsymbol{\beta}} = \mathbf{0}$ for the whole set of coefficients or H_0: $\hat{\beta}_m = 0$ for an individual component in $\hat{\boldsymbol{\beta}}$. To test the null hypothesis for all elements in $\hat{\boldsymbol{\beta}}$, the partial likelihood ratio statistic is

$$\begin{aligned} \Lambda_p &= 2 \log L_p(\boldsymbol{\beta}) - 2 \log L_p(\mathbf{0}) \\ &= -2\left[\log L_p(\mathbf{0}) - \log L_p(\boldsymbol{\beta})\right], \end{aligned} \tag{5.22}$$

where

$$\log L_p(\mathbf{0}) = -\sum_{i=1}^{d} \log(n_i).$$

In survival analysis, Equation (5.22) is generally referred to as the *minus two log partial likelihood ratio statistic*, often used for testing model fitness of the Cox model.

The statistic Λ_p is asymptotically distributed as $\chi^2_{(M)}$ as well. Consequently, the corresponding p-value can be obtained from the distribution which, in turn, provides information for testing the H_0 hypothesis. Specifically, if Λ_p is associated with a p-value smaller than α, the null hypothesis about $\hat{\boldsymbol{\beta}}$ should be rejected; otherwise, the null hypothesis is to be accepted.

The $100(1-\alpha)$ % partial likelihood based confidence interval for $\hat{\boldsymbol{\beta}}$ can be approximated by applying Equation (5.22), defined as

$$\Lambda_p = \left[2\log L_p(\boldsymbol{\beta}) - 2\log L_p(0)\right] \le \chi^2_{(1-\alpha\alpha)} \tag{5.23}$$

The above three main tests on the null hypothesis of the estimated regression coefficients generally yield fairly close statistics and therefore usually lead to the same testing conclusion. In most cases, the Wald and the likelihood ratio tests are more conservative than the score test. The Wald test is frequently used to test the statistical significance of an individual or a subset of coefficients, whereas the log partial likelihood ratio test provides a highly efficient statistic for the model fit of the Cox model. There are some other model fit statistics, such as Akaike's information criterion (AIC) and Schwartz's Bayesian criterion (SBC), used in the Cox model. These modified statistics generally yield fairly close scores, as does the partial likelihood ratio test, so are not particularly described in this text.

The variance of the hazard ratio can be estimated using the delta method. If covariances in $\hat{\boldsymbol{\beta}}$ are weak, the univariate approximation $V[g(X)] \approx [g'(\mu)]^2\sigma^2$ can be applied to transform the variance of the regression coefficient for a given covariate to the variance of its hazard ratio. As the derivative of exp(X) is still exp(X), the variance of the hazard ratio for covariate x_m can be approximated by

$$V(HR_m) \approx \left[\text{dexp}\left(\hat{\beta}_m\right)\right]^2 V\left(\hat{\beta}_m\right) = \left[\exp\left(\hat{\beta}_m\right)\right]^2 V\left(\hat{\beta}_m\right). \tag{5.24}$$

Therefore, the variance of the hazard ratio is simply the square of the hazard ratio multiplied by the variance of $\hat{\beta}_m$. The standard error of the hazard ratio is approximated by the square root of $V(HR_m)$, based on which the confidence interval of the hazard ratio can be easily calculated. Given the nonlinearity after transformation, however, this confidence interval is not symmetric. Accordingly, some statisticians suggest that the confidence interval of the hazard ratio should be computed by exponentiation of the two ending points of the confidence interval for β_m (Klein and Moeschberger, 2003).

As the reader might be aware, the inference and the estimation of the partial likelihood parameters are much like the general maximum likelihood procedure described in Chapter 4. Here, Cox develops an innovative likelihood function that eliminates the baseline functional parameters and derives the maximum likelihood estimates $\hat{\boldsymbol{\beta}}$ that are completely analogous to analytic results from the complete likelihood function (Kalbfleisch and Prentice, 2002). With the baseline hazard function canceling out of the likelihood function, the partial likelihood perspective provides substantial convenience and flexibility to the researcher who is doubtful of the validity of an observed parametric distribution in survival times.

5.2 Estimation of the Cox hazard model with tied survival times

The original Cox model is based on the assumption that there are no tied observations in survival data. This assumption, however, is not realistic in most survival datasets because ties in failure times frequently occur, particularly when a discrete time scale is used and the size of a random sample is large. In many observational surveys, events are reported during intervals (such as weeks, months, or years), making it extremely demanding to obtain data with exact event times. When two or more individuals experience a particular event at the same time, ordering their shared survival time is difficult. As a result, the application of the original Cox model is restricted by the difficulty in finding survival data without tied observations. Some statisticians, including Cox himself, have developed a number of approaches to handle ties in estimating the Cox model (Breslow, 1974; Cox, 1972; Efron, 1977; Kalbfleisch and Prentice, 1973).

This section describes four approximation methods for handling ties, in the order of their respective publication years. Then I compare advantages and disadvantages of these approximation approaches. Lastly, I provide an empirical illustration to demonstrate how to apply these methods when using the Cox model.

5.2.1 The discrete-time logistic regression model

In his original article on the proportional hazard model, Cox (1972) proposes to handle tied survival times by adapting the partial likelihood function to a discrete-time regression model, given by

$$\frac{h(t;\boldsymbol{x})\mathrm{d}t}{1-h(t;\boldsymbol{x})\mathrm{d}t}=\exp(\boldsymbol{x}'\boldsymbol{\beta})\frac{h_0(t)\mathrm{d}t}{1-h_0(t)\mathrm{d}t}. \tag{5.25}$$

If T is a continuous distributional function, Equation (5.25) reduces to Equation (5.1). If event times are considered a step function, however, the above equation becomes a logistic regression function, as can be identified from its formation.

Let $t_1 < t_2 < \cdots < t_{n'}$ be the distinct failure times, d_i be the number of events at t_i, and $\mathcal{D}(t_i)$ be the set of individuals sharing tied event time t_i. Given discrete event times, the contribution to the partial likelihood function becomes

$$\frac{\exp({}^{\backprime}\boldsymbol{s}_i'\boldsymbol{\beta})}{\sum_{l\in\mathcal{R}_{d_i}(t_i)}\exp[{}^{\backprime}\boldsymbol{s}_l'\boldsymbol{\beta}]}, \tag{5.26}$$

where

$${}^{\backprime}\boldsymbol{s}_i=\sum_{j\in\mathcal{R}_i}\boldsymbol{x}_{\mathrm{j}},$$

and the nonitalicized j represents jth person in $\mathcal{D}(t_i)$. Note that when there are tied observations, the notation i no longer can be used to indicate an individual and an event time simultaneously; therefore, in the following text the nonitalic letter j is used to indicate an individual at a tied event time.

The vector $`\boldsymbol{s}_i$ is the sum of the covariate values for individuals who fail at the discrete time t_i, represented by $\mathcal{D}(t_i)$. As the reader familiar with generalized linear regression might recognize, Equation (5.26) displays a typical logistic regression model, somewhat inconsistent with the proportional hazard function proposed by Cox himself. Additionally, in this logistic regression model, $\boldsymbol{\beta}$ includes an intercept factor, whereas the intercept cancels out in the partial likelihood function. Hence, this discrete-time function essentially represents a replacement of the Cox model (Kalbfleisch and Prentice, 1973, 2002).

The likelihood function for the above logistic model is given by

$$L_p^{\text{discrete}}(\boldsymbol{\beta}) = \prod_{i=1}^{n'} \frac{\exp(`\boldsymbol{s}_i'\boldsymbol{\beta})}{\sum_{l \in \mathcal{R}_{d_i}(t_i)} \exp(`\boldsymbol{s}_l'\boldsymbol{\beta})}. \tag{5.27}$$

Accordingly, the partial log-likelihood function is

$$\log L_p^{\text{discrete}}(\boldsymbol{\beta}) = -\sum_{i=1}^{n'} `\boldsymbol{s}_i'\boldsymbol{\beta} - \sum_{i=1}^{n'} \log\left[\sum_{l \in \mathcal{R}_{d_i}(t_i)} \exp(`\boldsymbol{s}_l'\boldsymbol{\beta})\right]. \tag{5.28}$$

Maximization procedures for the above log-likelihood function are the same as the maximum partial likelihood estimator described in Subsection 5.1.3. As commented by Kalbfleisch and Prentice (2002), the discrete-time logistic partial likelihood is difficult computationally if the number of ties is large. Additionally, the parameters specified in this logistic model do not have exactly the same interpretation as those in the Cox model.

5.2.2 Approximate methods handling ties in the proportional hazard model

The complete solution of handling tied survival times is to consider all possible orders of tied observations in likelihoods, as proposed by Kalbfleisch and Prentice (1973, 2002). As it accounts for all ordering arrangements and then takes the average contribution, this approximation method is generally referred to as the *exact partial likelihood* or the *average partial likelihood method*.

Mathematically, the full set of all possible orders for d_i is simply a matter of $[d_i \times (d_i - 1) \times (d_i - 2) \times \ldots]$ commutations, mathematically denoted by $d_i!$. For example, if there are three individuals with tied survival time at t_i, we have $3! = 6$ possible orders; if there are five tied observations, there are $5! = 120$ commutations; and so forth. Here, I write the set of $d_i!$ as $\mathcal{Q}_i$ with elements $(`p_1, `p_2, \ldots, `p_{d_i})$, following the notation of Kalbfleisch and Prentice (1973). The average partial likelihood contribution at t_i is then defined as

$$\frac{1}{d_i!}\exp\left[\left(\sum_{l \in \mathcal{D}_i} \boldsymbol{x}_l\right)'\boldsymbol{\beta}\right]\left\{\sum_{`p \in \mathcal{Q}_i} \prod_{r=1}^{d_i}\left[\sum_{l \in \mathcal{R}(t_i, `p, r)} \exp(\boldsymbol{x}_l'\boldsymbol{\beta})\right]\right\}^{-1}. \tag{5.29}$$

The average partial likelihood function for all survival times is proportional to the product of likelihoods across all t_i values ($i = 1, 2, \ldots, n'$), given by

$$L_p^{\text{exact}}(\boldsymbol{\beta}) \propto \prod_{i=1}^{n'} \left(\exp\left[\left(\sum_{l \in \mathcal{D}_i} \boldsymbol{x}_l \right)' \boldsymbol{\beta} \right] \left\{ \sum_{p \in \mathcal{Q}_i} \prod_{r=1}^{d_i} \left[\sum_{l \in \mathcal{R}(t_i, p, r)} \exp(\boldsymbol{x}_l' \boldsymbol{\beta}) \right] \right\}^{-1} \right). \tag{5.30}$$

Clearly, in the above exact partial likelihood function, the denominator involves all ordering arrangements at each risk set, whereas the numerator adds up the covariates of all individuals who experience the event at t_i.

Essentially, Equation (5.30) takes tremendous similarities with the discrete-time logistic regression method because both approaches use all ties without explicit ordering. The exact method, however, may slightly overestimate $\boldsymbol{\beta}$ because it assumes ties without genuine ordering in tied survival times. If a superficial tie covers up some unobservable ordering, the value of the denominator in Equation (5.30) may be underestimated, thus leading to overestimation of the overall partial likelihood. Additionally, this partial likelihood method is computationally cumbersome and tedious if there are a substantial number of ties at given observed survival times.

Breslow (1974) provides a much simpler method to handle ties. Specifically, this method is a tremendous simplification of Equation (5.26), given by

$$L_p^{\text{Breslow}}(\boldsymbol{\beta}) = \prod_{i=1}^{n'} \left[\frac{\exp\left[\left(\sum_{l \in \mathcal{D}_i} \boldsymbol{x}_l \right)' \boldsymbol{\beta} \right]}{\left[\sum_{l \in \mathcal{R}(t_i)} \exp(\boldsymbol{x}_l' \boldsymbol{\beta}) \right]^{d_i}} \right]. \tag{5.31}$$

In Equation (5.31), the numerator considers the sum of covariates over the d_i individuals who fail at t_i, whereas the denominator is simplified as, compared to the exact approximation, the sum of the partial hazard function in the risk set $\mathcal{R}(t_i)$ raised to the power d_i. Clearly, the Breslow approximation method accounts for the contributions of d_i events simply by multiplying the conditional probabilities over all events at t_i.

The Efron (1977) approximation method advances the Breslow method by proposing the following approximation:

$$L_p^{\text{Efron}}(\boldsymbol{\beta}) = \prod_{i=1}^{n'} \frac{\exp\left[\left(\sum_{l \in \mathcal{D}_i} \boldsymbol{x}_l \right)' \boldsymbol{\beta} \right]}{\prod_{r=0}^{d_i - 1} \left[\sum_{l \in \mathcal{R}(t_i)} \exp(\boldsymbol{x}_l' \boldsymbol{\beta}) - \frac{r-1}{d_i} \sum_{l \in \mathcal{D}_i} \exp(\boldsymbol{x}_l' \boldsymbol{\beta}) \right]}. \tag{5.32}$$

In Equation (5.32), Efron reduces weight of the denominator by introducing ordering into the partial likelihood function. Some statisticians consider the Efron method to be a more accurate approximation than both the exact and the Breslow methods after conducting some simulations (Hertz-Picciotto and Rockhill, 1997). This method is considered to be particularly preferable when sample size is small either from the outset or due to heavy censoring.

Notice that the above three partial likelihood functions have the same numerator, so that their differences reside completely in the way of specifying the denominator of the partial likelihood. In each of those estimators, $\boldsymbol{\beta}$ and the variances can be efficiently and consistently estimated by expanding the maximum partial likelihood estimator. When there are no tied survival times, the three partial likelihood functions converge to Equation (5.11).

Of the above three approximations, the exact or average likelihood method provides a complete partial likelihood function, arguably yielding the least amount of bias in $\hat{\boldsymbol{\beta}}$. Nevertheless, this method is computationally difficult when there are heavy ties in survival data. In the dataset of older Americans used for illustrative purposes in this book, the number of months since the baseline survey is used as the time scale, so that there are very heavy ties at many observed event times. In such circumstances, the application of the exact method is cumbersome and unnecessary. Consider 20 tied observations at a particular month: you need 20! steps to compute the likelihood for just one event time!

By contrast, the Breslow (1974) approximation method provides a much simpler approach and therefore becomes a popular first choice in analyzing tied survival data. Specifically, the Breslow approximation is used as default in many statistical software packages including SAS. This method, however, is considered to have some distinct limitations and weaknesses. Compared to the exact and the Efron approximation methods, the denominator in the Breslow likelihood function is slightly overweighed by failed individuals, so that $\hat{\boldsymbol{\beta}}$ may be biased toward zero. Furthermore, when $\boldsymbol{\beta}$ deviates considerably from zero, the Breslow method is thought to be a poor approximation. While some statisticians consider the Efron method to perform better than the other two approximations (Hertz-Picciotto and Rockhill, 1997), Kalbfleisch and Prentice (2002) contend that both the Breslow and the Efron estimators are subject to asymptotic bias under a grouped continuous Cox model. So far, there is no consensus about which method is the most appropriate approach in analyzing tied survival data.

Below, through an empirical example, I further discuss the similarities and differences in the results generated from these three approximation methods.

5.2.3 Illustration on tied survival data: Smoking cigarettes and the mortality of older Americans

In the present illustration, I conduct a study on the association between smoking cigarettes and the mortality of older Americans, using survival data of older Americans from the baseline survey to the end of 2004. The variable 'smoking cigarettes' is defined as a dichotomous variable with 1 = current or past smoker and 0 = else, given the variable name 'Smoking.' In addition to age and educational attainment, I add gender as a control variable. Because older men and women usually have different mortality rates and smoking behaviors, an individual's gender may confound the association between smoking cigarettes and survival. As conventionally applied, gender is measured dichotomously with 1 = female and 0 = male. The three control variables are rescaled to be centered at sample means, named, respectively, 'Age_mean,' 'Female_mean,' and 'Educ_mean.' The centered variable of gender represents the propensity score of being a female or the proportion of women for a population group. My working null hypothesis is that smokers have the same mortality rate as do nonsmokers after adjusting for these potential confounders. As planned, I want to estimate and compare three sets of regression coefficients of smoking cigarettes on the hazard function, using the exact, the Breslow, and the Efron approximation methods, respectively.

The PROC PHREG procedure is applied to fit the three Cox models on the survival data of older Americans. As mentioned in Section 5.1, the Cox model does not specify an intercept factor, so only the estimates of regression coefficients are obtained. As the Weibull hazard rate model is a proportional hazard function, I also apply the PROC LIFEREG procedure to derive the corresponding Weibull estimates for comparative purposes. Below is the SAS program for estimating the regression coefficients of three Cox models in an 11–12 year period (the code for the Weibull model is not included given a detailed description in Chapter 4).

SAS Program 5.1:

```
......

data new;
 set pclib.chapter5_data;

Status = 0;
if death=1 then Status = 1;

proc SQL;
  create table new as
  select *, age-mean(age) as age_mean,
    female-mean(female) as female_mean,
    educ-mean(educ) as educ_mean
  from new;
quit;

proc phreg data = new;
  model duration*Status(0) = smoking age_mean female_mean educ_mean / ties = EXACT ;
run;

proc phreg data = new;
  model duration*Status(0) = smoking age_mean female_mean educ_mean / ties = EFRON ;
run;

proc phreg data = new;
  model duration*Status(0) = smoking age_mean female_mean educ_mean / ties = BRESLOW ;
run;
```

SAS Program 5.1 specifies three Cox models with each using a specific approximation method to handle survival data with heavy ties. The SAS PROC SQL procedure creates three means-centered covariates as control variables, and then they are saved into the temporary SAS data file for further analysis. The TIES = <method> option specifies which the approximate likelihood function is used to handle tied survival times.

The resulting output file is fairly sizable because the information of all three separate Cox models is reported. Therefore, I select only to display results of the first model, using the exact method, as follows.

SAS Program Output 5.1:

The PHREG Procedure

Model Information

Data Set	WORK.NEW
Dependent Variable	duration
Censoring Variable	status
Censoring Value(s)	0
Ties Handling	EXACT

Number of Observations Read	2000
Number of Observations Used	2000

Summary of the Number of Event and Censored Values

Total	Event	Censored	Percent Censored
2000	950	1050	52.50

Model Fit Statistics

Criterion	Without Covariates	With Covariates
-2 LOG L	11348.893	11015.399
AIC	11348.893	11023.399
SBC	11348.893	11042.825

Testing Global Null Hypothesis: BETA=0

Test	Chi-Square	DF	Pr > ChiSq
Likelihood Ratio	333.4943	4	<.0001
Score	328.0644	4	<.0001
Wald	334.5104	4	<.0001

Analysis of Maximum Likelihood Estimates

Parameter	DF	Parameter Estimate	Standard Error	Chi-Square	Pr > ChiSq	Hazard Ratio
smoking	1	0.42041	0.10136	17.2023	<.0001	1.523
age_mean	1	0.08483	0.00519	266.9936	<.0001	1.089
female_mean	1	-0.42618	0.06670	40.8300	<.0001	0.653
educ_mean	1	-0.02238	0.00875	6.5512	0.0105	0.978

In SAS Program Output 5.1, the information on the dataset, the dependent variable, the censoring status variable, and the censoring value, is reported first. The 'Tied Handling: EXACT' statement indicates the use of the exact method for estimating regression coefficients of the four covariates. Given a long period of observation (11–12 years), 950 out of 2000 individuals are deceased (actual events) and the remaining 1050 older persons are right censored. The Model Fit Statistics section displays three indicators of model fitness, with their values being very close, obviously generating the same conclusion about model fitting. All three tests in the 'Testing Global Null Hypothesis: BETA = 0' section demonstrate that the null hypothesis $\hat{\boldsymbol{\beta}} = \mathbf{0}$ should be rejected. For example, the chi-square of the likelihood ratio test is 333.49 with 4 degrees of freedom, which is very strongly statistically significant ($p < 0.0001$).

In the table of 'Analysis of Maximum Likelihood Estimates,' the regression coefficient of 'Smoking' is 0.4204 ($SE = 0.1014$), statistically significant at $\alpha = 0.05$ ($\chi^2 = 17.2023$; $p < 0.0001$). Exponentiation of this regression coefficient generates the hazard ratio between smokers and nonsmokers, as presented in the last column. The estimate of this hazard ratio is 1.523, suggesting that the mortality rate for current or past smokers is about 52 % higher than among those who never smoke, other covariates being equal. The regression coefficients of the three control variables are all statistically significant. Age is positively associated with the hazard rate, with a hazard ratio of 1.089 ($\beta_2 = 0.0848$; $\chi^2 = 266.99$; $p < 0.0001$), as expected. Likewise, older women's mortality is about 35 % lower than among their male counterparts, given a hazard ratio of 0.65 ($\chi^2 = 40.83$; $p < 0.0001$). Educational attainment is negatively and significantly linked to the mortality of older Americans with a hazard ratio of 0.978 ($\beta_4 = -0.0224$; $\chi^2 = 6.5512$; $p = 0.0105$). In other words, one additional year in education would lower the mortality of older Americans by 2–3 %, other variables being equal.

The results for the other three hazard models have tremendous similarities. Table 5.1 presents the parameter estimates and the hazard ratios derived from all four models, from which the analytic results of these methods can be compared and assessed.

Table 5.1 Maximum likelihood estimates from three approximation methods and Weibull model: older Americans ($n = 2000$).

Explanatory variable	Parameter estimate	Standard error	Chi-square	p-value	Hazard ratio
Cox regression with exact method (likelihood ratio $\chi^2 = 333.49$; $p < 0.0001$)					
Smoking	0.4204	0.1014	17.2023	<0.0001	1.523
Age_mean	0.0848	0.0052	266.9936	<0.0001	1.089
Female_mean	−0.4262	0.0667	40.8300	<0.0001	0.653
Educ_mean	−0.0224	0.0088	6.5512	0.0105	0.978
Cox regression with Efron method (likelihood ratio $\chi^2 = 333.49$; $p < 0.0001$)					
Smoking	0.4204	0.1014	17.2022	<0.0001	1.523
Age_mean	0.0848	0.0052	266.9943	<0.0001	1.089
Female_mean	−0.4262	0.0667	40.8297	<0.0001	0.653
Educ_mean	−0.0224	0.0088	6.5509	0.0105	0.978
Cox regression with Breslow method (likelihood ratio $\chi^2 = 331.42$; $p < 0.0001$)					
Smoking	0.4189	0.1014	17.0786	<0.0001	1.520
Age_mean	0.0845	0.0052	265.2549	<0.0001	1.088
Female_mean	−0.4248	0.0667	40.5680	<0.0001	0.654
Educ_mean	−0.0230	0.0088	6.4900	0.0108	0.978
Weibull hazard rate model (−2 log likelihood = 4207.88; $p < 0.0001$)					
Smoking	0.4213	0.1018	17.1500	<0.0000	1.524
Age_mean	0.0849	0.0054	241.3300	<0.0000	1.089
Female_mean	−0.4239	0.0672	39.7200	<0.0001	0.654
Educ_mean	−0.0225	0.0087	6.5800	<0.0001	0.978

As Table 5.1 presents, even with heavy ties, the three approximation methods generate almost identical regression coefficient estimates and model fit statistics, especially between the exact and the Efron methods. As the simplest approximation, the Breslow method is shown to be a highly efficient and consistent perspective to handle tied survival times on this dataset. Not surprisingly, the Weibull proportional hazard model yields extremely close estimates of regression coefficients to those derived from the three partial likelihood functions. Because the estimation is based on the full likelihood, the Weibull hazard model has a much higher model fit statistic than the three partial likelihood models. Therefore, when the information on the intercept factor is needed, the Weibull regression should be the first choice to model the proportional hazard function.

Although the Brelow method proves an efficient and consistent approximation in this illustration, I have reason to believe that when the sample size is small, the Breslow method does not perform as well as the other two approximation approaches (Hertz-Picciotto and Rockhill, 1997; Kalbfleisch and Prentice, 2002). Given this limitation, caution must apply in selecting an approximation method when the sample size is exceptionally small (e.g., the number of events is smaller than 25). My personal recommendation is that when analyzing large-scale survival data, the application of the simple Breslow method is good enough to yield efficient, robust, and consistent estimates of regression coefficients. When the sample size is too small, as is often the case in clinical trials, the Efron method should be the choice. If a full likelihood function is needed, the Weibull model is appropriate as this parametric perspective provides similar estimates of regression coefficients with an intercept estimate.

5.3 Estimation of survival functions from the Cox proportional hazard model

Although it provides a simple, efficient way to estimate regression coefficients, the Cox model is a partial likelihood perspective in which the baseline hazard rate is an unspecified nuisance function and thereby is not parameterized. Therefore, some useful lifetime indicators, such as the survival rate or the cumulative hazard function, are not directly obtainable from analytic results of the partial likelihood. In the meantime, researchers are often interested in comparing some complete lifetime functions for assessing the effect of a particular covariate on the risk of experiencing an event. Here, a statistically significant relative risk on the hazard rate may not necessarily translate into strong differences in the hazard rate itself because such differentials also depend on the magnitude of the baseline hazard rate (Liu, 2000; Teachman and Hayward, 1993). Consider, for example, a hazard ratio of 1.5: this relative risk can come either from the ratio of 0.3 over 0.2 or from the ratio of 0.003 over 0.002. While the first case suggests a very strong difference in the hazard rate, the second ratio implies an ignorable disparity. Therefore, it is inappropriate for the researcher to reach a final conclusion about the effect of a covariate just by looking at the hazard ratio (Liu, 2000).

One useful approach to demonstrate a covariate's effect is to compare survival functions between two or more population subgroups or on some selected covariate values. Comparing group-wise cumulative hazard functions is equally informative. Some statisticians have developed approximation methods for estimating the survival function and other related lifetime indicators from the Cox model estimates. In this section, I describe two popular methods in this area: the Kalbfleisch–Prentice method (1973) and the Breslow approach (1972), both based on the discrete step function of survival. Lastly, I provide an empirical example to demonstrate how to estimate group-wise survival curves from results of a Cox model using SAS programming.

5.3.1 The Kalbfleisch–Prentice method

The Kalbfleisch–Prentice method (1973) starts with defining the conditional probability of survival in the interval (t_{i-1}, t_i) for the baseline population, given by

$$s_i = \exp\left[-\int_{i-1}^{i} h_0(u)\,\mathrm{d}u\right], \tag{5.33}$$

where s_i is the baseline conditional probability in (t_{i-1}, t_i). By definition, the baseline probability of survival at t_i is simply the product of a series of conditional probabilities prior to t_i:

$$S_0(t_i) = \prod_{j=0}^{i-1} s_j. \tag{5.34}$$

According to Equation (5.4), the survival function with covariate vector $\boldsymbol{x}$ can be written as

$$S(t_i; \boldsymbol{x}) = [S_0(t_i)]^{\exp(\boldsymbol{x}'\boldsymbol{\beta})} = \left(\prod_{j=0}^{i-1} s_j\right)^{\exp(\boldsymbol{x}'\boldsymbol{\beta})}. \tag{5.35}$$

The conditional probability that an individual with covariate vector $\boldsymbol{x}_i$ survives from a particular event beyond t_i, given survival just prior to t_i, can be written as

$$\frac{[S_0(t_{i+1})]^{\exp(\boldsymbol{x}'\boldsymbol{\beta})}}{[S_0(t_i)]^{\exp(\boldsymbol{x}'\boldsymbol{\beta})}} = s_i^{\exp(\boldsymbol{x}'\boldsymbol{\beta})}. \tag{5.36}$$

Likewise, the conditional probability that the individual with covariate vector $\boldsymbol{x}_i$ experiences an event of interest in interval (t_i, t_{i+1}), given survival just prior to t_i, is

$$\frac{[S_0(t_i)]^{\exp(\boldsymbol{x}'\boldsymbol{\beta})} - [S_0(t_{i+1})]^{\exp(\boldsymbol{x}'\boldsymbol{\beta})}}{[S_0(t_i)]^{\exp(\boldsymbol{x}'\boldsymbol{\beta})}} = 1 - s_i^{\exp(\boldsymbol{x}'\boldsymbol{\beta})}. \tag{5.37}$$

As the contribution to the likelihood of an individual with covariates $\boldsymbol{x}$ who fails at t_i is $S(t_{i-1}; \boldsymbol{x}) - S(t_i; \boldsymbol{x})$ and the contribution of a censored observation at t_i is simply $S(t_i; \boldsymbol{x})$, an approximate joint likelihood function can be written as

$$\prod_{i=0}^{n'} \left\{ \prod_{l \in \mathcal{D}_i} \left[1 - s_l^{\exp(\boldsymbol{x}'\boldsymbol{\beta})}\right] \right\} \prod_{l' \in \mathcal{R}_i - \mathcal{D}_i} s_{l'}^{\exp(\boldsymbol{x}'\boldsymbol{\beta})}, \tag{5.38}$$

which is to be maximized with respect to $s_1, s_2, \ldots, s_{n'}$ and $\boldsymbol{\beta}$, or simply to $s_1, s_2, \ldots, s_{n'}$, with estimates $\hat{\boldsymbol{\beta}}$ from the partial likelihood function.

Differentiating the log of Equation (5.38) with respect to s_i gives the maximum likelihood estimate of s_i by solving the following equation:

$$\sum_{l \in \mathcal{D}_i} \frac{\exp\left(\mathbf{x}_l'\hat{\boldsymbol{\beta}}\right)}{1 - \hat{s}_l^{\exp\left(\mathbf{x}_l'\hat{\boldsymbol{\beta}}\right)}} = \sum_{l \in \mathcal{R}(t_i)} \exp\left(\mathbf{x}_l'\hat{\boldsymbol{\beta}}\right) \tag{5.39}$$

If there are no ties ($d_i = 1$ for all $i = 1, 2, \ldots, \tilde{d}$), the conditional probability of survival is

$$\hat{s}_i = \left[1 - \frac{\exp\left(\mathbf{x}_i'\hat{\boldsymbol{\beta}}\right)}{\sum_{l \in \mathcal{R}(t_i)} \exp\left(\mathbf{x}_l'\hat{\boldsymbol{\beta}}\right)}\right]^{\exp\left(\mathbf{x}_i'\hat{\boldsymbol{\beta}}\right)}. \tag{5.40}$$

If there are tied observations, an iterative solution for (5.40) is required. Kalbfleisch and Prentice (1973) suggest that a suitable starting value for the iteration should be

$$\hat{s}_{i0} = \exp\left[\frac{-d_i}{\sum_{l \in \mathcal{R}(t_i)} \exp\left(\mathbf{x}_l'\hat{\boldsymbol{\beta}}\right)}\right], \tag{5.41}$$

where $\hat{s}_{i0}$ is expected to approximate $\hat{s}_i$ very closely if the number of distinct event times is large.

Consequently, the baseline survival probability can be easily estimated. If there are no ties, then

$$\hat{S}_0(t) = \prod_{t_i < t} \hat{s}_i = \prod_{t_i < t} \left[1 - \frac{\exp\left(\mathbf{x}_i'\hat{\boldsymbol{\beta}}\right)}{\sum_{l \in \mathcal{R}(t_i)} \exp\left(\mathbf{x}_l'\hat{\boldsymbol{\beta}}\right)}\right]^{\exp\left(\mathbf{x}_i'\hat{\boldsymbol{\beta}}\right)}. \tag{5.42}$$

Clearly, the above equation is essentially a discrete step function with $\hat{S}_0(t)$ for $t < t_1$ and $\hat{S}_0(t) = 0$ if $t > t_n$ unless there are censored times after t_n.

When $\hat{\boldsymbol{\beta}}$ in the above equation, $\exp\left(\mathbf{x}_i'\hat{\boldsymbol{\beta}}\right) = 1$ and

$$\sum_{l \in \mathcal{R}(t_i)} \exp\left(\mathbf{x}_l'\hat{\boldsymbol{\beta}}\right) = n_i,$$

then

$$\hat{s}_i = \frac{n_i - 1}{n_i}. \tag{5.43}$$

Consequently, Equation (5.42) reduces to

$$\hat{S}_0(t) = \prod_{t_i < t} \frac{n_i - 1}{n_i}. \tag{5.44}$$

Therefore, the above Kalbfleisch and Prentice (1973) method is essentially an extension of the Kaplan–Meier estimator without ties, described in Chapter 2.

With the baseline survival function $S_0(t)$ estimated, the baseline cumulative hazard function is given by

$$\hat{H}_0(t) = -\log \hat{S}_0(t) = -\sum_{t_i < t} \log \hat{s}_i. \tag{5.45}$$

Given the estimates of the baseline hazard and the baseline cumulative hazard functions, the step survival and the cumulative hazard functions, given covariate vector $\boldsymbol{x}_i$, can be readily derived:

$$\hat{S}(t; \boldsymbol{x}_i) = \left[\hat{S}_0(t)\right]^{\exp(\boldsymbol{x}_i'\boldsymbol{\beta})}, \tag{5.46}$$

$$\hat{H}(t; \boldsymbol{x}_i) = \hat{H}_0(t)\exp\left(\boldsymbol{x}_i'\hat{\boldsymbol{\beta}}\right). \tag{5.47}$$

The above procedures generate the survival function and the cumulative hazard function, conditional on $\boldsymbol{x}$, as two discrete step functions. If there are ties, Equations (5.46) and (5.47) require an iterative solution, and the estimation then becomes fairly tedious.

Kalbfleisch and Prentice (1973) also propose an approach to estimate a continuous estimate of the survival function by connecting a sequence of straight lines across the log transformed step function at all t_i values; this approach, however, is not well integrated in the formation of the Cox regression.

5.3.2 The Breslow method

Given the complexity of the Kalbfleisch–Prentice method, Breslow (1972) provides a much simpler and more user-friendly approach to estimate the survival function in the Cox model. It starts with the following approximate equation on the baseline hazard rate at t_i, denoted by h_i:

$$\hat{h}_i = \frac{d_i}{t_i - t_{i-1}}\left[\sum_{l \in \mathcal{R}(t_i)} \exp\left(\boldsymbol{x}_l'\hat{\boldsymbol{\beta}}\right)\right]^{-1}. \tag{5.48}$$

According to the definition given in Chapter 2, this approximate of the baseline hazard rate is actually the average hazard rate in interval (t_{i-1}, t_i), namely, the interval-specific discrete rate divided by the unit of the interval. Accordingly, the baseline conditional probability of experiencing a particular event can be written as

$$\hat{q}_i = \frac{d_i}{\sum_{l \in \mathcal{R}(t_i)} \exp\left(\boldsymbol{x}_l'\hat{\boldsymbol{\beta}}\right)}, \tag{5.49}$$

where the denominator can be understood as the model-based estimate of n_i because it counts the exposure to the risk at t_i.

As mentioned in Chapter 1, in a step function it is valid to view the conditional probability of event q_i as an approximate to h_i because in a step function all hazard rates between t_{i-1} and t_i are 0. Given the equation $S(t) = \exp[-H(t)]$, the baseline survival function at t_i can be estimated from

$$\hat{S}_0(t) = \prod_{t_i < t} \exp\left[\frac{-d_i}{\sum_{l \in \mathcal{R}(t_i)} \exp\left(\boldsymbol{x}_l'\hat{\boldsymbol{\beta}}\right)}\right]. \tag{5.50}$$

Likewise, the baseline cumulative hazard function is given by

$$\hat{H}_0(t) = -\log \hat{S}_0(t) = \sum_{t_i < t}\left[\frac{d_i}{\sum_{l \in \mathcal{R}(t_i)} \exp\left(\boldsymbol{x}_l'\hat{\boldsymbol{\beta}}\right)}\right]. \tag{5.51}$$

Given the estimates of the baseline hazard function and the resulting baseline cumulative hazard function, the full survival function and the cumulative hazard function can be estimated by applying Equations (5.46) and (5.47).

Just like the Kalbfleisch–Prentice method equivalent to the Kaplan–Meier estimator, the Breslow method on the survival function is essentially based on the Nelson–Aalen estimator. More specifically, Equation (5.50) is equivalent to Equation (2.6) when $\boldsymbol{\beta} = 0$ because the denominator becomes n_i.

As it is much simpler and equally efficient compared to the Kalbfleisch–Prentice method, the Breslow estimator on the survival function becomes a first-choice method to estimate survival curves from results of the Cox model.

5.3.3 Illustration: Comparing survival curves for smokers and nonsmokers among older Americans

In this illustration, I follow up the example presented in Subsection 5.2.3. Although the hazard ratio of smoking cigarettes is as high as 1.523, there is not enough evidence to conclude that this relative risk reflects a substantively meaningful difference in the risk of death because it is just a ratio of two absolute rates. Given this concern, in the present analysis I want to compare the survival curves between smokers and nonsmokers throughout the whole observation period, using results of the Cox model. A distinct separation between the two curves would suggest the 'meaningful' significance of the hazard ratio. As the Brelow approximation method for estimating the regression coefficients is the simplest approach that derives almost identical estimates, I use the third regression in SAS Program 5.1 as the final model. In estimating the two survival curves, values of the three control variables – 'Age_mean, 'Female_mean,' and 'Educ_mean' – are fixed as 0 (sample means), so that survival curves for smokers and nonsmokers can be compared effectively (Fox, 1987; Liu, 2000). As a result, the model-based baseline survival function actually describes the expected survival rate for nonsmokers. For smokers, the survival function can be estimated by

$$\hat{S}(t;\text{smokers}) = \left[\hat{S}_0(t)\right]^{\exp(\hat{b}_1)}.$$

For a further comparison, I also generate the same set of survival curves from analytic results of the Weibull model to examine whether the discrete and the continuous survival perspectives yield different survival curves.

Below is the SAS program for estimating the two discrete survival curves.

SAS Program 5.2:

```
......

data group;
  length Id $30;
  input smoking age_mean female_mean educ_mean Id $12-61;
  datalines;
  0.00 0.00 0.00 0.00 smoking = 0
  1.00 0.00 0.00 0.00 smoking = 1
  ;

ods graphics on;
proc phreg data = new plot(overlay) = survival;
  model duration*Status(0) = smoking age_mean female_mean educ_mean
        / ties = BRESLOW ;
  baseline covariates = group out = pred1 survival=_all_ / rowid = Id;
run;
ods graphics off;
```

In SAS Program 5.2, I use the results of the Cox model to create two predicted survival curves, one for smokers and one for nonsmokers. First, a temporary dataset 'GROUP' is created to specify values of covariates for predicting the two survival functions. As specified, the first group is nonsmokers and the second smokers, with values of the three control variables fixed at zero. Using ODS Graphics, the PROC PHREG procedure plots two survival curves for group = 0 and group = 1, respectively, according to the specification saved in the dataset 'GROUP.' The option PLOTS(OVERPLAY)=SURVIVAL tells SAS to overlay both survival curves in the same plot. In the MODEL statement, the TIES = BRESLOW option specifies the use of the Breslow approximation method to handle tied survival data (this option can be omitted because RESLOW serves as default in SAS). The COVARIATES=GROUP option specifies that the dataset GROUP contains the set of covariates in the Cox model. The ROWID=ID option identifies the curves in the plot. The option SURVIVAL=_ALL_ requests that the estimated survival function, standard error, and lower and upper confidence limits be output into the SAS dataset specified in the OUT=PRED1 option.

The resulting plot is displayed in Figure 5.1, which plots the evolution of the survival curves for, respectively, smokers and nonsmokers, derived from the Breslow approximation method on estimating the survival function. The plot displays distinct separation between the two survival curves, reflecting strong negative effects of smoking cigarettes on the survival probability. As I specify a long observation period with more than 130 time points, the step function approximates a continuous survival curve; therefore the area between the two survival curves approximates the extra person-months lived by nonsmokers as compared to the expected life among smokers. Thus, it can safely be concluded now that the hazard ratio of smoking cigarettes is substantively meaningful after adjusting for confounding effects.

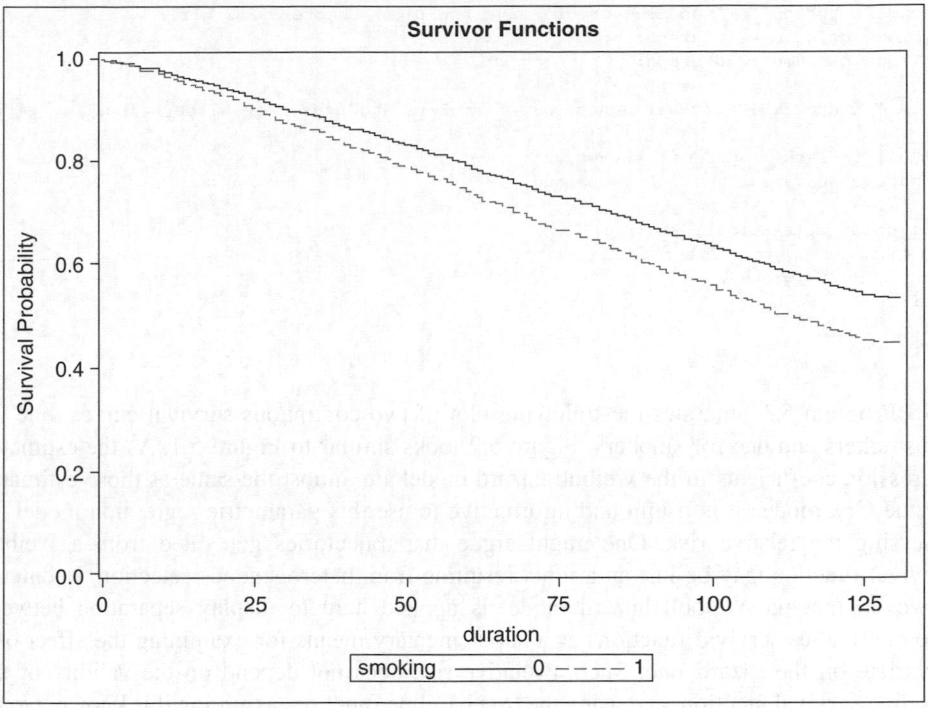

Figure 5.1 Estimated survival functions for smokers and nonsmokers.

Next, I generate two corresponding continuous survival curves using the regression coefficient of 'Smoking' from the Weibull hazard model (see SAS Program Output 5.1).

SAS Program 5.3:

```
options ls=80 ps=58 nodate;
ods select all;
ods trace off;
ods listing;
title1;
run;

data Weibull_smoking;
  do group = 1 to 2;
  do t = 0 to 130;
  if group = 1 then sr = exp(-exp(-6.9969)  *  (t**1.3237));
  if group = 2 then sr = exp(-exp(-6.9969 + 0.4213)*(t**1.3237));
  output;
  end;
  end;
run;

proc format;
  value group_fmt 1 = 'Nonsmokers'
        2 = 'Smokers';
run;
```

```
filename outgraph '<a subdirectory to save the plot>\Chapter5_332.gif';
goptions gsfname = outgraph;
goptions gsfname = outgraph;

Title "Figure 5.2. Survival functions of smokers and nonsmokers: the Weibull model";

symbol1 c=black i=splines l=1 v=plus;
symbol2 c=red i=splines l=2 v=diamond;

proc gplot data=Weibull_smoking;
  format group group_fmt.;
  plot sr*t = group ;
run;;
run;
quit;
```

SAS Program 5.3 generates the following plot of two continuous survival curves, one for nonsmokers and one for smokers. Figure 5.2 looks similar to Figure 5.1. As the estimated regression coefficients in the Weibull hazard model are almost the same as those estimated for the Cox model, it is useful and informative to use this parametric regression model for assessing the relative risk. One might argue that trajectories generated from a Weibull survival function may be just an artifact resulting from heterogeneous selection. I contend, however, that the Weibull hazard model is applied here to display separation between two continuous survival functions as a supplementary means for examining the effect of a covariate on the hazard rate. Such a relative risk does not depend on the validity of the baseline survival function, and using the true baseline function, assuming it is known, would lead to a similar separation of survival curves, thereby generating the same conclusion. If

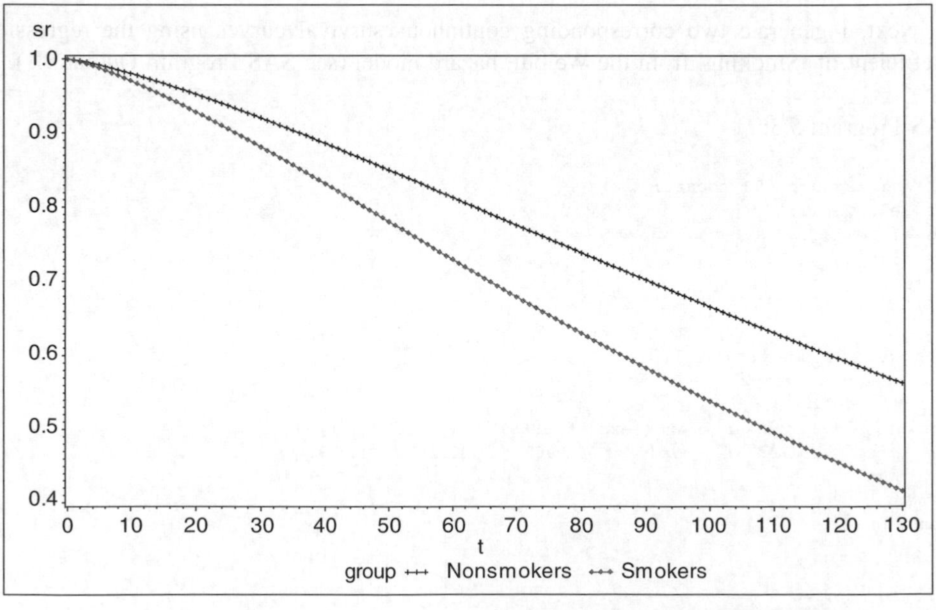

Figure 5.2 Survival functions of smokers and nonsmokers: Weibull model.

the presumed bias in the baseline hazard function truly exists, the step function generated from the Cox model should be subject to the same source of bias. At least, the area between the two Weibull survival curves displays more accurate differentials in survival times than does the Cox model.

In most situations, application of the Cox model is efficient enough to derive group-specific survival curves for large samples, as proved by Andersen *et al.* (1993) and Fleming and Harrington (1991) using the martingale central limit theorem, which will be described in Chapter 6. If the analyst needs to calculate the exact probability difference between two or more survival curves and perform a significance test, the Weibull hazard model is suggested for use.

5.4 The hazard rate model with time-dependent covariates

In previous sections, I described basic specifications of the Cox model and several refined Cox-type methods. All those regression models assume covariate values to be fixed throughout all study time, usually fixed at baseline. Variables thus specified are generally referred to as the *time-independent covariates*. This fixed-value assumption is valid for such demographic factors as sex, race/ethnicity, age at first marriage for ever-married persons, and, arguably, educational attainment among older persons. For some other variables, however, their values may change along the course of a particular life event, in turn posing potential threats to the validity of the time-independent assumption on covariates. Marital status among older persons, for example, varies over time due to high mortality, so that the mortality rate is not only a function of marital status at baseline but it may also be affected by its variations over time. The social environment, individual attitude and behavior, and many health indicators (e.g., blood pressure, cholesterol level, serum glucose), have the same time-varying characteristic. When used as explanatory factors in constructing a survival model, such time-varying variables are called the *time-dependent covariates*.

In this section, I first describe two categories of time-dependent variables, followed by specification of the hazard model using time-dependent variables as covariates and the estimating procedures. An empirical illustration is provided on the association between time-dependent marital status and the mortality of older Americans.

5.4.1 Categorization of time-dependent covariates

In the presence of time-dependent covariates, the covariate vector $\boldsymbol{x}$ is denoted by $\boldsymbol{x}(t)$ containing a set of variables $[x_1(t), \ldots, x_M(t)]$. Generally, the vector $\boldsymbol{x}(t)$ can be used to represent both time-independent and time-dependent covariates. If x_m is a time-independent covariate, $x_m(t) \equiv x_m(0)$, as a special case of $x_m(t)$; if it is a time-dependent covariate, $x_m(t)$ denotes the value of covariate x_m just prior to t. Theoretically, $x_m(t)$ as a time-dependent covariate is supposed to be known at every possible time point of an observation period. For some variables, however, measuring their values at every possible time point is unrealistic. A common practice is to measure values of such a time-dependent covariate at time intervals and then choose the measure closest to a specific survival time into analysis.

Here, I use $\tilde{x}(t)$ to indicate values of time-dependent covariates closest to t, mathematically defined as

$$\tilde{x}(t)=[x(\tilde{t}):0\leq\tilde{t}\leq t].$$

It must be borne in mind that a time-dependent covariate may be closely associated with other time-dependent variables because they tend to vary interactively along the course of survival processes, in turn implying the existence of complicated mechanisms among those variables. For example, currently smoking cigarettes generally predicts the death rate, but in the course of a lifetime event, the presence of a serious disease may influence cigarette smoking behavior, thus confounding the association between smoking cigarettes and mortality (Fisher and Lin, 1999). If currently smoking cigarettes and the severity of disease are used as time-dependent covariates simultaneously, it is very likely that both covariates will not display any significant effects on mortality due to the existence of colinearity. Considerable caution, therefore, must be exercised in using several time-dependent covariates simultaneously unless interactions among covariates are well understood.

Kalbfleisch and Prentice (2002) divide time-dependent covariates into two categories: external and internal. *External time-dependent covariates* are those whose values apply to all individuals thus not directly related to an individual's survival process. Although such time-dependent covariates can influence the hazard rate over time, its future variations are not affected by the occurrence of a particular event. One distinct example in social science is collective efficacy in the community, defined as the linkage of mutual trust and solidarity among neighbors (Sampson, Raudenbush, and Earls, 1997). This factor acts as a time-dependent variable given its frequent variations over time and the potential impact on an individual's attitude, behavior, and practice. Such an environmental variable, however, is external to an individual's survival mechanisms and thereby are not under direct observation of a particular study. In biomedical research, a prominent instance of external time-dependent covariates is the influence of the climate change on the rate of contracting bronchitis. Seasonal weather variation affects the rate of bronchitis, but its future progress is completely independent of an individual's survival from this disease.

Mathematically, an external time-dependent covariate satisfies the condition (Kalbfleisch and Prentice, 2002)

$$\mathrm{P}\{T\in[u,u+\mathrm{d}u)|\boldsymbol{x}(u),T\geq u\}=\mathrm{P}\{T\in[u,u+\mathrm{d}u)|\boldsymbol{x}(t),T\geq u\}. \tag{5.52}$$

The above equation indicates that the future path of $\boldsymbol{x}$ to any time greater than u is external to survival processes.

In contrast, the *internal time-dependent covariate* refers to a variable whose value is generated from time to time by an individual and thereby carries information on the hazard rate. Given such internal effects, time-dependent variables require periodic observation. There are many examples for an internal time-dependent covariate, such as marital status, cigarette smoking behavior, alcohol consumption, blood pressure, the presence and severity of a serious disease, and the like. In the field of military medicine, active-duty soldiers change deployments periodically, in turn affecting the prevalence and incidence of various psychiatric disorders among family members. As changes in a covariate's value are closely associated with an individual's survival process, ignoring such subject-specific variations can lead to the loss of important information.

It does not mean, however, that all subject-specific time-dependent covariates are internally time dependent. Age, for example, is a typical time-dependent variable that changes continuously over time. Nevertheless, it progresses simultaneously with time, thus not requiring direct observation. Technically, age even should not be considered an external time-dependent covariate because its time-dependent effect would simply cancel out in the partial likelihood function. As a result, fixing the value of age at baseline generates exactly the same regression coefficient as using it as a time-dependent covariate. Other age-related covariates, such as duration since first marriage, have the same property.

5.4.2 The hazard rate model with time-dependent covariates

The proportional hazard model with time-dependent covariates, as an extension of the Cox model, is defined by

$$h_i(t) = h_0(t)\exp\left[\boldsymbol{x}_i(t)'\boldsymbol{\beta}\right], \tag{5.53}$$

where the vector $\boldsymbol{x}(t)$, indicated earlier, may consist of both time-independent and time-dependent covariates. For analytic convenience, Equation (5.53) is sometimes written as

$$h_i(t) = h_0(t)\exp\left[\sum_{m=1}^{M} x_{im}(t)\beta_m\right], \tag{5.54}$$

where M is the number of covariates considered in the Cox model, among which some are time dependent and the others time independent.

Assuming censoring to be noninformative, the partial likelihood function with time-dependent covariates is

$$L_p(\boldsymbol{\beta}) = \prod_{i=1}^{d} \frac{\exp\left[\sum_{m=1}^{M} x_{im}(t_i)\beta_m\right]}{\sum_{l\in\mathcal{R}(t_i)} \exp\left[\sum_{m=1}^{M} x_{lm}(t_l)\beta_m\right]}. \tag{5.55}$$

Accordingly, the log-likelihood function is

$$\log\left[L_p(\boldsymbol{\beta})\right] = \sum_{i=1}^{d}\left(\sum_{m=1}^{M} x_{im}(t_i)\beta_m - \log\left\{\sum_{l\in\mathcal{R}(t_i)} \exp\left[\sum_{m=1}^{M} x_{lm}(t_l)\beta_m\right]\right\}\right). \tag{5.56}$$

As the standard procedure, the estimation of $\boldsymbol{\beta}$ is based on the partial likelihood score function, given by

$$\tilde{\boldsymbol{U}}(\boldsymbol{\beta}) = \sum_{i=1}^{d}\left(\boldsymbol{x}_i(t_i) - \frac{\sum_{l\in\mathcal{R}(t_i)_i} \exp\left[\boldsymbol{x}_l(t_i)'\boldsymbol{\beta}\right]\boldsymbol{x}_l(t_i)}{\sum_{l\in\mathcal{R}(t_i)} \exp\left[\boldsymbol{x}_l(t_i)'\boldsymbol{\beta}\right]}\right). \tag{5.57}$$

The vector $\hat{\boldsymbol{\beta}}$ can be estimated by solving $\tilde{\boldsymbol{U}}(\boldsymbol{\beta})=\mathbf{0}$. The variance–covariance matrix of $\hat{\boldsymbol{\beta}}$ can be obtained by the inverse of the observed information matrix, denoted by $\boldsymbol{I}^{-1}\left(\hat{\boldsymbol{\beta}}\right)$, where

$$\boldsymbol{I}\left(\hat{\boldsymbol{\beta}}\right)=\sum_{i=1}^{d}\left(\frac{\sum_{l\in\mathcal{R}(t_i)_i}\exp\left[\boldsymbol{x}_l(t_i)'\hat{\boldsymbol{\beta}}\right]\boldsymbol{x}_l(t_i)\boldsymbol{x}_l(t_i)'}{\sum_{l\in\mathcal{R}(t_i)}\exp\left[\boldsymbol{x}_l(t_i)'\hat{\boldsymbol{\beta}}\right]}\right.$$

$$\left.-\frac{\left\{\sum_{l\in\mathcal{R}(t_i)_i}\exp\left[\boldsymbol{x}_l(t_i)'\hat{\boldsymbol{\beta}}\right]\boldsymbol{x}_l(t_i)\right\}\left\{\sum_{l\in\mathcal{R}(t_i)_i}\exp\left[\boldsymbol{x}_l(t_i)'\hat{\boldsymbol{\beta}}\right]\boldsymbol{x}_l(t_i)\right\}'}{\sum_{l\in\mathcal{R}(t_i)}\exp\left[\boldsymbol{x}_l(t_i)'\hat{\boldsymbol{\beta}}\right]}\right). \tag{5.58}$$

With respect to a time-dependent covariate, time is taken into account in measuring its value, so that its effect on the hazard rate is no longer multiplicative or proportional. Consider, for example, the hazard ratio for two individuals, whose values of covariate x_m differ at time t while values of all other covariates are the same and time independent. Let j^* and l^* denote two individuals; the hazard ratio for those two individuals can be written as

$$\frac{h_{j^*}(t)}{h_{l^*}(t)}=\exp\left\{b_m\left[x_{j^*m}(t)-x_{l^*m}(t)\right]\right\},\quad j^*\neq l^*. \tag{5.59}$$

As both $x_{j^*m}(t)$ and $x_{l^*m}(t)$ are random over time, $[x_{j^*m}(t)-x_{l^*m}(t)]$ is a function of t, suggesting that this hazard ratio is not constant along the life course. For this reason, the hazard model with time-dependent covariates can be used as a tool to check proportionality of a covariate's effects, which will be further discussed in the next chapter.

With time-dependent covariates included in survival analysis, the hazard model becomes much more complicated both technically and substantively (Fisher and Lin, 1999). Without an extensive understanding of the interrelationship between the survival outcomes and a given time-dependent covariate, the estimated regression coefficient of a time-dependent covariate can lead to misleading conclusions. Consider the example of the association between smoking cigarettes and the mortality of older persons. If current cigarette smoking behavior is specified as a time-dependent covariate, then it is most likely that all deaths would be identified as nonsmokers in the time period just prior to death. Consequently, a misleading conclusion would be derived from the regression coefficient of smoking cigarettes: nonsmokers are more likely to die than smokers, other variables being equal. Obviously, specifying cigarettes smoking as a time-dependent covariate confounds the true relationship between smoking behavior and survival among older persons. Here, both current cigarette smoking status just prior to dying and the occurrence of death are the consequences of worsening health, thereby highlighting a misspecified time-dependent covariate in smoking cigarettes.

In terms of the above example, we may combine information on current and past smoking behaviors to define a smoker, as I did in some of the previous examples. Nevertheless, cigarette smoking behavior thus specified does not distinctively depend on time, particularly among older persons, because those who stop smoking cigarettes before or during a study are still considered smokers. As a result, defining cigarette smoking behavior as a time-independent covariate serves as a more appropriate choice. The above example indicates that whether a hazard rate model should involve any time-dependent covariates needs to be guided by extensive knowledge of the mechanisms involved in the time-varying processes of covariates. If an unclear and vague time-dependent function is misspecified, an underlying hazard model can yield disastrous results (Fisher and Lin, 1999).

5.4.3 Illustration: A hazard model on time-dependent marital status and the mortality of older Americans

In this illustration, I reanalyze the effect of marital status on the mortality of older Americans, replacing the time-independent variable 'Married' with a corresponding time-dependent covariate. In Chapter 4, I examined this association for two observation intervals, 12 months and 48 months, adjusting for the confounding effects of age and educational attainment. The results did not display a significant effect of current marriage on the mortality of older Americans. This lack of association might be due to a relatively short observation interval, during which the impact of marital status on the hazard rate cannot be captured. In the present illustration, therefore, I extend the observation period from baseline to the end of the AHEAD Wave VI survey (the end of 2004), yielding an 11–12-year observation period. Given a much extended interval, I specify marital status as a time-dependent covariate, evaluated at six time points (1993, 1995, 1998, 2000, 2002, and 2004). At each time point, marital status is indexed dichotomously: 1 = 'currently married' and 0 = else, with its variable name given as 'Married $\tilde{t}$,' where $\tilde{t} = 1,2,\ldots,6$. Age, gender, and educational attainment are used as the control variables, with centered measures, 'Age_mean,' 'Female_mean,' and 'Educ_mean,' considered in the regression analysis.

As marital status is measured repeatedly over a series of unequally spaced time points, I use some conditional statements to capture the appropriate value for an individual in each risk set. Specifically, I first define six time variables, time1 to time6, operationally defined as the number of months elapsed from the baseline survey to each follow-up investigation. Given this definition, I let time1 = 0, time2 = 24, time3 = 60, time4 = 84, time5 = 108, and time6 = 132. Marital status in the hazard rate model is used as a time-dependent variable, named 'Married_time,' with its value determined via the conditional statements displayed in the following SAS program.

SAS Program 5.4:

```
......
proc phreg data = new ;
  model duration*Status(0) = married_time age_mean female_mean educ_mean /
    ties = BRESLOW;
```

```
  array married{*} married1-married6;
  array time{*} time1-time6;
  time1 = 0; time2 = 24; time3 = 60; time4 = 84; time5 = 108; time6 = 132;
  if duration < time[2] then married_time = married[1];
  else if duration >= time[6] then married_time = married[6];
  else do i = 1 to 5;
    if time[i] <= duration < time[i+1] then married_time = married[i];
  end;
run;

proc phreg data = new ;
  model duration*Status(0) = married age_mean female_mean educ_mean / ties = BRESLOW ;
run;
```

SAS Program 5.4 specifies that an individual's marital status value, 0 or 1, is assigned according to his or her survival time, actual or censored. If an individual's survival time is located between time1 and time2 (24 months), the value of marital status at baseline is assigned. If it is equal to or greater than time6 (132 months), then the individual's marital status is measured at time6. For other situations, I ask SAS to assign the value of marital status at the beginning of a time interval during which the individual's death or censoring takes place. For comparison, I also estimate a Cox model with time-independent covariate 'Married' in SAS Program 5.4. From differences in the estimated regression coefficients and the model fit statistics, the importance of creating a time-dependent covariate for marital status can be evaluated. The results of the first model are presented below.

SAS Program Output 5.2:

Summary of the Number of Event and Censored Values

Total	Event	Event with Missing	Censored	Percent Censored
2000	864	86	1050	52.50

Testing Global Null Hypothesis: BETA=0

Test	Chi-Square	DF	Pr > ChiSq
Likelihood Ratio	326.5593	4	<.0001
Score	317.0191	4	<.0001
Wald	323.5435	4	<.0001

Analysis of Maximum Likelihood Estimates

Parameter	DF	Parameter Estimate	Standard Error	Chi-Square	Pr > ChiSq	Hazard Ratio
married_time	1	-0.22918	0.08009	8.1881	0.0042	0.795
age_mean	1	0.08074	0.00570	200.5965	<.0001	1.084
female_mean	1	-0.56492	0.07518	56.4661	<.0001	0.568
educ_mean	1	-0.02117	0.00924	5.2424	0.0220	0.979

In SAS Program Output 5.2, the information on the dataset, the dependent variable, the censoring status variable, and the censoring value statements, is not presented because it is exactly the same as previously reported. By involving a time-dependent covariate, there are 86 missing cases, 864 events (deaths), and 1050 censored observations. All three tests in the 'Testing Global Null Hypothesis: BETA = 0' section suggest that the null hypothesis $\hat{\boldsymbol{\beta}} = \mathbf{0}$ should be rejected, given a very strong statistical significance for each statistic ($p < 0.0001$).

In the table of 'Analysis of Maximum Likelihood Estimates,' the regression coefficient of 'Married_time' is −0.2292 ($SE = 0.0810$), statistically significant at $\alpha = 0.05$ ($\chi^2 = 8.1881$; $p = 0.0042$). The hazard ratio of this time-dependent variable, 0.795, suggests that the mortality rate for currently married persons is about 20 % lower than among those who are not currently married, other covariates being equal. The regression coefficients of the three control variables are all statistically significant, with values close to those previously reported. Therefore, for a long observation period, currently married older persons are shown to have significantly lower mortality than their counterparts not currently married, after adjusting for confounders.

Unfortunately, when time-dependent covariates are included, the survival curves for the currently married and currently not married cannot be estimated in SAS. Such survival functions, however, can be approximated by using the Cox model with all covariates fixed at baseline. Below are the results from the second model in SAS Program 5.4.

SAS Program Output 5.3:

Testing Global Null Hypothesis: BETA=0

Test	Chi-Square	DF	Pr > ChiSq
Likelihood Ratio	327.6730	4	<.0001
Score	315.3265	4	<.0001
Wald	321.5530	4	<.0001

Analysis of Maximum Likelihood Estimates

Parameter	DF	Parameter Estimate	Standard Error	Chi-Square	Pr > ChiSq	Hazard Ratio
married	1	-0.25749	0.07548	11.6369	0.0006	0.773
age_mean	1	0.07627	0.00549	193.2284	<.0001	1.079
female_mean	1	-0.53572	0.07187	55.5603	<.0001	0.585
educ_mean	1	-0.01856	0.00887	4.3840	0.0363	0.982

In SAS Program Output 5.3, the model fit statistics are very close to those generated from the hazard model with marital status used as a time-dependent covariate. For example, the likelihood ratio test of the time-independent model is 327.67 compared to 326.56 estimated for the time-dependent hazard model. Obviously, the difference in this statistic is not statistically significant, indicating the use of the time-dependent marital status variable to be unnecessary. There are some variations in the four parameter estimates, but such differences are not sizable and therefore can be ignored.

From the results reported in SAS Program Output 5.3, two survival curves, one for married and one for not married, are created from the same SAS procedure displayed in

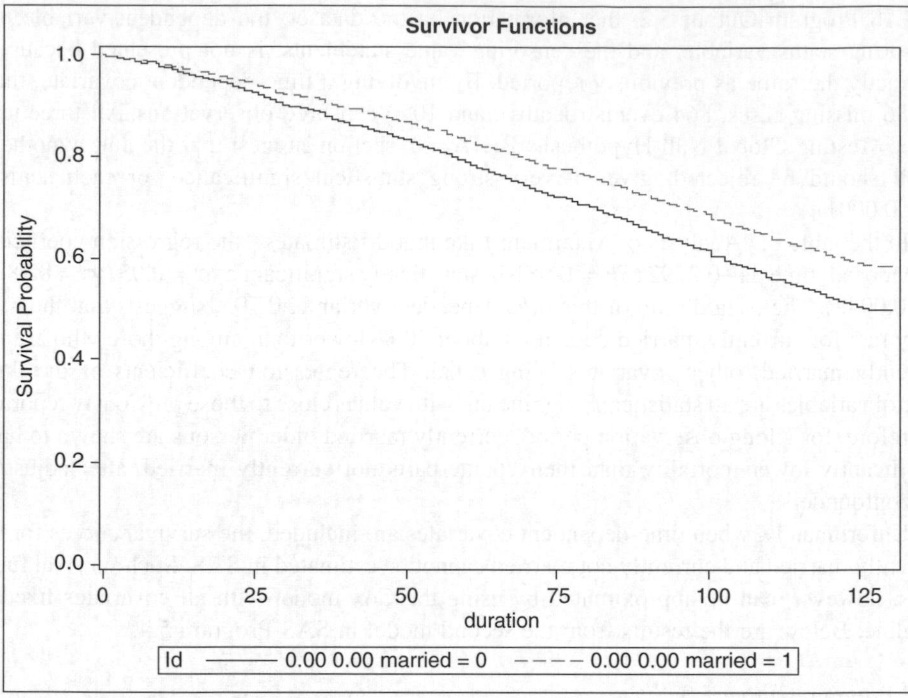

Figure 5.3 Estimated survival functions for currently married and currently not married.

SAS Program 5.2. Figure 5.3 displays distinct separation between the two survival curves, highlighting strong positive effects of current married life on the survival probability. As indicated earlier, the step function approximates a continuous survival curve given a long observation interval, so that the area between the two curves can be used for approximating the probability difference in survival. In view of the sizable separation displayed in Figure 5.3, the hazard ratio of 'Married' is associated with substantively meaningful differences in the probability of survival along the life course, exhibiting a strong impact of married life on the mortality of older Americans, other variables being equal.

As the hazard model involving one or more time-dependent covariates cannot be used to estimate the survival function, it is informative to use the Cox model without time-dependent covariates for plotting group-specific survival functions, even if the hazard model with time-dependent covariates fits survival data statistically better.

5.5 Stratified proportional hazard rate model

So far, the Cox model and its refinements have been described on the assumption that all individuals are subject to a common baseline hazard function, with population heterogeneity primarily reflected in the multiplicative predictor $\exp\left(\hat{\boldsymbol{\beta}}\boldsymbol{x}\right)$; that is, all subjects with the same x's are assumed to have an equivalent predicted hazard rate, given implicit random variation inherent in the unspecified baseline hazard function. This assumption is not always justified because some subpopulations can be subject to a very different distribution of the baseline hazard, thus making the proportionality assumption sometimes questionable. The cohort effect, for example, is a well-documented factor for differences in the distribution of survival times among older persons (Vaupel, Manton, and Stallard, 1979).

If the assumption of proportionality is violated for a given covariate, one popular approach is to stratify on this covariate, fitting a proportional hazard model for each stratified group. Consequently, this covariate no longer serves as a covariate but is used as a stratification factor. This stratifying technique, referred to as the *stratified Cox model*, permits the underlying hazard function to vary across two or more well-defined strata and thus can yield more efficient regression coefficients of other covariates. Additionally, the stratified hazard model can be used to make graphic checks for the proportional hazards hypothesis; that is, if the proportionality assumption does not hold, a set of stratified log–log survival functions (the log transformation of the cumulative hazard function) will not be parallel.

This section describes the stratified Cox proportional hazard model. As the estimating steps follow the standard procedures described in Section 5.1, I only introduce the basic equations of this technique. An empirical illustration is provided on the association between smoking cigarettes and the mortality of older Americans using age group as a stratification factor.

5.5.1 Specifications of the stratified hazard rate model

The general approach for the stratified proportional hazard rate model is to stratify on a specific covariate that is believed to be nonproportional and then to apply the proportional hazard model for each stratified group. Suppose individuals are assigned to K well-defined and mutually exclusive strata. In stratum k, where $k = 1, \ldots, K$, the proportional hazard rate model with covariate vector $\boldsymbol{x}$ is

$$h_k(t;\boldsymbol{x}_k) = h_{0k}(t)\exp(\boldsymbol{x}'\boldsymbol{\beta}), \tag{5.60}$$

where h_{0k} is the unspecified baseline hazard function for stratum k. As the above specification is actually a standard Cox model for individuals in the same stratum, Equation (5.60) is referred to as the *stratified Cox proportional hazard model*.

According to Equation (5.60), all individuals in stratum k are subject to a common baseline hazard function, whereas individuals in other strata are not. In the formulation of the Cox model, however, differences in the baseline hazard function across strata are unspecified because the primary purpose for applying the stratified Cox model is to derive more efficient regression coefficients. Because $\boldsymbol{\beta}$ in Equation (5.60) is not specific to stratum k, the stratified Cox model assumes consistent proportional hazards for other covariates across all strata. In other words, while the baseline hazard function varies from stratum to stratum, the regression coefficients and the hazard ratios of other covariates are assumed to be identical. Statistical models in which covariate effects vary over strata will be described in the next chapter.

For each stratum, the partial likelihood function is specified in the same fashion as described in Section 5.1. Specifically, the partial likelihood function for stratum k is

$$L_{kp}(\boldsymbol{\beta}) = \prod_{i=1}^{d_k} \frac{\exp(\boldsymbol{x}'_{ki}\boldsymbol{\beta})}{\sum_{l \in \mathcal{R}(t_{ki})} \exp(\boldsymbol{x}'_{kl}\boldsymbol{\beta})}, \tag{5.61}$$

where d_k is the number of events that occur in stratum k and t_{ki} is the ith observed event time in stratum k. Similarly, $\mathcal{R}(t_{ki})$ represents the corresponding risk set at event time t_{ki} and $\boldsymbol{x}_{ki}$ is the covariate vector with respect to stratum k. Accordingly, the log partial likelihood function is given by

$$\log L_{kp}(\boldsymbol{\beta}) = \sum_{i=1}^{d_k} \left\{ \boldsymbol{x}'_{ki}\boldsymbol{\beta} - \sum_{i=1}^{d_j} \log\left[\sum_{l \in \mathcal{R}(t_{ki})} \exp(\boldsymbol{x}'_{kl}\boldsymbol{\beta}) \right] \right\}. \tag{5.62}$$

Given the specification of the partial likelihood function for each stratum, the complete stratified partial likelihood is simply the combination of all contributions from K strata to the likelihood:

$$L_p^{\text{stratified}}(\boldsymbol{\beta}) = \prod_{k=1}^{K} L_{kp}(\boldsymbol{\beta}). \tag{5.63}$$

Accordingly, the complete stratified partial log-likelihood function is given by

$$\log L_p^{\text{stratified}}(\boldsymbol{\beta}) = \sum_{k=1}^{K} \log L_{kp}(\boldsymbol{\beta}). \tag{5.64}$$

The partial derivative of the complete log-likelihood function is obtained by summing the partial derivatives across all strata, and then the complete log partial likelihood function is maximized with respect to $\boldsymbol{\beta}$. The score test, the Wald, and the likelihood ratio test statistics can be readily obtained from using the procedures described in previous sections.

Although the heterogeneous baseline hazard functions are unspecified in estimating the regression coefficients, graphic checks can be made to evaluate whether or not those baseline hazard functions are proportional to each other. As the log–log survival function is the log transformation of the cumulative hazard rate, it is plausible to compare stratum-specific log–log survival curves with all covariates set at zero. If they are roughly parallel, it can be inferred that the baseline hazard rates across strata tend to be proportional and therefore using the stratified Cox model is unnecessary. In contrast, if they are not parallel at all, the baseline hazard functions of different strata differ nonmultiplicatively, in turn suggesting that the inclusion of an underlying stratification factor in the Cox model, as a covariate, would violate the proportional hazards assumption.

5.5.2 Illustration: Smoking cigarettes and the mortality of older Americans with stratification on three age groups

In this illustration, I follow up the example presented in Subsection 5.3.3. Although the distinct separation of two survival curves, one for older smokers and one for nonsmokers, displays the substantive importance of the hazard ratio for the variable 'Smoking' (1.523), this result might be somewhat biased because the effect of smoking cigarettes could be inappropriately adjusted by misspecifying the effect of age as multiplicative. Older persons at various age ranges are of different birth cohorts surviving from a rigorous 'selection of the fittest' process, so they may not necessarily be subject to a common baseline hazard function.

In this illustration, I want to estimate the effect of smoking cigarettes on the mortality of older Americans by stratifying on different age groups. In particular, I identify three age groups: younger than 75 years of age (young old), 74–84 years (old old), and 85 years or over (oldest old), all measured at baseline. The observation period is still from the baseline survey to the end of the year 2004. Among 2000 older Americans in the dataset, 923 persons are young old (46.15 %; termed 'Group I'), 884 are the old old (44.20 %; 'Group II'), and the remaining 193 older persons are oldest old (9.65 %; 'Group III'). The numbers of deaths in the three age groups are, respectively, 309, 485, and 156 persons. The estimating procedures are exactly the same as described in Subsection 5.3.3, except for the stratification procedure. In estimating the survival curves for older smokers and nonsmokers in each age group, values of the remaining two control variables – 'Female_mean' and 'Educ_mean' – are fixed as 0 (sample means). The SAS program for estimating this stratified proportional hazard model is displayed below.

SAS Program 5.5:

```
......

if age < 75 then age_group = 1;
  else if age < 85 then age_group = 2;
  else age_group = 3;

......

data group;
  length Id $30;
  input smoking female_mean educ_mean Id $12-61;
  datalines;
  0.00 0.00 0.00 0.00 smoking = 0
  1.00 0.00 0.00 0.00 smoking = 1
  ;

ods graphics on;
proc phreg data = new plot(overlay)=survival;
  model duration*Status(0) = smoking female_mean educ_mean / ties = BRESLOW ;
  strata age_group;
  baseline covariates = group out = pred1 survival=_all_ / rowid = Id;
run;
ods graphics off;
```

In SAS Program 5.5, I first create a stratification factor 'Age_group,' according to the aforementioned classification. The DATA statement and the SAS PROC SQL procedure are mostly the same as those of previous examples and are therefore not presented. I continue to use the TIES = BRESLOW option as the approximation method to handle tied survival times. In the PROC PHREG statement, I add a STRATA AGE_GROUP statement to tell SAS that a Cox model is fitted on each age group. The results of the stratified proportional hazard model are used to create two predicted survival curves for each stratum, one for older smokers and one for nonsmokers. A temporary dataset 'GROUP' is created to specify values of covariates for predicting the two survival functions for each stratum. Using ODS Graphics, the PROC PHREG procedure plots two survival curves for group = 0 and group = 1, respectively. The option PLOTS(OVERPLAY) = SURVIVAL tells SAS to overlay both survival curves in the same plot. Because of stratification on age, SAS generates three sets of survival curves, with each attaching to an age group. In the BASELINE statement, the options are exactly the same as previously presented.

The analytic results of the above stratified Cox model are shown in the following SAS output file.

SAS Program Output 5.4:

Summary of the Number of Event and Censored Values

Stratum	age_group	Total	Event	Censored	Percent Censored
1	1	923	309	614	66.52
2	2	884	485	399	45.14
3	3	193	156	37	19.17
Total		2000	950	1050	52.50

Testing Global Null Hypothesis: BETA=0

Test	Chi-Square	DF	Pr > ChiSq
Likelihood Ratio	65.2319	3	<.0001
Score	70.3170	3	<.0001
Wald	69.3868	3	<.0001

Analysis of Maximum Likelihood Estimates

Parameter	DF	Parameter Estimate	Standard Error	Chi-Square	Pr > ChiSq	Hazard Ratio
smoking	1	0.37484	0.10133	13.6846	0.0002	1.455
female_mean	1	-0.43271	0.06672	42.0592	<.0001	0.649
educ_mean	1	-0.02732	0.00878	9.6828	0.0019	0.973

In SAS Program Output 5.4, the 'Summary of the Number of Event and Censored Values' statement matches the data reported previously. All three tests in the 'Testing Global Null Hypothesis: BETA = 0' section demonstrate that the null hypothesis $\hat{\boldsymbol{\beta}} = \mathbf{0}$ should be rejected. Nevertheless, the chi-square values from the three tests, each with three degrees of freedom, are substantially lower than those generated from the Cox model using age as a covariate. For example, the chi-square value of the likelihood ratio is 65.23, much lower than the corresponding test statistic of 331.42 for the overall Cox model. As Kalbfleisch and Prentice (2002) caution, when stratification is used unnecessarily, some loss of efficiency is encountered.

In the table of 'Analysis of Maximum Likelihood Estimates,' the regression coefficient of 'Smoking' is 0.3748 ($SE = 0.1013$), statistically significant at $\alpha = 0.05$ ($\chi^2 = 13.68; p = 0.0002$) and close to the estimate obtained from the Cox model using age as a covariate ($\beta_1 = 0.4189$; $SE = 0.1014$; $\chi^2 = 17.08$; $p < 0.0001$). The hazard ratio of smoking cigarettes is 1.455, also

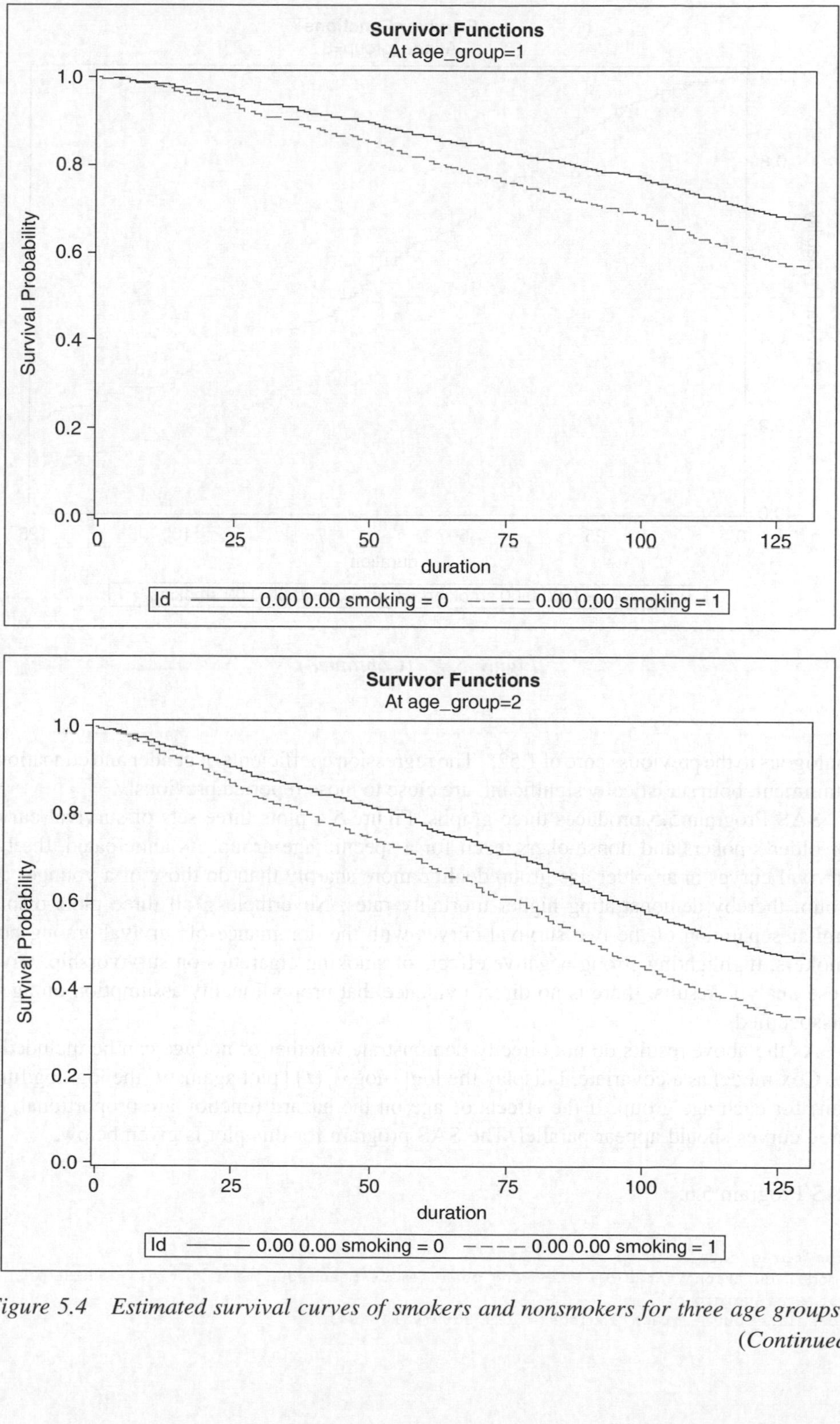

Figure 5.4 Estimated survival curves of smokers and nonsmokers for three age groups.

(Continued)

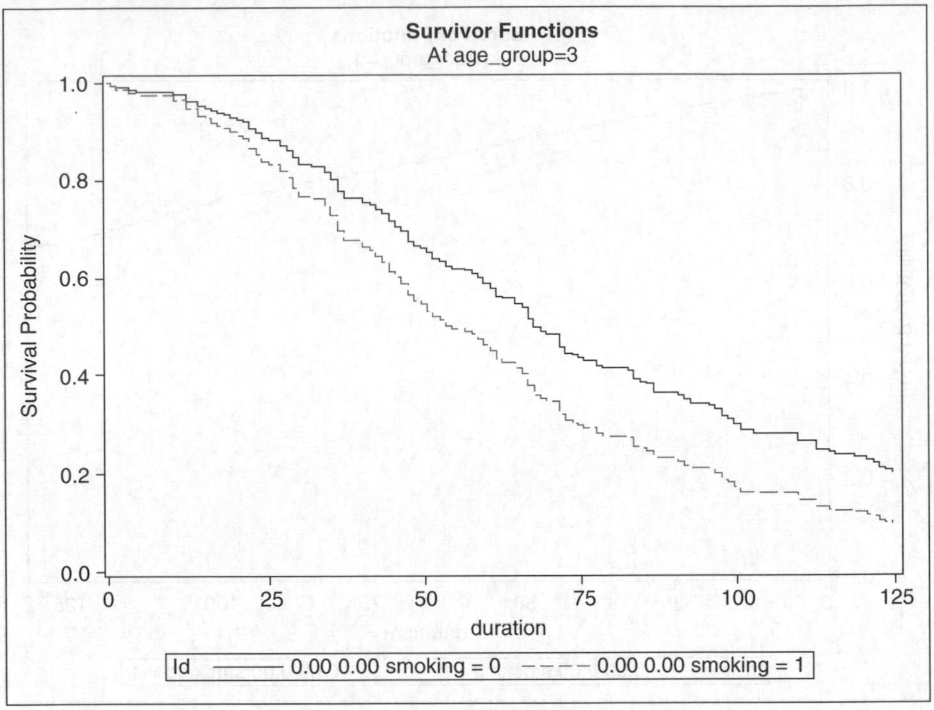

Figure 5.4 (*Continued*)

analogous to the previous score of 1.523. The regression coefficients of gender and educational attainment, both statistically significant, are close to those reported previously.

SAS Program 5.5 produces three graphs. Figure 5.4 plots three sets of survival curves for older smokers and nonsmokers, each for a specific age group. As anticipated, the two survival curves in an older age group decline more sharply than do those of a younger age group, thereby demonstrating higher mortality rates. Nevertheless, all three plots display similar separation of the two survival curves with the dominance of survival among nonsmokers, highlighting strong negative effects of smoking cigarettes on survivorship. Given these analytic results, there is no direct evidence that proportionality assumption on age is misspecified.

As the above results do not directly demonstrate whether or not age can be included in the Cox model as a covariate, I display the $\log\left[-\log\hat{S}_{0j}(t)\right]$ plot against t (the log–log function) for each age group. If the effects of age on the hazard function are proportional, the three curves should appear parallel. The SAS program for this plot is given below.

SAS Program 5.6:

```
......
proc phreg data = new ;
  model duration*Status(0) = smoking_mean female_mean educ_mean / ties = BRESLOW ;
  strata age_group;
  baseline out = graph loglogs = lls survival = s ;
run;
```

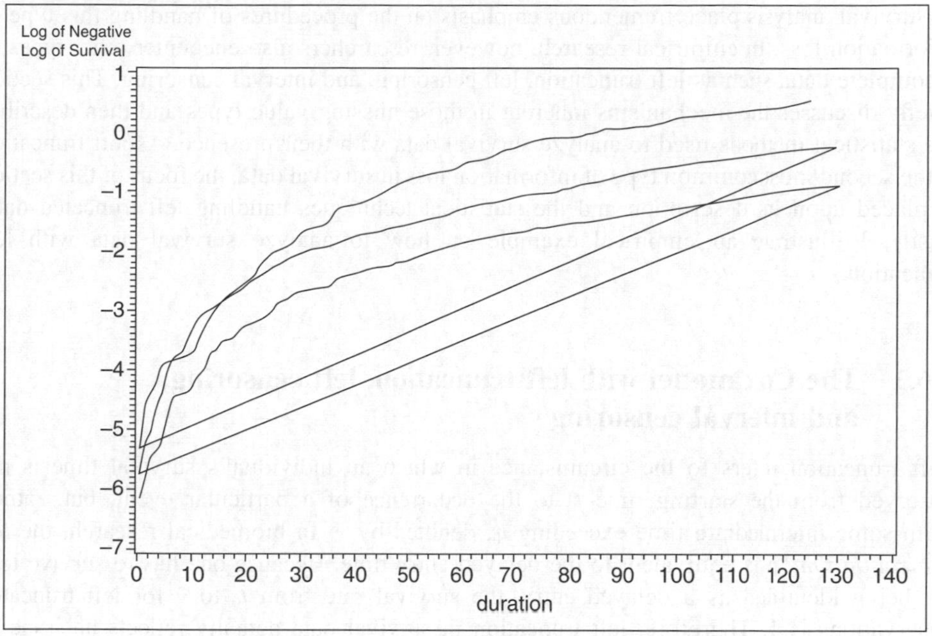

Figure 5.5 Log–log plot of three age groups.

```
proc gplot data = graph;
  plot lls * duration;
  Title "Figure 5.5. Log minus log plot of three age groups";
  symbol1 interol = join color = black line = 1;
  symbol2 interol = join color = black line = 2;
  symbol3 interol = join color = black line = 3;
run;
```

SAS Program 5.6 generates three log–log survival curves in one plot. In the PROC SQL procedure, not presented here, the variable 'Smoking' is rescaled to be centered about its sample mean, named 'Smoking_mean.' Consequently, the three baseline log–log survival curves in fact display the log-transformed cumulative hazard function for three age groups with values of all covariates fixed at sample means. Therefore, the proportionality hypothesis on age can be evaluated effectively. The resulting plot is presented in Figure 5.5, which displays three log–log survival curves with distinct separations that appear approximately parallel over time. Therefore, this graph provides some evidence that age can be considered a covariate in the Cox model for producing more efficient regression coefficients and model fit statistics. Proportionality of other covariates can be examined by plotting log–log survival curves over two or more well-defined strata.

5.6 Left truncation, left censoring, and interval censoring

Previous sections describe the Cox model and its refinements, assuming the presence of noninformative right censoring. As indicated in Chapter 1, right censoring is the most frequently encountered censoring type in survival analysis and, as a result, all textbooks of survival analysis place tremendous emphasis on the procedures of handling this type of information loss. In empirical research, however, researchers also encounter other types of incomplete data, such as left truncation, left censoring, and interval censoring. This section briefly discusses the mechanisms inherent in those missing value types and then describes the statistical methods used to analyze survival data with their presence. As left truncation is the second most common type of information loss in survival data, the focus of this section is placed upon its description and the statistical techniques handling left truncated data. Lastly, I illustrate an empirical example on how to analyze survival data with left truncation.

5.6.1 The Cox model with left truncation, left censoring, and interval censoring

Left truncation refers to the circumstance in which an individual's survival time is not observed from the starting time t_0 to the occurrence of a particular event, but, rather, from some intermediate time exceeding t_0, denoted by $\tilde{v}$. In biomedical research, the *left truncation time* $\tilde{v}$ is equivalent to the delayed entry time. Because one has to survive to $\tilde{v}$ for being identified as a delayed entry, the survival rate from t_0 to $\tilde{v}$ for left truncated observations is 1. Therefore, left truncation in survival data actually reflects an issue of selection bias, particularly since left truncated observations are selected by an intermediate process from the time origin to $\tilde{v}$. Methodologically, those who are left truncated should have an event time defined as $T \geq t \mid \tilde{v}$, instead of $T \geq t$. If a particular event time T_i is conditional on $\tilde{v}$, this lifetime is left truncated. When left truncated observations are counted into all the risk sets from t_0 to t, the hazard rate is underestimated because the denominator of the partial likelihood function is overrepresented by involving the left truncated observations whose left truncation time exceeds the observation time. For those left truncated with $T > \tilde{v} > t$, it is already known that all of them survive to $\tilde{v} > t$ and thereby are not at risk at t. If left truncation is associated with certain covariates, then regression coefficients of those covariates may be subject to some bias, with extent depending on how left truncated observations are distributed.

Left truncation is frequently observed in demographical research. As Andersen *et al.* (1993) comment, the construction of a classical life table is based on survival data of individuals within some well-specified age intervals; thus they are left truncated at the beginning of the interval. For this reason, a classical life table only reflects survival processes for a 'synthetic' cohort combining a series of left truncated survival data, rather than of a real birth cohort in the life course. In biomedical studies, left truncation arises when a researcher introduces some intermediate event as the eligible condition for further analysis of a lifetime event, thus yielding a unique survival pattern for those who have experienced that intermediate event (Klein and Moeschberger, 2003). In clinical trials, some patients may not have entered a particular study at the time of origin until some weeks or months later; without any adjustments, including them in the analysis for the entire study period can result in erroneous outcomes.

Statisticians believe that it is relatively easy to handle left truncation if the delayed entry time $\tilde{v}$ is conditionally independent of T with its distribution depending on parameters $\boldsymbol{x}$. If left truncation tends to be random, which I believe is often the case, then the partial likelihood given $T > t > \tilde{v}$ is unbiased when those with left truncation times exceeding t are excluded from the estimation process (Andersen *et al.*, 1993). Consequently, estimation of the Cox model with left truncated data only needs to modify the delayed event time in the risk set, given by

$$\mathcal{R}(t) = (r|\tilde{v} < t < T).$$

With this modification, the Cox model can be readily applied to analyze left truncated survival data with a redefined entry time.

Left censoring, briefly discussed in Chapter 1, points to the situation in which a time point is known to be before the start of a particular study but unknown about its exact location. While left truncation is often associated with a selection process, left censoring usually occurs randomly. One popular approach to handle left censoring is to reverse the time scale, using the difference between a large time value (the maximum time point observed) and the original survival time as the event time. By performing this reversion, the left censored survival data become right censored, thereby facilitating the estimation of the Cox model with limited functional adjustments (Ware and DeMets, 1976). Sometimes, survival data consist of both left and right censored survival times, referred to as *double censoring*, and its presence would considerably complicate the estimation of the variance–covariance matrix of the survival function. Given its relative rarity, however, I do not describe further the statistical techniques of handling double censoring in this text. The interested reader is referred to Klein and Moeschberger (2003) and Turnbull (1974).

Interval censoring, described extensively in Chapters 1 and 4, points to the condition in which the exact timing for the occurrence of a particular event is not observed and, instead, the researcher only knows that the actual survival time T_i falls in a time interval (t_{i-1}, t_i). In fact, in survival data with a longitudinal growth design, event times are mostly interval censored because the occurrence of a particular event is usually identified by the status change between two successive time points. When time intervals are narrowly spaced, T_i can be approximated by using the midpoint of an interval, as widely applied by demographers. In Section 4.6, an empirical illustration on the parametric regression model provides strong evidence that when a time interval for an observed event is reasonably limited, the use of the midpoint as the time scale is appropriate and statistically efficient, deriving unbiased parameter estimates. This conclusion also applies to the estimation of the Cox model. When the interval is large, however, regular inference of survival processes might overlook some important information on survival variations within intervals, thus causing some bias in parameter estimates.

5.6.2 Illustration: Analyzing left truncated survival data on smoking cigarettes and the mortality of unmarried older Americans

In this illustration, I analyze the association between smoking cigarettes and the mortality of older Americans who are not currently married prior to death. Specifically, I apply the Cox model to estimate the regression coefficient of 'Smoking' on the hazard function, excluding currently married persons in the risk sets, and then I compare the survival curves between unmarried smokers and unmarried nonsmokers. In estimating this model, I continue to use the centered measures of age, gender, and educational attainment as the control variables. When calculating the two survival curves, I set the values of those centered variables at 0 (sample means) for an effective comparison. Among those not currently married in the course of the study, some are unmarried at baseline and others are identified as not currently married only in subsequent waves of investigation. As an older person has to survive to a later time to change his or her marital status, those who become unmarried in follow-up surveys are systematically selected and left truncated. As indicated above, the direct application of the Cox model on left truncated data underestimates the hazard rate because individuals who become unmarried at a later time than t are improperly included in the risk set $\mathcal{R}(t)$. Thus, the risk set for estimating the relative risk of death needs to be adjusted by only including those who are unmarried prior to t and are still at risk. In other words, those who become unmarried later than t should be excluded from the risk set at t.

For analytic simplicity and convenience and without loss of generality, I assume currently unmarried persons would not become married in the course of the study, an assumption not unreasonable for older persons. Below is the SAS program to estimating the Cox model adjusting for left truncation.

SAS Program 5.7:

```
......
if married1 = 0 or married2 = 0 or married3 = 0 or married4 = 0 or married5 = 0 or
married6 = 0
 then not_married = 1;
 else not_married = 0;

 time1 = 0; time2 = 24; time3 = 60; time4 = 84; time5 = 108; time6 = 132;
 if married1 = 0 then t1 = time1;
 else if married1 = 1 and married2 = 0 then t1 = time2;
 else if married1 = 1 and married2 = 1 and married3 = 0 then t1 = time3;
 else if married1 = 1 and married2 = 1 and married3 = 1 and married4 = 0 then t1 =
  time4;
 else if married1 = 1 and married2 = 1 and married3 = 1 and married4 = 1 and
  married5 = 0 then t1 = time5;
 else if married1 = 1 and married2 = 1 and married3 = 1 and married4 = 1 and
  married5 = 1 and married6 =0 then t1 = time6;
 else t1 = 0;
......
data group;
 length Id $30;
 input smoking age_mean female_mean educ_mean Id $12-61;
 datalines;
 0.00 0.00 0.00 0.00 smoking = 0
 1.00 0.00 0.00 0.00 smoking = 1
 ;

ods graphics on;
proc phreg data = new plot(overlay)=survival; where not_married = 1;
 model duration*Status(0) = smoking age_mean female_mean educ_mean / entry = t1 ;
 baseline covariates = group out = pred1 survival=_all_ / rowid = Id;
run;
ods graphics off;
```

In SAS Program 5.7, I first create a dichotomous variable 'not_married,' with 1 = not married at any time of the observation period and 0 = married throughout the observation interval.

Next, I construct an entry time variable called 't1' redefining the origin of time for the occurrence of a death. Specifically, I define six time variables, time1 to time6, operationally defined as the number of months elapsed from the baseline survey to each follow-up survey. Given this definition, I let time1 = 0, time2 = 24, time3 = 60, time4 = 84, time5 = 108, and time6 = 132. The value of t1, the entry time, is determined via the conditional statements in SAS Program 5.7. If an individual is identified as currently not married at the baseline survey, t1 is set at 0, indicating the absence of left truncation. If the individual is married at baseline but not currently married at the first follow-up survey, t1 = 24, indicating a left truncation time of 24. Likewise, if the individual is married both at baseline and at the first follow-up but identified as currently not married at the second follow-up survey (Wave III), t1 is 60, and so forth. Obviously, for those who become unmarried later than t_0, t1 is the left truncation time $\tilde{v}$; therefore, by using this new origin of time, an event time can be properly adjusted.

A temporary dataset 'GROUP' is created again to specify values of covariates used for predicting the two survival functions, one for smokers and one for nonsmokers. As previously noted, the three control variables are fixed at zero, representing sample means. Using ODS Graphics, the PROC PHREG procedure plots two survival curves for group = 0 and group = 1 according to the specification saved in the dataset 'GROUP.' In the MODEL statement, the ENTRY = t1 option is now added to specify left truncated survival data. Here, the interval (t1, DURATION) specifies the at-risk time span, thereby taking left truncation time into consideration. Consequently, only those with $\tilde{v} < t < T$ are included in each risk set $\mathcal{R}(t)$. The options included in this procedure are interpreted previously.

The results of this Cox model with left truncated data are shown below.

SAS Program Output 5.5:

Summary of the Number of Event and Censored Values

Total	Event	Censored	Percent Censored
1214	568	646	53.21

Testing Global Null Hypothesis: BETA=0

Test	Chi-Square	DF	Pr > ChiSq
Likelihood Ratio	132.0691	4	<.0001
Score	136.6246	4	<.0001
Wald	137.3406	4	<.0001

Analysis of Maximum Likelihood Estimates

Parameter	DF	Parameter Estimate	Standard Error	Chi-Square	Pr > ChiSq	Hazard Ratio
smoking	1	0.41272	0.13479	9.3750	0.0022	1.511
age_mean	1	0.07271	0.00693	110.1823	<.0001	1.075
female_mean	1	-0.45409	0.09962	20.7774	<.0001	0.635
educ_mean	1	-0.01064	0.01160	0.8409	0.3591	0.989

SAS Program Output 5.5 shows that excluding those who are married throughout the study period and missing cases, 1214 observations are used in estimating this Cox model, among whom 568 persons are dead and 646 are right censored. Again, all three tests in the 'Testing Global Null Hypothesis: BETA = 0' section demonstrate that the null hypothesis $\hat{\boldsymbol{\beta}} = \mathbf{0}$ should be rejected.

In the table of 'Analysis of Maximum Likelihood Estimates,' the regression coefficient of 'Smoking' is 0.4127 ($SE = 0.1348$), statistically significant at $\alpha = 0.05$ ($\chi^2 = 9.38$; $p = 0.0022$), analogous to the estimate obtained from the Cox model including all individuals ($\beta_1 = 0.4189$; $SE = 0.1014$; $\chi^2 = 17.08$; $p < 0.0001$). Such a similarity indicates that marital status is not a modifier on the association between smoking cigarettes and the mortality of older Americans. The hazard ratio of 'Smoking' among unmarried persons is 1.511, very close to the score of 1.523 estimated for the entire sample. The regression coefficients of age and gender, both statistically significant, are also similar to those reported previously. Educational attainment does not have a statistically significant impact on the hazard rate.

SAS Program 5.7 also produces the graph in Figure 5.6, which plots two survival curves for, respectively, unmarried smokers and unmarried nonsmokers, derived from the Breslow method on estimating the survival function. With similar estimates of regression coefficients, the plot below is analogous to Figure 5.1, displaying distinct separation between the two survival curves. Therefore, the hazard ratio of 'Smoking' among unmarried older Americans is associated with significant differences in the survival probability between older smokers and nonsmokers, other covariates being equal. As marital status does not modify the association between smoking cigarettes and mortality, I expect married older Americans have the same pattern of survival differences displayed by Figure 5.6.

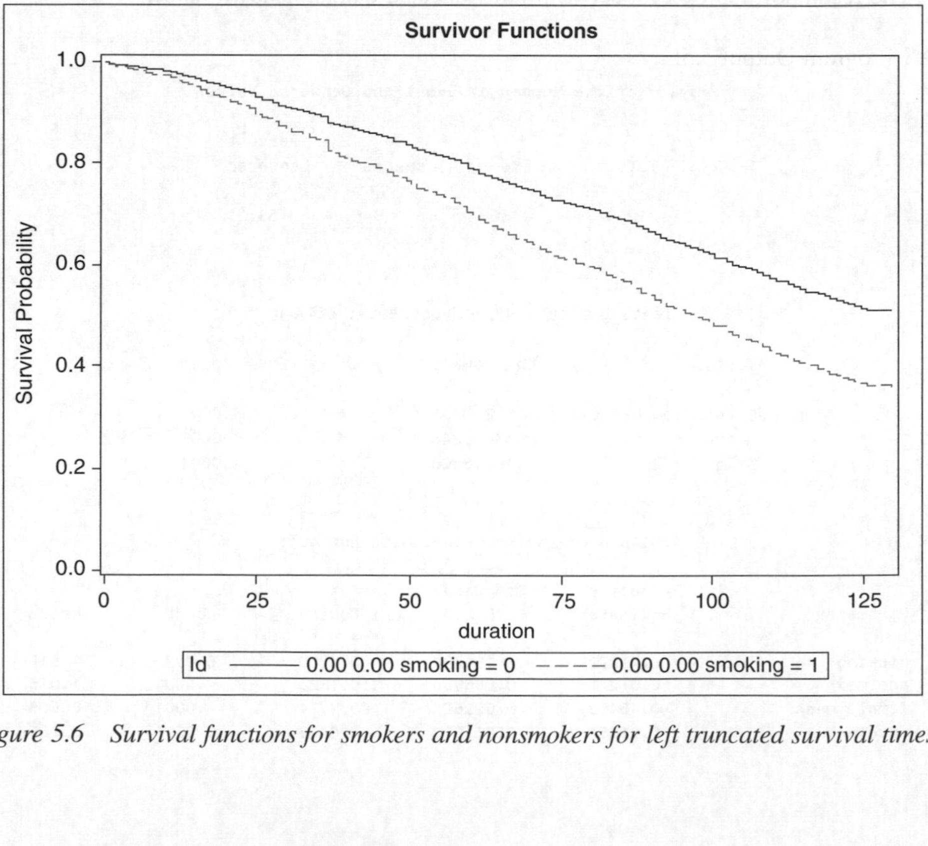

Figure 5.6 Survival functions for smokers and nonsmokers for left truncated survival times.

It may be useful to present the influence of left truncation on estimating the hazard function by using the stratified Cox model. To illustrate this influence, I create a stratification factor 'NOT_MARRIED_NEW,' with 1 = 'becoming unmarried after t_0' and 0 = 'unmarried at baseline.' The first group is left truncated, whereas the second is a regular right censored subsample. I first estimate a Cox model stratifying on this new variable without adjusting for left truncation. If left truncation impacts on the estimation of the Cox model, the survival curve for those becoming married after t_0 will tend to be relatively flat because those with left truncation times exceeding t values are all included in the risk set at t_i. Accordingly, this survival curve would deviate markedly from the survival curve for those unmarried at baseline. The SAS program for this stratified Cox model is presented below.

SAS Program 5.8:

```
......
if married1 ne 0 and not_married = 1 then not_married_new = 1;
  else if married1 = 0 then not_married_new = 0;
  else not_married_new = .;
......
proc phreg data = new ; where not_married = 1 ;
  model duration*Status(0) = smoking_mean age_mean female_mean educ_mean / ties =
    BRESLOW ;
  strata not_married_new ;
  baseline out = graph loglogs = lls survival = s ;
run;

proc gplot data = graph;
  plot lls * duration;
  Title "Figure 5.7. Log minus log plot of old and new singles";
  symbol1 interpol = join color = black line = 1;
  symbol2 interpol = join color = black line = 2;
run;
```

In SAS Program 5.8, I first create the stratification factor 'NOT_MARRIED_NEW' according to the above classification. When this variablc is 1, the survival time is left truncated because the individual has to survive to a given time point, later than t_0, when he or she becomes unmarried. The MODEL statement is conventional, thus indicating the partial likelihood function unadjusted. Given the STRATA NOT_MARRIED_NEW statement, SAS Program 5.8 generates two log–log survival curves in one plot, one for those unmarried at baseline and one for those who become unmarried later than the baseline survey and therefore left truncated. Figure 5.7 displays the result, with two log–log survival curves for those unmarried at baseline and those who become unmarried in later times. The left, upper log–log curve comes from the right censored subsample who are unmarried at baseline and thus unbiased, whereas the right, lower curve derives from the left truncated data. As can be well recognized, for those becoming unmarried after the baseline survey, the cumulative hazard rate prior to month 24 is 0 because all of them have to survive to at least 24 months later to be identified as a 'newly unmarried.' As those with left truncation times exceeding t values are mistakenly included in the risk sets, the underestimation of the log–log survival function for the left truncated stratum is obvious. The two log–log curves are uncommonly separated to an unexpected extent and the curve for the left truncated group looks strangely rectangularized. Without adjusting for left truncation,

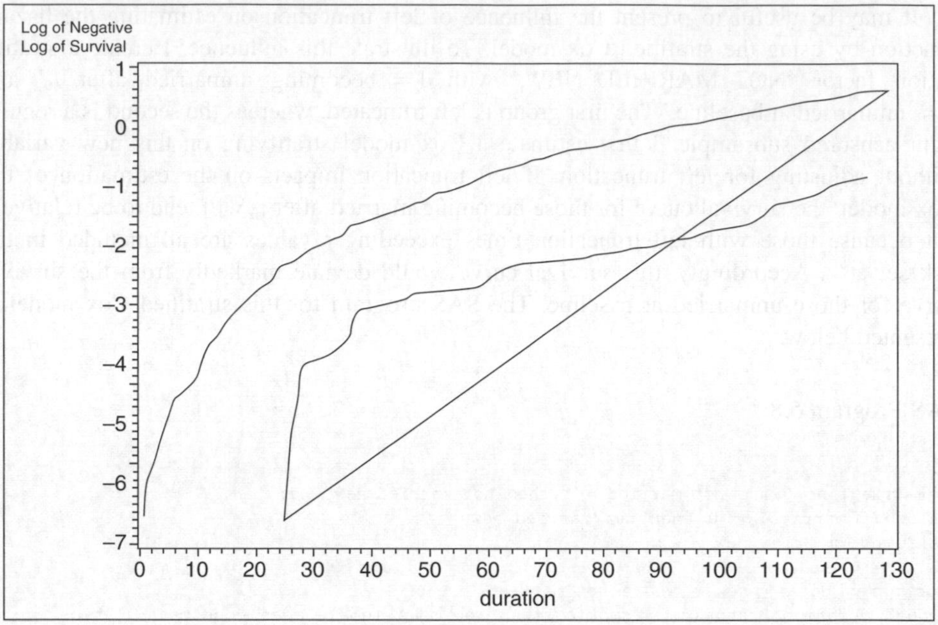

Figure 5.7 Log–log plot of old and new singles.

therefore, the application of the Cox model would inevitably yield erroneous survival differences.

To correct for the bias from left truncation, the following SAS program excludes those whose left truncation times exceed t values from the risk sets.

SAS Program 5.9:

```
......
proc phreg data = new ; where not_married = 1 ;
  model duration*Status(0) = smoking_mean female_mean educ_mean / entry = t1 ;
  strata not_married_new ;
  baseline out = graph loglogs = lls survival = s ;
run;

proc gplot data = graph;
  plot lls * duration;
  Title "Figure 5.8. Adjusted log minus log plot of unmarried persons";
  symbol1 interpol = join color = black line = 1;
  symbol2 interpol = join color = black line = 2;
run;
```

SAS Program 5.9 specifies that any contribution to the partial likelihood must satisfy the condition that the truncation time has been exceeded. Consequently, the selection bias caused by left truncation is corrected. Figure 5.8 demonstrates the result of such correction and shows that underestimation of the relative risk is corrected after taking the delayed entry into consideration. Now, the event time T and the left truncation time $\tilde{v}$ appear independent of each other, agreeing with the general belief. The two log–log survival curves now appear

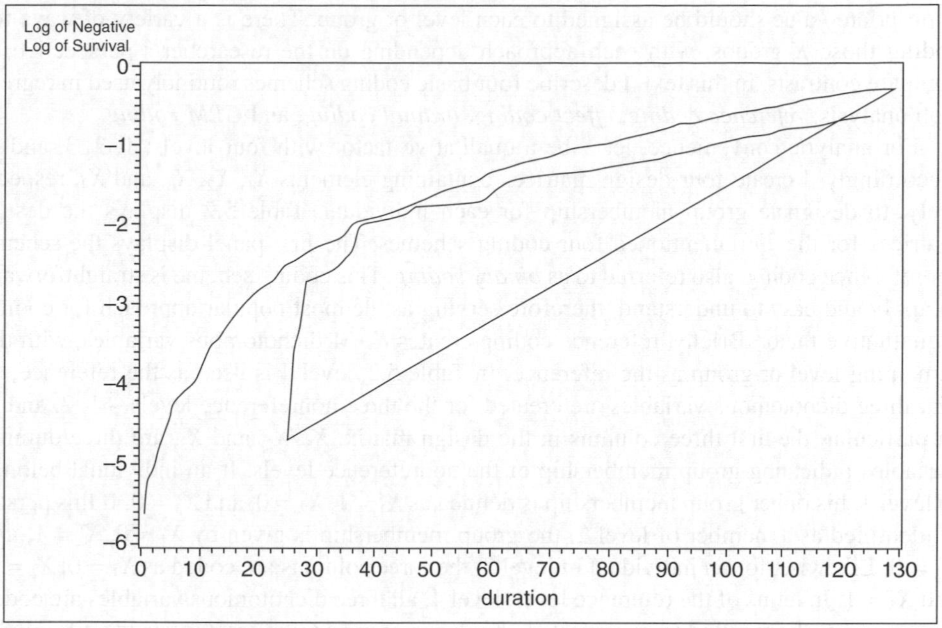

Figure 5.8 Adjusted log–log plot of unmarried persons.

parallel following the same survival pattern, except for the first 24 months, where the risk of dying for those becoming unmarried at later waves is 0.

5.7 Qualitative factors and local tests

In conducting a regression analysis, researchers often need to examine the effects of qualitative factors, represented by two or more nominal categories. For a dichotomous covariate, testing its effect on a lifetime outcome variable can be performed simply by looking at the estimated regression coefficient, the standard error, and the *p*-value. For a qualitative factor with more than two categories, however, just examining the results of the global tests does not provide an entire answer to the question on its effect because the factor involves a subset of $\boldsymbol{x}$, rather than a single variable. As qualitative factors are frequently used as covariates in survival analysis, it is essential for the reader to comprehend statistical techniques and estimating procedures of local tests in the Cox model.

This section first introduces several basic coding schemes for creating a qualitative factor taking more than two values. Then I describe statistical inference for local tests on the statistical significance of the estimated regression coefficients associated with a single qualitative factor. Lastly, an empirical illustration is provided on the effects of four educational groups on the mortality of older Americans, treating educational attainment as a qualitative factor.

5.7.1 Qualitative factors and scaling approaches

When a qualitative factor with K categories ($K > 2$) is used as a predictor in the Cox model, first this factor needs to be classified into K mutually exclusive levels or groups and then an appropriate value should be assigned to each level or group. There is a variety of ways for coding those K groups, with each approach depending on the researcher's perspective to compare contrasts. In this text, I describe four basic coding schemes routinely used in regression analysis: *reference coding*, *effect coding*, *ordinal coding*, and *GLM coding*.

For analytic convenience, let X be a qualitative factor with four levels: 1, 2, 3, and 4. Accordingly, I create four design matrices containing elements X_1, X_2, X_3, and X_4, respectively, to designate group membership for each individual. Table 5.2 displays the design matrices for the aforementioned four coding schemes. The first panel displays the scheme for reference coding, also referred to as *binary coding*. This coding scheme is straightforward to apply and easy to understand, therefore serving as the most popular approach for coding a qualitative factor. Briefly, reference coding creates $K - 1$ dichotomous variables, with the remaining level or group as the reference. In Table 5.2, level 4 is used as the reference, so that three dichotomous variables are created for the three nonreference levels – 1, 2, and 3. In particular, the first three columns in the design matrix, X_1, X_2, and X_3, are three dummy variables indicating group membership of the nonreference levels. If an individual belongs to level 1, his or her group membership is defined as $X_1 = 1, X_2 = 0$, and $X_3 = 0$. If this person is identified as a member of level 2, the group membership is given by $X_1 = 0, X_2 = 1$, and $X_3 = 0$. Likewise, for an individual in level 3, the three columns are coded as $X_1 = 0, X_2 = 0$, and $X_3 = 1$. In terms of the reference level, level 4, all three dichotomous variables are coded 0. Therefore, the fourth dummy variable, X_4, does not need to be created for identifying the

Table 5.2 Coding schemes for classification factor ***X***.

Group in X	Design matrix			
	X_1	X_2	X_3	X_4
Reference coding				
1	1	0	0	—
2	0	1	0	—
3	0	0	1	—
4	0	0	0	—
Effect coding				
1	1	0	0	—
2	0	1	0	—
3	0	0	1	—
4	−1	−1	−1	—
Ordinal coding				
1	0	0	0	—
2	1	0	0	—
3	1	1	0	—
4	1	1	1	—
GLM coding				
1	1	0	0	0
2	0	1	0	0
3	0	0	1	0
4	0	0	0	1

membership of the reference group. Within the construct of this coding scheme, the estimated regression coefficient of X_1, X_2, or X_3 estimates the main effect of each nonreference group relative to the effect of the reference level. In the Cox model, for example, a hazard ratio of 1.5 for X_1 indicates that members in group 1 are 1.5 times as likely to experience a particular event as those in level 4, other covariates being equal. Additionally, the difference between two of those estimated regression coefficients displays the main effect of one nonreference membership relative to the other.

The second panel in Table 5.2 presents the scheme for effect coding. This coding scheme is analogous to reference coding, except the code for the reference group. Three dichotomous variables are created for the three nonreference levels 1, 2, and 3, in the same fashion as reference coding. For the reference group, all three dichotomous variables are coded −1, instead of 0. Therefore, the fourth dummy variable, X_4, does not need to be specified for effect coding either. Given this coding scheme, the estimated regression coefficient of X_1, X_2, or X_3 estimates the difference in the main effect of each nonreference group relative to the average effect of all four levels. Consider the Cox model again: a hazard ratio of 1.5 for X_1, given effect coding, indicates an average member in group 1 to be 1.5 times as likely to experience a particular event as is expected for the whole population.

The third coding scheme presented in Table 5.2 is ordinal coding. Under this coding scheme, all three dummy variables are coded 0 for the membership of level 1, used as a control level. With one level up, the value of 1 is added to the membership code successively; as a result, a member in level 4 is assigned to value 1 for each of X_1, X_2, or X_3. Like the above two coding schemes, the fourth dummy variable, X_4, does not need to be created for ordinal coding. The estimated regression coefficient of X_1, X_2, or X_3, using ordinal coding, displays the effect difference between two successive levels. For example, a hazard ratio of 1.5 for X_3 suggests an average member in group 3 to be 1.5 times as likely to experience a particular event as those of level 2, other covariates being equal.

The last coding scheme is used in general linear regression modeling, as its name readily indicates. It is the only coding scheme presented in Table 5.2 that requires a code for the fourth dummy variable. Codes for the first three design matrices are analogous to the reference or effect coding scheme, with the value 1 assigned to a member of the fourth level. Using this coding scheme, the main effect for each of the first three dummy variables presents the effect difference between a nonreference group and the reference level. Operationally, the GLM coding scheme is a reference cell coding, deriving exactly the same estimates of the main effects as the reference coding.

There are some more complicated coding schemes, such as orthogonal contrast coding and polynomial coding. The orthogonal contrast coding is widely used in sociological and economic studies, applied for testing some specific uncorrelated hypotheses by creating uncorrelated variables for a qualitative factor. Statisticians have also developed some mathematically oriented orthogonalization schemes to account for multicollinearity incurred from correlation among multiple covariates for a particular qualitative factor. For more details on those complicated coding schemes, the interest reader is referred to Davis (2010), Hardy and Reynolds (2004), and SAS (2009).

5.7.2 Local tests

In the Cox model, the local tests are based on the null hypothesis on a subset of the coefficient vector $\boldsymbol{\beta}$ with null hypothesis H_0: $\boldsymbol{\beta}_a = \mathbf{0}$, where $\boldsymbol{\beta} = (\boldsymbol{\beta}_a', \boldsymbol{\beta}_b')'$. Specifically, $\boldsymbol{\beta}_a$ is defined as a $\hat{q}\times 1$ vector of β values and, accordingly, $\boldsymbol{\beta}_b$ is an $(M-\hat{q})\times 1$ vector containing coefficients of the remaining covariates.

Analogous to inference for the global test, the local test on the above null hypothesis uses the estimates derived from maximization of the partial likelihood function. Let $\hat{\boldsymbol{\beta}}=\left(\hat{\boldsymbol{\beta}}_a',\hat{\boldsymbol{\beta}}_b'\right)'$ be the decomposed maximum likelihood estimator of $\boldsymbol{\beta}$. Accordingly, the information matrix $\boldsymbol{I}\left(\hat{\boldsymbol{\beta}}\right)$ can also be partitioned into

$$\boldsymbol{I}\left(\hat{\boldsymbol{\beta}}\right)=-\begin{pmatrix}\boldsymbol{I}_{11} & \boldsymbol{I}_{12}\\ \boldsymbol{I}_{21} & \boldsymbol{I}_{22}\end{pmatrix}, \tag{5.65}$$

where $\boldsymbol{I}_{11}$ is the $\hat{q}\times\hat{q}$ submatrix of the second partial derivative of the minus log likelihood with respect to $\boldsymbol{\beta}_a$, $\boldsymbol{I}_{22}$ is the $(M-\hat{q})\times(M-\hat{q})$ submatrix of the second derivatives with respect to $\boldsymbol{\beta}_b$, and $\boldsymbol{I}_{12}$ and $\boldsymbol{I}_{21}$ are the matrices of mixed second derivatives.

Given Equation (5.65), the Wald test can be used with respect to $\hat{\boldsymbol{\beta}}_a$, given by

$$\chi^2_{\text{Wald}}=\left(\hat{\boldsymbol{\beta}}_a\right)'\left[\boldsymbol{I}_{11}\left(\hat{\boldsymbol{\beta}}_a\right)\right]^{-1}\left(\hat{\boldsymbol{\beta}}_a\right). \tag{5.66}$$

Given the large-sample approximation theory, this statistic is distributed as chi-square with $\hat{q}$ degrees of freedom under the null hypothesis; therefore H_0: $\boldsymbol{\beta}_a=\mathbf{0}$ can be statistically tested, given the value of $\chi^2_{(1-\alpha;q)}$.

Similarly, the other two test statistics can be readily defined for the local test on $\hat{\boldsymbol{\beta}}_a$. Let $\hat{\boldsymbol{\beta}}_b(\mathbf{0})$ be the partial maximum likelihood estimates of $\boldsymbol{\beta}_b$ with values in $\boldsymbol{\beta}_a$ all set at 0. The partial likelihood ratio test on H_0: $\boldsymbol{\beta}_a=\mathbf{0}$ is then given by

$$\chi^2_{\text{LR}}=2\left\{\left[\log L_p\left(\hat{\boldsymbol{\beta}}\right)\right]-\log L_p\left[\mathbf{0},\hat{\boldsymbol{\beta}}_b\left(\boldsymbol{\beta}_a=\mathbf{0}\right)\right]\right\}, \tag{5.67}$$

which also has a chi-square distribution with $\hat{q}$ degrees of freedom. Given the critical value of $\chi^2_{\text{LR},\alpha}$, the null hypothesis that $\boldsymbol{\beta}_a=\mathbf{0}$ can be tested by the partial likelihood ratio statistic described in Section 5.1.

In terms of the score statistic, let $\tilde{\boldsymbol{U}}_a\left[\mathbf{0},\hat{\boldsymbol{\beta}}_b\left(\boldsymbol{\beta}_a=\mathbf{0}\right)\right]$ be the $\hat{q}\times 1$ vector of scores for $\boldsymbol{\beta}_a$, evaluated at the hypothesized values of $\boldsymbol{\beta}_a=\mathbf{0}$ and at the restricted partial maximum likelihood estimator for $\boldsymbol{\beta}_b$. Then the score statistic is

$$\chi^2_{\text{SC}}=\tilde{\boldsymbol{U}}_a\left[\mathbf{0},\hat{\boldsymbol{\beta}}_b\left(\boldsymbol{\beta}_a=\mathbf{0}\right)\right]'\left\{\boldsymbol{I}_{11}\left[\mathbf{0},\hat{\boldsymbol{\beta}}_b\left(\boldsymbol{\beta}_a=\mathbf{0}\right)\right]\right\}^{-1}\tilde{\boldsymbol{U}}_a\left[\mathbf{0},\hat{\boldsymbol{\beta}}_b\left(\boldsymbol{\beta}_a=\mathbf{0}\right)\right], \tag{5.68}$$

which, like the other two test statistics, has a large-sample chi-square distribution with $\hat{q}$ degrees of freedom under the null hypothesis. Clearly, a local test on a subset of the coefficient vector $\boldsymbol{\beta}$ is simply the localized realization of the global test (Klein and Moeschberger, 2003).

Attaching to a specific coding scheme, local tests can be performed using a linear combination of parameters. For the Wald test, for example, a matrix of $\hat{q}$ linear combinations can be applied to test the null hypothesis with respect to $\boldsymbol{\beta}_a$. Let $\tilde{\boldsymbol{C}}$ be a vector of contrasts for the ith linear combination of $\boldsymbol{\beta}$ with elements $(c_{i1}, c_{i2}, \ldots, c_{iM})$. The null hypothesis is given by

$$\text{H}_0:\tilde{\boldsymbol{C}}'\boldsymbol{\beta}=\mathbf{0}. \tag{5.69}$$

From the large-sample theory, the Wald test statistic can be written as

$$\left(\tilde{C}'\hat{\beta}\right)'\left[\tilde{C}I^{-1}\left(\hat{\beta}\right)\tilde{C}'\right]^{-1}\left(\tilde{C}'\hat{\beta}\right), \tag{5.70}$$

which is distributed asymptotically as chi-square under the null hypothesis, as mentioned above.

Consider, for example, the qualitative factor with four levels, described above. After applying the reference coding scheme, three dummy variables are created – X_1, X_2, and X_3 (level 4 is used as the reference group, so X_4 does not need to be specified). The application of the Cox model generates the estimates of the main effects of those three dichotomous variables, denoted by b_1, b_2, and b_3, respectively, together with a robust variance–covariance estimator matrix. Suppose that I want to test the null hypothesis on the contrast between b_1 and b_3, given by H_0: $b_1 = b_3$. Then Equation (5.70) can be applied to test the statistical significance of this contrast, given by

$$\chi^2_W = \frac{(b_1 - b_3)^2}{\hat{V}(b_1) + \hat{V}(b_3) - 2\text{cov}(b_1 b_3)},$$

which has a chi-square distribution with one degree of freedom under the null hypothesis. Given the value of α, the significance of the contrast between b_1 and b_3 can be evaluated. Significance tests for other contrasts can be conducted in the same fashion.

5.7.3 Illustration of local tests: Educational attainment and the mortality of older Americans

In previous illustrations, I assume the effects of an older American's educational attainment to be a continuous function on mortality. On certain occasions, it may be more interesting to examine the variation in the death rate by several well-defined educational groups, classifying years of education into distinct categories. In this illustration, I specify educational attainment as a qualitative factor, categorizing older Americans into four educational groups – middle school or lower, high school, college, and higher than college. Here, I want to examine the associations of these four educational levels with the mortality of older Americans, using survival information from the baseline survey to the end of 2004. The null hypothesis of this analysis is that the mortality rate in each of these four educational groups does not differ from any of the others.

Of 2000 older persons in the dataset, 480 are identified as middle school graduates or lower, 944 received education in high school, 457 were in college, and the remaining 119 persons had an education level higher than college. Accordingly, I create a qualitative factor of educational attainment, named 'Educ_group,' with 1 = middle school or lower, 2 = high school, 3 = college, and 4 = more than college. Then this factor is included in the Cox model to replace the continuous variable 'Educ.' Three centered covariates, 'Married_mean,' 'Age_mean,' and 'Female_mean,' are used as control variables in the analysis. Below is the SAS program for estimating this proportional hazard model.

SAS Program 5.10:

```
......
if educ < 9 then educ_group = 1;
  else if educ < 13 then educ_group = 2;
  else if educ < 17 then educ_group = 3;
  else educ_group = 4;
```

```
proc phreg data = new ;
 class educ_group ;
 model duration*Status(0) = educ_group married_mean age_mean female_mean ;
run;
```

In SAS Program 5.10, I first create the variable 'Educ_group,' using the classification indicated earlier. In the PROC PHREG procedure, the CLASS EDUC_GROUP statement specifies the variable 'Educ_group' as a classification factor, with its effects on the mortality modeled as the regression coefficients of three dichotomous covariates. As reference coding is applied as default in the SAS PROC PHREG procedure, the highest value of Educ_group, representing 'higher than college,' is used as the reference level. The following output tables display some of the results from SAS Program 5.10.

SAS Program Output 5.6:

Class Level Information

Class	Value	Design Variables		
educ_group	1	1	0	0
	2	0	1	0
	3	0	0	1
	4	0	0	0

Testing Global Null Hypothesis: BETA=0

Test	Chi-Square	DF	Pr > ChiSq
Likelihood Ratio	333.8392	6	<.0001
Score	316.2930	6	<.0001
Wald	324.8221	6	<.0001

Type 3 Tests

Effect	DF	Wald Chi-Square	Pr > ChiSq
educ_group	3	9.4744	0.0236
married_mean	1	12.2753	0.0005
age_mean	1	199.5799	<.0001
female_mean	1	60.0868	<.0001

Analysis of Maximum Likelihood Estimates

Parameter		DF	Parameter Estimate	Standard Error	Chi-Square	Pr > ChiSq	Hazard Ratio	Label
educ_group	1	1	0.43256	0.16908	6.5449	0.0105	1.541	educ_group 1
educ_group	2	1	0.47551	0.16408	8.3987	0.0038	1.609	educ_group 2
educ_group	3	1	0.35007	0.17176	4.1541	0.0415	1.419	educ_group 3
married_mean		1	-0.26381	0.07530	12.2753	0.0005	0.768	
age_mean		1	0.07791	0.00552	199.5799	<.0001	1.081	
female_mean		1	-0.56012	0.07226	60.0868	<.0001	0.571	

In SAS Program Output 5.6, the Class Level Information section indicates the use of reference coding, with group 4 as the reference level. All three tests in the 'Testing Global Null Hypothesis: BETA = **0**' section demonstrate that the null hypothesis $\hat{\boldsymbol{\beta}} = \mathbf{0}$ should be rejected. The 'Type 3 Tests' table shows that the qualitative factor 'Educ_group' is locally statistically significant; that is, at least two of the four educational groups differ significantly in the mortality rate, other covariates being equal.

In the table of 'Analysis of Maximum Likelihood Estimates,' all the regression coefficients of the three dichotomous variables for 'Educ_group' are statistically significant, with each hazard ratio considerably greater than 1 (1.54, 1.61, and 1.42, respectively). These hazard coefficients and the hazard ratios suggest that members in each of the lower three educational groups are expected to have significantly higher mortality rates than those with an education higher than college. The three regression coefficients, however, differ slightly among themselves. The regression coefficients of the three control variables are all statistically significant, with values close to those previously reported.

Before proceeding with the local test on the contrasts of the three estimated regression coefficients, it is necessary to consider whether the effects of educational attainment depend on some other covariates. The presence of a significant interaction would change the test procedure tremendously and complicate the interpretation of the analytic results. In this analysis, I want to check whether education effects are uniform between currently married and currently not married persons. To test this interactive effect, marital status needs to be specified as a classification factor in the Cox model. Therefore, instead of using the centered covariate 'Married_mean,' I use the dichotomous variable 'Married' to construct an interaction term between education and marital status. Below is the SAS program, using Educ_group, Married, Educ_group × Married, and the two remaining control variables as covariates.

SAS Program 5.11:

```
......
proc phreg data = new ;
  class educ_group married ;
  model duration*Status(0) = educ_group married educ_group*married age_mean
     female_mean ;
run;
```

The CLASS statement now specifies two classification factors – Educ_group and Married. An interaction term between Educ_group and Married is created for assessing whether the effects of an older person's education on mortality depends on marital status. Consequently, three additional regression coefficients are estimated, presented below.

SAS Program Output 5.7:

```
                    The PHREG Procedure

           Testing Global Null Hypothesis: BETA=0

            Test                 Chi-Square    DF    Pr > ChiSq

            Likelihood Ratio       337.3597     9        <.0001
            Score                  319.9922     9        <.0001
            Wald                   326.8846     9        <.0001


              Analysis of Maximum Likelihood Estimates

                                    Parameter     Standard
Parameter                     DF     Estimate        Error    Chi-Square    Pr > ChiSq

educ_group           1         1      0.37332      0.20789        3.2247        0.0725
educ_group           2         1      0.30891      0.19595        2.4855        0.1149
educ_group           3         1      0.16471      0.20630        0.6374        0.4246
married              0         1     -0.17407      0.35442        0.2412        0.6233
educ_group*married 1 0         1      0.31359      0.37437        0.7016        0.4022
educ_group*married 2 0         1      0.49307      0.36517        1.8231        0.1769
educ_group*married 3 0         1      0.54644      0.38008        2.0669        0.1505
age_mean                       1      0.07802      0.00552      200.0903        <.0001
female_mean                    1     -0.56000      0.07252       59.6225        <.0001
```

In SAS Program Output 5.7, values of all three tests in the 'Testing Global Null Hypothesis: BETA = **0**' section are very close to those in the model without the interaction term. For example, the chi-square of the partial likelihood ratio test here is 337.36 with 9 degrees of freedom, compared to 333.84 with 6 degrees of freedom estimated for the model without the interaction. Obviously, the difference in the partial likelihood ratio statistic between the two Cox models is not statistically significant with 3 degrees of freedom (337.36 − 333.84 = 3.52; $p > 0.10$). The other two tests, the score and the Wald, yield the same testing results.

In the table of 'Analysis of Maximum Likelihood Estimates,' none of the three estimated regression coefficients for the interaction term between education and marital status is statistically significant. Furthermore, with three additional covariates, the regression coefficients of the three nonreference educational groups are not statistically significant, an indication of model misspecification compared to the estimates derived from the previous model. Consequently, the Cox model without the interaction is a better choice.

Given the results on statistical significance of the interaction between education and marital status, now I can comfortably perform the local tests on the coefficient contrasts among the three lower educational groups. The following SAS program is provided for this step.

SAS Program 5.12:

```
......
proc phreg data = new ;
  class educ_group ;
  model duration*Status(0)  = educ_group married_mean age_mean female_mean  ;
```

```
  contrast 'Middle school vs High School' educ_group 1 -1 ;
  contrast 'Middle School vs College' educ_group 1 0 -1 ;
  contrast 'High school vs College' educ_group 0 1 -1 ;
run;
```

In SAS Program 5.12, I use the CONTRAST statement to perform local tests on three null hypotheses: (1) H_0: $b_1 - b_2 = 0$; (2) H_0: $b_1 - b_3 = 0$; and (3) H_0: $b_2 - b_3 = 0$. I specify three contrasts – 'middle school' versus 'high school,' 'middle school' versus 'college,' and 'high school' versus 'college.' The point estimates of the three relative risks are $\exp(0.4755 - 0.4326) = 1.04$, $\exp(0.3501 - 0.4326) = 0.92$, and $\exp(0.3501 - 0.4755) = 0.88$, respectively. While the partial likelihood ratio test and the Wald statistic can both be applied for testing the three null hypotheses, the asymptotic chi-square distribution of the Wald statistic is used in SAS, with results displayed below.

SAS Program Output 5.8:

Contrast Test Results

Contrast	DF	Wald Chi-Square	Pr > ChiSq
Middle school vs High school	1	0.2923	0.5888
Middle school vs College	1	0.7465	0.3876
High school vs College	1	2.1534	0.1423

SAS Program Output 5.8 demonstrates that none of the three contrasts is statistically significant. It is now safe to conclude that while members in the lower three educational groups each have significantly higher mortality than those with an education higher than college, there are no distinct differences among themselves, other covariates being equal.

5.8 Summary

The Cox model, including the original perspective and later advancements, is the most widely applied regression models in survival analysis. Because of its simplicity, robustness, and efficiency, the Cox model becomes a very popular means to analyze the effects of covariates on the hazard function. Given the proportional hazards assumption, the application of this model has almost covered all applied disciplines, ranging from clinical trials to criminological research, from the analysis of social networks to studies of health services utilization. The development of various refined methods, such as time-dependent covariates and the stratified proportional hazard model, further widens the applicability of the Cox model, particularly in situations where the proportionality assumption in the Cox model is violated.

According to some researchers, one distinct limitation of the Cox model is the restriction of sample size. As the partial likelihood function is essentially based on the number of events, the application of the Cox model requires a much larger sample size than does a parametric regression model, particularly when categorical covariates are used or when an event of interest does not occur frequently. Therefore, the Cox model is thought not to be highly suitable for analyzing survival data with a small sample size or for dynamic events that rarely take place. Andersen, Bentzon, and Klein (1996) contend, however, that the Cox model can produce reliable estimates of survival probabilities with a small sample size. Through a Monte Carlo simulation study, these authors conclude that even with a sample size of 50 and with 25–50 % censoring, the Cox model still performs well and fits the survival data pretty nicely.

In some special situations, the use of parametric survival models is preferred (Allison, 2010; Johansen, 1983). Some advanced techniques in survival analysis, like structural equation modeling, need statistical information on the variation in the baseline hazard function. For example, with the addition or the elimination of one or more covariates, the added or purged effects are not only reflected in the estimated regression coefficients but they may also cause a change in the value of the intercept. Obviously, the Cox model cannot derive such a structural change, thereby making it difficult to derive additional estimators. In these circumstances, a parametric regression model with a complete likelihood function, like the Weibull proportional hazard model, can be used to replace the Cox model, as will be discussed further in Chapter 8.

6

Counting processes and diagnostics of the Cox model

As described in Chapter 5, maximization of the partial likelihood function derives efficient, robust, and consistent estimates of the coefficient vector $\boldsymbol{\beta}$ in the Cox model. In essence, the Cox model describes a stochastic counting process of survival over time without referring to an underlying probability distribution. As a result, it offers a flexible perspective for further advancement of survival models. More recently, some statisticians have solidified the Cox model by developing a unique counting system, referred to as *counting processes*, combining elements in the large sample theory, the martingale theory, and the stochastic integration theory (Aalen, 1975; Andersen *et al.*, 1993; Andersen and Gill, 1982; Fleming and Harrington, 1991). This counting process approach, given its tremendous flexibility and the attachment to the traditional probability theory, provides a powerful tool to describe some complex stochastic processes in survival analysis, such as regression residuals of the proportional hazard model and the occurrence of repeated events.

Once the Cox model is fitted with survival data, regression diagnostics are necessary for verifying whether the statistical model fits the data appropriately or meets the proportional hazards assumption. In linear regression models, such assessment of model adequacy is generally focused on checking linearity, normality, homogeneity of variance, independence of errors, and the like. With respect to survival analysis, regression diagnostics become more complicated because an individual's hazard rate is regression derived without an observed value, and heavy censoring regularly exists in survival data. Some general principles in this area, however, are universal for all regression models, and the Cox model is no exception. Standard diagnostic techniques, such as deviation of the expected value from the observed, the overall model fitness, and identification of influential observations, also need to be performed in survival analysis. Through certain functional transformations, advanced methods of regression diagnostics have been developed and used in the Cox model, with some applying formulations of counting processes.

In this chapter, I first introduce basic specifications of counting processes and the martingale theory. Then five types of residuals in the Cox model are described, which is

Survival Analysis: Models and Applications, First Edition. Xian Liu.

followed by three sections on, respectively, assessment of the proportional hazards assumption, inspection of the functional form for a covariate, and identification of influential observations from results of the Cox model, with each giving an empirical illustration. Lastly, I summarize the chapter with comments on these extended techniques attaching to the Cox model.

6.1 Counting processes and the martingale theory

As it provides a highly flexible and powerful counting system, counting processes and the martingale theory have seen increasing popularity in the past two decades. Inevitably, therefore, the counting process formulation is occasionally used in this book when I describe certain martingale-type techniques, as is seen in much of this chapter and some of the later chapters. This section provides a brief introduction of this unique counting system. In particular, I first describe the basic formulation of counting processes and then present specifications of the martingale theory and the martingale central limit theorems. Lastly, I respecify the Cox model and the partial likelihood inference with the counting process formulation for helping the reader further comprehend this system. To describe counting processes and martingales accurately, I use the original mathematical notations and functions specific to this work as much as possible. For the mathematical notations or symbols applied previously for other mathematical and statistical concepts or functions, I use the regular, nonitalicized fonts to avoid notational confusion.

6.1.1 Counting processes

In the Cox model, survival processes are expressed as a function of three key lifetime indicators – t_i, δ_i, and $\boldsymbol{x}_i$. Analogous to such expressions, a survival event in counting processes is formulated as following a triple $\{\mathrm{N}_i(t), \mathrm{Y}_i(t), \mathbf{Z}_i(t)\}$ of counting paths. Specifically, the nonitalicized $\mathrm{N}_i(t)$ is the number of observed events in (0, t), defined as

$$\mathrm{N}_i(t) = \mathrm{I}(T_i \le t, \delta_i = 1), \tag{6.1}$$

where δ_i is the 0/1 (1 = event, 0 = censored) censoring indicator as previously defined; in the counting process formulation, it can be written as

$$\delta_i(t) = \mathrm{I}(T_i \le C_i).$$

As a count variable, $\mathrm{N}_i(t)$ is specified as a right-continuous and piecewise constant step function, with jumps of size +1. Given a single event, it is defined as a stochastic process with $\mathrm{N}(0) = 0$ and $\mathrm{N}(t) < \infty$, with probability summing to one. Consequently,

$$\mathrm{N}(t) = \sum_i \mathrm{N}_i(t) = \sum_{t_i \le t} \delta_i$$

The count Y in the triple denotes the number at risk just before t for failing in the interval (t, t + dt), given by

$$\mathrm{Y}_i(t) = \mathrm{I}\{\tilde{T}_i \ge t\}, \tag{6.2}$$

where $Y_i(t)$ is a left-continuous process and

$$\tilde{T}_i = \min\{T_i, C_i\}.$$

Therefore,

$$\mathrm{Y}(t) = \sum_i \mathrm{Y}_i(t)$$

is the number of individuals at risk at t. The last component in the triple, $\mathbf{Z}$, is the covariate vector, equivalent to $\boldsymbol{x}$ in the Cox model. In counting processes, it is often specified as time dependent, written as $\mathbf{Z}(t)$.

Given the above specifications, counting processes are based on the prior history about survival, censoring, and covariates, referred to as a *filtration*, denoted by $\{\mathcal{F}_t; t \geq 0\}$. Mathematically, $\{\mathcal{F}_t; t \geq 0\}$ is the sub-σ-algebra of the σ-algebra $\mathcal{F}$, continuous if $\mathcal{F}_{t+} = \mathcal{F}_t$:

$$\mathcal{F}_t = \sigma\{\mathrm{N}_i(\mathrm{s}), \mathrm{Y}_i(\mathrm{s}+), \mathbf{Z}_i(\mathrm{s}), i = 1, \ldots, n; 0 \leq \mathrm{s} \leq t\}, \quad t > 0, \tag{6.3}$$

where the nonitalicized $\sigma\{\cdot\}$ is the *sigma algebra* generated from the random processes specified in the brace.

The corresponding limit of $\mathcal{F}_t$ from the left is referred to as $\mathcal{F}_{t-}$, defined as the σ-algebra generated by the stochastic process $\{\mathrm{N}(t), \mathrm{Y}(t), \mathbf{Z}(t)\}$ on $[0, t)$. In other words, $\mathcal{F}_{t-}$ indicates the values of $\tilde{T}_i$ and δ_i for all i values such that $\tilde{T}_i < t$, or otherwise just the information that $\tilde{T}_i \geq t$ (Andersen *et al.*, 1993). Note that for any $\mathrm{s} \leq t$, $\mathcal{F}_\mathrm{s} \subset \mathcal{F}_t$, so that $\mathcal{F}$ is increasing.

Let T and C be nonnegative, independent random variables and T is a continuous function; thus its distribution has a density. Given $F(t) = \mathrm{P}\{T \leq t\}$ and $S(t) = 1 - F(t)$ (note that F and $\mathcal{F}$ are different functions), the intensity function at t, denoted by $\lambda(t)$, is defined as

$$\lambda(t) = \lim_{\Delta t \to 0} \frac{\Pr\{t \leq T < t + \Delta t | T \geq t, C \geq T\}}{\Delta t}. \tag{6.4}$$

Clearly, the intensity function in the counting processes formulation, given a single event, is equivalent to the hazard function given that T is independent of C.

Given a limited time interval $[0, \tau)$ where $\tau < \infty$ is a fixed value, the intensity function for individual i at t can be expressed as the probability of an increment in N_i over the infinitesimal time interval $[t, t + \mathrm{d}t)$ conditional on the process history just prior to t:

$$\lambda(t)\mathrm{d}t = \Pr\{\mathrm{dN}(t)\} = \mathrm{E}\{\mathrm{dN}(t) | \mathcal{F}_{t-}\}, \tag{6.5}$$

where $\mathrm{dN}_i(t)$ is the infinitesimal change in the process $\mathrm{N}(t)$ over $[t, t + \mathrm{d}t)$. Assuming no ties, $\mathrm{dN}_i(t) = 1$ for event occurrence and $\mathrm{dN}_i(t) = 0$ otherwise. Therefore, the intensity function acts as a random variable through dependence on the random variables in $\mathcal{F}_{t-}$.

Because the value of $\mathrm{Y}_i(t)$, 0 or 1, is the discrete realization of the σ-algebra $\mathcal{F}_{t-}$ for individual i, Equation (6.5) can be written as

$$\begin{aligned} \mathrm{E}\{\mathrm{dN}_i(t) | \mathcal{F}_{t-}\} &= \mathrm{E}\{\mathrm{dN}_i(t) | \mathrm{Y}_i(t)\} \\ &= \Pr\{t \leq T_i < t + \mathrm{d}t,\ C_i \geq t | \mathrm{Y}_i(t)\} \\ &= \mathrm{Y}_i(t)\lambda(t)\mathrm{d}t. \end{aligned} \tag{6.6}$$

The third equation in (6.6) is an expected value, generally referred as the *compensator* of $N_i(t)$ with respect to the filtration $\mathcal{F}_t$. Individually, if the event has not occurred prior to t, the intensity rate is $\lambda(t)$; if it has already occurred, the intensity rate is 0 at t because individual i is no longer at risk at t. Therefore, $\{Y_i(t), t \geq 0\}$ is also referred to as the at-risk process.

The integrated intensity process for individual i, denoted by the nonitalicized $\Lambda_i(t)$, is given by

$$\Lambda_i(t) = \int_0^t \lambda_i(u)\mathrm{d}u = \int_0^t \mathrm{Y}_i(u)\lambda_i(u)\mathrm{d}u, \quad t \geq 0. \tag{6.7}$$

For a single event, $\Lambda(t)$ is equivalent to the cumulative hazard function defined previously and reflects the information on the prior history of counting processes (the definition of $\Lambda(t)$ for a repeatable event is discussed in Chapter 7). Given the filtration $\mathcal{F}_{t-}$, $Y(t)$ is fixed; therefore

$$\mathrm{E}[\Lambda(t)|\mathcal{F}_{t-}] = \mathrm{E}[\mathrm{N}(t)|\mathcal{F}_{t-}] = \Lambda(t). \tag{6.8}$$

Therefore, in the counting process system, $\Lambda(t)$, given $\mathcal{F}_{t-}$, is a predictable compensator because it is fixed, not random.

For analytic convenience, the intensity function is often expressed in terms of differential of the integrated intensity process, given by

$$\lambda_i(t)\mathrm{d}t = \mathrm{d}\Lambda_i(t). \tag{6.9}$$

Given the definition of $\Lambda(t)$, the intensity function for $N_i(t)$ with covariate vector $Z_i(t)$ can be written as a regression model:

$$\mathrm{Y}_i(t)\mathrm{d}\Lambda\{t, \mathbf{Z}_i(t)\} = \mathrm{Y}_i(t)\exp[\mathbf{Z}_i'(t)\boldsymbol{\beta}]\mathrm{d}\Lambda_0(t). \tag{6.10}$$

Given the flexibility of Equation (6.10), the above specification can be used to model counting processes of repeated events, as will be extensively described and discussed in Chapter 7.

6.1.2 The martingale theory

The processes $Y_i(t)$ and $\mathbf{Z}_i(t)$ are said to be *adapted* to the filtration $\mathcal{F}_t$ because their values are specified by $\mathcal{F}_{t-}$, thereby $\mathcal{F}_t$ measurable for each $t \in [0, \tau]$. Therefore, given the right continuous counting processes of $N_i(t)$, the left continuous functions $Y_i(t)$ and $Z_i(t)$ are predictable with respect to $\mathcal{F}_t$, which, in turn, highlights the intensity rate to be a deterministic function. According to the *Doob–Meyer decomposition theorem*, the observed event count $N_i(t)$ can be expressed as the summation of a systematic compensator, represented by Equation (6.10), and a random component, called 'the counting process martingale M':

$$\mathrm{N}_i(t) = \int_0^t \mathrm{Y}_i(u)\exp[\mathbf{Z}_i'(u)\boldsymbol{\beta}]\mathrm{d}\Lambda_0(u) + \mathrm{M}_i(t), \tag{6.11}$$

where the nonitalicized $M_i(t)$ is a counting process martingale, defined as a stochastic process in which the expected value for individual i at time t, given its process history $\mathcal{F}_{t-}$, is equal to its value at some earlier time s.

The martingale is mathematically defined as $\{M(t), 0 \leq t \leq \tau\}$ with respect to the filtration $\{\mathcal{F}_t\}$. From Equation (6.11), the martingale can be easily deduced by

$$M_i(t) = N_i(t) - \int_0^t Y_i(u) \exp[\mathbf{Z}_i'(u)\boldsymbol{\beta}] d\Lambda_0(u), \tag{6.12}$$

where $M_i(t)$ is the difference over $(0, t)$ between the observed number of events for individual i and the expected value of the cumulative intensity rate derived from a regression model.

As defined, a martingale must satisfy the following property:

$$E[M(t)|\mathcal{F}_s] = M(s), \quad \text{for all } s \leq t \leq \tau, \tag{6.13}$$

which implies

$$E[dM(t)|\mathcal{F}_{t-}] = 0, \quad \text{for all } t \in (0, \tau]. \tag{6.14}$$

If the equality '=' in Equations (6.13) and (6.14) are replaced by the inequality '≥', the process is defined as a *submartingale* or a *local martingale* with respect to $\mathcal{F}_t$. Likewise, when the inequality is reversed as '≤', M is called a *supermartingale*. Given the nature of survival processes, a counting process $N_i(t)$ is a nondecreasing step function and thus is a submartingale. Additionally, a martingale $M(t)$ is said to be *square integrable* if $V[M(t)] < \infty$, where $V[M(t)]$ is its variance.

From the above two equations, a martingale can be viewed as the discrete random walk in a typical Markovian process, conditional on its prior history $\mathcal{F}_{t-}$. Therefore we have $\Sigma M_i(t) = 0$ for any t. Additionally, as it is a stochastic process without drift and all increments are uncorrelated, a martingale also satisfies the following properties asymptotically (Andersen *et al.*, 1993; Barlow and Prentice, 1988; Therneau, Grambsch, and Fleming, 1990):

$$\text{cov}[M(t), M(t+u) - M(t)] = 0, \quad \text{for all } t \in (0, \tau], \tag{6.15}$$

$$\text{cov}[M_i(t), M_{i'}(t)] = 0, \quad \text{for } i, i' = 1, \ldots, n \text{ and } i \neq i'. \tag{6.16}$$

These two equations indicate that the martingale increment in any t is uncorrelated and that any two right continuous $\mathcal{F}_t$-measurable martingales at any t are conditionally independent of each other. Two martingales are said to be *orthogonal martingales* if they satisfy these two conditions.

A martingale, however, has positive autocorrelation given the $\mathcal{F}_{t-}$-measurable value because, given the independence of martingale increments,

$$\text{cov}[M(t+u), M(t)] = V[M(t)], \quad \text{for all } t \in (0, \tau].$$

Additionally,

$$E[M^2(t)|\mathcal{F}_s] = E\{[M(t) - M(s)]^2 + M^2(t)|\mathcal{F}_s\} \geq M^2(s), \quad \text{for all } s \leq t.$$

As a result, the variance of a martingale tends to increase over t. Obviously, these two properties do not agree with the random process of ordinary residuals, thereby bringing some difficulty in the decomposition of counting processes.

Differentiation of Equation (6.11) provides a better statistical perspective for the decomposition of counting processes. Let the compensator of the counting process be $\Lambda_i(t)$ because it is the compensator of the $N_i(t)$ process. Then the differentiated counting process is

$$dN_i(t) = d\Lambda_i(t) + dM_i(t). \tag{6.17}$$

Conditional on prior history $\mathcal{F}_{t-}$, the component $dM_i(t)$ is independent of $d\Lambda_i(t)$ with mean 0 and zero autocorrelation, though not satisfying the condition of equal variance. As a result, a differentiated martingale, in many ways, behaves like an ordinary residual of linear regression models with mean 0 and without autocorrelation.

The variance of M(t), denoted V[M(t)] and conditional on $\mathcal{F}_t$, is a submartingale, so that it can also be decomposed into a compensator and a martingale with M(0) = 0 and E[M(t)] = 0. The compensator component, denoted by $\langle M\rangle(t)$ or $\langle M, M\rangle(t)$ and generally referred to as the *predictable variation* process (Andersen *et al.*, 1993; Kalbfleisch and Prentice, 2002), is

$$\langle M\rangle(t) = \int_0^t \mathrm{var}[dM(u)|\mathcal{F}_{u-}], \tag{6.18}$$

with its differentiated form

$$d\langle M\rangle(t) = \mathrm{var}[dM(t)|\mathcal{F}_t]. \tag{6.19}$$

Behaving as a counting process martingale, $d\langle M\rangle(t)$ can be well decomposed according to the Doob–Meyer decomposition theorem, given by

$$d\langle M\rangle(t) = \mathrm{var}[dN(t) - d\Lambda(t)], \tag{6.20}$$

where dN(t) is a Poisson random variable with variance $\Lambda(t)$. As a consequence, the predictable variation for a counting process martingale is identical to the compensator for the counting process N(t). Using a regression formulation, $\langle M\rangle(t)$ can be written by

$$\langle M\rangle(t) = \Lambda(t) = \int_0^t Y_i(u)\exp[\mathbf{Z}_i'(u)\boldsymbol{\beta}]d\Lambda_0(u). \tag{6.21}$$

Given the above equation, $\langle M\rangle(t)$ can be viewed as an unbiased estimator of V[M(t)]. Correspondingly, a *predictable covariation* process, denoted by $\langle M_1, M_2\rangle(t)$, where M_1 and M_2 are two martingales, can be defined in the same rationale. Specifically, with $\langle M_1, M_2\rangle(0) = 0$ and, $E\langle M_1, M_2\rangle(t) < \infty$ and if $d\langle M_1, M_2\rangle(t) = \mathrm{cov}\{dM_1(t), dM_2(t)|\mathcal{F}_{t-}\}$, there exists a predictable covariation process for two martingales M_1 and M_2. M_1M_2 is a martingale if and only if $\langle M_1, M_2\rangle \equiv 0$. This process is important in specifying a covariance matrix for a set of martingales, as will be discussed in Chapter 7.

Another simpler estimator of V[M(t)] is the *quadratic variation process*, denoted by [M] (t) and also referred to as the *optional variation process*, a simple statistical function based on observed data. Let the interval [0, t] be partitioned into J subintervals such that $0 = t_0 < t_1 < \cdots < t_J = t$. Then [M]($t$) is defined by

$$[M](t) = \sum_{s \le t} [\Delta M(s)]^2, \tag{6.22}$$

where $s = 0, t_1, \ldots, t_J$ and $\Delta M(s) = M(s) - M(s-)$.

Because N(t) is a jump function with jump size +1, [M](t) jumps correspondingly with the counting process. Therefore, a counting process martingale with a continuous compensator satisfies [M.](t) = N.(t), indicating that [M](t) is a submartingale with ⟨M⟩(t) as its compensator. When M(t) has continuous sample paths, [M](t) = ⟨M⟩(t).

6.1.3 Stochastic integrated processes as martingale transforms

Let M(t) be a zero mean and square-integrable martingale and H be a predictable stochastic process, both with respect to the filtration $\mathcal{F}_t$. Then the process U(t) is defined as

$$\{U(t), 0 \le t \le \tau\} = \int_0^t H(u) dM(u). \tag{6.23}$$

Clearly, the process U(t) is also a square-integrable martingale if H(t) is bounded. This martingale transform can be readily verified given Equation (6.14):

$$\begin{aligned} E[dU(t)|\mathcal{F}_{t-}] &= E[H(t)dM(t)|\mathcal{F}_{t-}] \\ &= H(t)E[dM(t)|\mathcal{F}_{t-}] \\ &= 0. \end{aligned}$$

The component H(t) can be taken outside the expectation because it is predictable and fixed by the σ-algebra $\mathcal{F}_{t-}$. The specification of this martingale transform H(t) is important because, in survival analysis, many estimators, such as the Kaplan–Meier, the Nelson–Aalen, and the partial likelihood score functions, can be expressed as stochastic integration processes.

It follows then that the predictable and quadratic processes for U(t) can also be transformed from those of M(t), given by

$$\langle U \rangle(t) = \int_0^t H^2(u) d\langle M \rangle(u), \tag{6.24}$$

$$[U](t) = \int_0^t H^2(u) d[M](u). \tag{6.25}$$

These martingale transforms are orthogonal martingales if M(t) are orthogonal martingales with respect to a common filtration $\{\mathcal{F}_t, t \ge 0\}$.

The above specifications can be used to model a number of integrated functions. A simple example is the Nelson–Aalen estimator, which can be formulated by using the martingale theory. Specifically, for nonzero Y(t), the conditional probability at t can be expressed as

$$\frac{dN(t)}{Y(t)} = \lambda(t)dt + \frac{dM(t)}{Y(t)}. \tag{6.26}$$

Let J(t) = I{Y(t) > 0} be the number of observations at risk where $Y(t) = \sum_i Y_i(t)$ and let 0/0 be 0. Then, the Nelson–Aalen estimator can be written as

$$\hat{\Lambda}(t) = \int_0^t \frac{J(u)}{Y(u)} dN(u), \quad 0 \le t \le \tau. \tag{6.27}$$

As the counting process $\hat{\Lambda}(t)$ has the compensator

$$\Lambda^*(t) = \int_0^t J(u)\lambda(u)du, \quad 0 \le t \le \tau, \tag{6.28}$$

the function $\hat{\Lambda}(t) - \Lambda^*(t)$ is a martingale transform with mean 0, with the filtration $\{\mathcal{F}_t, t \ge 0\}$ given by

$$\begin{aligned}\hat{\Lambda}(t) - \Lambda^*(t) &= \int_0^t \frac{J(u)}{Y(u)}[dN(u) - Y(u)\lambda(u)du] \\ &= \int_0^t H(u)dM(u).\end{aligned}$$

Therefore, $\hat{\Lambda}(t) - \Lambda^*(t)$ is a martingale. Given Equation (6.24), the martingale transform $\hat{\Lambda}(t) - \Lambda^*(t)$ has variance

$$\langle \hat{\Lambda} - \Lambda^* \rangle(t) = \int_0^t \left[\frac{J(u)}{Y(u)}\right]^2 d\langle M \rangle(u).$$

The above inference indicates that the probability of an event occurrence at t is the sum of the predictable intensity rate and a random process. For large samples, the observed conditional probability tends to have continuous sample paths and, correspondingly, a predictable variation process tends to converge to a deterministic function. As a result, the bias in $\hat{\Lambda}(t)$ tends to be asymptotically negligible with an increase in sample size, thereby verifying the robustness of the Nelson–Aalen estimator. Some other stochastic integration processes, such as the Kaplan–Meier and the logrank test estimators, can also be assessed as martingale transforms (Andersen *et al.*, 1993; Fleming and Harrington, 1991), with their asymptotic processes mathematically proved by using the martingale central limit theorems described below.

6.1.4 Martingale central limit theorems

Suppose that normalized sums of orthogonal martingales converge weakly to a time-transformed *Wiener process* W(t) as the number of summed martingales increases. As defined, the process W(t) satisfies the following three characteristics:

(1) W(0) = 0;

(2) W(t) has independent increments with distribution $W(t) - W(s) \sim N(0, t - s)$ for $0 \le s \le t$;

(3) W(t) is an almost surely continuous martingale with W(0) = 0 and quadratic variation $[W(t)W(t,)] = t$.

Given the above three conditions, W(t) behaves as a Gaussian process if it has continuous sample paths, following the Brownian motion.

If f is a measurable nonnegative function and $V(t)=\int_0^t f^2(u)du$, then $\int f dW$ is a process satisfying the three characteristics, with

$$\mathrm{var}\left[\int_0^t f(u)dW(u)\right]=V(t). \tag{6.29}$$

If W(t) is a multivariate process, then let $\{W_1, \ldots, W_K\}$ be a K-variate independent Gaussian process with independent increments and $f_1, \ldots, f_K$ be K measurable nonnegative functions satisfying $V_\kappa(t)=\int_0^t f_\kappa^2(u)du<\infty$, for all $t>0$ and $\kappa = 1, \ldots, K$. The above specification is used to establish the weak convergence of a square-integrable martingale $U^{(n)}$, defined below, to the Wiener process.

Let $U^{(n)}(t)=\sum_{i=1}^n \int_0^t H_i^{(n)}(u)\, dM_i^{(n)}(u)$ be the sum of n orthogonal martingale transforms, where the superscript (n) indicates the dependence on sample size n (Fleming and Harrington, 1991). As a square-integrable martingale transform, the process $U^{(n)}(t)$, given that H(t) is bounded, satisfies the above three conditions for the W(t) process. Consequently, the process $U^{(n)}(t)$ can be viewed as a large-sample K-variate normal distribution, denoted by $U_1^{(n)}(t),\ldots,U_K^{(n)}(t)$. Then, define

$$U_{i,\kappa}^{(n)}(t)=\int_0^t H_{i,\kappa}^{(n)}(u)dM_{i,\kappa}^{(n)}(u), \tag{6.30}$$

$$U_\kappa^{(n)}(t)=\sum_{i=1}^n \int_0^t H_{i,\kappa}^{(n)}(u)dM_{i,\kappa}^{(n)}(u), \tag{6.31}$$

where $i = 1, \ldots, n$; $\kappa = 1, \ldots, K$. Also, for any $\epsilon > 0$ (size of jumps, say), define

$$U_{i,\kappa,\epsilon}^{(n)}(t)=\int_0^t H_{i,\kappa}^{(n)}(u)I\{|H_{i,\kappa}^{(n)}(u)|\geq\epsilon\}dM_{i,\kappa}^{(n)}(u), \tag{6.32}$$

$$U_{\kappa,\epsilon}^{(n)}(t)=\sum_{i=1}^n U_{i,\kappa,\epsilon}^{(n)}(t). \tag{6.33}$$

According to the specifications of $U^{(n)}$, the above four processes are local square-integrable martingales with independent increments.

The martingale central limit theorem about the homogeneous process $U^{(n)}$ considers conditions when $U^{(n)}$ approaches a normal limit as $n \to \infty$. If the process $U_1, U_2, \ldots, U_K$ are local square-integrable martingales, zero at time 0, with continuous sample paths, then the $\{U_1, U_2, \ldots, U_K\}$ behave like independent Gaussian processes, with independent increments and $\mathrm{var}\{U_i(t)\} = V(t)$. Given $V(t) < \infty$, all $t > 0$, and $n \to \infty$, the above conditions lead to the following two characteristics:

$$\langle U^{(n)}\rangle(t)\xrightarrow{P}V(t) \tag{6.34}$$

and

$$\langle U_\epsilon^{(n)}\rangle(t)\xrightarrow{P}0, \quad \text{for any } \epsilon>0. \tag{6.35}$$

Then, it can be concluded that

$$\mathrm{U}^{(n)} \Rightarrow \mathrm{U}^{\infty} \equiv \int \mathrm{f}\, \mathrm{dW} \text{ on } \mathbb{D}(0,\infty) \text{ as } n \to \infty, \tag{6.36}$$

where W is the Brownian motion defined in the Wiener process and the sign ⇒ denotes weak convergence over the relative interval.

The martingale central limit theorem about the multivariate process $\{\mathrm{U}_1, \mathrm{U}_2, \ldots, \mathrm{U}_\mathrm{K}\}$ is just an extension of the above specifications on the univariate distribution. If the three conditions for the standard W(t) process hold and $n \to \infty$, then

$$\left\langle \mathrm{U}_\kappa^{(n)} \right\rangle (t) \xrightarrow{\mathrm{P}} \int_0^t \mathrm{f}_\kappa^2(u)\, \mathrm{d}u, \tag{6.37}$$

$$\left\langle \mathrm{U}_{\kappa,\varepsilon}^{(n)} \right\rangle (t) \xrightarrow{\mathrm{P}} 0, \quad \text{for any } \varepsilon > 0, \tag{6.38}$$

$$\left(\mathrm{U}_1^{(n)}, \ldots, \mathrm{U}_\mathrm{K}^{(n)}\right) \Rightarrow \mathrm{U}^{\infty} \equiv \left(\int \mathrm{f}_1 \mathrm{dW}_1, \ldots, \mathrm{f}_\mathrm{K} \mathrm{dW}_\mathrm{K}\right) \text{ in } [\mathbb{D}(0,\tau)]^\mathrm{K} \quad \text{as } n \to \infty. \tag{6.39}$$

As $\mathrm{U}_1^{(\infty)}(t), \ldots, \mathrm{U}_\mathrm{K}^{(\infty)}(t)$ are defined as K independent Brownian motion processes, the covariance between $\mathrm{U}_\kappa^{(n)}$ and $\mathrm{U}_{\kappa'}^{(n)}$, where $\kappa \neq \kappa'$, has the property

$$\left\langle \mathrm{U}_\kappa^{(n)}, \mathrm{U}_{\kappa'}^{(n)} \right\rangle (t) \xrightarrow{\mathrm{P}} 0 \text{ as } n \to \infty \text{ for any } \kappa \neq \kappa'. \tag{6.40}$$

The above martingale central limit theorems literally state that when jumps of a martingale converge to a multivariate normal distribution, its sample paths or trajectory tend to an asymptotically transformed Wiener process with mean 0 and variance–covariance vector $\boldsymbol{V}(t)$. Then the variation process becomes deterministic given multivariate normality $[0, \boldsymbol{V}(t)]$.

The aforementioned seven equations compose the martingale central limit theorems when $\mathrm{U}_1^{(\infty)}(t), \ldots, \mathrm{U}_\mathrm{K}^{(\infty)}(t)$ are independent processes. Theorems about dependent time-transformed Brownian motion processes are not included in this book. For mathematical proofs of the theorems, the reader is referred to Fleming and Harrington (1991) and Rebolledo (1980).

Some statisticians have utilized the martingale central limit theorem to develop refined estimators in survival analysis (Andersen and Gill, 1982; Prentice, Williams, and Peterson, 1981). For example, if $\{\mathrm{M}_1(\cdot), \ldots, \mathrm{M}_n(\cdot)\}$ are orthogonal martingales in a partial likelihood regression model, the score function $\tilde{\boldsymbol{U}}(\boldsymbol{\beta}_0,\cdot)$, defined in Chapter 5, is a local martingale; hence it follows directly from the martingale central limit theorems that

$$\sqrt{n}\tilde{\boldsymbol{U}}(\boldsymbol{\beta}_0,\cdot) \to N(0, \boldsymbol{\Sigma}),$$

where Σ is the variance–covariance matrix for $\tilde{\boldsymbol{U}}(\boldsymbol{\beta}_0,\cdot)$. Consequently, $\hat{\boldsymbol{\beta}}$ has asymptotical normality, denoted by

$$\sqrt{n}\left(\hat{\boldsymbol{\beta}} - \boldsymbol{\beta}_0,\cdot\right) \to N\left(0, \boldsymbol{\Sigma}^{-1}\right).$$

In some specific counting processes, $\{\mathrm{M}_1(\cdot), \ldots, \mathrm{M}_n(\cdot)\}$ are not martingales given the existence of dependence in survival times. On those occasions, the martingale central limit theorem described above is not directly applicable for estimating a hazard model, so some adjustments are needed for correctly formulating various stochastic processes, especially of $\boldsymbol{V}(t)$, as will be discussed in Chapter 7.

6.1.5 Counting process formulation for the Cox model

As Andersen *et al.* (1993) contend, the Cox model can be viewed as a special case of counting processes as it sequentially counts the number of events according to the rank order of event times. Given the counting process formulation and the powerful martingale theory, counting processes can be readily used to specify the Cox model and its asymptotic stochastic properties. For example, the score function $\tilde{U}(\boldsymbol{\beta}_0,\cdot)$, the partial derivatives of the log partial likelihood, is basically a local martingale, for which the martingale central limit theorem applies.

Let $N_i \equiv \{N_i(t),\ t \geq 0\}$ be the number of observed events experienced over time t for individual i, with $N_i(0) = 0\}$, and the sample paths of the process are step functions. The hazard function for individual i at time t, given an underlying nuisance function λ_0, can be specified as a counting process:

$$\lambda_i(t) = \lambda_0(t)\exp[\mathbf{Z}_i'(t)\boldsymbol{\beta}], \tag{6.41}$$

where $\boldsymbol{\beta}$ is an $M \times 1$ vector of regression coefficients. By definition, $Y_i(t) = 1$ is specified until the occurrence of a particular event or of censoring and $Y_i(t) = 0$ otherwise.

The partial likelihood for n independent triples $\{N_i, Y_i, Z_i\}$, where $i = 1, \ldots, n$, is given by

$$L_p(\boldsymbol{\beta}) = \prod_{i=1}^{n}\prod_{t\geq 0}\left\{\frac{Y_i(t)\exp[\mathbf{Z}_i'(t)\boldsymbol{\beta}]}{\sum_l Y_l(t)\exp[\mathbf{Z}_l'(t)\boldsymbol{\beta}]}\right\}^{dN_i(t)}. \tag{6.42}$$

Equation (6.42) is basically analogous to the formation of the Cox model but using a different system of terminology. Likewise, in the counting process formulation the log partial likelihood function is

$$\log L_p(\boldsymbol{\beta}) = \sum_{i=1}^{n}\int_0^{\infty} Y_i(t)[\mathbf{Z}_i'(t)\boldsymbol{\beta}] - \log\left\{\sum_l Y_l(t)\exp[\mathbf{Z}_l'(t)\boldsymbol{\beta}]\right\} dN_i(t). \tag{6.43}$$

As routinely applied, the estimator $\hat{\boldsymbol{\beta}}$ in the partial likelihood function is defined as the solution to the equation

$$\tilde{U}(\boldsymbol{\beta}) = \frac{\partial}{\partial}\log L_p(\boldsymbol{\beta}) = 0,$$

where $\tilde{U}(\boldsymbol{\beta}) = (\partial \log L_p/\partial\beta_1, \ldots, \partial \log L_p/\partial\beta_M)'$. Then the total score statistic at time t is given by

$$\tilde{U}(\boldsymbol{\beta},\infty) = \sum_{i=1}^{n}\int_0^{\infty}\{\mathbf{Z}_i(t) - \bar{\mathbf{Z}}(\boldsymbol{\beta},t)\}dN_i(t), \tag{6.44}$$

where the second term within the brace represents the expected covariate vector over a given risk set, defined as

$$\bar{\mathbf{Z}}(\boldsymbol{\beta},t)=\frac{\sum_{l=1}^{n}\mathrm{Y}_l(t)\mathbf{Z}_l(t)\exp[\mathbf{Z}_l'(t)\boldsymbol{\beta}]}{\sum_{l=1}^{n}\mathrm{Y}_l(t)\exp[\mathbf{Z}_l'(t)\boldsymbol{\beta}]}.$$

As $\mathrm{dN}(t)$ is a submartingale, the score function with respect to $\boldsymbol{\beta}$ can be expressed as a martingale transform in the form of Equation (6.23):

$$\tilde{\boldsymbol{U}}(\boldsymbol{\beta},\infty)=\sum_{i=1}^{n}\int_0^{\infty}\{\mathbf{Z}_i(t)-\bar{\mathbf{Z}}(\boldsymbol{\beta},t)\}\mathrm{dM}_i(t), \tag{6.45}$$

where

$$\mathrm{M}_i(t)=\mathrm{N}_i(t)-\int_0^t \mathrm{Y}_i(u)\exp[\mathbf{Z}_i'(u)\boldsymbol{\beta}]\mathrm{d}\Lambda_0(u).$$

As discussed in Chapter 5, the score function in the Cox model can be conveniently expressed in terms of a permutation test based on residuals computed for the regression on covariates, rather than on the regression coefficients. Here, using the counting process formulation to express the score function provides a flexible instrument to specify some complex refinements in the hazard model, such as the asymptotic variance estimators for handling clustered survival data in the Cox model, as will be described extensively in Chapter 7.

If the N counting process satisfies conditions of the martingale central limit theorem, the $\{\mathrm{M}_1(.), \ldots, \mathrm{M}_n(.)\}$ series are orthogonal martingales; then $\boldsymbol{\beta}$ can be estimated using the conventional estimators (Andersen and Gill, 1982). The case in which the M_i series do not behave as orthogonal martingales will be discussed in Chapter 7.

Given that $\{\mathrm{M}_1(.), \ldots, \mathrm{M}_n(.)\}$ are martingales, the information matrix, which is the minus second partial derivatives of the log partial likelihood function with respect to $\boldsymbol{\beta}$, can be used to approximate $\boldsymbol{V}(t)$, given by

$$\boldsymbol{I}(\boldsymbol{\beta},\infty)=\sum_{i=1}^{n}\int_0^{\infty}\{\tilde{\mathbf{Z}}(\boldsymbol{\beta},t)-\bar{\mathbf{Z}}(\boldsymbol{\beta},t)\}\mathrm{dN}_i(t), \tag{6.46}$$

where

$$\tilde{\mathbf{Z}}(\boldsymbol{\beta},t)=\frac{\sum_{l=1}^{n}\mathrm{Y}_l(t)\mathbf{Z}_l(t)^{\otimes 2}\exp[\mathbf{Z}_l'(t)\boldsymbol{\beta}]}{\sum_{l=1}^{n}\mathrm{Y}_l(t)\exp[\mathbf{Z}_l'(t)\boldsymbol{\beta}]}.$$

Given the above inference, statistical tests on the null hypothesis that H_0: $\boldsymbol{\beta}=\boldsymbol{\beta}_0$ can be based on the estimated values $\hat{\boldsymbol{\beta}}$. According to the martingale central limit theorem, $\sqrt{n}\left(\hat{\boldsymbol{\beta}}-\boldsymbol{\beta}_0\right)$

has approximately a multivariate normal distribution with mean 0 and covariance matrix $n\boldsymbol{I}^{-1}(\boldsymbol{\beta}_0)$, which can be estimated by $n\hat{\boldsymbol{I}}^{-1}\left(\hat{\boldsymbol{\beta}}\right)$. Subsequently, the three test statistics – the score, the Wald, and the partial likelihood ratio tests – can be readily derived using procedures described in Chapter 5.

Expressed in terms of the counting process formulation, the above specifications take a tremendous resemblance to the corresponding formulas in the Cox model. The counting process formulation, however, describes counts at observed times, thereby permitting multiple jumps for an individual as a step function. As a result, this system provides a more flexible perspective to describe repeated events and the proportional rates/means function. The Cox model in the counting process formulation can be estimated in SAS by specifying a semi-closed time interval; given a single event, however, the procedure derives exactly the same results as the conventional Cox approach.

6.2 Residuals of the Cox proportional hazard model

In linear regression models, it is straightforward to compute residuals from the difference between the observed and the expected values for a continuous outcome variable. In the case of the Cox model, however, the hazard rate is unobservable because the outcome data are binary and censored. The same issue also exists for some other generalized linear models such as the logistic and the probit regressions. This lack of adequate information makes computation of regression residuals challenging in the Cox model, in turn prompting the development of a number of residual types for assessing the adequacy of the proportional hazards model. In principle, a considerable deviation from an observed rate transform reflects inadequate specification of the relative risk, thereby alerting the researcher to reconsider the analytic strategy on the model specification.

In this section, I describe five residuals that have been widely used in survival analysis: the Cox and Snell (1968), the Schoenfeld (1982) and the scaled Schoenfeld (Grambsch and Therneau, 1994), the martingale (Andersen *et al.*, 1993; Fleming and Harrington, 1991), the score (Therneau, Grambsch, and Fleming, 1990), and the deviance (Therneau, Grambsch, and Fleming, 1990) residuals. Lastly, I provide an illustration to demonstrate how to derive various types of residuals using SAS programming.

6.2.1 Cox–Snell residuals

The Cox–Snell residual is originally developed to define residuals associated with different model functions, including the log-linear regression. Let the link function of a regression model be $g(\cdot)$ and the outcome variable be Y. Then, for individual i, a regression model can be expressed by

$$Y_i = g_i\left(\hat{\boldsymbol{\beta}}, \varepsilon_i\right), \tag{6.47}$$

where $\hat{\boldsymbol{\beta}}$ contains the ML estimates of regression coefficients and ε_i is the residual for individual i. Equation (6.47) has a unique solution for ε_i, given by

$$\varepsilon_i = g_i^{-1}\left(Y_i, \hat{\boldsymbol{\beta}}\right), \tag{6.48}$$

where $g^{-1}(\cdot)$ is the inverse link function of $g(\cdot)$.

In the case of a log-linear regression, Equation (6.47) can be expanded to

$$Y_i = \exp\left(\boldsymbol{x}_i'\hat{\boldsymbol{\beta}} + \varepsilon_i\right) = \exp\left(\boldsymbol{x}_i'\hat{\boldsymbol{\beta}}\right)\exp(\varepsilon_i). \tag{6.49}$$

Let $\tilde{r}_i = \exp(\varepsilon_i)$ be a transform from the additive residual ε_i. It follows that the transformed residuals of this log-linear regression can be readily specified from Equation (6.49):

$$\tilde{r}_i = \left[\exp\left(\boldsymbol{x}_i'\hat{\boldsymbol{\beta}}\right)\right]^{-1} Y_i, \tag{6.50}$$

where $\tilde{r}_1, \ldots, \tilde{r}_n$ are multiplicative residuals transformed from ε_i, which should have a lognormal distribution with mean $\exp(\sigma^2/2)$ and variance $\exp[2\sigma^2 - \exp(\sigma^2)]$ if ε_i is normally distributed with mean 0 and variance σ^2. We can also say that if the mean of $\tilde{r}_1, \ldots, \tilde{r}_n$ is assumed to be 1, ε_i does not have a normal distribution with zero expectation unless $\sigma^2 = 0$.

While developed prior to the publication of the Cox model, the Cox–Snell residual has been borrowed to specify residuals of the semi-parametric proportional hazard model. If the equation $h_i(t) = \hat{h}_0(t)\exp\left(\boldsymbol{x}_i'\hat{\boldsymbol{\beta}}\right)$ reflects the true hazard rate for individual i at time t, the integrated hazard rate, the cumulative hazard function, is considered to be a random variable evaluated at survival time t_i ($i = 1, \ldots, n'$). The parametric form $H_0(t) = t$ yields a unit exponential distribution. This distribution is referred to as the *unit exponential function*. Given this specification, the estimated cumulative hazard function, represented by $\hat{H}_i(t_i) = \hat{H}_0(t_i)\exp\left(\boldsymbol{x}_i'\hat{\boldsymbol{\beta}}\right)$, should behave approximately as a censored sample with the unit exponential distribution. Therefore, the Cox–Snell residual for a step function is simply given by

$$\tilde{r}_i^{\text{Cox-Snell}} = \hat{H}_0(t_i)\exp\left(\boldsymbol{x}_i'\hat{\boldsymbol{\beta}}\right), \tag{6.51}$$

where the baseline cumulative hazard rate at t_i, $\hat{H}_0(t_i)$, can be obtained from applying the Breslow estimator defined by Equation (5.51). Given a unit exponential distribution of residuals, the expected cumulative hazard function should display an upward straight line from the origin. Therefore, if the model is fitted correctly, the Cox–Snell residuals should be narrowly scattered around a straight line, behaving approximately as a censored sample with a unit exponential distribution.

The validity of the Cox–Snell residuals is based on the assumption of a unit exponential distribution for survival times, so that the expected straight line of the cumulative hazard function only applies to the special case of the exponential function. For other distributional functions, another transform should be specified (Cox and Snell, 1968). For example, if the true form is $H_0(t) = t^{\tilde{p}}$, a Weibull function, then the Cox–Snell residuals would be misspecified. Even if deviations from the unit exponential distribution demonstrate an unbiased set of random errors, the Cox–Snell residuals are not associated with a numeric statistic that can be used to assess analytically whether the residuals are statistically significant under the null hypothesis.

6.2.2 Schoenfeld residuals

Schoenfeld (1982) proposes an approach to calculate residuals from a different direction. Specifically, such residuals, formally called the *Schoenfeld residuals*, are defined specifically for the proportional hazard model, with computations performed within the context of the

Cox model. Like the specification of the partial likelihood, the derivation of the Schoenfeld residual does not depend on time but, rather, on the rank order of survival times. For fully comprehending this residual type, the reader might want to review general inference on the Cox model, described in Chapter 5, before proceeding with the following description.

Let d be the total number of events, ordered by event time, and $\mathcal{R}(t_i)$ the risk set at t_i. In the Cox model, the coefficient vector $\boldsymbol{\beta}$ can be estimated by maximizing the partial likelihood function:

$$L_p(\boldsymbol{\beta}) = \prod_{i=1}^{d} \frac{\exp(\boldsymbol{x}_i'\boldsymbol{\beta})}{\sum_{l \in \mathcal{R}(t_i)} \exp(\boldsymbol{x}_l'\boldsymbol{\beta})}. \tag{6.52}$$

From Equation (6.52), $\boldsymbol{x}_i$ can be viewed as a random variable with expected value

$$\mathrm{E}[\boldsymbol{x}_i | \mathcal{R}(t_i)] = \frac{\sum_{l \in \mathcal{R}(t_i)} \boldsymbol{x}_l \exp(\boldsymbol{x}_l'\boldsymbol{\beta})}{\sum_{l \in \mathcal{R}(t_i)} \exp(\boldsymbol{x}_l'\boldsymbol{\beta})}. \tag{6.53}$$

Notice that for analytic simplicity and without loss of generality, the above specifications are based on the assumption of no tied observations.

As described in Chapter 5 (and also in Section 6.1 using the counting process formulation), the maximum likelihood estimate of $\boldsymbol{\beta}$ is a solution to

$$\sum_{l=1}^{d} \{\boldsymbol{x}_i - \mathrm{E}[\boldsymbol{x}_i | \mathcal{R}(t_i)]\} = \mathbf{0}.$$

Given the above partial likelihood estimator, Schoenfeld (1982) defines the partial residual at t_i as a vector $\hat{\tilde{\boldsymbol{r}}}_i = \left(\hat{\tilde{r}}_{i1}, \ldots, \hat{\tilde{r}}_{iM}\right)'$, where

$$\hat{\boldsymbol{r}}_i^{\text{Schoen}} = \boldsymbol{x}_i - \mathrm{E}[\boldsymbol{x}_l | \mathcal{R}(t_i)].$$

Therefore, the Schoenfeld residuals are the differences between the covariate vector for the individual at event time t_i and the expectation of the covariate vector over the risk set $\mathcal{R}(t_i)$. Because it comes from the covariate vector $\boldsymbol{x}$, the Schoenfeld residual is an $M \times n$ matrix, computing a series of individual-specific residual values corresponding to each of the M covariates considered in the Cox model. Consequently, each residual needs to be evaluated separately, corresponding to a given covariate. Given the simplicity of the formulation, the variance–covariance matrix of the Schoenfeld residuals at event time t_i, denoted by $\hat{\boldsymbol{V}}\left(\hat{\tilde{\boldsymbol{r}}}_i\right)$, can be easily estimated. Notice that, as in Equation (6.52), $\boldsymbol{x}_i$ represents the covariate vector for an event at t_i; Schoenfeld does not define this type of residual for censored observations.

Let $\tilde{\boldsymbol{U}}_i$ be an $M \times M$ score matrix with the (m, m')th element being $\partial \tilde{r}_{im} / \partial \beta_{m'}$ evaluated at $\hat{\boldsymbol{\beta}}$, and let $\tilde{\boldsymbol{U}} = \sum_{i \in d} \tilde{\boldsymbol{U}}_i$. Using a Taylor expansion series, the Schoenfeld residual can be written by

$$\hat{\boldsymbol{r}}_i^{\text{Schoen}} = \boldsymbol{r}_i^{\text{Schoen}} + \tilde{\boldsymbol{U}}_i\left(\hat{\boldsymbol{\beta}}\right) + 0_{\mathrm{p}}\left(n^{-1}\right), \tag{6.54}$$

where $0_p(n^{-1})$, by definition, indicates the set of $\hat{\tilde{r}}_i$ to converge to 0 in probability as n tends to a large number.

When the score statistic is substituted for $\hat{\boldsymbol{\beta}}$, we have

$$\hat{\tilde{\boldsymbol{r}}}_i^{\text{Schoen}} = \tilde{\boldsymbol{r}}_i^{\text{Schoen}} + \tilde{\boldsymbol{U}}_i \tilde{\boldsymbol{U}}^{-1} \sum_{l \in D} \tilde{\boldsymbol{r}}_l^{\text{Schoen}} + 0_p\left(n^{-1}\right). \tag{6.55}$$

Equation (6.55) displays the dependence of $\hat{\tilde{\boldsymbol{r}}}_i^{\text{Schoen}}$ on $\hat{\boldsymbol{\beta}}$.

Grambsch and Therneau (1994) consider it statistically more efficient to standardize the Schoenfeld residuals by using the coefficients and the variance matrix from a standard time-independent Cox model fit, given by

$$\hat{\tilde{\boldsymbol{r}}}_i^{*,\text{Schoen}} = \frac{\hat{\tilde{\boldsymbol{r}}}_i^{\text{Schoen}}}{\hat{V}\left(\tilde{\boldsymbol{r}}_i^{\text{Schoen}}\right)}. \tag{6.56}$$

It is recognizable that Equation (6.56) is the standard formulation for computing a standardized score. Such standardized scores, contained in the vector $\hat{\tilde{\boldsymbol{r}}}_i^{*,\text{Schoen}}$, are referred to as the *weighted*, or the *scaled, Schoenfeld residuals*.

Grambsch and Therneau (1994) found through some empirical analyses that the variance–covariance matrix $\hat{\boldsymbol{V}}\left(\hat{\tilde{\boldsymbol{r}}}_i^{\text{Schoen}}\right)$ varies slowly and remains quite stable over time until the last few event times, so that computation of $\hat{\boldsymbol{V}}\left(\hat{\tilde{\boldsymbol{r}}}_i^{\text{Schoen}}\right)$ at each observed event time is not necessary. As a result, the inverse of $\hat{\boldsymbol{V}}\left(\hat{\tilde{\boldsymbol{r}}}_i^{\text{Schoen}}\right)$ can be approximated by the inverse of the observed information matrix, given by

$$\hat{\tilde{\boldsymbol{r}}}_i^{*,\text{Schoen}} = \boldsymbol{I}^{-1}\left(\hat{\boldsymbol{\beta}}\right)\hat{\tilde{\boldsymbol{r}}}_i^{\text{Schoen}}. \tag{6.57}$$

As a result, the scaled, or the weighted Schoenfeld residuals can be conveniently obtained from the analytic results of the Cox model. Because its plot against the rank order of survival times can display deviations from proportional hazards, the scaled Schoenfeld residuals can be used to assess the time trend of proportionality for a specific covariate, as will be discussed further in next section.

6.2.3 Martingale residuals

The specification of martingale residuals is based on the counting process formulation, so I use the terminology used in Section 6.1. In the system of counting processes, the intensity function is given by

$$\Pr\{\mathrm{dN}_i(t)\} = \mathrm{E}\{\mathrm{dN}_i(t) | \mathcal{F}_{t-}\} = \lambda(t)\mathrm{d}t, \tag{6.58}$$

where $\mathcal{F}_{t-}$ is the process history prior to t about survival, censoring, and covariates. The integrated intensity processes, denoted by $\Lambda(t)$, is given by

$$\Lambda(t) = \int_0^t \lambda(u)\mathrm{d}u, \quad t \geq 0. \tag{6.59}$$

$\Lambda(t)$ is equivalent to the cumulative hazard function for a single event per individual.

The intensity function or the hazard rate for the $N_i(t)$ counting process can be more conveniently expressed in terms of $\Lambda(t)$, as also indicated in Section 6.1:

$$Y_i(t)d\Lambda\{t, \mathbf{Z}_i(t)\} = Y_i(t)\exp[\mathbf{Z}_i'(t)\boldsymbol{\beta}]d\Lambda_0(t), \tag{6.60}$$

where Λ_0 is the baseline integrated intensity function or, for a single event per individual, the baseline cumulative hazard function.

The observed event count $N_i(t)$ can be written as the summation of a compensator and a martingale process:

$$N_i(t) = \int_0^t Y_i(u)\exp\left[\mathbf{Z}_i'(u)\hat{\boldsymbol{\beta}}\right]d\Lambda_0(u) + M_i(t), \tag{6.61}$$

where, as defined earlier, $M_i(t)$ is a martingale given the σ-algebra $\mathcal{F}_{t-1}$:

$$\hat{M}_i(t) = N_i(t) - \int_0^t Y_i(u)\exp\left[\mathbf{Z}_i'(u)\hat{\boldsymbol{\beta}}\right]d\hat{\Lambda}_0(u), \tag{6.62}$$

where $\hat{M}_i(t)$ is estimated as the difference over $(0, t)$ between the observed number and the expected number of events from a regression model for individual i. As defined, such martingale residuals have the property that $\sum \hat{M}_i(t) = 0$ for any t because

$$\begin{aligned}\sum_{i=1}^n \hat{M}_i(t) &= \sum_{i=1}^n \left\{N_i(t) - \int_0^t Y_i(u)\exp\left[\mathbf{Z}_i'(u)\hat{\boldsymbol{\beta}}\right]d\hat{\Lambda}_0(u)\right\} \\ &= \sum_{i=1}^n \left(\int_0^t dN(u) - \int_0^t Y_i(u)\exp\left[\mathbf{Z}_i'(u)\hat{\boldsymbol{\beta}}\right]\left\{\frac{\sum_{i=1}^n dN(u)}{\sum_{l=1}^n Y_l(u)\exp\left[\mathbf{Z}_l'(u)\hat{\boldsymbol{\beta}}\right]}\right\}d\hat{\Lambda}_0(u)\right) \\ &= 0.\end{aligned}$$

Also, as two martingales $\langle \hat{M}_i, \hat{M}_{i'} \rangle = 0$, then $E(\hat{M}_i) = \text{cov}(\hat{M}_i, \hat{M}_{i'}) = 0$ asymptotically (Andersen *et al.*, 1993; Barlow and Prentice, 1988; Therneau, Grambsch, and Fleming, 1990). Given these properties, in many ways the martingale residuals resemble the ordinary residuals of linear regression models. Because $N_i(t)$ is a binary count for a single event per individual, however, the distribution of the martingale residuals is not symmetric. Because $N_i(t)$ is 0 or 1 for a single event, for the Cox model without time-dependent covariates the martingale residual reduces to

$$\hat{M}_i(t) = \delta_i - \hat{\Lambda}_0(t_i)\exp\left(\mathbf{Z}_i'\hat{\boldsymbol{\beta}}\right), \tag{6.63}$$

where $\hat{\Lambda}_0(t_i)$ is the estimated baseline cumulative hazard function at the observed survival time t_i.

In logic, Equation (6.63) defines a martingale when the Cox model is correctly specified, so the adequacy of the Cox model can be graphically assessed by the martingale residuals in the presence of censoring. In reality, however, when the survival time is an actual survival time ($\delta_i = 1$), the martingale residual is positive; when it is a censored time ($\delta_i = 0$), the martingale residual is negative. Consequently, individuals with early failure times tend to have positive residuals along the life course because they experience the event too early. Likewise, those with large values of failure times yield more negative scores because the event occurs too late. For survival data with heavy censoring, the majority of martingale residuals are negative, though scattered about zero. Furthermore, in the martingale residuals the Type I right censored observations would be clustered below zero at the ending limit of a given observation interval. Such loss of balance led to the development of more symmetrically distributed martingale transforms.

6.2.4 Score residuals

The martingale residual provides a natural specification of deviations in the counting processes formulation. When Equation (6.63) is applied to the Cox model, the Breslow (1974) method can be used to estimate the baseline cumulative hazard function $\hat{\Lambda}_0(t_i)$. The advantage of using the martingale residuals is that departures from the expected values can be evaluated at every observed survival time for the overall fit of the Cox model.

Therneau, Grambsch, and Fleming (1990) advance the martingale residuals by considering a Kolmogorov-type test based on the cumulative sum of residuals. For the Cox model in which $\hat{\Lambda}_0(t_i)$ is unspecified, the partial derivative of the log partial likelihood L_p with respect to a single covariate β_m can be written as

$$\left[\frac{\partial \log L_p}{\partial \beta_m}\right]_{\beta=b} = \sum_{i=1}^{n}\int_0^\infty [\mathrm{Z}_{im}(u) - \bar{\mathrm{Z}}_m(b,u)]\,\mathrm{dN}_i(u), \tag{6.64}$$

where

$$\bar{\mathrm{Z}}_m(b,u) = \frac{\sum_{i=1}^{n}\mathrm{Y}_i(u)\exp\left[\mathbf{Z}_i'(u)\hat{\boldsymbol{\beta}}\right]\mathrm{Z}_{im}(u)}{\sum_{i=1}^{n}\mathrm{Y}_i(u)\exp\left[\mathbf{Z}_i'(u)\hat{\boldsymbol{\beta}}\right]}. \tag{6.65}$$

Equation (6.65) is the weighted mean of the covariate over the risk set at time u, as indicated in Chapter 5 and in Section 6.1.

Given the specification of martingale residuals, Equation (6.64) can be rewritten as

$$\begin{aligned}\left[\frac{\partial \log L_p}{\partial \beta_m}\right]_{\beta=b} &= \sum\int_0^\infty [\mathrm{Z}_{im}(u) - \bar{\mathrm{Z}}_m(b,u)]\mathrm{dM}_i(u) \\ &\equiv \sum \mathrm{L}_{im}(b,\infty).\end{aligned} \tag{6.66}$$

The first equality in Equation (6.66) follows the specification of the score function when evaluated at $\boldsymbol{\beta} = \boldsymbol{b}$. As a result, the score process for individual i at time t can be formally defined by the vector

$$\mathbf{L}_i(\boldsymbol{\beta},t) = \int_0^t [\mathbf{Z}_i(u) - \bar{\mathbf{Z}}(\boldsymbol{\beta},u)]\mathrm{dM}_i(\boldsymbol{\beta},u). \tag{6.67}$$

The vector $\hat{\mathbf{L}}_i \equiv \mathbf{L}_i\left(\hat{\boldsymbol{\beta}},\infty\right)$, the first partial derivatives of the log partial likelihood function, defines the score residual for individual i.

In particular, assuming covariate x_m to be time independent, the score residual at a specific survival time is

$$\begin{aligned} \mathrm{L}_{im}(\boldsymbol{\beta},t) = \delta_i \mathrm{Y}_i(t)\left[\mathrm{Z}_{im} - \bar{\mathrm{Z}}_m(t_i)\right] \\ - \sum_{t_b \le t}\left[\mathrm{Z}_{im} - \bar{\mathrm{Z}}_m(t_b)\right]\mathrm{Y}_i(t_b)\exp\left(\mathbf{Z}_i'\hat{\boldsymbol{\beta}}\right)\left[\hat{\Lambda}_0(t_b) - \hat{\Lambda}_0(t_{b-1})\right], \end{aligned} \tag{6.68}$$

where $t_b = t_0 < t_1 < \cdots < t_d$ are the ordered actual survival times. Consequently, for individual i ($i = 1, 2, \cdots, n$), the score process for the mth covariate is specified.

The score residuals are useful to evaluate the influence of each individual on each individual parameter estimate. The overall score residual for an observation can also be obtained by summing the component residuals within the observation. Technically, the score residuals are simply the modification of the Schoenfeld residuals by applying the martingale theory. As the development of this method is based on martingales, the score residuals are generally viewed as a martingale-based transform. The reader interested in learning more details of this residual type might want to read Barlow and Prentice (1988).

6.2.5 Deviance residuals

Although the martingale residuals are useful for providing information on model adequacy, one inherent limitation in the specification is the marked skewness of random departures. Given the 0–1 observed value for the outcome variable in the Cox model, the martingale residual does not follow the theory of normality, therefore causing difficulty in analyzing its impact. As indicated above, this is a common problem of specifying random disturbances encountered in all generalized linear models. One popular perspective to handle skewness in qualitative outcome data is to transform a nonnormal distribution to a distribution 'as normal as possible' (Box and Cox, 1964; McCullagh and Nelder, 1989; Sakia, 1992).

Therneau, Grambsch, and Fleming (1990) use the *deviance score*, a statistic widely used in econometrics, to measure residuals. Specifically, the deviance is defined as

$$\tilde{D} = 2\left[\log L(\text{saturated}) - \log L\left(\hat{\boldsymbol{\beta}}\right)\right]. \tag{6.69}$$

where the saturated model indicates a perfect regression model that has no random errors (each individual has his or her own $\hat{\boldsymbol{\beta}}$ vector). While $\tilde{D}$ is distributed as χ^2 with $(n - M)$ degrees of freedom, its square root approximates a normal distribution, thereby possessing potentials to derive a more efficient residual type.

The nuisance parameter $h_0(t)$ in the Cox model is assumed to be constant across the saturated model and the reduced proportional hazard model with $\hat{\boldsymbol{\beta}}$. Let $\tilde{\boldsymbol{g}}_i$ be the individual-specific estimate of $\boldsymbol{\beta}$. The deviance with $\mathbf{Z}_i$ (including time-independent covariates only) and known Λ_0 is extended as

$$\begin{aligned} \tilde{D} = 2\sup\sum\Big\{\int\left[\log\exp(\mathbf{Z}_i'\tilde{\boldsymbol{g}}_i) - \log\exp\left(\mathbf{Z}_i'\hat{\boldsymbol{\beta}}\right)\right]d\mathrm{N}_i(u) \\ - \int \mathrm{Y}_i(u)\left[\exp(\mathbf{Z}_i'\tilde{\boldsymbol{g}}_i) - \exp\left(\mathbf{Z}_i'\hat{\boldsymbol{\beta}}\right)\right]d\Lambda_0(u)\Big\}. \end{aligned} \tag{6.70}$$

After some transformation, Equation (6.70) leads to the estimator of the deviance residual $\tilde{D}_i$ as a transform of the martingale residual:

$$\tilde{D}_i = \text{sign}\left(\hat{\text{M}}_i\right)\sqrt{2\left\{-\hat{\text{M}}_i - \text{N}_i(\infty)\log\left[\frac{\text{N}_i(\infty) - \hat{\text{M}}_i}{\text{N}_i(\infty)}\right]\right\}}, \qquad (6.71)$$

where sign(·) is the sign function. Mathematically, the use of the sign function guarantees $\tilde{D}_i$ to take the same sign as the martingale residual, the square root shrinks large martingale residuals, and the logarithmic transformation makes martingale residuals close to 0 (Fleming and Harrington, 1991). Consequently, the deviance residuals, while taking the same signs as martingale residuals, are more symmetrically distributed around 0 than the martingale residuals, providing tremendous convenience for assessing the model adequacy. In the presence of light censoring, the deviance scores against the linear predictor $\mathbf{Z}_i'\hat{\boldsymbol{\beta}}$ should approximate a normal distribution.

For the Cox model, the deviance residual reduces to

$$\tilde{D}_i^{\text{Cox}} = \text{sign}\left(\hat{\text{M}}_i\right)\sqrt{2\left[-\hat{\text{M}}_i - \delta_i \log\left(\delta_i - \hat{\text{M}}_i\right)\right]}. \qquad (6.72)$$

Equation (6.72) indicates that the deviance residual is a transform of the martingale residuals; therefore it is also classified as a martingale-based statistic.

6.2.6 Illustration: Residual analysis on the Cox model of smoking cigarettes and the mortality of older Americans

In the present illustration, I calculate residuals from results of the Cox model on the association between smoking cigarettes and the mortality of older Americans, using the same survival information as presented in Subsection 5.7.3. The purpose of this diagnostic analysis is to assess departures of model estimates from the observed survival data, thereby generating information on the adequacy of the Cox model. Specifically, I obtain four types of residuals from analytic results of the Cox model on smoking cigarettes and mortality – the martingale, the deviance, the score, and the Schoenfeld residuals. In the Cox model, the four covariates – smoking cigarettes, age, gender, and educational attainment – are measured as centered variables, with names given as, respectively, 'Smoking_mean,' 'Age_mean,' 'Female_mean,' and 'Educ_mean.'

The PROC PHREG procedure is applied to generate those residuals. First, I request SAS to include the four residuals in the OUTPUT statement by specifying an OUT = OUT_RES temporary dataset. Then I ask SAS to plot those residual scores by using the PROC SGPLOT procedure. Below is the SAS program for the work.

SAS Program 6.1:

```
......

proc phreg data = new noprint ;
  model duration*Status(0) = smoking_mean age_mean female_mean educ_mean ;
  output out = out_res XBETA = XB RESMART = Mart RESDEV = Dev RESSCO =
```

```
   Scosmoking_mean Scoage_mean Scofemale_mean Scoeduc_mean RESSCH =
   Schsmoking_mean Schage_mean Schfemale_mean Scheduc_mean;
run;

Title "Figure 6.1a. Martingale residuals";
proc sgplot data = out_res ;
 yaxis grid;
 refline 0 / axis = y ;
 scatter y = Mart x = xb ;
run;

Title "Figure 6.1b. Deviance residuals";
proc sgplot data = out_res ;
 yaxis grid;
 refline 0 / axis = y ;
 scatter y = Dev x = xb ;
run;

Title "Figure 6.1c. Score residuals against Age_mean";
proc sgplot data = out_res ;
 yaxis grid;
 refline 0 / axis = y ;
 scatter y = Scoage_mean x = duration ;
run;

Title "Figure 6.1d. Schonfeld residuals against Age_mean";
proc sgplot data = out_res ;
 yaxis grid;
 refline 0 / axis = y ;
 scatter y = Schage_mean x = duration ;
run;
```

SAS Program 6.1 specifies a classical PROC PHREG model by adding an OUTPUT statement. The keywords XBETA, RESMART, RESDEV, RESSCO, and RESSCH specify the linear predictor, the martingale, the deviance, the score, and the Schoenfeld residuals, respectively. The first three new variables are identified as XB, MART, and DEV. As the score and the Schoenfeld residuals are designed to display a series of individual-specific residual values corresponding to each covariate, the keyword RESSCO or RESSCH is followed by the variable names of the four covariates considered in the Cox model. Given the nature of the illustration, in this example I only plot the score and the Schoenfeld residuals corresponding to the covariate Age_mean. As residuals on the entire model, the martingale and the deviance residuals are plotted against the linear predictor XB for displaying their distributions. The score and the Schoenfeld residuals, on the other hand, are plotted against the rank order of survival times to demonstrate the time trend of proportionality for Age_mean. These four residuals are then output into the temporary data file OUT_RES. The Breslow approximation method, as default in SAS, is used to handle survival data with tied survival times. The four residual plots are generated by four PROC SGPLOT steps with each defining a specific type of residual, as shown in Figure 6.1, which includes four residual plots against the linear predictor $\boldsymbol{x}_i'\hat{\boldsymbol{\beta}}$ for the martingale and the deviance residuals or against the rank order of survival times for the score and the Schoenfeld residuals, from which the pattern of residuals can be evaluated. The first plot, Figure 6.1a, shows the martingale residuals. The linear predictor has a range between −3 and 2 since all covariates in the Cox model are centered about means. As expected, the martingale residuals are skewed given the single event setting and heavy right censoring in the dataset. Nevertheless, these residuals are concentrated around zero, highlighting a fairly decent fit of the model. In this plot, an outlier can be easily identified with a value below −3.

Figure 6.1b demonstrates deviance residuals against the linear predictor. Here, the logarithms, as discussed in Subsection 6.2.4, derive impact on narrowing the range of residuals, thereby making the plot look more balanced. Compared to the martingale residual, the deviance residuals are more intensely scattered around zero, with the outlier, identified in Figure 6.1a, nearly vanishing. Because of heavy censoring, however, a large quantity of residuals are clustered near zero, thus disturbing the expected normal approximation.

The score residuals corresponding to the covariate Age_mean, as another martingale transform and displayed in Figure 6.1c, look randomly distributed against the rank order of survival times, with the vast majority of the scores narrowly scattered around zero. Most significantly, no distinct outliers can be identified in this plot.

The last plot, Figure 6.1d, presents the Schoenfeld residuals corresponding to the covariate Age_mean. Obviously, these age-specific residuals are independent of survival times as they are scattered randomly around zero without displaying any systematic pattern. As a result, the effect of age is not shown to depart from the proportional hazards assumption in the Cox model. Because the Schoenfeld residuals are not defined for censored observations, Figure 6.1d only plots residuals for those who died in the observation period. Therefore, as a modification of the Schoenfeld residual, the score residuals are obviously preferable to show a complete, more refined set of residuals.

From the above evaluation of four residual plots, it may be appropriate to conclude that there is no evidence of model misspecification on individual observations, both overall and with specific regard to age. All four residual types behave as expected, without revealing a distinct trend of model inadequacy. Additionally, only one distinct outlier can be identified. Therefore, I have reason to believe that the underlying Cox model is adequately applied for analyzing the association between smoking cigarettes and the mortality of older Americans. Even so, in the presence of heavy censoring, it seems very difficult to find a highly efficient residual transform that can display an explicit and normally distributed random process as generated in linear regression models.

6.3 Assessment of proportional hazards assumption

In Chapter 5, I discussed the use of some simple graphical checks on the proportional hazards assumption. Specifically, if two or more stratum-specific log–log survival curves, with all covariates set at zero, are approximately parallel, it can be inferred that the baseline hazard rates across strata tend to be proportional. If not, the effects of the stratification factor on the hazard function are probably not multiplicative over time, thereby displaying violation of the proportionality hypothesis. Such graphical checks, however, do not provide sufficient information on nonproportionality because they are not associated with an explicit and unambiguous statistical criterion on observed deviations from a proportional effect. Some statisticians have developed more refined techniques for checking the proportionality assumption of the Cox model, based on various methodological perspectives (Andersen, 1982; Arjas, 1988; Gill and Schumacher, 1987; Lagakos and Schoenfeld, 1984; Lin, Wei, and Ying, 1993; Storer and Crowley, 1985; Struthers and Kalbfleisch, 1986).

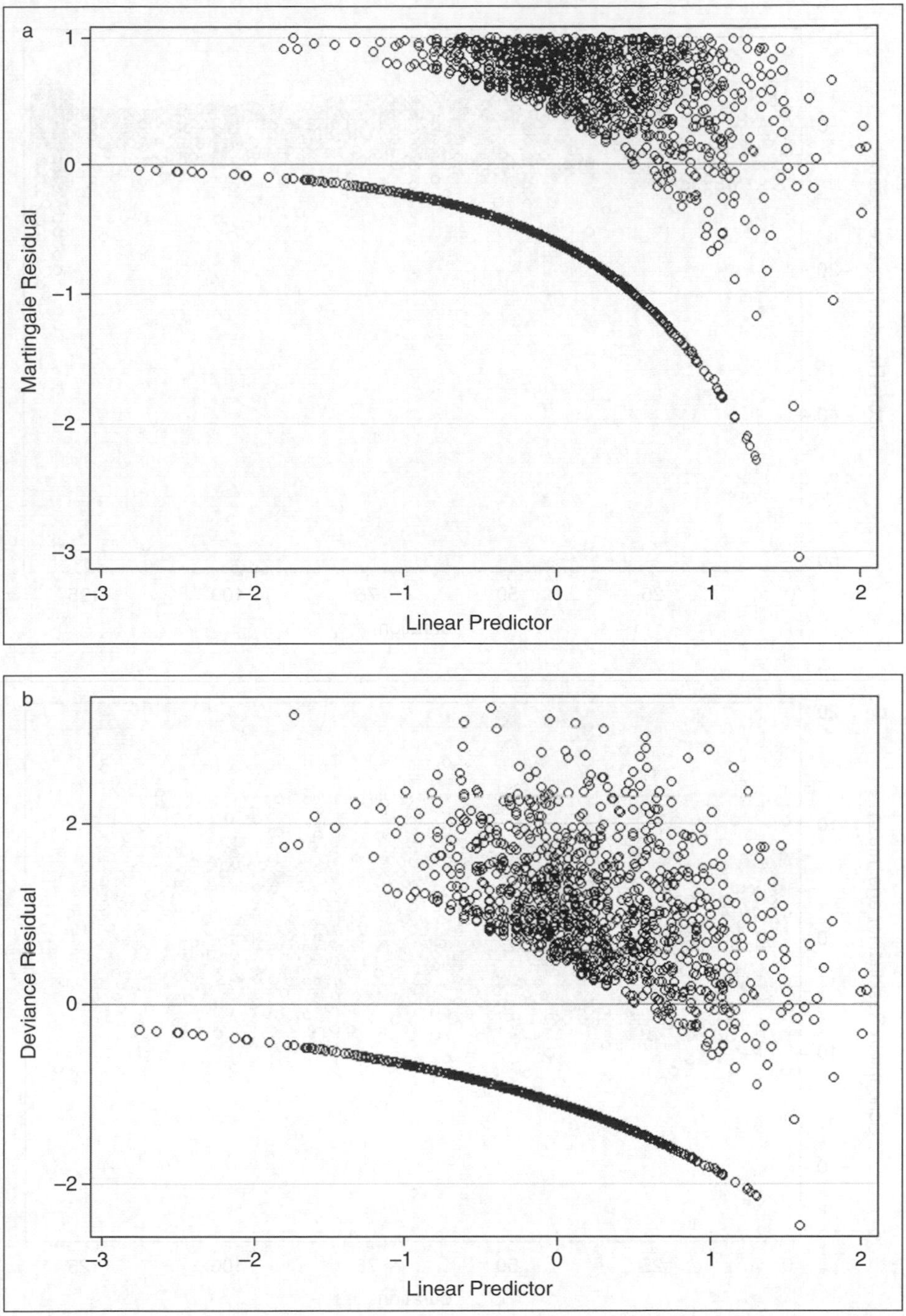

Figure 6.1 a Martingale residuals. b Deviance residuals.

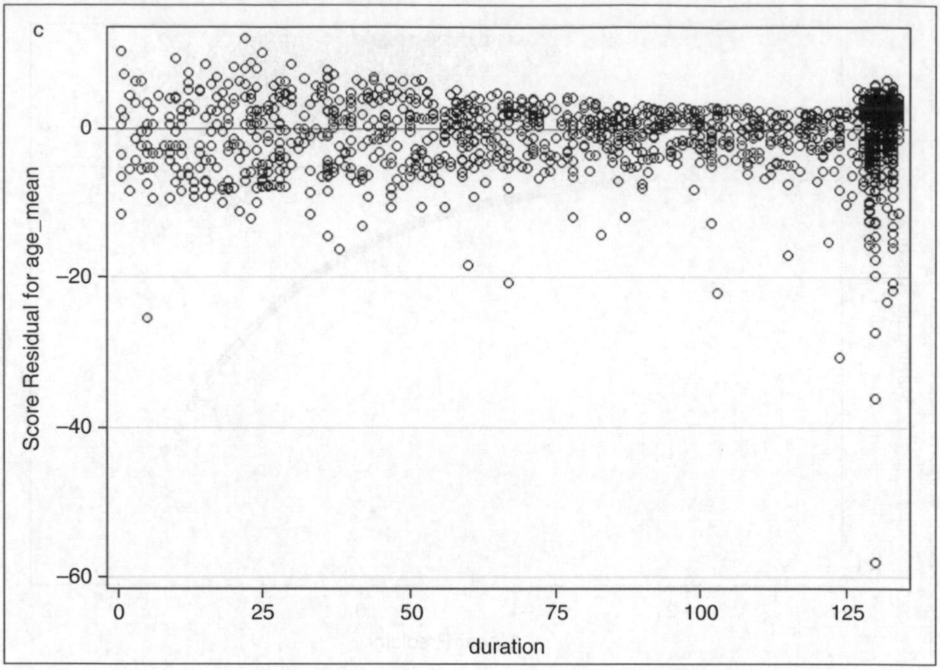

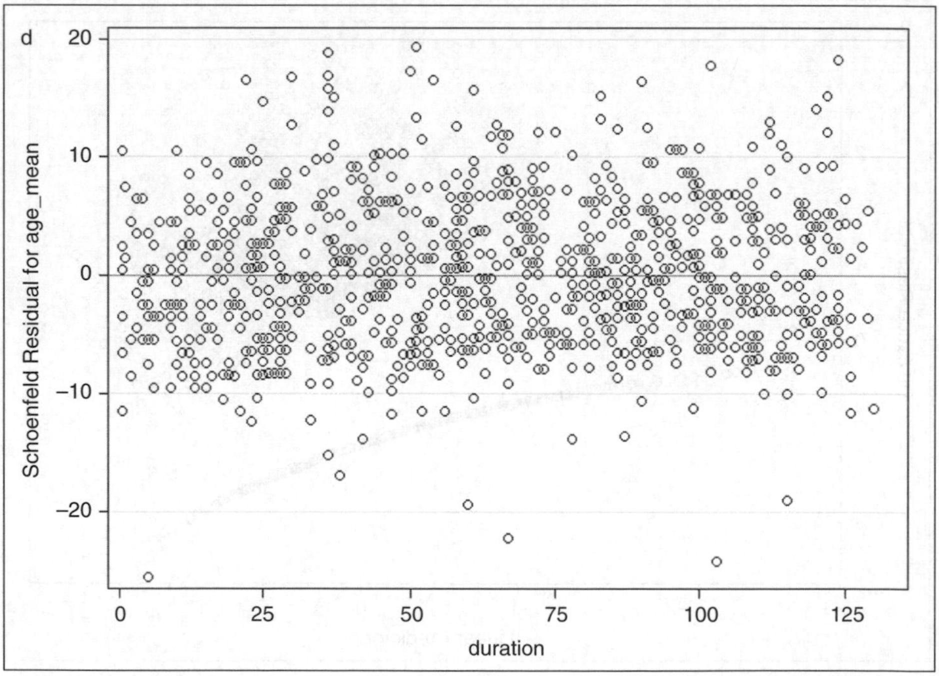

Figure 6.1 (*Continued*) *c Score residuals against Age_mean. d Schonfeld residuals against Age_mean.*

In this section, I introduce five methods in this regard: (1) checking proportionality by adding a time-dependent variable, (2) the Andersen plots, (3) checking proportionality with the scaled Schoenfeld residuals, (4) the Arjas plots, and (5) checking the proportional hazards assumption with cumulative sums of martingale-based residuals. Lastly, I provide an empirical illustration on testing the proportionality assumption in the Cox model, using survival data of older Americans.

6.3.1 Checking proportionality by adding a time-dependent variable

The Cox model is based on the assumption that the hazard ratio of a given covariate x_m is independent of time. This assumption is violated if the hazard ratio changes significantly over time, thus highlighting the absence of a constant multiplicative effect. From this logic, a straightforward approach to check the validity of the proportionality assumption is to compare two Cox models, one specifying x_m as a single covariate with time-independent effects and one adding a time-dependent interaction term ($x_m \times t$) with the assumption that the effect of x_m varies over time. While the first regression is a standard Cox model, the second model can be written by

$$h(t|x_m, \boldsymbol{x}_r) = h_0(t)\exp[x_m\beta_1 + (x_m \times t)\beta_2 + \boldsymbol{x}_r'\boldsymbol{\beta}_r], \tag{6.73}$$

where β_2 measures the time-dependent effect of x_m and $\boldsymbol{x}_r$ is the vector of other covariates, used as controls.

In practice, the estimation of Equation (6.73) may encounter some specification problems, so some functional adjustments are needed. First, the distribution of t may not necessarily be linearly associated with log hazards, thus causing some numeric instability. As widely applied in survival and longitudinal data analyses, using $\log t$ to replace t can considerably improve stability in the estimation process (Collett, 2003). Second, the two covariates, x_m and $x_m \times t$, come from the same source of variability; therefore they tend to be highly correlated, thus affecting the efficiency of the model fit. Using the centered log time for t, defined as $[\log t - \text{mean}(\log t)]$, can substantially reduce multicollinearity in longitudinal data (Hedeker and Gibbons, 2006). Accordingly, Equation (6.73) can be adjusted by

$$h(t|x_m, \boldsymbol{x}_r) = h_0(t)\exp\{x_m\beta_1 + x_m[\log t - \text{mean}(\log t)]\beta_2 + \boldsymbol{x}_r'\boldsymbol{\beta}_r\}. \tag{6.74}$$

By performing a significance test on the time-dependent component of x_m, the validity of the proportionality assumption on x_m can be statistically assessed. In particular, the Wald test can be used for testing the null hypothesis H_0: $\beta_2 = 0$, given a chi-square distribution. If β_2 is not statistically significant, the addition of the time-dependent component $\{x_m[\log t - \text{mean}(\log t)]\}$ should be viewed as redundant. In this situation, as the multiplicative effect of x_m does not depend on time, the 1-unit hazard ratio of x_m is $\exp(\beta_1)$.

If it is statistically significant, however, the value of β_2 reflects the extent to which the hazard ratio of x_m increases ($\beta_2 > 0$) or decreases ($\beta_2 < 0$) over time. Then, the proportional hazards assumption on the effects of x_m should be considered violated. The 1-unit hazard ratio of x_m then becomes

$$HR(x_m|t) = \frac{h_0(t)\exp\{(x_{m0}+1)\beta_1 + (x_{m0}+1)[\log t - \text{mean}(\log t)]\beta_2 + \mathbf{x}_r'\hat{\boldsymbol{\beta}}_r\}}{h_0(t)\exp\{x_{m0}\hat{\beta}_1 + x_{m0}[\log t - \text{mean}(\log t)]\hat{\beta}_2 + \mathbf{x}_r'\hat{\boldsymbol{\beta}}_r\}}$$
$$= \frac{\exp\{(x_{m0}+1)\hat{\beta}_1 + (x_{m0}+1)[\log t - \text{mean}(\log t)]\hat{\beta}_2\}}{\exp\{x_{m0}\hat{\beta}_1 + x_{m0}[\log t - \text{mean}(\log t)]\hat{\beta}_2\}}$$
$$= \exp\left[\hat{\beta}_1 - \text{mean}(\log t)\hat{\beta}_2\right] t^{\hat{\beta}_2}, \tag{6.75}$$

where $\exp(\hat{\beta}_1)$ is the hazard ratio at the mean survival time because $\log t$ is centered. At other time points, the hazard ratio varies significantly if the value of β_2 is sizable, thereby highlighting misspecification of the proportionality assumption in the Cox model.

More formally, statistical testing on the proportional hazards assumption can be executed by using the partial likelihood ratio test. With respect to the above-mentioned two Cox models, the score of the log partial likelihood ratio test is

$$G_{\beta_2} = -2\times\left[\log L_p\left(\hat{\beta}_1, \hat{\beta}_2, \hat{\boldsymbol{\beta}}_r; t, x_m, \mathbf{x}_r\right) - \log L_p\left(\hat{\beta}_1, \hat{\boldsymbol{\beta}}_r; x_m, \mathbf{x}_r\right)\right], \tag{6.76}$$

where G_{β_2} is the partial likelihood ratio statistic for the time-dependent effect of x_m, distributed as χ^2 with one degree of freedom. In the bracket on the right of Equation (6.76), the first term is the log partial likelihood ratio statistic for the time-dependent model, whereas the second is for the standard Cox model. If $G_{\beta_2} < \chi^2_{(1-\alpha;1)}$, the model is not statistically improved by adding the time-dependent component $\{x_m[\log t - \text{mean}(\log t)]\}$; hence the proportional hazards assumption is not violated. If $G_{\beta_2} > \chi^2_{(1-\alpha;1)}$, the addition of the time-dependent variable significantly increases the quality of the overall fit, so the null hypothesis on the proportional effects of covariate x_m should be rejected.

On most occasions, I expect the above two test statistics, the Wald and the partial likelihood ratio tests, to yield the same result on the significance of the time-dependent effect. Specifically, the Wald statistic checks the statistical significance of a single parameter estimate, whereas the partial likelihood ratio test is based on the entire model fit. In certain circumstances, however, the two tests can generate statistics that designate different test results. These test statistics, in turn, would provide ambiguous information about statistical significance of nonproportionality in the Cox model. For example, one statistic is associated with a p-value greater than α, whereas the other is less than α. If such a situation happens, the results generated from the partial likelihood ratio test are recommended as the final criterion.

When applying this numeric method, however, we must consider the potential problems in the specification of a time-dependent covariate. As stated in Chapter 5, without extensive knowledge about the mechanisms involved in a time-dependent process, the estimated effect of a time-dependent covariate can imply other interrelationships, thereby leading to misleading conclusions. Additionally, a sizable effect on the hazard ratio may not necessarily translate into strong effects on the hazard rate itself and, consequently, some graphical checks are useful to aid in the interpretation of numeric results.

6.3.2 The Andersen plots for checking proportionality

The Andersen (1982) plots are somewhat similar to the graphical checks described in Chapter 5 (Section 5.5). Suppose that $M + 1$ covariates are considered and that $\boldsymbol{x} = (x_1, \ldots, x_M)'$ is included in a proportional hazard model. The covariate x_{M+1} is the independent variable under assessment concerning whether its effects on the hazard rate are proportional over time. Given such, the null hypothesis for a statistical test is

$$\mathrm{H}_0 : h_0(t; x_{M+1})\exp(\boldsymbol{x}'\boldsymbol{\beta}) = h_0(t)\exp(\boldsymbol{x}'\boldsymbol{\beta} + x_{M+1}\beta_{M+1}). \tag{6.77}$$

As discussed in Chapter 5, checking the proportionality assumption for a single covariate can be performed by stratifying on this covariate, fitting a proportional hazard model for each stratum, and then combining them by assuming a common coefficient vector $\boldsymbol{\beta}$. In stratum k, where $k = 1, \ldots, K$, the proportional hazard model with covariate vector $\boldsymbol{x}$ is

$$h_k(t; \boldsymbol{x}_k) = h_{0k}(t)\exp(\boldsymbol{x}'\boldsymbol{\beta}), \tag{6.78}$$

where h_{0k} is the baseline hazard function for stratum k. Graphical checks can be made to evaluate whether the K baseline hazard functions are proportional to each other. As the log–log survival function is actually the log transformation of the cumulative hazard rate, it is informative to compare stratum-specific log–log survival curves with all covariates set at zero. In Chapter 5, I provided an empirical illustration on how to perform this method.

Based on the graphical check on a plot of $\log\hat{H}_k(t)$ versus t, Andersen (1982) proposes a unique graphical checking method for the proportionality assumption in the Cox model. Let $K = 2$ be a binary variable for variable x_{M+1}, observed at time points $t_1, \ldots, t_n$. Then, if the proportional hazards assumption holds, a plot of $\hat{H}_2(t_1), \ldots, \hat{H}_2(t_n)$ versus $\hat{H}_1(t_1), \ldots, \hat{H}_1(t_n)$ should be approximately a straight line through the origin. Accordingly, the slope of the line should approximate the regression coefficient of x_{M+1} if the Cox model is valid. In contrast, considerable deviations of this plot from a straight line would suggest that the proportionality assumption may be violated. For $K > 2$ in x_{M+1}, each pair of $\hat{H}_k(t_1), \ldots, \hat{H}_k(t_n)$ versus $\hat{H}_1(t_1), \ldots, \hat{H}_1(t_n)$, where $k \neq 1$ may be plotted to assess the adequacy of the proportional hazards assumption on this added covariate. Such graphical checks are known as the Andersen plots. As Gill and Schumacher (1987) summarize, the shape of such a plot demonstrates the direction of deviations from the proportionality assumption. If the hazard ratio increases over time, the Andersen plot should appear convex; if the hazard ratio decreases over time, the plot should appear concave.

Andersen (1982) also attempts to develop some numeric tests to support the results of the graphical checks, using the stratification perspective. Specifically, t is divided into a number of time intervals and the stratum-specific baseline hazard function is assumed to be constant in each of those intervals. Given those additional assumptions, statistical tests on the proportionality assumption in the Cox model become very tedious and can easily come across some specification problems. Therefore, I do not present this numeric method in this text. The interested reader on this numeric method is referred to Andersen's (1982) article.

6.3.3 Checking proportionality with scaled Schoenfeld residuals

Grambsch and Therneau (1994) proposed the use of scaled Schoenfeld residuals to check the proportional hazards assumption in the Cox model. First, for a single covariate x_m, they expand the proportional hazards by adding a time-varying coefficient, given by

$$\beta_m(t) \equiv \beta_m + \beta_m g_m(t), \tag{6.79}$$

where $g_m(t)$ is defined as a predictable process, which can take various functional forms. Accordingly, the ith scaled Schoenfeld residual corresponding to x_m, represented by Equation (6.56), is also expanded about $\beta_m(t_i) = \beta_m$, given by

$$\tilde{r}_{im}^{*,\text{Schoen}} = \frac{\tilde{r}_{im}^{\text{Schoen}}(\beta_m)}{V(\beta_m, t_i)}. \tag{6.80}$$

Therefore, within this context, the scaled Schoenfeld residual is evaluated with respect to $\beta_m(t_i)$ rather than to β_m itself.

Assuming g to vary about 0 and $\boldsymbol{G}_i = \boldsymbol{G}(t_i)$ to be an $M \times M$ diagonal matrix with the mmth element being $g_m(t_i)$, the expected value of the Schoenfeld residual can be expressed by

$$\mathrm{E}\left[\tilde{\boldsymbol{r}}_i^{\text{Schoen}}(\boldsymbol{\beta})\right] \approx V(\boldsymbol{\beta}, t_i)\boldsymbol{G}(t_i)\overline{\boldsymbol{\theta}}. \tag{6.81}$$

Because the scaled Schoenfeld residual is defined as $\tilde{\boldsymbol{r}}_i^{*,\text{Schoen}} = \tilde{\boldsymbol{r}}_i^{*,\text{Schoen}}(\boldsymbol{\beta}) = V^{-1}(\boldsymbol{\beta}, t_i)\tilde{\boldsymbol{r}}_i^{\text{Schoen}}(\boldsymbol{\beta})$, the expected value of the scaled Schoenfeld residual is

$$\mathrm{E}\left(\tilde{\boldsymbol{r}}_i^{*,\text{Schoen}}\right) \approx \boldsymbol{G}_i\overline{\boldsymbol{\theta}}, \tag{6.82}$$

with variance

$$V\left(\tilde{\boldsymbol{r}}_i^{*,\text{Schoen}}\right) = V^{-1}(\boldsymbol{\beta}, t_i). \tag{6.83}$$

The score test can be performed on the null hypothesis that H_0: $\beta_m(t_i) = \beta_m$. As $\overline{\theta}_m$ can be viewed as the time-dependent component of $\beta_m(t)$, given the functional form of $g_m(t)$, Equation (6.82) can be more conventionally written as

$$\mathrm{E}\left(\tilde{r}_{im}^{*,\text{Schoen}}\right) \approx \beta_m(t_i) - \beta_m, \tag{6.84}$$

where $\beta_m(t_i)$ is the regression coefficient of covariate x_m at observed time t_i and $\hat{\beta}_m$ is the estimate of β_m from the Cox model.

Grambsch and Therneau (1994) suggest that as the variance matrix of $\boldsymbol{x}(t)$ is stable over time (also discussed in Section 6.2), a smoothed scatter plot of the values of $\tilde{r}_{im}^{*,\text{Schoen}} + \beta_m$ against t_i can be used to track the nonproportionality of $\beta_m(t)$. Specifically, a horizontal line of $\tilde{r}_{im}^{*,\text{Schoen}} + \beta_m$ versus t_i suggests the hazard ratio of x_m to be constant, in turn reflecting the validity of the proportional hazards assumption. By contrast, if the line of $\tilde{r}_{im}^{*,\text{Schoen}} + \beta_m$ versus t_i deviates considerably from horizontality, the Cox proportional hazard model may be misspecified. As also suggested by Grambsch and Therneau (1994), a smoothed line can be drawn to supplement the interpretation of analytic results.

This graphical check has some advantages for use. It is intimately linked to the scaled Schoenfeld residual, so that computation of this graphical check is handy and the resulting plot is easy to comprehend. In particular, a plot can be readily drawn with the estimated regression coefficient of a given covariate plus the scaled Schoenfeld residuals. As a coarse graphical approach, however, this test does not make distinct improvements in checking the proportionality assumption compared to other traditional graphical checking methods. Additionally, it is not associated with a numeric statistic that can be used to perform more rigorous statistical testing on the proportionality hypothesis.

6.3.4 The Arjas plots

Another popular graphical method for checking the proportional hazards assumption in the Cox model is using the Arjas (1988) plots. Specifically, the Arjas plots are designed to make direct comparisons between observed and estimated event frequencies without adding a time-dependent variable. Therefore, this method is not based on the estimation of alternative models and only involves parameter estimates already derived from the partial likelihood procedure.

According to Arjas (1988), the application of the stratified Cox model is subject to two types of defects: (1) an influential covariate may be deleted from the model (this defect has been discussed in Section 5.5 of this book) and (2) the stratified Cox model is based on the assumption of a common baseline hazard for all individuals, so that the individuals are stratified according to the baseline hazard. These two defects can seriously influence the efficiency of the Cox model, thus making it difficult to perform a graphical check correctly on the validity of the proportionality hypothesis. Accordingly, he proposes to test the proportionality assumption directly from the proportional hazard model including all $(M + 1)$ covariates.

Practically, deriving the Arjas plots can be performed by taking the following steps. First, divide n individuals into K strata of the $(M + 1)$th covariate according to the research interest of a particular study or previous findings. If the $(M + 1)$th covariate is a continuous variable, classify the sample respondents into a few categories according to an existing theory or results from a previous empirical analysis. Second, calculate the estimated cumulative hazard rate at each observed survival time for each stratum using the parameter estimates obtained from the Cox model. Third, compute the cumulative number of actual events at each survival time for each stratum. Fourth, plot the estimated cumulative hazard rate at each actual survival time along the y axis against the corresponding observed cumulative number of events on the x axis for each stratum. Eventually, discrepancies between the estimated cumulative hazard rate and the empirical data can display whether the estimated hazard rates of those strata are scattered randomly or systematically too high or too low.

In particular, if the proportionality assumption for the $(M + 1)$th covariate holds, the stratum-specific plots should be approximately linear with various slopes, so that the discrepancy between the estimated and the observed should be a martingale. If all stratum-specific plots are closely clustered around a 45-degree line, then adding the $(M + 1)$th covariate to the Cox model is unnecessary because the variable does not contribute additional information into the Cox model. Likewise, if those stratum-specific curves are separated in a nonlinear fashion, it can be inferred that the proportional hazards assumption for the

$(M + 1)$th covariate is violated. Between two stratum-specific curves, if the curve for the first stratum is concave and the second curve convex, the hazard ratio between the two strata would increase over time. Obviously, this checking approach is somewhat similar to the graphical check using the scaled Schoenfeld residuals.

The Arjas plots have the advantage that the plots are derived from an integrated proportional hazard model, rather than from several stratified models. Therefore, this graphical approach increases the statistical power of the assessment. These plots are particularly useful when the baseline hazard function tends to be common across all strata. If there is strong evidence on distinct differences in the baseline hazard function, however, using this graphical check is inappropriate; under such circumstances, the Andersen plots are preferred.

6.3.5 Checking proportionality with cumulative sums of martingale-based residuals

This graphical and numeric method is based on the martingale theory, so I use the counting processes terminology for its description. In principle, the application of the martingale residuals and their transforms, described in Section 6.1, can detect departures from the proportionality assumption by plotting the score process versus follow-up times. Just looking at such residuals, however, is not clear enough to make a firm conclusion about the validity of the proportional hazards assumption because considerable residual deviations can occur even when the model is correctly specified. Accordingly, it is essential to develop a martingale transform that can be used both for a graphical check and as a summary statistic with a known distribution, thereby providing additional information on whether the null hypothesis on the proportional hazards should be accepted or rejected.

Lin, Wei, and Ying (1993) propose a combined method for the assessment of the Cox model based on the cumulative sums of martingale residuals and the transforms. The rationale of this method is that the failure of the proportionality assumption in the Cox model would be reflected by deviations of observed martingale residuals from some standardized martingale transforms with a known distribution.

Specifically, they first group the martingale-based residuals cumulatively with respect to follow-up times and/or covariate values. Then they develop the following two classes of multiparameter Wiener stochastic processes:

$$\mathrm{W_z}(t,\mathbf{z}) = \sum_{i=1}^{n} \mathrm{f}(\mathbf{Z}_i)\mathrm{I}(\mathbf{Z}_i \le \mathbf{z})\hat{\mathrm{M}}_i(t), \tag{6.85}$$

$$\mathrm{W_r}(t,\mathrm{r}) = \sum_{i=1}^{n} \mathrm{f}(\mathbf{Z}_i)\mathrm{I}(\mathbf{Z}_i'\boldsymbol{\beta} \le \mathrm{r})\hat{\mathrm{M}}_i(t), \tag{6.86}$$

where $\mathrm{f}(\cdot)$ is a known smooth function, $\mathbf{z} = (\mathrm{z}1, \ldots, \mathrm{z}_M)' \in \mathcal{R}^M$, and $(Z_i \le z)$ means that all the M covariates in $\mathbf{Z}_i$ are not larger than the respective components of $\mathbf{z}$. The distributions of these two stochastic processes under the proportionality hypothesis can be approximated by the distributions of certain zero-mean Gaussian processes, assuming a known stochastic structure of the martingale process $\mathrm{M}_i(t)$. In particular, a standardized process $\mathrm{N}_i(u)\mathrm{G}_i$ is recommended given $\langle \mathrm{M}_i \rangle(t) = \mathrm{E}[\mathrm{N}_i(t)]$ (Fleming and Harrington, 1991), where $(\mathrm{G}_1, \ldots, \mathrm{G}_n)$ are the standard normal variables that are independent of the triple $(T_i, \delta_i, \mathbf{Z}_i)$. Given a zero-mean Gaussian distribution, these two standardized processes should fluctuate randomly around zero. Consequently, each observed martingale process can be plotted along with a number of realizations from simulation using an estimator of W_z. Observed patterns of residuals can then be compared, both graphically and numerically, under the null distribution. The resulting graphical plots and the attached numeric statistics, in turn, enable the researcher to assess more objectively whether the observed residual pattern deviates significantly from random fluctuations.

In particular, given the definition of the martingale residuals, formulated by Equation (6.62), the empirical score process $\tilde{\boldsymbol{U}}(\hat{\boldsymbol{\beta}},t)=\left[\tilde{U}_1(\hat{\boldsymbol{\beta}},t),\ldots,\tilde{U}_M(\hat{\boldsymbol{\beta}},t)\right]$ can be viewed as a transform of the martingale residuals, given by

$$\tilde{\boldsymbol{U}}(\hat{\boldsymbol{\beta}},t)=\sum_{i=1}^{n}\mathbf{Z}_i\hat{\mathrm{M}}_i(t). \tag{6.87}$$

The standardized empirical score process for the mth component of $\mathbf{Z}$, denoted by $\tilde{U}_m^*(t)$, is

$$\tilde{U}_m^*(t)=\sup\left\{\left[\boldsymbol{I}^{-1}(\hat{\boldsymbol{\beta}})_{mm}\right]^{1/2}\tilde{U}_m^*(\hat{\boldsymbol{\beta}},t)\right\},\quad m=1,\ldots,M. \tag{6.88}$$

where $\boldsymbol{I}^{-1}(\hat{\boldsymbol{\beta}})_{mm}$ represents the diagonal elements in the inverse of the observed information matrix.

This standardized test statistic $\tilde{U}_m^*(t)$, under the null hypothesis that the proportional hazards assumption holds, is a special case of $W_z(t, \mathbf{z})$ with $\mathbf{z}=\infty$ and $f(\cdot)=\cdot$. Given the Taylor series expansion, it can be approximated by

$$\begin{aligned}\tilde{U}_m^*(t)=\left[\boldsymbol{I}^{-1}(\hat{\boldsymbol{\beta}})_{mm}\right]^{1/2}&\left\{\sum_{l=1}^{n}\mathrm{I}(T_l\le t)\delta_l\left[\mathbf{Z}_{ml}-\bar{\mathbf{Z}}_m(\hat{\boldsymbol{\beta}},t)\right]\mathrm{G}_l\right.\\&-\sum_{k=1}^{n}\int_0^t \mathrm{Y}_k(u)\exp(\mathbf{Z}_k'\hat{\boldsymbol{\beta}})\mathbf{Z}_{mk}\left[\mathbf{Z}_k-\bar{\mathbf{Z}}(\hat{\boldsymbol{\beta}},u)\right]'\mathrm{d}\hat{\Lambda}_0(u)\\&\left.\times\boldsymbol{I}^{-1}(\hat{\boldsymbol{\beta}})\sum_{l=1}^{n}\delta_l\left[\mathbf{Z}_l-\bar{\mathbf{Z}}(\hat{\boldsymbol{\beta}},T_l)\right]\mathrm{G}_l\right\},\end{aligned} \tag{6.89}$$

where $\bar{\mathbf{Z}}_m(\hat{\boldsymbol{\beta}},t)$ is the mth component of $\bar{\mathbf{Z}}(\hat{\boldsymbol{\beta}},t)$. As the standardized score converges to a zero-mean Gaussian process, the resulting p-values are valid asymptotically regardless of the covariance structure.

Given the above empirical score process, the proportional hazards assumption for the mth covariate, according to Lin, Wei, and Ying (1993), can be assessed by plotting a dozen or so realizations of the simulated $\tilde{U}_m^*(t)$ on the same graph as the observed $\tilde{U}_m^*(t)$, thereby checking whether the observed scores fit in the null distribution samples. Additionally, given Equation (6.89), this graphical method can be supplemented by applying a Kolmogorov-type supremum test. The test statistic is

$$\sup_t\left\|\tilde{U}_m^*(\hat{\boldsymbol{\beta}},t)\right\|$$

or

$$\sup_t \sum_{m=1}^{m} \left[I^{-1}\left(\hat{\beta}\right)_{mm} \right]^{1/2} \left| \tilde{U}_m^*\left(\hat{\beta}, t\right) \right|.$$

Lin, Wei, and Ying (1993) contend that such test scores are consistent against the nonproportional hazards alternative, in which the effects of one or more covariates are not time independent. Given the value of α, the researcher can make a decision on whether or not the proportional hazards assumption in the Cox model is valid. Specifically, if the p-value of the Kolmogorov-type supremum test is smaller than α on a given covariate, it is appropriate to conclude with sufficient confidence that the proportionality assumption for this covariate is invalid.

This checking method is appealing in several aspects. First, it uses a standardized martingale transform that is distributed asymptotically as a zero-mean Gaussian process, so that it can be applied effectively to compare the expected and the observed martingales with a known distribution. Second, such a plot of martingale-typed residuals is linked with a Kolmogorov-type supremum test score, thus making a graphical check on the proportionality assumption in conjunction with a routine statistical test with a known distribution. Third, the development of this method provides a solid theoretical foundation for further refinements for handling other statistical issues encountered in survival analysis, as will be described in the next section and in Chapter 7.

6.3.6 Illustration: Checking the proportionality assumption in the Cox model for the effect of age on the mortality of older Americans

In Section 5.5, I displayed three log–log survival curves for three age groups: 70–74 years, 75–84 years, and 85 years or over. These survival curves present distinct separations and appear approximately parallel over time. Therefore, this graph provides some evidence that the effects of age on the mortality of older Americans are approximately proportional and thus can be considered a covariate in the Cox model. In Section 6.2, a plot of the Schoenfeld residuals corresponding to age also displays the effect of age to be independent of time. Those graphical checks, however, are crude in several aspects. First, in the stratified Cox model age is roughly divided into three groups, so that the proportionality within each age group cannot be assessed. Second, the stratified Cox model using three age groups as strata is poorly fitted and thus the graph derived from its results is not highly efficient (this issue is also discussed in Subsection 6.3.4). Third, it is difficult to conclude with sufficient confidence that the approximate parallel of the three log–log curves is statistically significant because a separation between two curves can also come from sampling errors. Lastly, the Schoenfeld residuals do not specify residuals for censored observations. Given these limitations, more refined methods should be applied to check the proportional hazards assumption further on the effects of age.

In the present illustration, I check the proportionality assumption on the effects of age by using two refined methods: (1) the checking approach with the addition of a time-dependent variable and (2) the graphical and numeric method using cumulative sums of the martingale-based residuals developed by Lin, Wei, and Ying (1993). The observation period is still from the baseline survey to the end of the year 2004. Three mean-centered variables – 'Age_mean,' 'Female_mean,' and 'Educ_mean' – are used as covariates with their values fixed at baseline.

As the first step, I illustrate the application of the first approach, which adds a time-dependent component to the effect of age. Specifically, a time-dependent variable is created – {Age_mean × [log t – mean(log t)]} – for checking the statistical significance of the time-dependent component on the effect of age. The working hypothesis on this numeric test is that the estimated regression coefficient of the time-dependent component of age is not statistically significant, thus validating the effect of age to be multiplicatively constant. The estimation procedure is exactly the same as described in Subsection 5.3.3, except for the addition of a time-dependent variable.

The SAS program for estimating this hazard model is given below.

SAS Program 6.2:

```
......
log_t = log(duration);
......
proc SQL;
  create table new as
  select *, age - mean(age) as age_mean,
    female - mean(female) as female_mean,
    educ - mean(educ) as educ_mean,
    log_t - mean(log_t) as logt_mean
  from new;
quit;

proc phreg data = new ;
  model duration*Status(0) = age_mean female_mean educ_mean age_t / ties = BRESLOW ;
  age_t = age_mean * logt_mean ;
run;
```

In SAS Program 6.2, I first create a variable log(t) to increase numeric stability in estimating the Cox model. Then, in the PROC SQL procedure, a mean-centered variable of log(t) is constructed for reducing collinearity. In the MODEL statement, the time-dependent variable, subsequently defined and named as 'Age_t,' is included in the regression, so that at each survival time, the individuals exposed to the risk of dying just before t are subject to two age dimensions. The Breslow method is applied again to handle tied observations. The following SAS output table displays parameter estimates.

SAS Program Output 6.1:

The PHREG Procedure

Analysis of Maximum Likelihood Estimates

Parameter	DF	Parameter Estimate	Standard Error	Chi-Square	Pr > ChiSq	Hazard Ratio
age_mean	1	0.09011	0.00483	347.8409	<.0001	1.094
female_mean	1	-0.41081	0.06644	38.2347	<.0001	0.663
educ_mean	1	-0.01963	0.00888	4.8920	0.0270	0.981
age_t	1	-0.09544	0.00656	211.6169	<.0001	0.909

In SAS Program Output 6.1, the estimated regression coefficients of all four covariates are statistically significant. In particular, the regression coefficient of the time-dependent variable 'Age_t' is –0.0954, with the Wald chi-square statistic very strongly statistically significant ($p < 0.0001$). The difference in the chi-square of the likelihood ratio test scores with or without the time-dependent variable, not presented here, is as high as 154.57 (470.56–315.99), also very strongly significant given one degree of freedom ($p < 0.0001$). Therefore, from the results of this test, the effect of age on the hazard function is shown to be a function of time. It is interesting to note that the main effect of age is positive, whereas the regression coefficient of the time-dependent component is negative, which, combined, highlights a decreasing trend over time in the hazard ratio of age. If such a decrease in the hazard ratio is sizable, it can be inferred that the proportional hazards assumption on age is invalid.

Closer examination on the hazard ratio of the time-dependent variable, however, suggests some caution in rejecting the null hypothesis on the proportional hazards of age. As the interaction of time is measured as log time, a hazard ratio of 0.91, though statistically significant, may not necessarily translate into a strong offsetting effect on proportional hazards. Given this concern, it is informative to display a plot that supports the absence of proportionality along the life course. Accordingly, next I illustrate Lin, Wei, and Ying's (1993) method with cumulative sums of the martingale-based residuals on the same data.

Below is the SAS program for using this method to check the proportionality assumption on the effects of age.

SAS Program 6.3:

```
......
ods graphics on ;
proc phreg data = new ;
  model duration*Status(0) = age_mean female_mean educ_mean / ties = BRESLOW ;
  assess ph / resample seed = 25 ;
run;
ods html close ;
```

In SAS Program 6.3, the MODEL statement does not include the time-dependent variable Age_t because this method is based on the martingale residual and its transforms, rather than on specifying an additional time-dependent covariate. The ASSESS statement tells SAS that the graphical and numeric methods of Lin, Wei, and Ying (1993) should be performed for checking the proportional hazards assumption and, as will be presented in next section, the adequacy of some other specifications in the Cox model. In particular, the PH option requests SAS to check the proportional hazards assumption for all covariates in the model. For each covariate, the observed score process component is plotted versus follow-up times along with 20 simulated patterns. The RESAMPLE option requests SAS to compute the Kolmogorov-type supremum test on 1000 simulated patterns. The last option in the ASSESS statement, the SEED = 25, specifies the number used to create simulated realizations for plots and the Kolmogorov-type supremum tests.

The plot in Figure 6.2 displays the graphical results of the proportional hazards assumption check for the covariate Age_mean. The standardized and the observed score processes are shown for covariate Age_mean, suggesting that in the early stage of the life course, the observed scores are consistently below zero, thus showing some systematic variability. Overall, however, the observed process tends to fluctuate randomly around zero, particularly at later survival

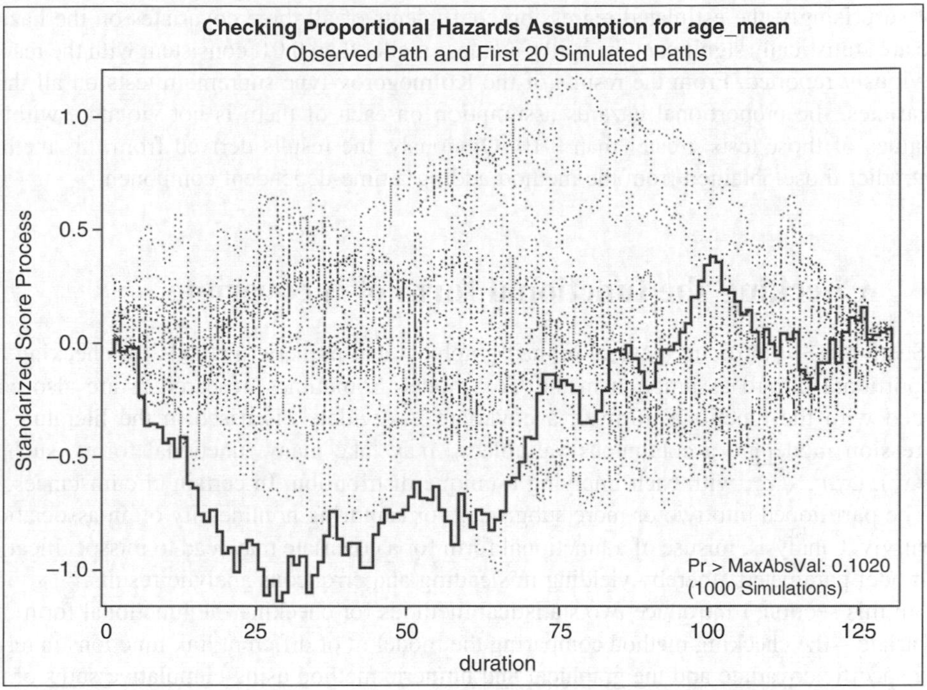

Figure 6.2 Checking the proportional hazards assumption for age.

times. Therefore, it seems that the null hypothesis on the proportionality assumption about age cannot be rejected. SAS Program 6.3 also generates graphical results for Female_mean and Educ_mean, not presented here, with both plots revealing proportional hazards.

The following SAS output tables present the numeric results of the regression coefficients and the Kolmogorov-type supremum tests for all the three covariates, also produced from SAS Program 6.3.

SAS Program Output 6.2:

The PHREG Procedure

Analysis of Maximum Likelihood Estimates

Parameter	DF	Parameter Estimate	Standard Error	Chi-Square	Pr > ChiSq	Hazard Ratio
age_mean	1	0.08228	0.00516	254.2103	<.0001	1.086
female_mean	1	-0.44312	0.06649	44.4090	<.0001	0.642
educ_mean	1	-0.02289	0.00876	6.8227	0.0090	0.977

Supremum Test for Proportionals Hazards Assumption

Variable	Maximum Absolute Value	Replications	Seed	Pr > MaxAbsVal
age_mean	1.1432	1000	25	0.1020
female_mean	0.9822	1000	25	0.2390
educ_mean	0.7734	1000	25	0.4600

Not surprisingly, the estimated regression coefficients of all three covariates on the hazard rate are statistically significant, with all p-values smaller than 0.01, consistent with the results previously reported. From the results of the Kolmogorov-type supremum tests on all three covariates, the proportional hazards assumption on each of them is not violated, with all p-values of those tests greater than 0.10. Obviously, the results derived from this method contradict those obtained from the method adding a time-dependent component.

6.4 Checking the functional form of a covariate

In Section 6.3, I introduce several refined graphical and numeric methods for checking the proportional hazard assumption in the Cox model. Sometimes, researchers are also concerned with the functional form of a covariate. As widely discussed in the literature on regression modeling, a continuous variable x_m may take many functional forms, such as $\log(x_m)$, $(x_m)^2$, $\sqrt{x_m}$, with each implying a unique distribution. In certain circumstances, x_m can be partitioned into two or more subgroups for capturing nonlinearity of an association. In survival analysis, misuse of a functional form for a covariate may lead to misspecification of model parameters, thereby yielding misleading and erroneous analytic results.

In this section, I introduce two statistical methods for checking the functional form of a covariate – the checking method comparing the model fit of different link functions in terms of a specific covariate and the graphical and numeric method using cumulative sums of the martingle-based residuals. An illustration is provided for checking the function form of age in the Cox model on the mortality of older Americans.

6.4.1 Checking model fit statistics for different link functions

Statistically, this method is simple, straightforward, and consistent with the corresponding approaches used for other linear or nonlinear regressions. Suppose we want to check the functional form of covariate x_m. First, the covariate vector $\boldsymbol{x}$ in the Cox model can be partitioned into two parts – x_m, the covariate under assessment, and $\boldsymbol{x}_r$, the vector of other covariates in $\boldsymbol{x}$. Assuming the proportional hazards for $\boldsymbol{x}_r$ to be valid and letting the true functional form of x_m be denoted by $\mathrm{f}(x_m)$, the correct Cox model should be written by

$$h(t|x_m, \boldsymbol{x}) = h_0(t)\exp[\mathrm{f}(x_m)\beta_1 + \boldsymbol{x}_r'\boldsymbol{\beta}_r], \tag{6.90}$$

where β_1 is the regression coefficient of $\mathrm{f}(x_m)$. On most occasions, $\mathrm{f}(x_m)$ is simply approximated by taking its natural form x_m or its mean-centered form (x_m minus mean(x_m)), assuming the variable to be linearly associated with the log hazards. If there is strong evidence against the assumption of such linearity, however, exploring an appropriate functional form of x_m becomes necessary.

Practically, we may create $\acute{n}$ regression models by using $\acute{n}$ different link functions of x_m for checking which functional form fits most closely with the log hazards. Suppose that x_m is independent of other covariates; an appropriate functional form of x_m can be determined by comparing the results of the Wald test statistic for those $\acute{n}$ Cox models. The regression having the highest Wald test score on the estimated regression coefficient among a variety of functional forms of x_m should be regarded as the most appropriate Cox model. Therefore, that specific functional form of x_m can be taken as the one closest to the true function $f(x_m)$.

Alternatively, the statistical testing on the functional form of x_m can be performed by using the partial likelihood ratio test. In particular, for two successive Cox models that specify two different functional forms of x_m, denoted by $f^{(\gamma-1)}$ and by $f^{(\gamma)}$, respectively, the partial likelihood ratio test score is given by

$$G_{\beta_1(\beta-1,\beta)} = -2\times\left\{\log L_p\left[\hat{\beta}_1^{(\gamma-1)},\hat{\boldsymbol{\beta}}_r\right]-\log L_p\left[\hat{\beta}_1^{(\gamma)},\hat{\boldsymbol{\beta}}_r\right]\right\}, \quad \gamma=1,\ldots \dot{w}, \tag{6.91}$$

where $\hat{\beta}_1^{(\gamma-1)}$ and $\hat{\beta}_1^{(\gamma)}$ are the estimated regression coefficients of x_m transforms from models with functional forms $f^{(\gamma-1)}$ and $f^{(\gamma)}$, respectively, and $G_{\beta_1(\gamma-1,\gamma)}$ is the partial likelihood ratio test statistic that reflects whether or not the functional form $f^{(\gamma)}$ gains statistical information as compared to the functional form $f^{(\gamma-1)}$, distributed as χ^2 with one degree of freedom. Within the brace on the right of Equation (6.91), the first term is the log partial likelihood ratio statistic for the model with functional form $f^{(\gamma-1)}$, whereas the second is the same statistic for the Cox model with functional form $f^{(\gamma)}$. If $G_{\beta_1(\gamma-1,\gamma)} < \chi^2_{(1-\alpha;1)}$, the specification of $f^{(\gamma)}$ does not improve the quality of the model fit, thereby suggesting that $f^{(\gamma)}$ should be dropped from further comparison and the function $f^{(\gamma-1)}$ should be retained. If $G_{\beta_1(\gamma-1,\gamma)} > \chi^2_{(1-\alpha;1)}$, the specification of the functional form $f^{(\gamma)}$ predicts the hazard rate statistically better than does the functional form $f^{(\gamma-1)}$; therefore this functional form should be retained for further comparison and, accordingly, $f^{(\gamma-1)}$ be dropped. Eventually, the most appropriate functional form of x_m can be determined statistically from those $\acute{n}$ candidates ordered by the level of complexity.

Sometimes, it is technically difficult to judge the validity of a specific functional form of a covariate simply from the above procedure. For example, other than several frequently used functional forms (e.g., $\log x_m$, $(x_m)^2$, $\sqrt{x_m}$), some high-order polynomial functions are occasionally used. Given the problem of correlation among the linear, quadratic, and high-order terms, centering x_m is necessary to reduce multicollinearity, thereby complicating the selection of an appropriate function form. Correlation between x_m and other covariates must also be considered, which can significantly complicate the selection process. Specifically, the existence of complex interrelationships among covariates can make the test results dubious. Perhaps due to these reasons, some statisticians recommend computing and plotting the martingale residuals to find a functional form that is closest to f (Klein and Moeschberger, 2003; Therneau, Grambsch, and Fleming, 1990). If the martingale plot with x_m as a covariate appears linear, no transformation of x_m is needed; if the plot appears nonlinear, then a transformation of x_m may be necessary. In the presence of heavy censoring, however, it is very infrequent to find a plot of the martingale residual or its transforms to be distributed linearly, as evidenced in Subsection 6.3.6.

6.4.2 Checking the functional form with cumulative sums of martingale-based residuals

This method for checking the functional form of a covariate is an integral part of the graphical and numeric approach described in Subsection 6.3.5. As previously discussed, it is difficult to derive a convincing conclusion about the validity of the proportional hazards assumption just by examining the martingale residuals and their transforms. The same problem exists for checking the functional form of a covariate. Lin, Wei, and Ying (1993) provide a less subjective approach by examining the two stochastic processes with a known distribution, specified by Equations (6.85) and (6.86). In terms of checking the functional form of covariate x_m, they propose to plot the partial-sum processes of the martingale residuals, written as

$$\mathrm{W}_m(\mathrm{z}) = \sum_{i=1}^{n} \mathrm{I}(\mathrm{Z}_{im} \le \mathrm{z})\hat{\mathrm{M}}_i, \quad m = 1, \ldots, M, \tag{6.92}$$

where $\mathrm{W}_m(\mathrm{z})$ is a special case of $\mathrm{W}_\mathrm{z}(t, \mathrm{z})$, specified in Equation (6.85), with $\mathrm{f}(\cdot) = 1$ and $z_{m'} = \infty(m' \neq m)$.

As indicated above, the null distribution of $\mathrm{W}_m(\cdot)$ can be approximated through simulating the corresponding zero-mean Gaussian process $\hat{\mathrm{W}}_m(\cdot)$ along with a dozen or so realizations. In the case of checking the functional form of covariate m, $\mathrm{W}_m(\mathrm{z})$ can be approximated by

$$\begin{aligned}\hat{\mathrm{W}}_m(\mathrm{z}) = \sum_{l=1}^{n} \delta_l \Bigg\{ \mathrm{I}(\mathrm{Z}_{lm} \le \mathrm{z}) - \frac{\sum_{i=1}^{n} \mathrm{Y}_i(T_l)\exp\left(\mathbf{Z}_i'\hat{\boldsymbol{\beta}}\right)\mathrm{I}(\mathrm{Z}_{im} \le \mathrm{z})}{\sum_{i=1}^{n} Y_i(\mathrm{T}_l)\exp\left(\mathbf{Z}_i'\hat{\boldsymbol{\beta}}\right)} \Bigg\} G_l \\ - \sum_{\bar{k}=1}^{n} \int_0^t Y_{\bar{k}}(u)\exp\left(\mathbf{Z}_{\bar{k}}'\hat{\boldsymbol{\beta}}\right)\mathrm{I}(\mathrm{Z}_{\bar{k}m} \le \mathrm{z})\left[\mathbf{Z}_{\bar{k}} - \bar{\mathbf{Z}}\left(\hat{\boldsymbol{\beta}}, u\right)\right]' \mathrm{d}\hat{\Lambda}_0(u) \\ \times \boldsymbol{I}^{-1}\left(\hat{\boldsymbol{\beta}}\right)\sum_{l=1}^{n} \delta_l \left[\mathbf{Z}_l - \bar{\mathbf{Z}}\left(\hat{\boldsymbol{\beta}}, T_l\right)\right]\mathrm{G}_l \Bigg\}.\end{aligned} \tag{6.93}$$

Consequently, if the null hypothesis about the functional form of x_m holds, $\hat{\mathrm{W}}_m(\cdot)$ should fluctuate randomly around zero. Accordingly, a natural numeric measure can be created:

$$\tilde{\mathrm{s}}_m = \sup_{\mathrm{z}} \left|\mathrm{w}_m(\mathrm{z})\right|, \tag{6.94}$$

where $\mathrm{w}_m(\cdot)$ is the observed value of the Gaussian approximate $\mathrm{w}_m(\cdot)$. This numeric score, $\tilde{\mathrm{s}}_m$, can be used to display whether or not the functional form of x_m is statistically suitable. Specifically, if the value of $\tilde{\mathrm{s}}_m$ is beyond a critical point, the underlying functional form of x_m is questionable; therefore, using another transform of x_m in the Cox model may be necessary. The p-value for the distribution of $\tilde{\mathrm{s}}_m$, under the null hypothesis, can be approximated by $\Pr\left(\hat{\tilde{\mathrm{S}}}_m \ge \tilde{\mathrm{s}}_m\right)$, where

$$\hat{\tilde{\mathrm{S}}}_m = \sup_{\mathrm{z}} \left|\hat{\mathrm{W}}_m(\mathrm{z})\right|.$$

The calculation of $\Pr\left(\hat{\tilde{S}}_m \geq \tilde{s}_m\right)$ is conditional on the triple $(T_i, \delta_i, \mathbf{Z}_i)$. Lin, Wei, and Ying (1993) showed that $\Pr\left(\hat{\tilde{S}}_m \geq \tilde{s}_m\right)$ converges to $\Pr\left(\tilde{S}_m \geq \tilde{s}_m\right)$ as n tends to ∞, consistent against incorrect functional forms for x_m if there is no additional model misspecification and if x_m is independent of other covariates.

6.4.3 Illustration: Checking the functional form of age in the Cox model on the mortality of older Americans

In this illustration, I check the functional form of age by using the two methods described above: (1) the method based on the partial likelihood ratio test and (2) the graphical and numeric approach using cumulative sums of the martingale-based residuals developed by Lin, Wei, and Ying (1993). The observation period is still the same as indicated in the previous example (from the outset of the baseline survey to the end of the year 2004). Three mean-centered variables – 'Age_mean,' 'Female_mean,' and 'Educ_mean' – are used as time-independent covariates. For applying the first method, I focus on comparing three functional forms of age – Age_mean (age – mean[age]), log(age), and age × age. Specifically, I want to know whether the second and the third functional forms significantly improve the overall fit of the Cox model by examining the partial likelihood ratio test statistics. The SAS program for estimating the three models are displayed below.

SAS Program 6.4:

```
......
proc SQL;
  create table new as
  select *, age - mean(age) as age_mean,
    log(age) as log_age,
    (age)**2 as age_2,
    female - mean(female) as female_mean,
    educ - mean(educ) as educ_mean
  from new;
quit;

proc phreg data = new ;
  model duration*Status(0) = age_mean female_mean educ_mean / ties = BRESLOW ;
run;

proc phreg data = new ;
  model duration*Status(0) = log_age female_mean educ_mean / ties = BRESLOW ;
run;

proc phreg data = new ;
  model duration*Status(0) = age_2 female_mean educ_mean / ties = BRESLOW ;
run;
```

In SAS Program 6.4, I create two additional functional forms of age – log(age) and $(\text{age})^2$ – using the PROC SQL procedure. Then, three Cox models are specified using those three different functional forms. In the MODEL statement of each model, age is considered in the regression with a unique functional form. The Breslow method is applied again to handle tied observations. The following output table displays the results of the overall test statistics on the three models.

SAS Program Output 6.3:

Testing Global Null Hypothesis: BETA=0

Test	Chi-Square	DF	Pr > ChiSq
Likelihood Ratio	315.9911	3	<.0001
Score	308.5743	3	<.0001
Wald	316.1353	3	<.0001

Testing Global Null Hypothesis: BETA=0

Test	Chi-Square	DF	Pr > ChiSq
Likelihood Ratio	317.4981	3	<.0001
Score	290.6365	3	<.0001
Wald	305.2581	3	<.0001

Testing Global Null Hypothesis: BETA=0

Test	Chi-Square	DF	Pr > ChiSq
Likelihood Ratio	312.3025	3	<.0001
Score	321.8433	3	<.0001
Wald	324.8013	3	<.0001

As shown in SAS Program Output 6.3, differences in the chi-square value of the likelihood ratio test score between the three models do not support the proposition that the specification of the second and the third functional forms of age significantly improve the overall fit of the Cox model. Changes in this test score are not statistically significant ($p > 0.05$), thus suggesting that the two additional functional forms of age do not have a better link with the hazard function. Among the three functional forms, the centered variable Age_mean is the natural and the most parsimonious transform of age.

As discussed above, however, this method does not necessarily provide sufficient information for deriving a convincing conclusion. Like the case in checking the proportionality assumption in the Cox model, a statistical method combining both graphical and numeric checks provides more insights for an appropriate functional form of a covariate. For this reason, next I apply Lin, Wei, and Ying's (1993) approach with cumulative sums of the martingale-based residuals. In particular, I start by using [age – mean(age)], represented by covariate Age_mean, as the functional form. Below is the SAS program for fitting this model.

SAS Program 6.5:

```
......
ods graphics on ;
proc phreg data = new ;
  model duration*Status(0) = age_mean female_mean educ_mean / ties = BRESLOW ;
  assess var = (age_mean) / resample seed = 25 ;
run;
ods html close ;
```

In SAS Program 6.5, I fit the Cox model with the covariate 'Age_mean,' using 'Female_mean' and Educ_mean' as controls. The Breslow method is used again to handle tied observations. As mentioned in Subsection 6.3.6, the ASSESS statement can be used to check the adequacy of some other specifications in the Cox model, including the capability of checking the functional form of a covariate. Accordingly, I use the VAR=(AGE_MEAN) option to create a plot of the cumulative martingale residuals against values of the covariate Age_mean. From this option, the functional form of this age transform can be assessed both visually and analytically. The RESAMPLE and SEED options are explained in Section 6.3.

SAS Program 6.5 yields an output table and a graph. I first review the result of the supremum test for this functional form of age, shown below.

SAS Program Output 6.4:

Supremum Test for Functional Form

Variable	Maximum Absolute Value	Replications	Seed	Pr > MaxAbsVal
age_mean	24.1452	1000	25	0.0850

SAS Program Output 6.4 displays that the *p*-value of Age_mean from the Kolmogorov-type supremum test, based on 1000 simulations, is 0.0850. Statistically, this *p*-value is marginal: if the value of α is set at 0.05, it can be said that the observed martingale process does not deviate significantly from the simulated realizations, so that using another transform of age seems unnecessary. If $\alpha = 0.10$, the observed process would be considered atypical compared to the normal simulations, which, in turn, suggests that a more appropriate functional form of age should be used to replace centered age. Therefore, a graphical check may be helpful to draw a more confident conclusion. The graph generated from SAS Program 6.5 is shown in Figure 6.3, which displays the plot of the observed cumulative martingale residual process for Age_mean, along with 20 simulated realizations from the null

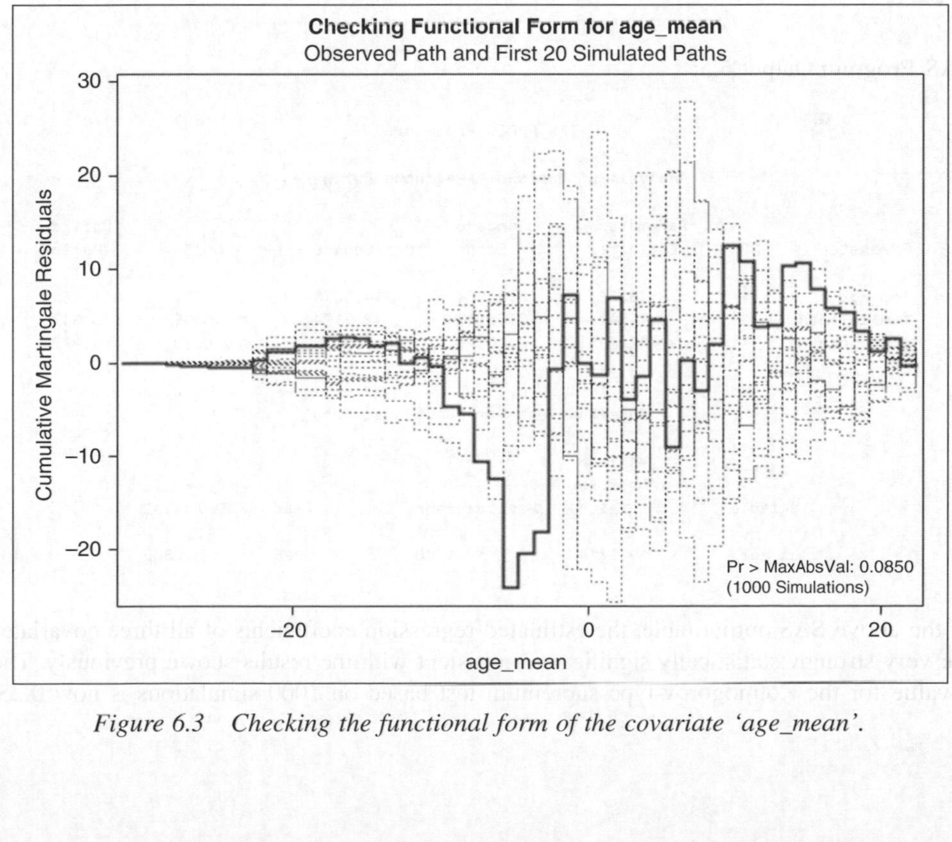

Figure 6.3 Checking the functional form of the covariate 'age_mean'.

distribution. According to this plot, the observed martingale residuals do not seem to fall off systematically from the null distribution, except at some survival times located in the middle range of Age_mean; therefore, using another transform of age seems unnecessary.

To ensure that [age – mean(age)] is the appropriate functional form of age in the Cox model, I perform some additional analyses by replacing this variable with the functional form log(age) in the Cox model. In particular, I want to check whether the cumulative martingale residual plot, obtained from the model using the new covariate Log_age as the transform of age, differs significantly from Figure 6.3. Below is the SAS program for this step.

SAS Program 6.6:

```
......
ods graphics on ;
proc phreg data = new ;
 model duration*Status(0) = log_age female_mean educ_mean / ties = BRESLOW ;
 assess var = (log_age) / crpanel resample seed = 25 ;
run;
ods html close ;
```

SAS Program 6.6 considers log(age) as the functional form of age. In the ASSESS statement, the CRPANEL option is added to request a panel of four plots for extensive checks, with each plotting the observed cumulative martingale residual process along with two simulated realizations. The following SAS output table presents the estimated regression coefficients of the three covariates and the result of the supremum test on covariate Log_age.

SAS Program Output 6.5:

The PHREG Procedure

Analysis of Maximum Likelihood Estimates

Parameter	DF	Parameter Estimate	Standard Error	Chi-Square	Pr > ChiSq	Hazard Ratio
log_age	1	6.46375	0.41354	244.3073	<.0001	641.460
female_mean	1	-0.43541	0.06647	42.9104	<.0001	0.647
educ_mean	1	-0.02289	0.00876	6.8278	0.0090	0.977

Supremum Test for Functional Form

Variable	Maximum Absolute Value	Replications	Seed	Pr > MaxAbsVal
log_age	19.9714	1000	25	0.2300

In the above SAS output table, the estimated regression coefficients of all three covariates are very strongly statistically significant, consistent with the results shown previously. The p-value for the Kolmogorov-type supremum test based on 1000 simulations is now 0.23,

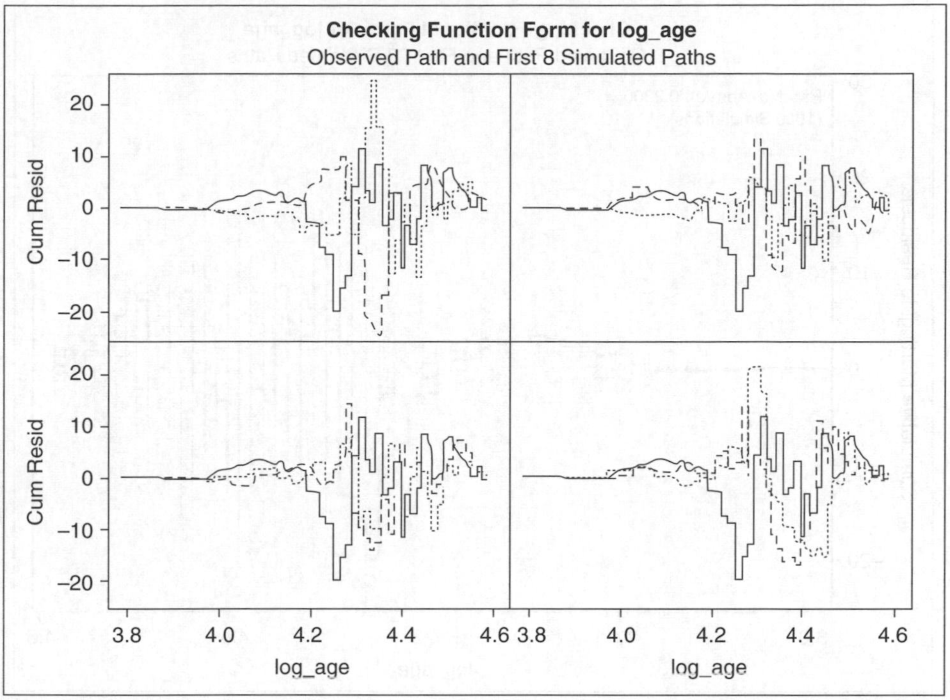

Figure 6.4 Panel plot of cumulative martingale residuals against log (age).

indicating that using additional functional forms of age is unnecessary for estimating the effects of age.

The plot in Figure 6.4 displays the panel with four plots, where the observed cumulative martingale process agrees nicely with each set of two realizations of the null distributions. The next graph further demonstrates this consistency, where Figure 6.5 displays a summary plot of the cumulative martingale residuals against log(age) generated from the VAR= option in the ASSESS statement. This graph plots the observed martingale score process for log(age) along with 20 realizations from the null distribution. In general, this graph appears consistent both with Figure 6.3 and with those in the panel plot. Obviously, either using Age_mean or using Log_age yields the same results on the overall fit of the Cox model and on the distribution of the martingale residuals. As a result, I now have sufficient confidence to conclude that using covariate Age_mean in the Cox model is most appropriate given the simplicity and parsimony attaching to this functional form. As in the survival data of older Americans, an older person's age is not highly correlated with gender and educational attainment, this conclusion seems valid and reliable. This conclusion is also in accordance with the result obtained from the method using the partial likelihood ratio test statistic.

6.5 Identification of influential observations in the Cox model

Another important aspect of regression diagnostics on the Cox model is identification of influential observations. In the literature of regression diagnostics, it is an essential statistical

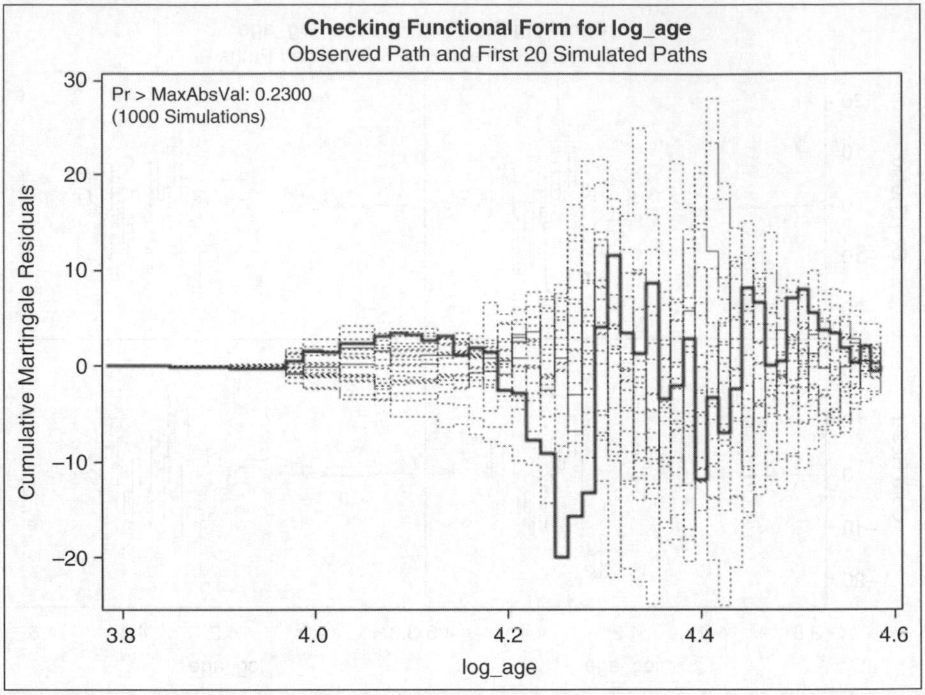

Figure 6.5 Cumulative martingale residuals against log(age).

step to ascertain particular observations that have extraordinary influences on analytic results of a linear or a nonlinear regression model. With regard to the Cox model, removal of such influential cases from the regression should be followed by substantially increased or decreased hazard rates. Identification of influential observations in survival data, however, is not an easy undertaking and differs markedly from conventional perspectives in several ways. Most significantly, the diagnostic techniques on survival data involve individuals at many survival times, rather than at a single data point. As a result, elimination of one individual may affect a series of risk sets, in turn magnifying its influence on parameter estimates. This unique impact is especially strong for those who experience a particular event late in an observation period. Given such characteristics, some of the conventional diagnostic measures, like the Cook's distance (Fox, 1991), would not perform appropriately in the Cox model. Identification of influential observations for the proportional hazard model thus calls for the development of more refined techniques.

This section describes two popular diagnostic methods for identifying influential observations in the Cox model – the likelihood displacement score (the *LD* statistic) and the *LMAX* standardized statistic. An illustration is provided for checking whether there are any influential observations in the Cox model on the mortality of older Americans.

6.5.1 The likelihood displacement statistic approximation

The Cox model is a log-linear regression model and therefore, like other relevant techniques involving a linear predictor, some observations can have an unduly impact on inferential procedures for deriving parameter estimates. Theoretically, such influential cases can be identified by changes in the estimated regression coefficients after deleting each observation in a sequence.

Let $\hat{\boldsymbol{\beta}}$ be the value of $\boldsymbol{\beta}$ that maximizes the log partial likelihood function and $\hat{\boldsymbol{\beta}}_{(-i)}$ be the same estimate of $\boldsymbol{\beta}$ when individual i is eliminated. For covariate x_m, the distance in the estimated regression coefficient after removing individual i, denoted $\bar{D}_{mi}$, is given by

$$\bar{D}_{mi} = \hat{\beta}_m - \hat{\beta}_{m(-i)}. \tag{6.95}$$

The above equation provides an exact measure for the absolute influence of deleting individual i from a regression model on the estimates of regression coefficients. By applying the likelihood ratio test with one degree of freedom, the significance of this influence can be statistically assessed. This likelihood ratio test is referred as the *likelihood displacement* (*LD*) statistic, given by

$$LD_i = 2\log L\left(\hat{\boldsymbol{\beta}}\right) - 2\log L\left[\hat{\boldsymbol{\beta}}_{(-i)}\right]. \tag{6.96}$$

The likelihood displacement statistic is distributed as chi-square under the null hypothesis that $\hat{\boldsymbol{\beta}}_{(-i)} = \hat{\boldsymbol{\beta}}$. Therefore, the observations having a strong impact on $\hat{\boldsymbol{\beta}}$ can be statistically identified, thus helping the researcher decide whether or not they should be removed from an estimation process.

When analyzing survival data, however, the use of this exact effect is not realistic. First, when the sample size is large, the checking process becomes extremely tedious and time-consuming. Consider, for example, a sample of 2000 observations: the analyst needs to create 2001 Cox models to identify which case or cases have an exceptionally strong impact on the estimation of regression coefficients. Second, unlike other types of generalized linear regression models, eliminating one observation from the Cox model would affect a series of risk sets. In particular, for those who experience a particular event early, less weight should be considered in the estimating process because their contributions to the partial likelihood function are relatively limited. In contrast, for individuals who have the event late, they are involved in more risk sets than others in likelihoods and thus should be given more weight. Hence, identifying influential observations in the Cox model involves a much more complicated procedure than in a common generalized linear regression model. If the distance score $\hat{\boldsymbol{\beta}} - \hat{\boldsymbol{\beta}}_{(-i)}$ can be statistically approximated by a scalar measure in the Cox model, influential observations can be identified without removing each case in sequence from the estimation process.

Cain and Lange (1984) developed a method to approximate Equation (6.95) by introducing weights into the partial likelihood function. Suppose that a weighted analysis is needed to identify influential observations in the Cox model, with individual i assigned weight w_i and all other observations given the weight 1. The approximation to Equation (6.95), based on the first-order Taylor series expansion about $w_i = 1$, is

$$\hat{\boldsymbol{\beta}} - \hat{\boldsymbol{\beta}}_{(-i)} \cong \frac{\partial \hat{\boldsymbol{\beta}}}{\partial w_i}. \tag{6.97}$$

This approximation is called the *infinitesimal jackknife approach* (Pettitt and Bin Raud, 1989). This derivative can be evaluated in terms of the score vector $\tilde{\boldsymbol{U}}\left[\hat{\boldsymbol{\beta}}(w_i), w_i\right]$.

The derivative of the log partial likelihood function with respect to $\boldsymbol{\beta}$ can be written as

$$\tilde{U}\left(\hat{\beta}\right) = \sum_{i=1}^{d} \tilde{U}_i = \sum_{i=1}^{d} \left[w_i \boldsymbol{x}_i - w_i \hat{\mathrm{E}}(\boldsymbol{x}|\mathcal{R}_i) \right], \tag{6.98}$$

where

$$\hat{\mathrm{E}}(\boldsymbol{x}|\mathcal{R}_i) = \frac{\sum_{l \in \mathcal{R}(t_i)} w_l \boldsymbol{x}_l \exp\left(\boldsymbol{x}_l' \hat{\boldsymbol{\beta}}\right)}{\sum_{l \in \mathcal{R}(t_i)} \mathrm{w}_l \exp\left(\boldsymbol{x}_l' \hat{\boldsymbol{\beta}}\right)}.$$

Let D_i be the set of individuals who experience a particular event before or at time t_i. After some algebra, the derivative of $\tilde{\boldsymbol{U}}$ with respect to w_i is

$$\frac{\partial \tilde{\boldsymbol{U}}}{\partial w_i} = \delta_i \left[\boldsymbol{x}_i - \hat{\mathrm{E}}(\boldsymbol{x}|\mathcal{R}_i) \right] - \sum_{i=1}^{D_i} \frac{w_i \exp\left(\boldsymbol{x}_i' \hat{\boldsymbol{\beta}}\right)}{\sum_{l \in \mathcal{R}_i} w_l \exp\left(\boldsymbol{x}_l' \hat{\boldsymbol{\beta}}\right)} \left[\boldsymbol{x}_i - \hat{\mathrm{E}}(\boldsymbol{x}|\mathcal{R}_i) \right]. \tag{6.99}$$

Equation (6.99) shows that the score vector $\tilde{\boldsymbol{U}}$ with respect to changes in w_i can be decomposed into two components. The first component is the Schoenfeld (1982) residual, defined as the difference between the covariate vector for individual i at time t and the expected values of the covariate vector at the same time. The second component measures the impact that changes in w_i have on all the risk sets including individual i. The second component increases in absolute magnitude with t because it is the sum of an increasing number of terms. Consequently, the second term plays an increasingly important role in estimating the regression coefficients as time progresses.

In Equation (6.99), D_i is fixed for censored patients between event times, so can be written as

$$\frac{\partial \tilde{\boldsymbol{U}}}{\partial w_i} = \delta_i \left[\boldsymbol{x}_i - \frac{\sum_{l \in \mathcal{R}_{tt}} \boldsymbol{x}_l \exp\left(\boldsymbol{x}_l' \hat{\boldsymbol{\beta}}\right)}{\sum_{l \in \mathcal{R}_{tt}} \exp\left(\boldsymbol{x}_l' \hat{\boldsymbol{\beta}}\right)} \right] - \exp\left(\boldsymbol{x}_i' \hat{\boldsymbol{\beta}}\right) \left\{ \frac{\boldsymbol{x}_i}{\sum_{l \in \mathcal{R}_{tt}} \exp\left(\boldsymbol{x}_l' \hat{\boldsymbol{\beta}}\right)} - \frac{\sum_{l \in \mathcal{R}_{tt}} \boldsymbol{x}_l \exp\left(\boldsymbol{x}_l' \hat{\boldsymbol{\beta}}\right)}{\left[\sum_{l \in \mathcal{R}_{tt}} \exp\left(\boldsymbol{x}_l' \hat{\boldsymbol{\beta}}\right) \right]^{2}} \right\} \tag{6.100}$$

Clearly, the above approximation evades the specification of w_i. As a result, such simplification facilitates the development of an approximation for the likelihood displacement statistic.

Consequently, when $w_i = 0$ and all w_l are unity ($l \neq i$), the regular Cox model can be applied to approximate the likelihood displacement statistic without fitting numerous regressions and deleting each individual in sequence. Cain and Lange (1984) suggest that with information of the triple (t, δ, $\boldsymbol{x}$) for each individual as well as of $\hat{\boldsymbol{\beta}}$ and the observed information matrix, an M vector of estimated influence for each individual can be produced.

Assuming the elimination of individual i not to change the values of the observed information matrix, Pettitt and Bin Raud (1989) proposed the following approximation of the likelihood displacement statistic for individual i:

$$\boldsymbol{LD}_i \approx \hat{\mathbf{L}}_i' \hat{\boldsymbol{I}}^{-1}\left(\hat{\boldsymbol{\beta}}\right) \hat{\mathbf{L}}_i, \tag{6.101}$$

where $\hat{\mathbf{L}}_i$ is the score residual vector of individual i, described in Subsection 6.2.4. The mth element of the LD_i vector, referred to as the *delta-beta statistic*, approximates the case influence on the estimated regression coefficient of covariate x_m after deleting individual i. More important, from the LD_i scores, a single measure of the LD statistic can be created by summing all component score residuals within an individual. This global influence statistic reflects the case influence on the overall fit of the Cox model.

The above LD statistic approximates the change in the estimated regression coefficients after deleting each individual from estimation of the Cox model, thus evading elimination of useful survival data. Empirically, both Collett (2003) and Klein and Moeschberger (2003) display remarkable agreement between the exact and the approximate LD statistics using some survival data with a small sample size.

6.5.2 LMAX statistic for identification of influential observations

Another innovative technique for identifying influential observations in the Cox model is the *LMAX* statistic, originally developed by Cook (1986) as a standardized diagnostic method for general regression modeling and later introduced and advanced into survival analysis by Pettitt and Bin Raud (1989). Specifically, this method maximizes the approximation to the $LD(w)$ statistic for changes standardized to the unit length.

Cook (1986) suggests the use of a standardized likelihood displacement statistic for more accurately measuring influences of particular cases in estimating a regression model. Given the likelihood displacement (LD) statistic, represented by Equation (6.96), Cook first defines a symmetric matrix $\mathbf{B}$, given by

$$\mathbf{B} = \mathbf{L}'\boldsymbol{I}\left(\hat{\beta}\right)^{-1}\mathbf{L}, \tag{6.102}$$

where $\mathbf{L}$ is the matrix with rows containing the score residual vector $\hat{\mathbf{L}}_i$. With $\mathbf{B}$ defined, Cook considers the direction of the $n \times 1$ vector $\tilde{\mathbf{l}}$ that maximizes $\tilde{\mathbf{l}}'\mathbf{B}\tilde{\mathbf{l}}$, and $\tilde{\mathbf{l}}$ is standardized to have unit length. Because the $M \times M$ matrix $\hat{\boldsymbol{I}}\left(\hat{\beta}\right)^{-1}$ is positive definite, the $n \times n$ symmetric matrix $\mathbf{B}$ is positive semi-definite with rank no more than M. The statistic $\tilde{\mathbf{l}}_{\max}$ corresponds to the unit length eigenvector of $\mathbf{B}$ that has the largest eigenvalue $\tilde{\gamma}_{\max}$. Then, $\tilde{\mathbf{l}}'_{\max}\mathbf{B}\tilde{\mathbf{l}}_{\max}$ maximizes $\tilde{\mathbf{l}}'\mathbf{B}\tilde{\mathbf{l}}$ and satisfies the equation

$$\mathbf{B}\tilde{\mathbf{l}}_{\max} = \ddot{\lambda}_{\max}\tilde{\mathbf{l}}_{\max} \quad \text{and} \quad \tilde{\mathbf{l}}'_{\max}\tilde{\mathbf{l}}_{\max} = 1,$$

where $\ddot{\lambda}_{\max}$ is the largest eigenvalue of $\mathbf{B}$ and $\tilde{\mathbf{l}}_{\max}$ is the eigenvector associated with $\ddot{\lambda}_{\max}$. The elements of $\tilde{\mathbf{l}}_{\max}$, standardized to unit length, measure the sensitivity of the model fit to each observation of the data. The absolute value of $\tilde{\mathbf{l}}_i$, the ith element in $\tilde{\mathbf{l}}_{\max}$, is used as the *LMAX* score for individual i. Given the unit length, the expected value of the squared *LMAX* statistic for each observation is $1/n$, where n is sample size, so that a value significantly greater than this expected figure indicates a strong influence on the overall fit of a regression model thereby being identified. If $M = 1$, the *LMAX* statistic is proportional to $\mathbf{L}'$ and $\ddot{\lambda}_{\max} = \boldsymbol{I}\left(\hat{\beta}\right)^{-1}\|\mathbf{L}\|$. When $M > 1$, an advantage of looking at elements of the *LMAX* statistic, rather than at the delta-beta statistics, is that each case has a single summary measure of influence.

As the *LMAX* score is a standardized statistic, it is highly useful to plot elements of *LMAX* scores against survival times and/or values of covariates. The standardization of $\tilde{\mathbf{l}}_{\max}$ to unit length means that the squares of the elements in $\tilde{\mathbf{l}}_{\max}$ sum to unity, so that signs of the elements of $\tilde{\mathbf{l}}_{\max}$ are not of concern. Accordingly, for $\tilde{\mathbf{l}}_i$, only the absolute value needs to be plotted. Observations that have most unduly influence on parameter estimates and the model fit can then be identified by examining the relative influence of the elements in $\tilde{\mathbf{l}}_{\max}$. If none of the observations has an undue impact on model inference, the plot of the elements of the *LMAX* scores should approximate a horizontal line.

6.5.3 Illustration: Checking influential observations in the Cox model on the mortality of older Americans

In the present illustration, I extend the example presented in Subsection 6.4.3. Specifically, I want to identify whether there are influential cases in terms of the overall fit of the Cox model on the mortality of older Americans, using the centered variables Age_mean, Female_mean, and Educ_mean as covariates. Both the *LD* and the *LMAX* statistics are applied for such identification, as against the rank order of survival times. Here, only the case influence on the overall model fit is considered, given the aforementioned advantage of using a single summary measure. Therefore, I do not examine the delta-beta statistic for each covariate. Additionally, I plot the elements of the *LMAX* statistic against values of a covariate – age, as recommended by Collett (2003) and Pattitt and Bin Raud (1989). The SAS program for generating the three *LD* and *LMAX* plots are displayed below.

SAS Program 6.7:

```
......

proc phreg data = new noprint ;
 model duration*Status(0) = age_mean female_mean educ_mean / ties = BRESLOW ;
 output out = out_case LD = LD LMAX = LMAX ;
run;

Title "Figure 6.6. Case influence against duration based on LD";
proc sgplot data = out_case ;
 yaxis grid;
 refline 0 / axis = y ;
 scatter y = LD x = duration ;
run;

Title "Figure 6.7. Case influence against duration based on LMAX";
proc sgplot data = out_case ;
 yaxis grid;
 refline 0 / axis = y ;
 scatter y = LMAX x = duration ;
run;

Title "Figure 6.8. Case influence against age based on LMAX";
proc sgplot data = out_case ;
 yaxis grid;
 refline 0 / axis = y ;
 scatter y = LMAX x = age ;
run;
```

In SAS Program 6.7, I first specify the Cox model on the mortality of older Americans, with Age_mean, Female_mean, and Educ_mean as covariates. In the PROC PHREG procedure, an OUTPUT statement is added for saving information needed for creating the three plots. The keyword LD specifies the approximate likelihood displacement for each individual. Similarly, the keyword LMAX tells SAS to derive the score of relative influence on the overall fit of the Cox model, standardized to unit length. Those two keywords identify two new variables – *LD* and *LMAX* – and they are then output into the temporary data file OUT_CASE. Lastly, I use the PROC SGPLOT procedure to generate the three plots, specifying different variables for axis y and axis x in each graph.

The first plot, displaying the likelihood displacement scores against the rank order of survival times, is displayed in Figure 6.6, where numerous values of the *LD* statistic are plotted against the duration of survival times, actual or censored. As can be easily identified, there is an outstanding case located near the end of the observation period. Additionally, there are some other observations obviously deviating markedly from the vast majority of the cases, though distant from the most outstanding case. In total, however, the influences of those observations on the overall fit of the Cox model seem small, considering the limited range of values of the *LD* statistics. Even for the most influential case, the value of the *LD* statistic is less than 0.10. As indicated earlier, when sample size is large, such an *LD* approximate is supposed to agree closely with the exact *LD* statistic. At least, I do not need to create $n + 1$ Cox models to identify those influential observations.

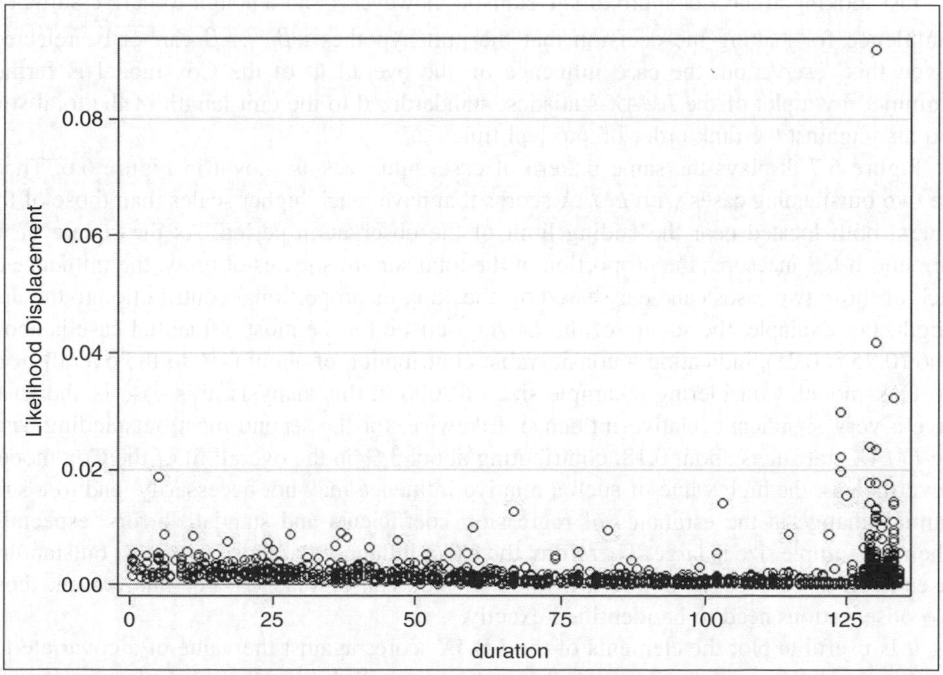

Figure 6.6 Case influence against duration based on LD.

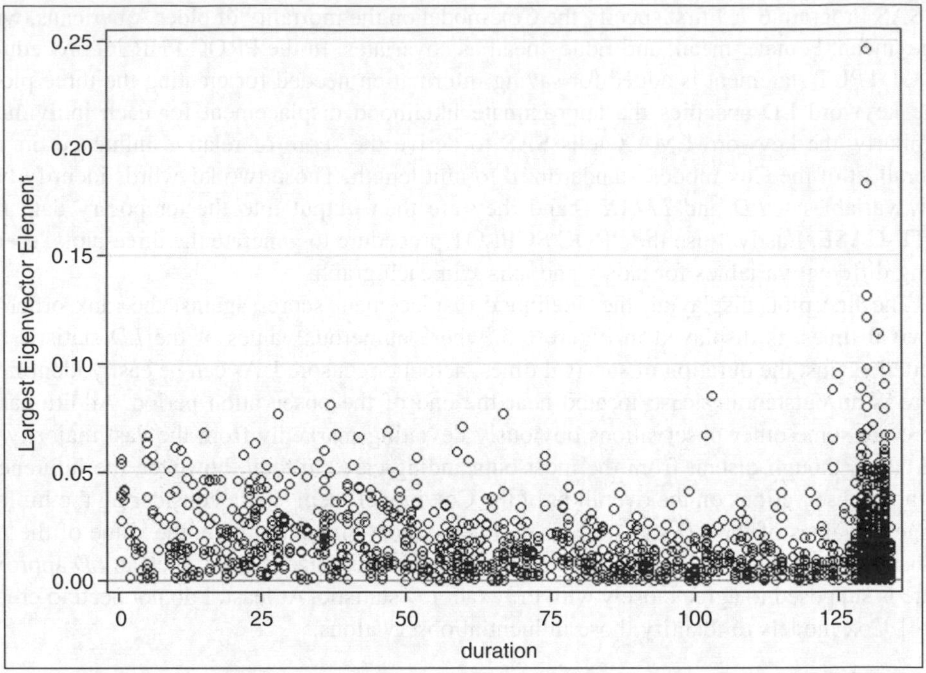

Figure 6.7 Case influence against duration based on LMAX.

Just looking at the *LD* approximate statistic, however, is not enough to derive sufficient confidence for making the decision that the null hypothesis $\hat{\boldsymbol{\beta}}_{(-i)} = \hat{\boldsymbol{\beta}}$ cannot be rejected. Given this reservation, the case influence on the overall fit of the Cox model is further examined by a plot of the *LMAX* statistics, standardized to the unit length of the total sum and also against the rank order of survival times.

Figure 6.7 displays the same pattern of case influences as shown in Figure 6.6. There are two outstanding cases with *LMAX* scores that have much higher scales than those of the others, both located near the ending limit of the observation period. As the square of an element in $\tilde{\mathbf{l}}_{\max}$ measures the proportion of the total sum of squares of unity, the influence of each of those two cases can be assessed by checking its proportional contribution to the unit length. For example, the square of the *LMAX* statistic for the most influential case is about 0.06 (0.25×0.25), indicating a considerable contribution of about 6 % to the overall fit of the Cox model. Considering a sample size of 2000 in this analysis, this case is shown to have a very significant relative influence. Likewise, for the second most outstanding case, the *LMAX* statistic is about 0.18, contributing about 3 % in the overall fit of the Cox model. Nevertheless, the high value of such a relative influence may not necessarily lead to a substantial change in the estimates of regression coefficients and standard errors, especially when the sample size is large. Therefore, the exact influences of those two most outstanding cases need to be checked before a firm conclusion can be reached. For this reason, those two observations need to be identified exactly.

It is useful to plot the elements of the *LMAX* scores against the value of a covariate for identifying the two most influential observations. I will display the third plot specified in SAS Program 6.7, a plot of the *LMAX* statistic against age, which can help us identify those two individuals.

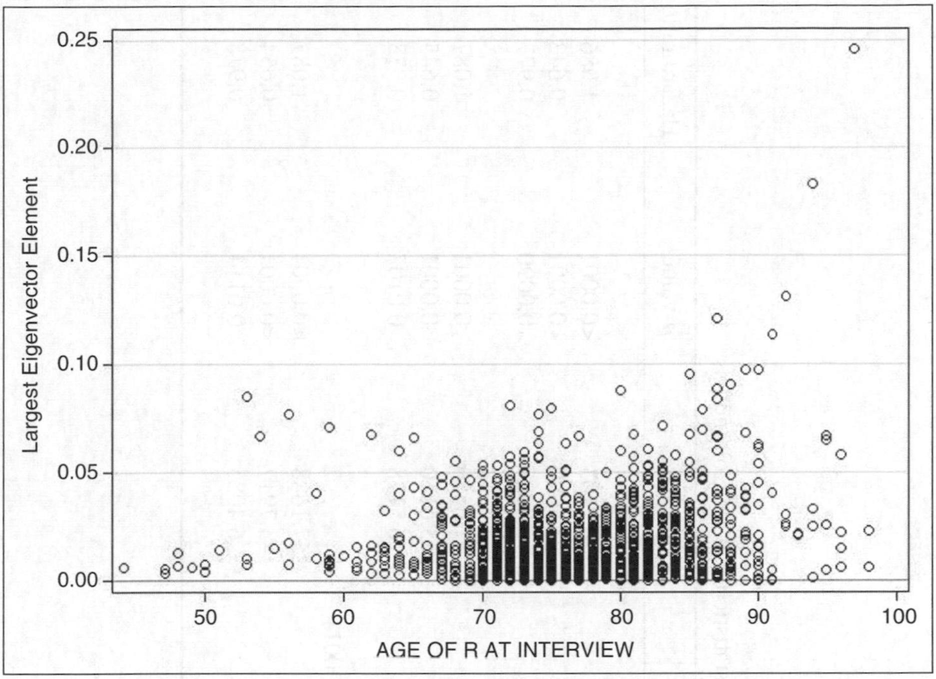

Figure 6.8 Case influence against age based on LMAX.

Figure 6.8 shows that the most influential cases are two individuals who are over 90 years of age at the baseline survey. After some additional graphical and numeric checks, those two observations are further identified. In particular, the most influential case is aged 97 years and the other one is aged 94, and both are female and right censored. With regard to educational attainment, one has 11 years of education and one has 13 years; thus both have education around the level of high school graduation. It can be inferred that compared to other cases, these two observations are so highly influential on the overall fit of the Cox model because both are expected to die early in the observation period at such old ages. In other words, it is their unexpected survival throughout the entire observation that yields very strong statistical impact on the inferential procedures.

Given the high proportional contribution of those two influential cases to the overall fit of the Cox model, it is necessary to check the exact likelihood displacement for both. Accordingly, I create two additional Cox models with each deleting one of those influential cases. The SAS program for this step is not presented here because the two models follow the standard procedures as previously exhibited, except removal of a single observation. Table 6.1 summarizes the results.

In Table 6.1, the first Cox model uses full data, with results previously reported. The second Cox model is fitted after removing the most influential case. The exact *LD* statistic, obtained from the formula $2\log L\left(\hat{\boldsymbol{\beta}}\right) - 2\log L\left[\hat{\boldsymbol{\beta}}_{(-i)}\right]$, is statistically significant with one degree of freedom and at $\alpha = 0.05$ ($LD = 6.15$, $p < 0.05$), indicating the most influential observation to make a strong statistical impact on the overall fit of the first Cox model. Likewise, the third Cox model is fitted after deleting the second most influential case, with the exact likelihood displacement statistic also statistically significant at the same criterion

Table 6.1 Maximum likelihood estimates and the likelihood displacement statistic for three Cox models.

Explanatory variable	Parameter estimate	Standard error	Chi-square	p-value	Hazard ratio
Cox model with full data (–2 LL = 13583.84; $p < 0.0001$)					
Age_mean	0.0823	0.0052	254.2103	<0.0001	1.086
Female_mean	–0.4431	0.0665	44.4090	<0.0001	0.642
Educ_mean	–0.0229	0.0088	6.8227	0.0090	0.977
Cox model deleting most influential case (–2 LL = 13577.69; $p < 0.0001$)					
Age_mean	0.0838	0.0052	257.6550	<0.0001	1.087
Female_mean	–0.4390	0.0665	43.6150	<0.0001	0.645
Educ_mean	–0.0224	0.0088	6.5178	0.0107	0.978
LD statistic	6.15 ($df = 1$; $p < 0.05$)				
Cox model deleting second most influential case (–2 LL = 13579.28; $p < 0.0001$)					
Age_mean	0.0833	0.0052	257.1688	<0.0001	1.087
Female_mean	–0.4399	0.0665	43.7917	<0.0001	0.654
Educ_mean	–0.0220	0.0088	6.4085	0.0114	0.978
LD statistic	4.56 ($df = 1$; $p < 0.05$)				

($LD = 4.56$, $p < 0.05$). In both the second and the third models, however, the parameter estimates, including the regression coefficients and the standard errors, do not vary noticeably at all after removing each of those two cases. The three sets of hazard ratios are almost identical. Obviously, deleting those two cases makes no genuine impact on the results of the model fit. Given such remarkable similarities of the estimated regression coefficients, I do not see any reason that the two influential cases should be eliminated from the Cox model, albeit their exceptionally strong statistical contributions. Indeed, for large samples, a strong relative influence of a few particular cases can be easily averaged out by the effects of the vast majority of the normal observations in the estimation process. Consequently, deleting any influential observation can hardly make an actual impact on the estimates of regression coefficients and standard errors.

6.6 Summary

In survival analysis, one of the most remarkable progresses in the past two decades is the application of counting processes, martingales in continuous time, and stochastic integration for the development of refined techniques. Attaching to this work, the martingale central limit theorem provides a strong theoretical foundation for verifying the efficiency and robustness of various statistical models based on counting processes. In this chapter, therefore, I first describe basic specifications of the counting process system, the martingale theory, and the stochastic integrated function as martingale transforms. The martingale central limit theorems are also presented. Additionally, given the close connection between counting processes and the partial likelihood perspective, I consider it helpful to respecify the Cox model as a stochastic counting process so that the reader can have a better comprehension of this popular regression model. It is worth noting here that in using this highly flexible counting system for developing advanced techniques, the score function, regarded as a martingale transform, plays an extremely important role in specifying various complex functions and distributions.

I perform the residuals analysis on the survival data of older Americans, describing five types of residuals widely used in survival analysis. Not surprisingly, these residuals do not display any signs of model inadequacy, as they are all scattered around zero, displaying a regular distributional pattern as shown by some other studies of this kind (Grambsch and Therneau, 1994; Schoenfeld, 1982; Therneau, Grambsch, and Fleming, 1990). Compared to linear regression models, however, these residuals do not behave explicitly enough to generate deterministic implications on the adequacy of the Cox model (Fleming and Harrington, 1991). Given the unobservable nature of the hazard function and the regular existence of heavy censoring, it is difficult to develop a residual that follows an unambiguous and known distribution. Thus, developing more efficient residuals in survival analysis remains a challenge to statisticians and other quantitative methodologists.

Compared to the residual-related diagnostic methods, the techniques for identification of influential observations on the overall fit of the Cox model are more mature. In Section 6.5, I described two popular approaches in this area, and interesting results are displayed in an empirical illustration. For large samples, the actual impact of influential cases is often found to be very limited, even though they may statistically affect the summary measure of the Cox model. The techniques for identifying the case influence are particularly useful for clinical trials and the observational studies characterized with a small sample size. Here, I recommend the following steps for identifying influential cases in survival analysis with small samples. First, identify the most influential observations by using the *LD* and *LMAX* approximations. Then examine the exact changes in the estimated regression coefficients and the overall model fit of the Cox model after deleting each of those cases. Following this strategy, a decision can be made regarding whether those cases should be removed in fitting the Cox model.

7

Competing risks models and repeated events

So far, I have described a large number of statistical models on censored survival times of a single process. Occasionally, an individual can be exposed to the risks of several events at any time. In such situations, an overall survival process entails different modes of failure, with each involving a unique survival mechanism. In analyzing the mortality of a human population, for example, the occurrence of a death can come from various causes, and each cause may involve a distinct pathological and physical system (Kalbfleisch and Prentice, 2002). While the presence of a serious or a chronic disease generally increases the risk of dying via some prognostic mechanisms, the mortality due to accidents may be associated closely with some demographic factors such as age, gender, and education. Because the actual failure for an individual usually occurs only once, the different event types are referred to as *competing risks*. Accordingly, the statistical techniques analyzing survival data with competing risks are called *competing risks models*.

Researchers also encounter survival data with recurrences of the same event. For some particular nonabsorbing survival processes, an individual can be subject to several survival times with regard to a single type of event within a limited observation period. There are many examples of such repeated events in various disciplines. An older person may be hospitalized or institutionalized several times within a single calendar year; a particular cancer may recur after each medical treatment; a drug user is likely to take drugs again after being released from a rehabilitative center; and so on. As a consequence, an individual can be observed more than once within a limited time range, thereby changing the primary unit of analysis from an 'individual' to a specific time 'episode.' Given the potential dependence of failure times between or among those person-specific observations, conventional statistical inference for fitting a survival model can result in biased parameter estimates and an erroneous model-based prediction (Clayton, 1978; Holt and Prentice, 1974; Hougaard, 2000; Wei, Lin, and Weissfeld, 1989). As a result, the assumption about conditional independence of survival times may not be justifiable, therefore calling for the development of more advanced techniques to address the statistical issues inherent in repeated events.

Survival Analysis: Models and Applications, First Edition. Xian Liu.

In this chapter, I first describe statistical inferences for fitting the competing risks hazard model, providing an empirical illustration on the effects of smoking cigarettes on the cause-specific death rates among older Americans. Second, this chapter surveys approaches for analyzing survival data with repeated events, also illustrated with an empirical example. In the summary section, I discuss merits and limitations of those survival models.

7.1 Competing risks hazard rate models

In this section, I define the latent failure times of different event types and describe the statistical conditions for developing a competing risks model. Then I introduce basic inferences and statistical procedures for estimating various competing risks models, both without and with covariates. The issue of dependence between or among failure times of different event types is also discussed. Lastly, I display an illustration of cigarette smoking behavior and the mortality of older Americans due to different causes.

7.1.1 Latent failure times of competing risks and model specifications

I assume that individual i is at risk of $\mathcal{K}$ event types, with each type having a corresponding survival time series, $T_{i1}, T_{i2}, \ldots, T_{i\mathcal{K}}$, where i = 1, . . . , n. Because the actual failure time, T_i, can be associated with only one of those $\mathcal{K}$ types, the multiple event time series describes a set of latent or potential failure times associated with $\mathcal{K}$ event risks. Accordingly, the actual survival time is given by

$$T_i = \min(T_{i1}, T_{i2}, \ldots, T_{i\mathcal{K}}), \tag{7.1}$$

where $T_{i\mathcal{K}}$ is the $\mathcal{K}$th latent survival time for individual i ($\mathcal{K}$ = 1, . . . , $\mathcal{K}$), assumed to be observable if he or she does not experience any of the other event types first.

As only one of $\mathcal{K}$ risk types can occur, I define a status indicator to denote which type of those risks actually occurs to individual i:

$$\delta_i = k \quad \text{if } T_i = T_{ik}, \quad k = 1, 2, \ldots, \mathcal{K}. \tag{7.2}$$

The value of δ_i can arbitrarily be assigned for a censored case (none of the $\mathcal{K}$ types has actually occurred). Thus, the survival information for a sample of n individuals can be conveniently denoted by (T_i, δ_i) if there are distinct competing risks.

I start the description of competing risks by specifying a joint survival function of $\mathcal{K}$ latent failure time series. If a vector of time-independent covariates x is considered, the joint probability of survival can be written by

$$S(t_1, t_2, \ldots, t_{\mathcal{K}}; \boldsymbol{x}) = \Pr(T_1 \geq t_1, T_2 \geq t_2, \ldots, T_{\mathrm{K}} \geq t_{\mathcal{K}}; \boldsymbol{x}). \tag{7.3}$$

Given the specification of the joint survival function, the overall survival rate, $S(t)$, can be expressed as a multivariate survival function, denoted by $S(t, t, \ldots, t)$. (Note that the term 'multivariate' here refers to the simultaneous variation in the survival probability as a function of multiple modes of failure, and is not linked to the term used in regression modeling.)

Therefore, in the presence of $\mathcal{K}$ event types, the overall survival probability is a multiple decrement function, a concept often used in life table techniques.

Under the condition that $T \geq t$, the type-specific survival function with respect to the $\mathcal{K}$th event type is defined as

$$S_{\mathscr{k}}(t; \boldsymbol{x}) = \Pr(T \geq t, \delta = \mathscr{k}; \boldsymbol{x}), \quad \mathscr{k} = 1, 2, \ldots, \mathcal{K}. \tag{7.4}$$

As the calculation of $S_K(t, \boldsymbol{x})$ depends on the condition that an individual must survive to time t and then experience the event type $\mathcal{K}$, this type-specific survival function is referred to as the *crude probability of survival* from event type $\mathcal{K}$ (Tsiatis, 1975). The marginal survival function for $T_{\mathcal{K}}$, defined as the survival function of the latent failure time series for event $\mathcal{K}$, is a different lifetime concept from Equation (7.4), given by

$$S_{\mathscr{k}}^{*}(t; \boldsymbol{x}) = \Pr(T_{\mathscr{k}} \geq t; \boldsymbol{x}) = S(0, \ldots, 0, t, 0, \ldots, 0; \boldsymbol{x}), \tag{7.5}$$

where t reflects the distribution of $T_{\mathcal{K}}$ regardless of the distributions of other latent time series. The marginal type-specific survival function is also called the *net probability of survival* from event type $\mathcal{K}$ (Prentice *et al.*, 1978; Tsiatis, 1975), given the assumption that only event type $\mathcal{K}$ operates in the survival process. Without the assumption that the latent failure times of all event types are mutually independent, a given set of the crude survival probabilities for event type $\mathcal{K}$ does not identify the corresponding net probabilities, as will be explained below.

The above specifications of the crude and the net survival functions indicate that a statistical model of latent survival times is unidentifiable without introducing additional assumptions because a given set of crude survival probabilities implies an infinite number of joint distributions. Consequently, modeling competing survival times needs to depend on some theoretically-based hypotheses about the stochastic processes of the joint distribution for the latent failure time series. For example, assuming the random variables $T_1, T_2, \ldots, T_{\mathcal{K}}$ to be mutually independent, $S_{\mathscr{k}}^{*}(t; \boldsymbol{x}) = S_{\mathscr{k}}(t; \boldsymbol{x})$, so that the overall, or joint, survival function at t can be conveniently expressed as the product of $\mathcal{K}$ type-specific crude functions or net survival functions:

$$S(t; \boldsymbol{x}) = \prod_{\mathscr{k}=1}^{\mathcal{K}} S_{\mathscr{k}}^{*}(t; \boldsymbol{x}) = \prod_{\mathscr{k}=1}^{\mathcal{K}} S_{\mathscr{k}}(t; \boldsymbol{x}), \quad \mathscr{k} = 1, 2, \ldots, \mathcal{K}. \tag{7.6}$$

The independence assumption for validating Equation (7.6), however, is found not to be directly verifiable, as will be discussed in Subsection 7.1.5.

At a first glance, it seems feasible to express the hazard rate for experiencing the $\mathcal{K}$th event type, denoted by $h_{\mathcal{K}}(t, \mathbf{x})$, as the minus derivative of the log net survival function with respect to the $\mathcal{K}$th event type, given by

$$h_{\mathscr{k}}^{*}(t; \boldsymbol{x}) = -\frac{\mathrm{d} \log S_{\mathscr{k}}^{*}(t; \boldsymbol{x})}{\mathrm{d}t}. \tag{7.7}$$

The hazard rate defined above is called the *net hazard function* for event type $\mathcal{K}$, given the consideration of a specific latent failure time system regardless of the other $\mathcal{K} - 1$ series. Such a marginal hazard rate, however, is not identifiable and cannot be estimated without making further assumptions, given the infinity of joint distributions of latent survival times

(Kalbfleisch and Prentice, 2002; Tsiatis, 1975). Therefore, Equation (7.7) cannot be used as the standard specification of the type-specific hazard function in competing risks analysis unless the $\mathcal{K}$ types of competing risks are truly independent of each other.

As indicated in Chapter 1, the hazard function can be specified in another perspective, which, in the context of competing risks, can be used to formulate the type-specific hazard function without introducing further assumptions, given by

$$\begin{aligned} h_{\mathcal{k}}(t;\boldsymbol{x}) &= \lim_{\Delta t \to 0} \frac{\Pr\{T \in (t, t+\Delta t], \delta = \mathcal{k} | T \geq t; \boldsymbol{x}\}}{\Delta t} \\ &= \left.\frac{-\partial \log S(t_1, \ldots, t_{\mathcal{K}}; \boldsymbol{x})}{\partial t_{\mathcal{k}}}\right|_{t_1 = \cdots = t_{\mathcal{K}} = t}, \quad \mathcal{k} = 1, \ldots, \mathcal{K}. \end{aligned} \tag{7.8}$$

The type-specific hazard function defined in Equation (7.8) depends on the condition that the actual survival time T is greater than or equal to t as it is evaluated at $t_1 = t_2 = \ldots = t_{\mathcal{K}} = t$. Corresponding to the crude survival function, $h_{\mathcal{K}}(t, \boldsymbol{x})$ is referred to as the *crude hazard function* for event type $\mathcal{K}$. This crude hazard function has tremendous appeal in the competing risks analysis because it is identifiable and can be estimated whatever is the joint distribution of latent survival times.

Because Equation (7.8) is so flexible that no further assumption is needed for its identifiability, it is more convenient to specify other lifetime functions of competing risks in terms of the crude hazard function (David, 1974). For example, the cumulative hazard function for the $\mathcal{K}$th event type at time t can be readily specified as

$$H_{\mathcal{k}}(t;\boldsymbol{x}) = \int_0^t h_{\mathcal{k}}(u;\boldsymbol{x})\mathrm{d}u. \tag{7.9}$$

Given the assumption on the independence of $T_1, T_2, \ldots, T_{\mathcal{K}}$, the overall hazard and the overall cumulative hazard functions are

$$h(t;\boldsymbol{x}) = \sum_{\mathcal{k}=1}^{\mathcal{K}} h_{\mathcal{k}}(t;\boldsymbol{x}), \tag{7.10}$$

$$H(t;\boldsymbol{x}) = \int_0^t h(u;\boldsymbol{x})\mathrm{d}u = \sum_{\mathcal{k}=1}^{\mathcal{K}} \left[\int_0^t h_{\mathcal{k}}(u;\boldsymbol{x})\mathrm{d}u\right]. \tag{7.11}$$

Likewise, assuming distinct failure types, the overall survival function can be expressed in terms of the type-specific crude hazard rates:

$$S(t;\boldsymbol{x}) = \exp[-H(t;\boldsymbol{x})] = \exp\left\{-\sum_{\mathcal{k}=1}^{\mathcal{K}} \left[\int_0^t h_{\mathcal{k}}(u;\boldsymbol{x})\mathrm{d}u\right]\right\}. \tag{7.12}$$

The probability density function of event time $T_{\mathcal{K}}$, defined as $f_{\mathcal{K}}(t, \boldsymbol{x})$, can be obtained from the hazard and the survival functions given the independence assumption:

$$f_{\mathcal{k}}(t;\boldsymbol{x}) = h_{\mathcal{k}}(t;\boldsymbol{x})S(t;\boldsymbol{x}). \tag{7.13}$$

Given the definition of the total probability and the independence assumption on T_1, $T_2, \ldots, T_{\mathcal{K}}$ and on right censoring, the overall p.d.f. of T is

$$f(t;\boldsymbol{x}) = \sum_{k=1}^{\mathcal{K}} f_k(t;\boldsymbol{x}). \tag{7.14}$$

With the survival and the density functions specified, the likelihood function can be created, which, in turn, can be applied to derive parameter estimates on a competing risks model. To minimize the influence of dependence among the latent failure time series, the construction of the likelihood function for competing risks should be based on the crude type-specific hazard function, given its flexibility without introducing the independence assumption (Prentice *et al.*, 1978).

7.1.2 Competing risks models and the likelihood function without covariates

When the random variables $T_1, T_2, \ldots, T_{\mathcal{K}}$ are truly independent, there is no problem of identifiability for making inference about the joint survival function by means of the type-specific survival functions. Assuming the distributions of $\mathcal{K}$ event time systems to be homogeneous among observations, the standard nonparametric techniques can be applied to estimate the lifetime measures with competing risks. Specifically, the standard Kaplan and Meier (1958) and the Nelson–Aalen (Nelson, 1972; Aalen, 1975) estimators can be used for estimating the multiple decrement survival function $S(t_1, t_2, \ldots, t_{\mathcal{K}})$ and the type-specific survival function $S_{\mathcal{K}}(t)$.

With respect to event type $\mathcal{K}$, survival times of n individuals can be rank ordered by

$$t_{1k} < t_{2k} < \cdots < t_n,$$

where $t_{i\mathcal{K}}(i = 1, 2, \ldots, n')$ represents the time at which event $\mathcal{K}$ or right censoring (including failures from other events) occurs to individual i. Because at time $t_{i\mathcal{K}}$ individuals with actual survival or censored times smaller than t_i have already exited, there is a specific number of survivors who remain exposed to the risk of the event just prior to $t_{i\mathcal{K}}$, denoted by $n_{i\mathcal{K}}$, where $n_{1\mathcal{K}} > n_{2\mathcal{K}} > \ldots > n_n$. As t_n is the lifetime for the last survivor in the rank list, $n_n = 1$. Let $d_{i\mathcal{K}}$ be the number of failures for the event type $\mathcal{K}$ at time $t_{i\mathcal{K}}$ ($d_{i\mathcal{K}} = 1$ if there are no tied cases). The Kaplan–Meier estimator for the type-specific probability of survival from event type $\mathcal{K}$ at time $t_{i\mathcal{K}}$ is given by

$$\hat{S}_k(t) = \prod_{t_{ik}<t} \left(\frac{n_{ik} - d_{ik}}{n_{ik}} \right). \tag{7.15}$$

The above estimated probability for event type $\mathcal{K}$ is the crude type-specific survival function, because individual i must survive to at least time $t_{i\mathcal{K}}$ to be counted in. This estimate is thus exactly the same as the estimate derived from the standard Kaplan–Meier estimator when all failures of other event types are treated as right censored. For this reason, the denominator in Equation (7.15), $n_{i\mathcal{K}}$, can be replaced by n_i if d_{ir}, where $r \neq \mathcal{K}$ is viewed as $c_{i\mathcal{K}}$.

Assuming the latent failure time series to be mutually independent and there are no ties between different event types, the overall survival function is defined as

$$\hat{S}(t)=\prod_{\ell=1}^{\mathcal{K}}\hat{S}_{\ell}(t)=\prod_{\ell=1}^{\mathcal{K}}\prod_{t_{i\ell}<t}\left(\frac{n_{i\ell}-d_{i\ell}}{n_{i\ell}}\right). \tag{7.16}$$

Therefore, the Kaplan–Meier estimator for the joint survival function can be specified as the product of $\mathcal{K}$ type-specific Kaplan–Meier functions. The computation is handy and simple as long as the event types are well specified and the independence assumption is valid.

Likewise, the Nelson–Aalen estimator of the cumulative hazard function for the $\mathcal{K}$th event type at time t is

$$\hat{H}_{\ell}(t)=\sum_{t_{i\ell}<t}\left(\frac{d_{i\ell}}{n_{i\ell}}\right). \tag{7.17}$$

By definition, the overall cumulative hazard rate at time t is the summation of all $\hat{H}_{\ell}(t)$ values over $\mathcal{K}$ event types, given the independence of $T_{i1}, T_{i2}, \ldots, T_{i\mathcal{K}}$:

$$\hat{H}(t)=\sum_{\ell=1}^{\mathcal{K}}\hat{H}_{\ell}(t)=\sum_{\ell=1}^{\mathcal{K}}\sum_{t_{i\ell}<t}\left(\frac{d_{i\ell}}{n_{i\ell}}\right). \tag{7.18}$$

As the Kaplan–Meier and the Nelson–Aalen estimators are both descriptive measures, it may be more interesting to present the likelihood function for competing risks under the independence assumption. For analytic convenience, here I specify an additional type-specific censoring indicator denoted by $\delta_{i\mathcal{K}}$, where $\delta_{i\mathcal{K}}=1$ if $T_{i\mathcal{K}}=t_i$ and $\delta_{i\mathcal{K}}=0$ if $T_{i\mathcal{K}}>t_i$. If the distribution of the type-specific survival function is known, the basic likelihood function, without involving any covariates, consists of a set of random variables indicating a surviving or censoring status for t_i:

$$\begin{aligned}L(t;\delta_{i1},\delta_{i2},\ldots,\delta_{i\ell})&=\prod_{\ell=1}^{\mathcal{K}}\prod_{i=1}^{n}[f_{\ell}(t_i)]^{\delta_{i\ell}}[S_{\ell}(t_i)]^{1-\delta_{i\ell}}\\&=\prod_{\ell=1}^{\mathrm{K}}\prod_{i=1}^{n}[h_{\ell}(t_i)]^{\delta_{i\ell}}\exp[-H_{\ell}(t_i)].\end{aligned} \tag{7.19}$$

In the presence of competing risks, the likelihood function $L(t, \delta_{i1}, \delta_{i2}, \ldots, \delta_{i\mathcal{K}})$ is the probability of a set of parameter values given n observed lifetime outcomes and $\mathcal{K}$ event types. It follows that, when $\delta_{i\mathcal{K}}=1$, $L_i(t, \delta_{i1}, \delta_{i2}, \ldots, \delta_{i\mathcal{K}})$ is the probability density for the occurrence of a $\mathcal{K}$th event. Likewise, when $\delta_{i\mathcal{K}}=0$, $L_i(t, \delta_{i1}, \delta_{i2}, \ldots, \delta_{i\mathcal{K}})$ is the marginal survival function for a censored time for the $\mathcal{K}$th type. This specification suggests that the likelihood contribution from an individual reflects the density if he or she is observed to experience a type-specific event, or it represents the type-specific survival function if the individual is censored. In either case, this individual's survival time, actual or censored, is accounted for in the likelihood series. Given the intimate interrelationships among lifetime indicators, the second equality in Equation (7.19) expresses the likelihood function of competing risks in terms of the type-specific crude hazard rate. This functional conversion is necessary in the analysis of competing risks in view of the aforementioned advantage of using the crude hazard rate for specifying a competing risks model.

Maximization of Equation (7.19) with respect to the model parameters yields the maximum likelihood (ML) estimates of the type-specific hazard rates, which, under the independence assumption, derive the density, and the survival functions. The detailed procedures of such maximization and estimation are standard, described extensively in some of the earlier chapters, and therefore they are not elaborated further here.

7.1.3 Inference for competing risks models with covariates

Given the independence assumption on the random lifetime variables $T_1, T_2, \ldots, T_{\mathcal{K}}$, statistical inference for fitting a competing risks model with covariates is simply the extension of the standard procedures for a single survival process. In particular, when covariates are considered, the lifetime process for individual i can be described as a function of a triple $\{t_i, \delta_i, \boldsymbol{x}_i\}$. Given the added assumption that right censoring is noninformative, the likelihood function for the $\mathcal{K}$th event type is

$$L(\boldsymbol{\beta}_{k}) = \prod_{i=1}^{n} h_{ik}(t_i, \boldsymbol{x}_i, \boldsymbol{\beta}_{k})^{\delta_{ik}} S(t_i, \boldsymbol{x}_i, \boldsymbol{\beta}_{k}), \tag{7.20}$$

where $\boldsymbol{\beta}_{\mathcal{K}}$ represents the coefficient vector on the $\mathcal{K}$th event type. Equation (7.20) is simply an extension of Equation (7.19) with the addition of parameter vector $\boldsymbol{\beta}_{\mathcal{K}}$. Therefore, the contribution of a given individual to the likelihood for event type $\mathcal{K}$ is exactly the same as the contribution in a general hazard model, where only failures of event type $\mathcal{K}$ are considered while all other observations are treated as right censored. As a result, the latent failure times of each event type can be modeled separately by maximizing $\mathcal{K}$ likelihood functions in sequence. As Prentice *et al.* (1978) comment, this specification provides a formal justification for applying the standard procedures, as long as separate hazard functions are identifiable.

Additionally, in Equation (7.20) the coefficient vector $\boldsymbol{\beta}$ is subscripted by $\mathcal{K}$, so that a unique set of coefficients is specified for each event type. This specification, highlighting a major difference from the stratified Cox model, is essential because otherwise the independence assumption about latent time series is violated, thus indicating the above competing risks model to be nonidentifiable.

Equation (7.20) can be more conveniently expressed in terms of the hazard function, given by

$$\begin{aligned} L(\boldsymbol{\beta}_{k}) &= \prod_{i=1}^{n} h_{ik}(t_i, \boldsymbol{x}_i, \boldsymbol{\beta}_{k})^{\delta_{ik}} \prod_{k=1}^{\mathcal{K}} S_{k}(t_i, \boldsymbol{x}_i, \boldsymbol{\beta}_{k}) \\ &= \prod_{i=1}^{n} h_{ik}(t_i, \boldsymbol{x}_i, \boldsymbol{\beta}_{k})^{\delta_{ik}} \prod_{k=1}^{\mathcal{K}} \exp\left[-\int_0^t h_{k}(u, \boldsymbol{x}, \boldsymbol{\beta}_{k})\,\mathrm{d}u\right] \\ &= \prod_{i=1}^{n} h_{ik}(t_i, \boldsymbol{x}_i, \boldsymbol{\beta}_{k})^{\delta_{ik}} \prod_{k=1}^{\mathcal{K}} \exp[-H_{k}(u, \boldsymbol{x}, \boldsymbol{\beta}_{k})]. \end{aligned} \tag{7.21}$$

This formulation is more feasible for statistical inference and estimation for a competing risks regression model. Because only one event can actually occur for each observation, the overall likelihood function can be partitioned by the number of actual events with respect to $\mathcal{K}$ outcomes, such that

$$L(\boldsymbol{\beta}_{k}) = \prod_{i=1}^{n_k} \prod_{k=1}^{\mathcal{K}} h_{ik}(t_i, \boldsymbol{x}_i, \boldsymbol{\beta}_k)^{\delta_{ik}} \exp[-H_k(u, \boldsymbol{x}, \boldsymbol{\beta}_k)]. \tag{7.22}$$

Given the above inference, the estimation of the competing risks model can be performed by involving $\mathcal{K}$ separate hazard models where failures of other event types are assumed to be right censored. This simple approach applies to both parametric and semi-parametric hazard models as long as the likelihood function can be expressed in terms of the type-specific crude hazard rates.

Consider, for example, the Weibull proportional hazard model for the $\mathcal{K}$th event type. This model is simply the standard formulation with respect only to the risk for event type $\mathcal{K}$, written as

$$h_k(t, \boldsymbol{x}) = \lambda_k \tilde{p}_k (\lambda_k t)^{\tilde{p}_k - 1} \exp(\boldsymbol{x}' \boldsymbol{\beta}_k). \tag{7.23}$$

Clearly, Equation (7.23) is a standard Weibull hazard model with regard to a particular event type. Therefore, the Weibull parameters $\lambda_{\mathcal{K}}$, $\tilde{p}_k$, and $\boldsymbol{\beta}_{\mathcal{K}}$ can be estimated by using the procedures described in Chapter 4, assuming failures of other event types to be right censored. Given the independence assumption on $T_{i1}, T_{i2}, \ldots, T_{i\mathcal{K}}$, the overall likelihood function of the Weibull model for $\boldsymbol{\beta}_1, \boldsymbol{\beta}_2, \ldots, \boldsymbol{\beta}_{\mathcal{K}}$ is

$$L(\lambda_k, \tilde{p}_k, \boldsymbol{x}) = \prod_{k=1}^{\mathcal{K}} \left\{ \prod_{i=1}^{n} \left[\lambda_k \tilde{p}_k (\lambda_k t)^{\tilde{p}_k - 1} \exp(\boldsymbol{x}' \boldsymbol{\beta}_k) \right]^{\delta_{ik}} \exp\left[-\exp(\boldsymbol{x}' \boldsymbol{\beta}_k) \lambda_k t^{\tilde{p}_k} \right] \right\}. \tag{7.24}$$

Therefore, the likelihood function for the overall Weibull model, given $\mathcal{K}$ competing risks, is the product of $\mathcal{K}$ standard type-specific likelihoods, with each estimating an independent set of parameter estimates.

Likewise, the standard partial likelihood estimator can be adapted to derive parameter estimates in the Cox competing risks model, given by

$$L_p(\boldsymbol{\beta}_1, \ldots, \boldsymbol{\beta}_{\mathcal{K}}) = \prod_{k=1}^{\mathcal{K}} \left[\prod_{i=1}^{d_k} \frac{\exp(\boldsymbol{x}'_{ik} \boldsymbol{\beta}_k)}{\sum_{l \in \mathcal{R}(t_{ik})} \exp(\boldsymbol{x}'_{lk} \boldsymbol{\beta}_k)} \right], \tag{7.25}$$

where $t_{i\mathcal{K}}$, $i = 1, 2, \ldots, d_{\mathcal{K}}$, represents $d_{\mathcal{K}}$ ordered failure times for event type $\mathcal{K}$, $\boldsymbol{x}_{i\mathcal{K}}$ is the corresponding covariate vector, and $\mathcal{R}(t_{i\mathcal{K}})$ is the $\mathcal{K}$th risk set just prior to time $t_{i\mathcal{K}}$. As a result, a separate, standard Cox model can be created for each event type, treating failures from other event types as right censored. The event-specific survival function can be estimated by using either the Kalbfleisch and Prentice (1973) or the Breslow (1974) approximation methods. Similarly, the overall survival function is obtainable by applying the multiple decrement approach as long as the independence assumption is valid.

One of the limitations of using the hazard model techniques is that the model actually consists of $\mathcal{K}$ separate regression processes, with each involving an independent estimation procedure; thus, the overall hazard model is not fitted by maximizing an approximation to the whole likelihood integrated over all type-specific parameters. Some prediction bias might be derived from such a perspective.

7.1.4 Competing risks model using the multinomial logit regression

Another approach used to analyze survival data of competing risks is the multinomial logit regression, a statistical method mostly applied by economists, demographers, and sociologists for modeling probabilities of discrete choices (Amemiya, 1981; Greene, 2003; Liao, 1994; Liu *et al.*, 1995; Long, 1997; Maddala, 1983). Specifically, the multinomial logit model is used to analyze nominal and unordered outcome variables, as associated with a set of explanatory factors. Given such features, this regression model is suitable for examining the lifetime outcomes in which an individual is at risk to more than one event type.

In the multinomial logit model, the qualitative outcome variable is denoted by 1, . . . , $\mathcal{K}+1$, and the estimation of the model parameters is performed on a series of linked logit components as linear functions of covariates. Compared to the hazard rate approach that models each event type separately, the multinomial logit model is statistically more efficient because it integrates information of all competing risks within one estimating process. As a result, this model derives smaller standard errors of estimated regression coefficients. The limitation of using the multinomial logit regression in survival analysis is the combination of all observations in a single risk set and, consequently, the risk interval is not particularly considered.

Let Y_i denote the value of the nominal variable representing $\mathcal{K}+1$ event types for individual i where the $\mathcal{K}+1$th level indicates actual censoring. The probability that $Y_i = \mathcal{K}(\mathcal{K} = 1, \ldots, \mathcal{K})$ for individual i, conditional on a covariate vector $\boldsymbol{x}_i$ and denoted by $P_{i\mathcal{K}}$, is given by

$$P_{ik} = \left[1 + \sum_{t=1}^{\mathcal{K}} \exp(\boldsymbol{x}_i'\boldsymbol{\beta}_t)\right]^{-1} \exp(\boldsymbol{x}_i'\boldsymbol{\beta}_k), \quad k = 1, \ldots, \mathcal{K}, \tag{7.26}$$

where $\boldsymbol{\beta}_{\mathcal{K}}$ is the vector of regression coefficients to be estimated, providing a set of the nonlinear effects on $P_{i\mathcal{K}}$ given values of $\boldsymbol{x}$. The $(\mathcal{K}+1)$th level, representing actual right censoring, is treated as the reference event type. In other words, $P_{\mathcal{K}+1}$ is defined as the residual probability, the estimation of which depends on the estimates of the probabilities for other event types, given the constraint that a set of mutually exclusive choice probabilities must sum to unity. More precisely, the reference probability, conditional on the covariate vector $\boldsymbol{x}_i$ and the coefficient matrix β, where $\boldsymbol{\beta} = (\boldsymbol{\beta}_1, \ldots, \boldsymbol{\beta}_{\mathcal{K}})'$, is defined by

$$P_{i,\mathcal{K}+1} = \left[1 + \sum_{t=1}^{\mathcal{K}} \exp(\boldsymbol{x}_i'\boldsymbol{\beta}_t)\right]^{-1}. \tag{7.27}$$

The inverse of the above probability function gives rise to the multinomial logit model combining $\mathcal{K}$ logit components, where each is linearly associated with the linear predictor $\boldsymbol{x}_i'\boldsymbol{\beta}_k$, given by

$$\log\left(\frac{P_{ik}}{P_{i,\mathcal{K}+1}}\right) = \boldsymbol{x}_i'\boldsymbol{\beta}_k, \quad k = 1, \ldots, \mathcal{K}. \tag{7.28}$$

The left side of the equation is defined as the $\mathcal{K}$th logit component.

The likelihood function for the multinomial logit model can be written as a joint probability, given by

$$L(\boldsymbol{\beta}_1, \boldsymbol{\beta}_2, \ldots, \boldsymbol{\beta}_{\mathcal{K}}) = \prod_{i=1}^{n} P_{i1}^{\delta_{i1}} P_{i2}^{\delta_{i2}} \cdots P_{i,\mathcal{K}+1}^{\delta_{i,\mathcal{K}+1}}, \tag{7.29}$$

where $\delta_{i\mathcal{K}}$ is 1 if the ith observation experiences the $\mathcal{K}$th event type and is 0 otherwise, and

$$P_{i\hat{k}} = MNL_{\hat{k}}^{-1}(\boldsymbol{x}_i'\boldsymbol{\beta}_1, \boldsymbol{x}_i'\boldsymbol{\beta}_2, \ldots, \boldsymbol{x}_i'\boldsymbol{\beta}_{\mathcal{K}}), \quad \hat{k} = 1, 2, \ldots, \mathcal{K}+1,$$

where *MNL* denotes the multinomial logit function. The estimation of $P_{\mathcal{K}+1}$ is given by $P_{\mathcal{K}+1} = 1 - P_1 - \ldots - P_{\mathcal{K}}$.

Taking log values on both sides of Equation (7.29) leads to

$$\log L(\boldsymbol{\beta}_1, \boldsymbol{\beta}_2, \ldots, \boldsymbol{\beta}_{\mathcal{K}}) = \sum_{i=1}^{n} \sum_{\hat{k}=1}^{\mathcal{K}+1} \delta_{i\hat{k}} \log(P_{i\hat{k}}). \tag{7.30}$$

Maximizing Equation (7.30) requires that this log likelihood function be differentiated with respect to β, and the ML estimates of $\boldsymbol{\beta}$ can be obtained by solving the following equation:

$$\frac{\partial \log L}{\partial(\boldsymbol{\beta})} = \sum_{i=1}^{n} \sum_{\hat{k}=1}^{\mathcal{K}+1} \delta_{i\hat{k}} P_{i\hat{k}}^{-1} \left[\frac{\partial P_{i\hat{k}}}{\partial(\boldsymbol{\beta}_{\hat{k}})}\right] = 0. \tag{7.31}$$

It is recognizable from the above equations that all $\mathcal{K}$ logit components are integrated within a single maximization process. Hypothesis testing on linear combinations of the model parameters can be performed by calculating the generalized Wald statistic, distributed approximately as chi-square under the null hypothesis that $\boldsymbol{\beta} = 0$. Statistically, differentiating Equation (7.31) with respect to $\mathcal{K}$ sets of $\boldsymbol{\beta}_{\mathcal{K}}$ involves a set of complex and tedious procedures. For detailed statistical inference, the interested reader is referred to Amemiya (1985), Greene (2003), Long (1997), and Maddala (1983).

Given the estimated regression coefficients for $\mathcal{K}$ event types, a critical issue about applying the multinomial logit model is the interpretation of parameter estimates. Although some researchers have attempted to interpret results of the multinomial logit model by displaying regression coefficients or odds ratios, such logit coefficients are in fact not highly useful for deriving substantively meaningful implications. In the presence of more than two nominal outcome types, the regression coefficients in the multinomial logit model do not necessarily bear any relationship to changes in the choice probabilities, thereby making their interpretations very difficult (Greene, 2003; Liao, 1994; Liu *et al.*, 1995). Because the probabilities for all event types, including right censoring, always sum to unity, the simultaneous structural variation in the probability distribution of more than two alternatives is indeed beyond what changes in a set of log odds can capture.

To present a covariate's effects in the multinomial logit model correctly, I propose to apply the discrete probability change approach (Long, 1997) for calculating the conditional effects on the probabilities of various event types. Consider the case of a continuous variable first. Specifically, I define $\left(\hat{P}_{\hat{k}} \,|\, \bar{\boldsymbol{x}}\right)$ as the marginalized estimate of $(P_{\mathcal{K}}|\boldsymbol{x})$ when all covariates are scaled at sample means. In the meantime, I let $\left(\hat{P}_{\hat{k}} \,|\, \bar{x}_m + 1, \bar{\boldsymbol{x}}_r\right)$ be another marginalized estimate of $(P_{\mathcal{K}}|\boldsymbol{x})$ when a continuous covariate of interest, denoted by x_m, is scaled at one unit greater than its sample mean and other covariates are fixed as sample means. The difference between $\left(\hat{P}_{\mathcal{k}}|\bar{x}_m+1,\bar{x}_r\right)$ and $\left(\hat{P}_{\mathcal{k}}|\bar{x}\right)$ is defined as the conditional effect of the continuous covariate x_m on the probability of experiencing event type $\mathcal{K}$, denoted by $\Delta\hat{P}_{\mathcal{k}x_m}$, written by

$$\Delta\hat{P}_{\mathcal{k}x_m}=\frac{\exp\left[\hat{\beta}_{\mathcal{k}m}(\bar{x}_m+1)+\bar{x}_r'\hat{\boldsymbol{\beta}}_{\mathcal{k}r}\right]}{1+\sum_{\mathcal{t}=1}^{\mathcal{K}}\exp\left[\hat{\beta}_{\mathcal{t}m}(\bar{x}_m+1)+\bar{x}_r'\hat{\boldsymbol{\beta}}_{\mathcal{t}r}\right]}-\frac{\exp\left(\bar{x}'\hat{\boldsymbol{\beta}}_{\mathcal{k}}\right)}{1+\sum_{\mathcal{t}=1}^{\mathcal{K}}\exp\left(\bar{x}'\hat{\boldsymbol{\beta}}_{\mathcal{t}}\right)},\tag{7.32}$$

where $\bar{x}$ is the vector containing sample means of all covariates and $\bar{x}_r$ represents the vector containing sample means of the covariates other than x_m.

If the effects of a dichotomous variable on the probabilities are analyzed, the 0–1 change in that covariate should be specified. Suppose that the covariate x_m is a dichotomous variable. Then, the conditional effect of covariate x_m on the probability of experiencing event type $\mathcal{K}$, denoted $\Delta\hat{P}_{\mathcal{k}x_m}$, is

$$\Delta\hat{P}_{\mathcal{k}x_m}=\frac{\exp\left(\hat{\beta}_{\mathcal{k}m}+\bar{x}_r'\hat{\boldsymbol{\beta}}_{\mathcal{k}r}\right)}{1+\sum_{\mathcal{t}=1}^{\mathcal{K}}\exp\left(\hat{\beta}_{\mathcal{t}m}+\bar{x}_r'\hat{\boldsymbol{\beta}}_{\mathcal{t}r}\right)}-\frac{\exp\left(\bar{x}_r'\hat{\boldsymbol{\beta}}_{\mathcal{k}r}\right)}{1+\sum_{\mathcal{t}=1}^{\mathcal{K}}\exp\left(\bar{x}_r'\hat{\boldsymbol{\beta}}_{\mathcal{t}r}\right)}.\tag{7.33}$$

Using one of the above two equations, the conditional effects of a given covariate on the probabilities of $\mathcal{K}$ event types can be estimated. Given the mathematical constraints that a set of choice probabilities always sum to unity and the corresponding conditional effects must sum to zero, the conditional effect of a covariate on the probability of not experiencing any event is defined as $\Delta\hat{P}_{\mathcal{K}+1,x_m}=-\left(\Delta\hat{P}_{1x_m}+\cdots+\Delta\hat{P}_{\mathcal{K}x_m}\right)$. Use of this discrete probability change approach can accommodate the inclusion of qualitative factors as covariates.

As in a step function the conditional probability is equivalent to the hazard rate, the hazard ratio of a given covariate, continuous or dichotomous, can be approximated by

$$HR_{\mathcal{k}m}\approx\frac{\left(\hat{P}_{\mathcal{k}1}|\bar{x}_m+1,\bar{x}_r\right)}{\left(\hat{P}_{\mathcal{k}0}|\bar{x}\right)}.\tag{7.34}$$

The rationale for using covariate means to calculate the conditional effects is well justified: as a probability is specified as a nonlinear function of both covariate values and logit coefficients, other covariates need to be fixed at sample means for representing a 'typical' population (Fox, 1987; Liu *et al.*, 1995; Long, 1997). Notice that the conditional effect is discrete and differs conceptually from a 'marginal' effect, which represents the slope of a probability function and actually has no bound in value (Petersen, 1985). Because they are scale dependent, such conditional effects might be sensitive to changes in covariate values (Greene, 2003; Long, 1997). Nevertheless, the logistic function approximates a straight line except for the two ends, so these effects do not tend to vary considerably within zones where most cases are located. The interested reader can sensitize themselves to the variation in the conditional effects by calculating the effects at different scales using selected values of covariates.

The variance–covariance matrix for the predicted probabilities, needed for testing the null hypothesis that $H_0 : \Delta P_{1x_m} = \cdots = \Delta P_{\mathcal{K}x_m} = \Delta P_{(\mathcal{K}+1)x_m} = 0$, can be obtained either from the bootstrapping approach or from the delta method. While the bootstrap techniques overlook the covariance structure of a multivariate distribution, the delta method yields the approximate variance–covariance matrix from transforming the corresponding variance matrix for the predicted logits.

Suppose that $\hat{\mathcal{L}}$ is a random vector of predicted logit components $\left(\hat{\mathcal{L}} = \hat{\mathcal{L}}_1, \hat{\mathcal{L}}_2, \ldots, \hat{\mathcal{L}}_{\mathcal{K}}\right)$ from Equation (7.28), with mean μ and variance–covariance matrix $\hat{V}\left(\hat{\mathcal{L}}\right)$, and $\hat{P} = g\left(\hat{\mathcal{L}}\right)$ is a transform of $\hat{\mathcal{L}}$ where g is the link function defined by Equation (7.26). The first-order Taylor series expansion of $g\left(\hat{\mathcal{L}}\right)$ yields an approximation of the mean

$$E\left[g\left(\hat{\mathcal{L}}\right)\right] \approx g(\mu), \tag{7.35}$$

and the variance–covariance matrix $\hat{V}\left(\hat{P}\right)$

$$V\left[g\left(\hat{\mathcal{L}}\right)\right] \approx \left[\frac{\partial g\left(\hat{\mathcal{L}}\right)}{\partial \hat{\mathcal{L}}}\bigg|\hat{\mathcal{L}} = \mu\right]' V\left(\hat{\mathcal{L}}\right)\left[\frac{\partial g\left(\hat{\mathcal{L}}\right)}{\partial \hat{\mathcal{L}}}\bigg|\hat{\mathcal{L}} = \mu\right]. \tag{7.36}$$

A more detailed description of the delta method is provided in Appendix A.

Given Equation (7.36), the variance–covariance matrix for a given set of predicted probabilities can be approximated and thus can be used to test the null hypothesis on the conditional effects. In view of the fact that a set of probabilities for $\mathcal{K} + 1$ alternatives must sum to unity and the corresponding conditional effects must sum to zero, the statistical significance of all conditional effects of a given covariate on a set of probabilities should be accepted if any one of them is statistically significant (Liu *et al.*, 1995).

Because a probability is not empirically observable for an individual, the logit function does not have an observed value, so the variance–covariance matrix for the predicted logit components is not directly obtainable from survival data. Here, I recommend a statistical method to obtain an approximate of the matrix. First, fit a multinomial logit model, with all covariates rescaled to be centered at sample means or at some selected values. Second, use the squared standard errors of $\mathcal{K}$ intercepts as the variances of the $\mathcal{K}$ logit components. Third, take values of the covariance between each pair of those intercepts as the off-diagonal elements in the matrix $\hat{V}\left(\hat{\mathcal{L}}\right)$. The rationale is that if covariates are centered at sample means, for example, the estimated intercepts represent the grand means of the logits, so that the variance–covariance matrix of these parameter estimates can be considered approximates of the variances and covariances for $\mathcal{K}$ sample means. The concrete procedure of this approximation method is described in Subsection 7.1.6, where an empirical illustration is provided.

7.1.5 Competing risks model with dependent failure types

It has been argued that the latent failure times of various event types are often interrelated, thereby suggesting the invalidity of the independence assumption. Such dependence is particularly observable in survival data with a clinical controlled trial design. For example, a new medical treatment can decrease the rate of death from one particular disease; at the same time, the side effects incurred from this treatment may enhance the mortality from another health condition. Obviously, the latent survival times associated with those diseases are mutually dependent, so the overall survival function is multivariate. In the presence of such correlation, neither the joint nor the marginal survival function is identifiable from the probability distribution of $(T, \delta, \boldsymbol{x})$ because there are an infinite number of joint distributions of potential survival times. When considerable dependence exists, only the crude type-specific hazard function is statistically estimable. Moreover, the hypothesis on independent survival times cannot be statistically tested with only one actual T series available.

Prentice *et al.* (1978) and Kalbfleisch and Prentice (2002) provide a simple illustration demonstrating that even if a parametric model with dependent risks is assumed for the net survival function and all parameters are estimable with that model, it is impossible to distinguish between the model with dependence and the model assuming independent competing risks. In particular, this illustration indicates two overall survival functions, one associated with the dependence assumption and one with the independence hypothesis, which turn out to be subject to the same set of the type-specific hazard functions and thus having the identical observable consequences. An important conclusion is then obtained: if a competing risks model is specified with a measure of dependence between or among the latent survival times, the hypothesis of dependence cannot be statistically tested from the empirical data, so that the model does not necessarily improve the quality of parameter estimates.

Even with such warnings, some statisticians and economists have attempted to develop statistical methods for handling dependence of latent survival time series. Heckman and Singer (1980) proposes the use of joint modeling for identifying marginal survival functions by linking the latent failure times by means of a dependence factor. Given the specification of this factor as a model covariate, the latent survival time systems are thought to be conditionally independent and, hence, more efficient, and less biased estimates of marginal survival functions can be obtained from this statistical perspective. The two-step parametric joint modeling, however, has been criticized given its restrictive assumptions, which are impossible to verify (Demirtas, 2004; Hedeker and Gibbons, 2006; Hogan, Roy, and Korkontzelou, 2004; Little and Rubin, 2002, Chapter 15; Liu *et al.*, 2010; Winship and Mare, 1992). With survival data based on the actual event time and the event type, the dependence of latent survival times cannot be captured and statistically tested by arbitrarily parameterizing dependence. Empirically, this selection approach is highly sensitive to minor deviations from its underlying assumptions, with the adjusting effect of the added dependence factor often found to be very limited (Liu *et al.*, 2010). Some other researchers suggest using a 'frailty' factor for addressing dependence of competing risks (Steele, Goldstein, and Browne, 2004). It is believed that with taking random effects into account, conditional independence of multiple modes of failure can be achieved, in turn ensuring the generation of unbiased parameter estimates. In Chapter 9, the frailty theory is described and discussed.

Another promising approach to detect dependence of latent failure times is to examine the correlation of certain time-dependent covariates between two event types. The rationale of this method is: if the effect of a common risk variable varies simultaneously over time for two event types, then the two series of latent times are likely to be interrelated due to some unobservable causal linkages. This method may be more relevant to medical studies where the physical and pathological causality between or among different diseases is more theoretically explainable. For example, if a time-dependent treatment variable has similar effects on the death rates from both lung cancer and leukemia, it may be reasonable to infer that this treatment has the same effectiveness on both diseases, so that survival times for patients of those two diseases are mutually dependent. It is difficult, however, to test the statistical implication of such correlation because high correlation is often observed even when the independence assumption is correctly assumed.

So far, the vast majority of competing risks analyses has been conducted using the independence hypothesis on type-specific failure times, which, I believe, is not unreasonable as long as the classification of event types derives from strong theoretical inference and previous findings. Even when dependence is identified, independent event categories can still be accomplished by suitably regrouping constituent causes of failure (David, 1974).

7.1.6 Illustration of competing risks models: Smoking cigarettes and the mortality of older Americans from three causes of death

In this illustration, I analyze the effects of smoking cigarettes on the death rate from three categories of primary causes – cancer, other serious diseases, and all remaining causes of death. In particular, the primary cause category 'cancer' includes all types of neoplasms and 'other serious diseases' consist of diabetes, heart disease, hypertension, and cerebrovascular illnesses. As the residual category, 'all remaining causes' are composed of infectious diseases, lung diseases, accidents and adverse effects, and the other primary causes. Accordingly, the variable of the event/censoring status indicator now contains four values: 0 = actually censored, 1 = death from cancer, 2 = death from other serious diseases, and 3 = death from all remaining causes. The observation period is defined as from the baseline survey to the end of the year 2004. Among 2000 older Americans in the mortality data, 1050 persons are actually censored, 103 died from cancer, 200 were deceased from other serious diseases, and the remaining 647 deaths occurred due to all remaining causes. Smoking cigarettes, as previously defined, is a dichotomous variable with 1 = current or past smoker and 0 = else, named 'Smoking.' For a full illustration of competing risks modeling, I apply both the hazard rate and the multinomial logit models to estimate the effects of smoking cigarettes on the three cause-specific death rates.

I start the analysis with the hazard rate model. For each cause category, a separate Cox model is created with deaths from the other two categories treated as right censored, assuming the three categories of primary causes of death to be mutually independent. I use the three mean-centered variables – 'Age_mean,' 'Female_mean,' and 'Educ_mean' – as controls in estimating each Cox model. Here, my primary interest is in examining whether or not smoking cigarettes has a similar impact on all three cause-specific death rates.

As the regression coefficient of smoking cigarettes and the corresponding hazard ratio may not necessarily display absolute differences in the hazard rate, I compare three sets of the cause-specific survival curves between smokers and nonsmokers, using the Brelow approximation method. Given that all control variables are centered at sample means, the baseline survival function describes the cause-specific survival function among nonsmokers. For smokers, the cause-specific survival function for event type $\mathcal{K}$ is estimated by

$$\hat{S}_{\mathcal{K}}(t;\text{smokers}) = \left[\hat{S}_{0\mathcal{K}}(t)\right]^{\exp\left(\hat{b}_{1\mathcal{K}}\right)}.$$

Under the independence assumption, these cause-specific survival curves are viewed as the estimated survival functions associated with $\mathcal{K}$ latent failure time series.

Below is the SAS program for estimating the three cause-specific Cox models.

SAS Program 7.1:

```
......
  length Id $30;
  input smoking age_mean female_mean educ_mean Id $12-61;
  datalines;
  0.00 0.00 0.00 0.00 smoking = 0
  1.00 0.00 0.00 0.00 smoking = 1
  ;

ods graphics on;
proc phreg data = new plot(overlay)=survival;
  model duration*Status(0, 2, 3) = smoking age_mean female_mean educ_mean / ties =
     BRESLOW ;
  baseline covariates = group out = pred1 survival=_all_ / rowid = Id;
run;
ods graphics off;

ods graphics on;
proc phreg data = new plot(overlay)=survival;
  model duration*Status(0, 1, 3) = smoking age_mean female_mean educ_mean / ties =
     BRESLOW ;
  baseline covariates = group out = pred1 survival=_all_ / rowid = Id;
run;
ods graphics off;

ods graphics on;
proc phreg data = new plot(overlay)=survival;
  model duration*Status(0, 1, 2) = smoking age_mean female_mean educ_mean /  ties =
     BRESLOW ;
  baseline covariates = group out = pred1 survival=_all_ / rowid = Id;
run;
ods graphics off;
```

In SAS Program 7.1, I specify three Cox models with each on a specific cause category of death. First, a temporary dataset 'GROUP' is created to specify values of covariates used for predicting two survival functions for each cause category. As previously indicated, the first group is nonsmokers and the second smokers, with values of the three control variables fixed at zero (sample means). Using the ODS Graphics, the PROC PHREG procedure plots two cause-specific survival curves for group = 0 and group = 1 for each Cox model, according to the specification saved in the dataset 'GROUP.' In each of the PROC PHREG procedures, censoring status is now redefined in the MODEL statement. For example, the first Cox model is created on the cancer-specific death rate, so that only deaths due to cancer are regarded as events and deaths from the other two causes are treated as right censored. Accordingly, I include values 0, 2, and 3 when specifying censoring, represented by the 'MODEL DURATION*STATUS(0, 2, 3)' statement. Similarly, in specifying the second and the third Cox models, the values within the parentheses are (0, 1, 3) and (0, 1, 2), respectively. The options in each PROC PHREG procedure were described previously.

The above SAS program generates information on model fit, parameter estimates, and the plots of survival curves for the three cause-specific Cox models. First, the results of the Cox model for cancer are displayed.

SAS Program Output 7.1a:

The PHREG Procedure

Model Information

Data Set	WORK.NEW
Dependent Variable	duration
Censoring Variable	status
Censoring Value(s)	0 2 3
Ties Handling	BRESLOW

Number of Observations Read	2000
Number of Observations Used	2000

Summary of the Number of Event and Censored Values

Total	Event	Censored	Percent Censored
2000	103	1897	94.85

Convergence Status

Convergence criterion (GCONV=1E-8) satisfied.

Model Fit Statistics

Criterion	Without Covariates	With Covariates
-2 LOG L	1544.117	1510.075
AIC	1544.117	1518.075
SBC	1544.117	1528.614

Testing Global Null Hypothesis: BETA=0

Test	Chi-Square	DF	Pr > ChiSq
Likelihood Ratio	34.0425	4	<.0001
Score	37.4503	4	<.0001
Wald	36.4019	4	<.0001

Analysis of Maximum Likelihood Estimates

Parameter	DF	Parameter Estimate	Standard Error	Chi-Square	Pr > ChiSq	Hazard Ratio
smoking	1	0.82869	0.25255	10.7666	0.0010	2.290
age_mean	1	0.04711	0.01577	8.9289	0.0028	1.048
female_mean	1	-0.68956	0.19794	12.1359	0.0005	0.502
educ_mean	1	-0.03534	0.02616	1.8251	0.1767	0.965

In SAS Program Output 7.1a, the information on the dataset, the dependent variable, the censoring status variable, and the censoring value is reported first. The censoring variable 'STATUS' contains three values. The 'Tied Handling: BRESLOW' statement indicates the use of the Breslow method for estimating regression coefficients of the four covariates. As indicated earlier, 103 out of 2000 individuals have died of cancer (actual events in this cause-specific analysis) and the remaining 1897 older persons either are right censored or died from other causes. The Model Fit Statistics table displays three indicators of model fitness. All three tests in the 'Testing Global Null Hypothesis: BETA = 0' section demonstrate that the null hypothesis $\hat{\boldsymbol{\beta}} = \mathbf{0}$ should be rejected. Because only a small portion of the actual events are under examination, the values of these test scores are much lower than those derived from the all-causes model (see Section 5.3).

In the table of 'Analysis of Maximum Likelihood Estimates,' the regression coefficient of 'Smoking' is 0.8287 ($SE = 0.2526$), statistically significant at $\alpha = 0.05$ ($\chi^2 = 10.7666$; $p = 0.001$). The estimate of its hazard ratio is 2.29, much higher than the all-cause estimate of 1.523, suggesting that the cancer-specific death rate among current or past smokers is about 2.3 times as high as the corresponding rate among nonsmokers, other covariates being equal. This high hazard ratio, however, may not necessarily lead to a greater difference in the hazard rate because the cause-specific baseline hazard function is unspecified. The regression coefficients of 'Age_mean' and 'Female_mean' are statistically significant, whereas the regression coefficient of 'Educ_mean' is not. Age is positively associated with the mortality from cancer, with a hazard ratio of 1.048 ($\beta_2 = 0.047$; $\chi^2 = 8.93$; $p = 0.0028$). Likewise, the older women's cancer-specific death rate is about 50 % lower than among their male counterparts when other covariates are adjusted, given a hazard ratio of 0.50 ($\chi^2 = 12.14$; $p = 0.0005$).

Some selected results of the second Cox model, predicting the death rate from other serious diseases, are presented below.

SAS Program Output 7.1b:

Testing Global Null Hypothesis: BETA=0

Test	Chi-Square	DF	Pr > ChiSq
Likelihood Ratio	76.1879	4	<.0001
Score	75.8220	4	<.0001
Wald	77.1783	4	<.0001

Analysis of Maximum Likelihood Estimates

Parameter	DF	Parameter Estimate	Standard Error	Chi-Square	Pr > ChiSq	Hazard Ratio
smoking	1	0.27658	0.22808	1.4705	0.2253	1.319
age_mean	1	0.08391	0.01096	58.6056	<.0001	1.088
female_mean	1	-0.47747	0.14336	11.0925	0.0009	0.620
educ_mean	1	-0.02425	0.01892	1.6421	0.2000	0.976

In SAS Program Output 7.1b, I only present the sections of 'Testing Global Null Hypothesis: BETA = 0' and 'Analysis of Maximum Likelihood Estimates.' As mentioned earlier, 200 older persons died from other serious diseases within the observation period. Although the null hypothesis $\hat{\boldsymbol{\beta}} = \mathbf{0}$ should be rejected given the results of all three global test statistics, the regression coefficient of 'Smoking' on this cause-specific death rate is not statistically significant ($\chi^2 = 1.47$; $p = 0.2253$). The regression coefficients of the three control variables on this specific cause category are similar to those on the cancer-specific mortality: age is positively and significantly associated with this cause-specific mortality ($\chi^2 = 58.61$; $p < 0.0001$) and women's mortality due to other serious diseases is considerably lower than among their male counterparts. The effect of education on this cause category remains statistically insignificant.

The following output table displays the same result sections for the Cox model on the death rate from all remaining causes.

SAS Program Output 7.1c:

Testing Global Null Hypothesis: BETA=0

Test	Chi-Square	DF	Pr > ChiSq
Likelihood Ratio	235.0531	4	<.0001
Score	229.1031	4	<.0001
Wald	235.3862	4	<.0001

Analysis of Maximum Likelihood Estimates

Parameter	DF	Parameter Estimate	Standard Error	Chi-Square	Pr > ChiSq	Hazard Ratio
smoking	1	0.37482	0.12721	8.6812	0.0032	1.455
age_mean	1	0.09072	0.00635	204.1184	<.0001	1.095
female_mean	1	-0.36884	0.08191	20.2774	<.0001	0.692
educ_mean	1	-0.01966	0.01066	3.3996	0.0652	0.981

The Cox model on the death rate from all remaining causes fits much better than the first and the second cause-specific models because there are 647 deaths from those remaining causes. Here, the regression coefficient of 'Smoking' is 0.3748 ($SE = 0.1272$), statistically significant ($\chi^2 = 8.68$; $p = 0.0032$). The hazard ratio is very close to the value estimated for the all-cause Cox model as the deaths from those remaining causes weigh heavily in total deaths. For the three control variables, the effects and the testing results are consistent with those generated from the above two Cox models.

As discussed previously, just looking at the regression coefficients and the hazard ratios of smoking cigarettes does not necessarily yield constructive policy implications, particularly since the relative risk needs to be combined with the baseline hazard function for fully demonstrating a covariate's effect on the hazard rate. From separation of two corresponding survival curves, the effect of smoking cigarettes on each cause-specific death rate can be effectively assessed. For this need, below I present three plots of survival curves, with each for a specific primary cause category of death, to graphically display the impact of smoking cigarettes on the cause-specific death rate of older Americans.

The first plot, Figure 7.1a, displays two cancer-specific survival curves, one for smokers and one for non-smokers. In Figure 7.1a, some separation is noted between the two cancer-specific survival curves; the degree of such separation, however, is not as dramatic as can be expected from a hazard ratio of 2.3. This plot provides very strong evidence that a high hazard ratio may not necessarily translate into a strong effect on the hazard rate itself, highlighting the importance of presenting the predicted survival curves for assisting in the interpretation of the analytic results in the Cox model.

Figure 7.1b displays the corresponding survival curves for smokers and nonsmokers with respect to the death rate from other serious diseases. Figure 7.1b shows that smoking cigarettes does not impact the death rate from other serious diseases. Besides the lack of statistical significance on the estimated regression coefficient of 'Smoking' shown in SAS Program Output 7.1b, the two survival curves for this cause category do not appear to separate at all, thereby indicating the absence of any meaningful influence from smoking cigarettes on the death rate due to other serious diseases.

The third plot presents the two survival curves from all remaining causes. Figure 7.1c plots the evolution of the two survival functions for all remaining causes. At most time points, nonsmokers are expected to have considerably higher chances of survival from those residual causes than do smokers, other covariates being equal. The separation of these two survival curves looks analogous to the pattern derived from the all-cause Cox model, shown in Section 5.3.

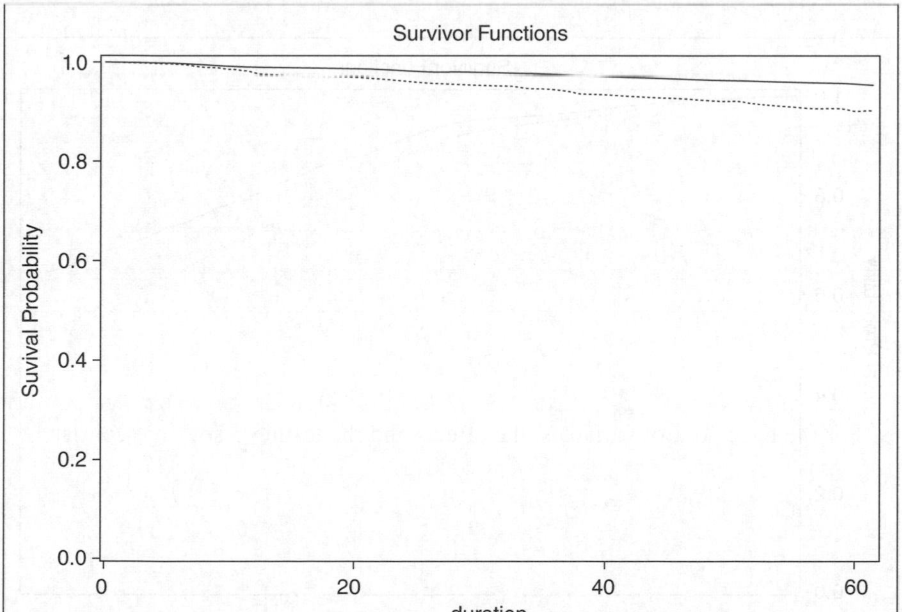

Figure 7.1a The probability of survival from cancer.

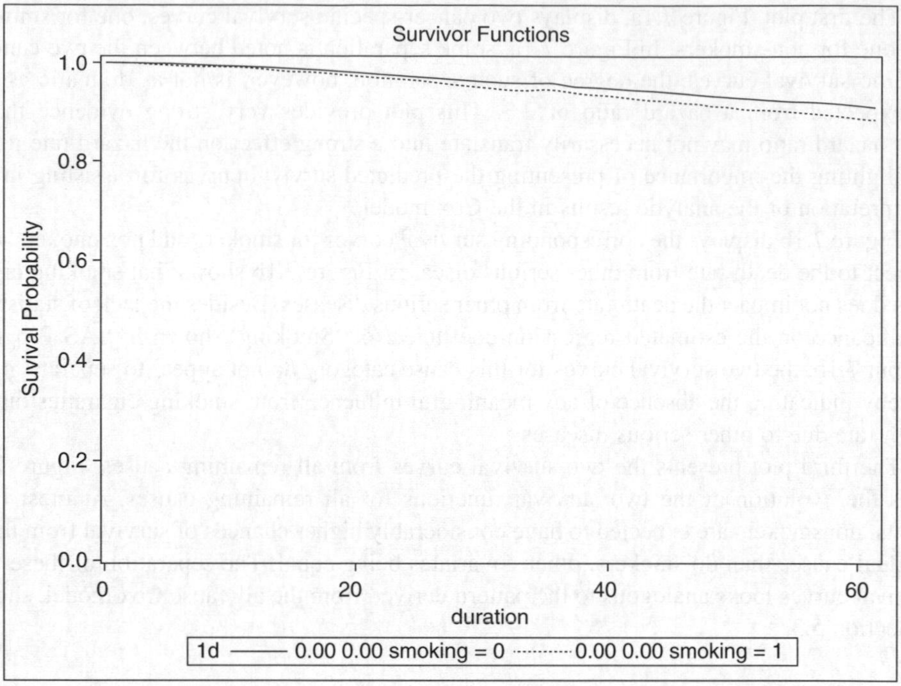

Figure 7.1b The probability of survival from other serious diseases.

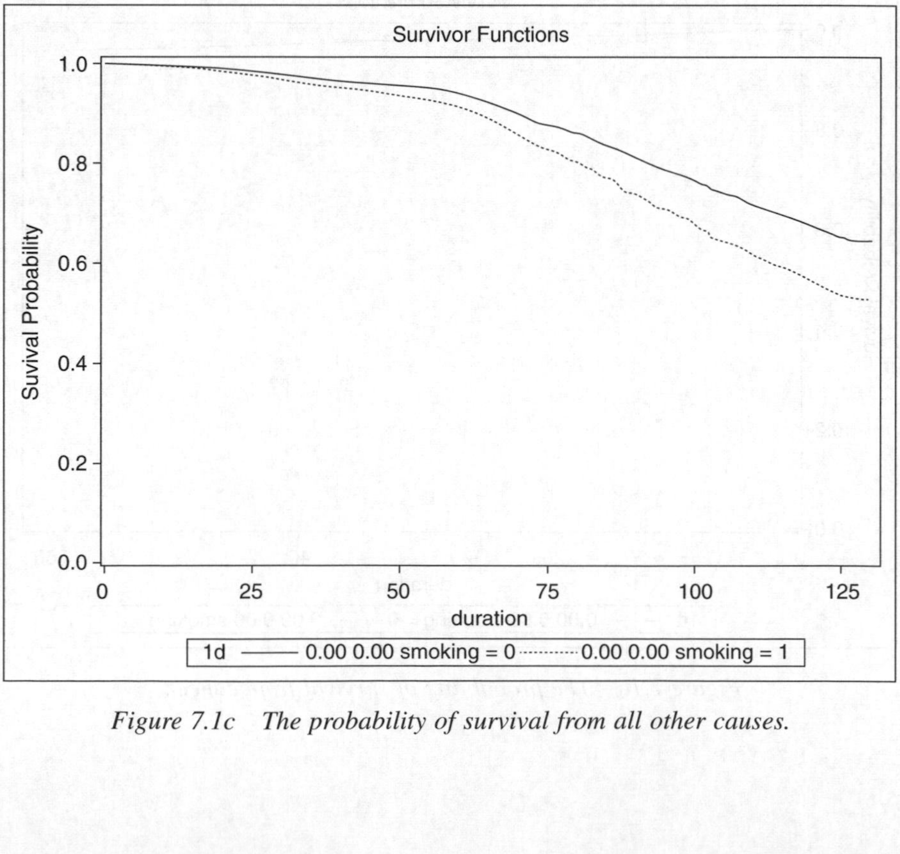

Figure 7.1c The probability of survival from all other causes.

Next, I use the multinomial logit model to estimate the effects of smoking cigarettes on the three cause-specific death rates. Other than the application of a different regression perspective, variable and data specifications remain exactly the same as for the three Cox models. The SAS PROC CATMOD procedure is applied for fitting the multinomial logit regression on the probabilities of four event types including right censoring, with 'Smoking' and the three mean-centered variables used as covariates. The following SAS program is written for this analytic step.

SAS Program 7.2:

```
......
if death = 0 then cause = 4;
  else if Z900 > 1 and Z900 < 7 then cause = 1;
  else if Z900 > 6 and Z900 < 12 then cause = 2;
  else cause = 3;

......
proc catmod data =new;
  direct smoking age_mean female_mean educ_mean;
  model cause = smoking age_mean female_mean educ_mean / covb ml maxiter = 100;
run;
```

In SAS Program 7.2, I first create a CAUSE variable. The variable Z900 is the original classification factor on the primary causes of death in the AHEAD mortality data. Because SAS treats the highest value of the qualitative dependent variable as the reference level, I assign value 4 to CAUSE if an individual survives throughout the entire observation period or is randomly censored during the observation interval. The three actual event types, 'dying from cancer,' 'dying from other serious diseases,' and 'dying from all remaining causes,' are given values 1, 2, and 3, respectively. The application of the PROC CATMOD procedure requires a DIRECT statement for listing covariates to be treated as quantitative variables; otherwise, all variables in the MODEL statement are viewed as qualitative factors. In this exercise, I include all covariates in the DIRECT statement because all of them, including 'Smoking,' should be analyzed quantitatively. The MODEL statement defines the relationship between the qualitative dependent variable CAUSE and the four covariates within the construct of a multinomial logistic regression. Specifically, given four response levels, three logit components are specified: $\log(P_1/P_4)$, $\log(P_2/P_4)$, and $\log(P_3/P_4)$, with each logit expressed as a linear function of the four covariates. Notice that this multinomial logit regression can also be estimated by using the PROC LOGISTIC procedure.

Some options are selected in the MODEL statement. The option COVB requests SAS to display the estimated covariance matrix of the parameter estimates, needed for approximating the variance–covariance matrix of the conditional effects and the hazard ratios. The option ML tells SAS to compute maximum likelihood estimates (MLE) using a Newton–Raphson algorithm (default in SAS). Given the selection of the ML estimator, the MAXITER=100 option specifies the maximum number of iterations used for the maximum likelihood estimation of the parameters.

SAS Program 7.2 produces the following analytic results.

SAS Program Output 7.2:

```
                    The CATMOD Procedure

                        Data Summary

Response             cause     Response Levels    4
Weight Variable      None      Populations      74
Data Set             NEW       Total Frequency  200
Frequency Missing    0         Observations     200


                     Response Profiles

                     Response    cause
                     -----------------
                         1         1
                         2         2
                         3         3
                         4         4


                 Maximum Likelihood Analysis

           Maximum likelihood computations converged.


           Maximum Likelihood Analysis of Variance

  Source              DF    Chi-Square    Pr > ChiSq
  ---------------------------------------------------
  Intercept            3        710.67        <.0001
  smoking              3         19.47        0.0002
  age_mean             3        206.13        <.0001
  female_mean          3         32.98        <.0001
  educ_mean            3          6.78        0.0794

  Likelihood Ratio   2E3       1789.57        1.0000
```

Analysis of Maximum Likelihood Estimates

Parameter	Function Number	Estimate	Standard Error	Chi-Square	Pr > ChiSq
Intercept	1	-2.4950	0.1241	404.32	<.0001
	2	-1.8135	0.0935	375.83	<.0001
	3	-0.5370	0.0567	89.78	<.0001
smoking	1	1.1171	0.2843	15.44	<.0001
	2	0.5741	0.2647	4.70	0.0301
	3	0.5323	0.1783	8.91	0.0028
age_mean	1	0.1091	0.0182	35.72	<.0001
	2	0.1483	0.0138	114.83	<.0001
	3	0.1221	0.00951	164.63	<.0001
female_mean	1	-0.8911	0.2126	17.57	<.0001
	2	-0.6813	0.1650	17.06	<.0001
	3	-0.4263	0.1122	14.43	0.0001
educ_mean	1	-0.0528	0.0285	3.42	0.0642
	2	-0.0432	0.0220	3.84	0.0499
	3	-0.0267	0.0152	3.07	0.0797

Covariance Matrix of the Maximum Likelihood Estimates

Row	Parameter		Col1	Col2	Col3
1	Intercept	1	0.01539597	0.00124187	0.00121458
2	Intercept	2	0.00124187	0.00875047	0.00121455
3	Intercept	3	0.00121458	0.00121455	0.00321157

In SAS Program Output 7.2, the SAS PROC CATMOD procedure provides a summary table first. The response variable is CAUSE, consisting of four levels, as listed in the 'Response Profiles' section. The results of model fit are presented in the 'Maximum Likelihood Analysis of Variance' table, showing that the overall effects of smoking cigarettes, age, and female on the three logit components are statistically significant, whereas the effect of education is marginally significant ($0.05 < p < 0.10$). The degree of freedom for each parameter is 3 because there are three values for the intercept and for each of the covariates corresponding to three logit components. The estimates and tests for individual parameters are presented in the table 'Analysis of Maximum Likelihood Estimates.' For each parameter, there are three estimates corresponding to the three logit components – $\log(P_1/P_4)$, $\log(P_2/P_4)$, and $\log(P_3/P_4)$ – respectively (Function Numbers 1, 2, 3). The results of this section are highly consistent with those reported in the ANOVA table: the parameter estimates for the intercept, smoking cigarettes, age, and female are all highly statistically significant; for education, however, only the effect on the second logit component is statistically significant. The last section, 'Covariance Matrix of the Maximum Likelihood Estimates,' displays the variance–covariance matrix of the intercepts on three logit components, which, as mentioned earlier, is used for calculating the variances and the pair-wise covariance of the conditional effects and hazard ratios for the variable 'Smoking.'

The regression coefficients of a covariate in the multinomial logit model are not highly intuitive because they may not necessarily reflect changes in the probabilities of the four event types. Consequently, the estimated regression coefficients of smoking cigarettes need to be transformed to the conditional effects and the hazard ratios for the interpretation of analytic results. Given the variable 'Smoking' defined as a dichotomous covariate, Equations (7.33) and (7.34) are applied to generate those transforms. First, using Equation (7.26) and the estimated regression coefficients reported in SAS Program Output 7.2, the baseline probabilities of the four event types reflect the estimates for nonsmokers (Smoking = 0 and the control variables are fixed as sample means), given by

$$\hat{P}_{10} = \frac{\exp(-2.4950)}{1+\exp(-2.4950)+\exp(-1.8135)+\exp(-0.5370)} = 0.0451,$$

$$\hat{P}_{20} = \frac{\exp(-1.8135)}{1+\exp(-2.4950)+\exp(-1.8135)+\exp(-0.5370)} = 0.0891,$$

$$\hat{P}_{30} = \frac{\exp(-0.5370)}{1+\exp(-2.4950)+\exp(-1.8135)+\exp(-0.5370)} = 0.3194.$$

By dentition, $\hat{P}_{40}$ is the residual to the sum of the predicted probabilities for the three cause categories of death, so that

$$\hat{P}_{40} = 1 - \hat{P}_{10} - \hat{P}_{20} - \hat{P}_{30} = 1 - 0.0451 - 0.0891 - 0.3194 = 0.5464.$$

Likewise, the four probabilities for smokers (Smoking = 1 and the control variables are fixed as sample means) are

$$\hat{P}_{11} = \frac{\exp(-2.4950+1.1171)}{1+\exp(-2.4950+1.1171)+\exp(-1.8135+0.5741)+\exp(-0.5370+0.5323)} = 0.0994,$$

$$\hat{P}_{21} = \frac{\exp(-1.8135+0.5741)}{1+\exp(-2.4950+1.1171)+\exp(-1.8135+0.5741)+\exp(-0.5370+0.5323)} = 0.1141,$$

$$\hat{P}_{31} = \frac{\exp(-0.5370+0.5323)}{1+\exp(-2.4950+1.1171)+\exp(-1.8135+0.5741)+\exp(-0.5370+0.5323)} = 0.3923.$$

$$\hat{P}_{41} = 1 - 0.0994 - 0.1141 - 0.3923 = 0.3942.$$

Using Equation (7.33), the conditional effects of smoking cigarettes on the probabilities of four event alternatives are

$$\Delta\hat{P}_{1,\text{Smoking}} = \hat{P}_{11} - \hat{P}_{10} = 0.0994 - 0.0451 = 0.0543,$$

$$\begin{aligned}\Delta\hat{P}_{2,\text{Smoking}} &= \hat{P}_{21} - \hat{P}_{20} = 0.1141 - 0.0891 = 0.0250,\\ \Delta\hat{P}_{3,\text{Smoking}} &= \hat{P}_{31} - \hat{P}_{30} = 0.3923 - 0.3194 = 0.0729,\\ \Delta\hat{P}_{4,\text{Smoking}} &= -\left(\Delta\hat{P}_{1,\text{Smoking}} + \Delta\hat{P}_{2,\text{Smoking}} + \Delta\hat{P}_{3,\text{Smoking}}\right)\\ &= -(0.0543 + 0.0250 + 0.0729) = -0.1522.\end{aligned}$$

Applying Equation (7.34) gives rise to the hazard ratios of smoking cigarettes:

$$HR_{1,\text{Smoking}} \approx \frac{\left(\hat{P}_{11}\right)}{\left(\hat{P}_{10}\right)} = \frac{0.0994}{0.0451} = 2.2040,$$

$$HR_{2,\text{Smoking}} \approx \frac{\left(\hat{P}_{21}\right)}{\left(\hat{P}_{20}\right)} = \frac{0.1141}{0.0891} = 1.2806,$$

$$HR_{3,\text{Smoking}} \approx \frac{\left(\hat{P}_{31}\right)}{\left(\hat{P}_{30}\right)} = \frac{0.3923}{0.3194} = 1.2282,$$

$$HR_{4,\text{Smoking}} \approx \frac{\left(\hat{P}_{41}\right)}{\left(\hat{P}_{40}\right)} = \frac{0.3942}{0.5464} = 0.7214.$$

The first two hazard ratios are fairly consistent with those derived from the corresponding Cox models (2.20, 1.28 versus 2.29, 1.32). The third hazard ratio differs in the absolute value from that of the third Cox model (1.23 versus 1.46) but both values are substantially greater than unity, thereby leading to the same conclusion concerning the effect of smoking cigarettes on the death rate due to all remaining causes. It is interesting to note that the conditional effect of smoking cigarettes on the probability of death from other serious diseases (CAUSE = 2) is the lowest of all four effects; in the meantime, it converts to a hazard ratio that is higher than the third hazard ratio. This phenomenon, once more, provides solid evidence that without checking the absolute difference between two hazard rates, a hazard ratio does not necessarily indicate the actual impact of a given covariate.

Statistical significance of the conditional effects and the hazard ratios can be tested by using the approximated variance–covariance matrix for the predicted probabilities, obtained by applying the delta method. Specifically, the first step is to approximate the variances and covariances for two sets of the predicted probabilities, one for smokers and one for nonsmokers, as transformed from the variance–covariance matrix of the intercepts on the three logit components. The transformation procedure is simple but tedious, described extensively in Appendix B.

Using the method described in Appendix B and the covariance matrix of the three intercepts presented in SAS Program Output 7.2, the variance–covariance matrix of the three predicted probabilities for nonsmokers is approximated as

$$\boldsymbol{V}\left(\hat{\boldsymbol{P}}_0\right) \approx \begin{pmatrix} 0.0000276 & -0.0000027 & -0.0000090 \\ -0.0000027 & 0.0000548 & -0.0000189 \\ -0.0000090 & -0.0000189 & 0.0001402 \end{pmatrix}.$$

The corresponding matrix for smokers can be obtained in the same fashion. First, the variance–covariance matrix of the three logit components is approximated by estimating a multinomial logit model with letting smokers = 0, nonsmokers = 1, and the values of the three controls fixed as sample means. The covariance matrix of the three intercepts for smokers is

Row	Parameter		Col1	Col2	Col3
1	Intercept	1	0.06772874	0.01521945	0.01439765
2	Intercept	2	0.01521945	0.06259528	0.01496414
3	Intercept	3	0.01439765	0.01496414	0.02848663

Using the transformation approach described in Appendix B, the variance–covariance matrix of the three predicted probabilities for smokers is approximated as

$$V\left(\hat{\boldsymbol{P}}_1\right) \approx \begin{pmatrix} 0.0004756 & -0.0000541 & -0.0002088 \\ -0.0000541 & 0.0005497 & -0.0002321 \\ -0.0002088 & -0.0002321 & 0.0013134 \end{pmatrix}.$$

Given the above two variance–covariance matrices for the predicted probabilities, the conditional effects of smoking cigarettes on the three cause-specific probabilities can be tested by using the Wald chi-square statistic. Let $\left(\hat{P}_{k} \,|\, \bar{\boldsymbol{x}}\right)$ be $\hat{P}_{k0}$ and $\left(\hat{P}_{k} \,|\, \bar{x}_m + 1, \bar{\boldsymbol{x}}_r\right)$ be $\hat{P}_{k1}$. Then, the following equation from the delta method is defined:

$$\chi^2_{W,k} = \frac{\left(\hat{P}_{k1} - \hat{P}_{k0}\right)^2}{\hat{V}\left(\hat{\mathrm{P}}_{k0}\right) + \hat{V}\left(\hat{P}_{k1}\right) - 2\,\mathrm{cov}\left(\hat{P}_{k0}\hat{P}_{k1}\right)}, \quad k = 1, \ldots, \mathcal{K}.$$

As predicted from the same parameter estimates and where all but one covariate have exactly the same values, $\hat{P}_{k0}$ and $\hat{P}_{k1}$ are subject to the same probability distribution. Therefore, the two random variables $P_{\mathcal{K}0}$ and $P_{\mathcal{K}1}$ should be very closely correlated. For analytic convenience, I assume them to be perfectly correlated. As a result, the above equation for calculating the Wald chi-square statistic becomes

$$\chi^2_{W,k} = \frac{\left(\hat{P}_{k1} - \hat{P}_{k0}\right)^2}{\hat{V}\left(\hat{P}_{k0}\right) + \hat{V}\left(\hat{P}_{k1}\right) - 2\sqrt{\hat{V}\left(\hat{P}_{k0}\right)\hat{V}\left(\hat{P}_{k1}\right)}}.$$

Given the above equation, the Wald chi-square statistics for the three conditional effects of smoking cigarettes are

$$\chi^2_{W,\Delta\hat{P}_1} = \frac{(0.0994 - 0.0451)^2}{0.0000276 + 0.0004756 - 2 \times \sqrt{0.0000276 \times 0.0004756}} = 10.7587,$$

$$\chi^2_{W,\Delta\hat{P}_2} = \frac{(0.1141 - 0.0891)^2}{0.0000548 + 0.0005497 - 2 \times \sqrt{0.0000548 \times 0.0005497}} = 2.4283,$$

$$\chi^2_{W,\Delta\hat{P}_3} = \frac{(0.3923 - 0.3194)^2}{0.0001402 + 0.0013134 - 2 \times \sqrt{0.0001402 \times 0.0013134}} = 8.9262.$$

Each Wald statistic is distributed asymptotically as chi-square with 1 degree of freedom under the null hypothesis, so that $\chi^2_{W,1}$ is statistically significant given $\alpha = 0.05$. The evaluation of $\Delta\hat{P}_4$, the residual effect, depends on the testing results of the three nonreference conditional effects. Given the constraint that a set of conditional effects must sum to zero, all four conditional effects of smoking cigarettes are considered statistically significant.

The variances of the three hazard ratios can be approximated by using the following ratio estimator, given perfect correlation between $P_{\mathcal{K}0}$ and $P_{\mathcal{K}1}$:

$$V\left(\frac{\hat{P}_{k1}}{\hat{P}_{k0}}\right) \approx \left(\frac{\hat{P}_{k1}^2}{\hat{P}_{k0}^4}\right)\hat{V}\left(\hat{P}_{k0}\right) + \left(\frac{1}{\hat{P}_{k0}^2}\right)\hat{V}\left(\hat{P}_{k1}\right) - 2\left(\frac{\hat{P}_{k1}}{\hat{P}_{k0}^3}\right)\sqrt{\hat{V}\left(\hat{P}_{k0}\right)\hat{V}\left(\hat{P}_{k0}\right)},$$

$$k = 1, \ldots, \mathcal{K}.$$

Given this equation, the variance for the hazard ratio of smoking cigarettes on the cancer-specific death rate is

$$\begin{aligned} V\left(\frac{\hat{P}_{11}}{\hat{P}_{10}}\right) &\approx \left(\frac{0.0994^2}{0.0451^4}\right) \times 0.0000276 + \left(\frac{1}{0.0451^2}\right) \times 0.0004756 \\ &\quad - 2 \times \left(\frac{0.0994}{0.0451^3}\right) \times \sqrt{0.0000276 \times 0.0004756} \\ &\approx 0.0514. \end{aligned}$$

Similarly,

$$\begin{aligned} V\left(\frac{\hat{P}_{21}}{\hat{P}_{20}}\right) &\approx \left(\frac{0.1141^2}{0.0891^4}\right) \times 0.0000548 + \left(\frac{1}{0.0891^2}\right) \times 0.0005497 \\ &\quad - 2 \times \left(\frac{0.1141}{0.0891^3}\right) \times \sqrt{0.0000548 \times 0.0005497} \\ &\approx 0.0246 \end{aligned}$$

and

$$\begin{aligned} V\left(\frac{\hat{P}_{31}}{\hat{P}_{30}}\right) &\approx \left(\frac{0.3923^2}{0.3194^4}\right) \times 0.0001402 + \left(\frac{1}{0.3194^2}\right) \times 0.0013134 \\ &\quad - 2 \times \left(\frac{0.3923}{0.3194^3}\right) \times \sqrt{0.0001402 \times 0.0013134} \\ &\approx 0.0046. \end{aligned}$$

The square roots of the above three variances approximate the standard errors for the three hazard ratios, which are 0.2267, 0.1568, and 0.0678, respectively. Given those approximates, the three hazard ratios of smoking cigarettes, estimated from the multinomial logit model, are all statistically significant, in turn indicating the statistical significance of the fourth hazard ratio. The standard error approximates for the first three hazard ratios are each smaller than the corresponding figures derived from the separate Cox models, which are 0.2526, 0.2281, and 0.1271, respectively (see SAS Program Output 7.1). Accordingly, a narrower confidence interval of each hazard ratio is accomplished. The decreased value of the standard error highlights the statistical advantage of applying the multinomial logit model over the hazard rate model when analyzing competing risks. The multinomial logit regression, however, does not build upon survival times, so survival curves cannot be produced from this model. Therefore, the competing risks hazard model and the multinomial logit regression each have their own respective strengths and limitations. Using both perspectives in an empirical study, as shown in this illustration, helps the analyst grasp a better understanding of a covariate's effects on a set of competing risks.

7.2 Repeated events

In survival data, repeated, or recurrent, events occur when an individual experiences repetitions of the same event within a specific observation interval. Such events are perhaps most frequently observed in biomedical research given the high rate of recurrent infections, multiple disease episodes, and the like. Among the widely cited examples are asthmatic attacks, recurrences of the same tumor, and bronchial infections (Kalbfleisch and Prentice, 2002). Repeated events are also observable in other settings, such as repetitions of criminal offenses, family violence recidivism, marital disruption, and the repair history of an automobile.

A number of statisticians have contributed to the development of refined models for analyzing survival data of repeated events (Andersen and Gill, 1982; Kelly and Lim, 2000; Lawless and Nadeau, 1995; Lee, Wei, and Amato, 1992; Lin, 1994; Lin *et al.*, 2000; Pepe and Cai, 1993; Prentice, Williams, and Peterson, 1981; Wei, Lin, and Weissfeld, 1989). These techniques share some common ground, and all are based on standard inference for fitting the proportional hazard model by combining all events within an integrated maximization process. Let T_{iq} be the actual event time for the qth time of experiencing the same event for individual i, where $q = 1, \ldots, \mathcal{Q}$, C_{iq} be the censored time with respect to the qth event for the same individual, and $t_{iq} = \min(T_{iq}, C_{iq})$ is the observation time. Then the partial likelihood function of a proportional hazard model with repeated events can be generally written as

$$L_p(\boldsymbol{\beta}) = \prod_{i=1}^{d} \prod_{q=1}^{\mathcal{Q}} \left\{ \frac{\exp\left[\boldsymbol{x}_{iq}(t)' \boldsymbol{\beta} \right]}{\sum_{l \in \mathcal{R}(t_i)} \exp\left[\boldsymbol{x}_{lq}(t)' \boldsymbol{\beta} \right]} \right\}. \tag{7.37}$$

Each of the refined hazard models with repeated events, however, depends on its own assumptions about the risk interval and within-persons dependence. Accordingly, they specify different risk sets of $\mathcal{R}(t_i)$ and propose dissimilar statistical approaches for adjusting the intrapersons correlation. As a result, the models handling repeated events are often found to yield substantially different results (Kelly and Lim, 2000). Given such variability, understanding the characteristics, the strengths, and the limitations of each model is essential for correctly employing those techniques to analyze survival data with repeated events.

In this section, I introduce the following five regression models handling repeated events: those of Andersen and Gill (1982), Prentice, Williams, and Peterson (1981) with total time and gap time, Wei, Lin, and Weissfeld (1989), and the proportional rates and means models (Lawless and Nadeau, 1995; Lin *et al.*, 2000; Pepe and Cai, 1993). In the survival analysis literature, the first four methods are generally referred to as *AG*, *PWP-CP*, *PWP-GT*, and *WLW* models, respectively, whereas the proportional means model is relatively new. An illustration is provided on the effects of a new medical treatment on repeated clinical visits by patients originally diagnosed with Posttraumatic Stress Disorder (PTSD).

7.2.1 Andersen and Gill model (AG)

Andersen and Gill (1982) consider it statistical feasible to extend the Cox model into the regression analysis on the intensity of a repeated event. Specifically, they provide a thorough derivation using the counting process formulation and the martingale theory for the description of event repetitions. From parameter estimates by maximizing the partial likelihood function, the integrated intensity processes, denoted by $\Lambda(t)$ in counting process terminology, can be obtained by a linear interpolation between failures times, given by

$$\hat{\Lambda}(t) = \sum_{T_i \le t} \left[\frac{\delta_i}{\sum\limits_{l \in \mathcal{R}(t_i)} \exp(\mathbf{Z}_l \boldsymbol{\beta})} \right]. \tag{7.38}$$

The above function is flexible enough to permit multiple events for an individual up to time t as its computation and, as can be seen from the equation, is not restricted to a single event. Therefore, by extending the Cox model, a joint likelihood $L(\beta, \Lambda)$ is proposed to model the intensity rate of a repeated event given past event history:

$$\lambda_{\mathbf{Z}}(t)\mathrm{d}t = \mathrm{E}\{\mathrm{dN}(t)|\mathcal{F}_{t-}\} = \lambda_0(t)\exp[\mathbf{Z}_i'(t)\boldsymbol{\beta}_0]\mathrm{d}t, \tag{7.39}$$

where $\lambda_0(t)$ is an arbitrary baseline intensity function, $\boldsymbol{\beta}_0$ is an $M \times 1$ vector of regression parameters, and $\mathcal{F}_{t-}$ is the σ-algebra generated from the process history prior to t about survival, censoring, and covariates, defined in Chapter 6. The covariate vector $\mathbf{Z}(t)$ is defined as time dependent for reflecting the influences of previous events on future recurrences.

Based on the Cox partial likelihood function, the regression coefficient $\boldsymbol{\beta}$ can be flexibly estimated over survival data of repeated events. Specifically, the log partial likelihood function can be written as

$$\log L_p(\boldsymbol{\beta}) = \sum_{i=1}^{n} \int_0^t \mathbf{Z}_i'(u)\boldsymbol{\beta}\, \mathrm{dN}_i(u) - \int_0^t \log\left\{\sum_{i=1}^{n} \mathrm{Y}_i(u)\exp[\mathbf{Z}_i'(u)\boldsymbol{\beta}]\right\} \mathrm{d}\bar{\mathrm{N}}(u), \tag{7.40}$$

where $\mathrm{N}_i(t)$, in the context of repeated events, is the number of events to time t for individual i and $\bar{\mathrm{N}} = \Sigma_{i=1}^{n} \mathrm{N}_i$ is the risk set for the occurrence of each jump (the first and the recurrent events). It is recognizable in Equation (7.40) that the AG approach sets up a restricted condition that permits only one contribution to the risk set for a given event.

As indicated in Chapter 5, the estimator $\hat{\boldsymbol{\beta}}$ in the partial likelihood function is defined as the solution to the equation

$$\tilde{U}(\boldsymbol{\beta}) = \frac{\partial}{\partial} \log L_p(\boldsymbol{\beta}) = \mathbf{0},$$

where $\tilde{U}(\boldsymbol{\beta}) = (\partial \log L_p / \partial\beta_1, \ldots, \partial \log L_p / \partial\beta_M)'$. Then the total score statistic at time t is given by

$$\tilde{U}(\beta, t) = \sum_{i=1}^{n} \int_0^t \{\mathbf{Z}_i(u) - \bar{\mathbf{Z}}(\beta, u)\} \mathrm{dN}_i(u), \tag{7.41}$$

where the second term within the brace represents, as also defined in Section 6.1, the expected covariate vector over a given risk set, defined as

$$\bar{\mathbf{Z}}_i(\beta, u) = \frac{\sum_{i=1}^{n} \mathrm{Y}_i(u)\mathbf{Z}_i(u)\exp[\mathbf{Z}_i'(u)\beta]}{\sum_{i=1}^{n} \mathrm{Y}_i(u)\exp[\mathbf{Z}_i'(u)\beta]}.$$

As described in Chapter 6, the score function with respect to β_0 can be expressed as a function of martingales:

$$\tilde{U}(\beta_0, t) = \sum_{i=1}^{n} \int_0^t \{\mathbf{Z}_i(u) - \bar{\mathbf{Z}}(\beta, u)\} \mathrm{dM}_i(u), \tag{7.42}$$

where

$$\mathrm{M}_i(t) = \mathrm{N}_i(t) - \int_0^t \mathrm{Y}_i(u)\exp[\mathbf{Z}_i'(u)\beta_0]\mathrm{d}\Lambda_0(u).$$

If the N counting process satisfies the intensity model given in Equation (7.39), the $\{\mathrm{M}_1(.), \ldots, \mathrm{M}_n(.)\}$ series are martingales from the martingale central limit theorem (Andersen and Gill, 1982). The case in which the M_i series do not behave as martingales is discussed in Subsections 7.2.3 and 7.2.4.

Given that $\{\mathrm{M}_1(.), \ldots, \mathrm{M}_n(.)\}$ are martingales, the Fisher information matrix, defined as the minus second partial derivatives of the log partial likelihood function with respect to β, can be specified as

$$I(\beta, t) = \sum_{i=1}^{n} \int_0^t \{\tilde{\mathbf{Z}}(\beta, u) - \bar{\mathbf{Z}}(\beta, u)\} \mathrm{dN}_i(u), \tag{7.43}$$

where

$$\tilde{\mathbf{Z}}(\beta, u) = \frac{\sum_{i=1}^{n} \mathrm{Y}_i(u)\mathbf{Z}_i(u)^{\otimes 2}\exp[\mathbf{Z}_i'(u)\beta]}{\sum_{i=1}^{n} \mathrm{Y}_i(u)\exp[\mathbf{Z}_i'(u)\beta]}.$$

The above counting process formulas describe counts at observation times, thereby permitting multiple jumps for an individual as a step function. Consequently, this system provides a more flexible perspective to the description of repeated events than does the classical Cox model.

Andersen and Gill (1982) contend that statistically the process $\sqrt{n}\left(\hat{\beta} - \beta_0\right)$ converges to a normal vector with mean 0 and the covariance matrix $I^{-1}\left(\hat{\beta}, t\right)$ for large samples. If this inference holds, the score, the Wald, and the likelihood ratio test statistics can be readily computed given the null hypothesis that all regression coefficients be zero, with each statistic distributed asymptotically as chi-square with M degrees of freedom.

Given the estimator $\hat{\boldsymbol{\beta}}$, the integrated intensity processes can be estimated as an actual count:

$$\hat{\Lambda}(t) = \int_0^t \frac{d\bar{N}[u]}{\sum_{i=1}^{n} Y_i(u)\exp(\mathbf{Z}_i \hat{\boldsymbol{\beta}})}. \tag{7.44}$$

Clearly, in terms of repeated events, the integrated intensity is no longer a cumulative probability function, but, rather, represents a mean of cumulative counts with $\hat{\Lambda}(t)$ allowed greater than unity, as will be further discussed later.

The above specifications permit recurrences of the same event for the same individual and therefore the Andersen–Gill model provides a flexible perspective for modeling repeated events. In an estimation of the AG model, the unit of analysis is an 'event episode' instead of a 'person.' Specifically, an individual who has experienced Q events should be assigned a block of observations, rather than a single unit, with $Q + 1$ observations input to the dataset for analysis. The event time for the qth observation of an individual is defined as the time elapsed from the occurrence of the $(q - 1)$th event to the occurrence of the qth event, where $q = 1, \ldots, Q$ (for the first event $q = 1$, the event time is the regular time interval from 0 to the occurrence of the event). For the $(Q + 1$th) event, the time interval represents a censored survival time. Such a specification of risk intervals is flexible because delayed entry is allowed as long as the entry time for a specific observation is known. Another unique characteristic of the AG model is that an individual is not counted in the risk set for the qth event until he or she experiences the $(q - 1)$th event. Technically, the AG intensity rate model does not differ significantly from a standard Cox model if each repeated event is viewed as a conditionally independent episode given covariates (Therneau and Grambsch, 2000). In general, this method is applicable when a common baseline hazard for repeated events can be theoretically and statistically justified.

The Andersen–Gill model does not particularly address the potential dependence of repeated events within individuals, assuming an individual's recurrent event to be conditionally independent of earlier events in the presence of certain theoretically-based time-dependent covariates. Under certain circumstances, such specification of time-dependent covariates, like the number of prior recurrences and given interactions, can considerably mitigate intraperson correlation, especially when analyzing large-scale survey data. Therefore, the AG method provides tremendous simplicity and analytic convenience for the modeling of repeated events (Kelly and Lim, 2000).

Empirically, however, the independence hypothesis cannot be verified by means of any statistical means and hence the assumption cannot be statistically tested. On many occasions of repeated events, particularly in clinical trial settings, such dependence is not able to be ignored, and the existence of such a latent factor may not be completely accounted for by the effects of measurable covariates. Given this, the strong assumption on the conditional independence of repeated events does not always conform to the correlation of event recurrences for the same individual, even when time-dependent covariates are considered. As a consequence, statistical adjustments on the independence assumption are often found necessary.

7.2.2 PWP total time and gap time models (PWP-CP and PWP-GT)

Prentice, Williams, and Peterson (1981) develop two useful hazard models for analyzing repeated events, generally referred to as the PWP total time (PWP-CP) and the PWP gap time (PWP-GT) models. Here, the total time refers to the time interval from time origin 0 to the occurrence of each event whereas the gap time counts the time elapsed between two successive events or from the occurrence of a recurrent event to the censored time for a censored case. Therefore, the two risk intervals are equal only for the first event. Conceptually, the total time describes a complete survival process from the start of an observation period, regardless of how many earlier events have actually occurred. In contrast, the gap time depends on the occurrence of a prior event, originating from the time of the immediately preceding event. Consider, for example, an individual who has experienced the same type of event twice before eventually being censored, with the first event occurring at time 4, the second at time 9, and right censoring taking place at time 14. With the total time, the individual is at risk to the two events at time intervals (0, 4] and (0, 9], respectively, and the censored survival time is counted as 14. On the other hand, the corresponding three gap times are (0, 4], (0, 5], and (0, 5], with the last interval as the censored gap time. It follows that the gap time of a recurrent event is actually nested within the corresponding total time for later recurrences. Both models use a stratified proportional hazard approach, treating the qth event as a unique stratum.

Let $N_i(t) = \{q(s): s \leq t\}$ be the number of events for individual i at time t, corresponding to the random survival times $T_{i1} < \ldots < T_{iQ}$, and $Z_i(t)$ be the covariate vector of the individual at t. For an individual with Q repeated events before being censored, $t_0 = 0$, t_q is the qth recurrent event time for $q = 1, \ldots, Q$, and t_{Q+1} is the censored time, equivalent to the specification in the Andersen–Gill model. The so-called PWP-CP and PWP-GT models are actually based on the two time scales described above, given by

$$\lambda[t|\mathrm{N}(t), \mathbf{Z}(t)] = \lambda_{0q}(t)\exp\left[\mathbf{Z}(t)'\boldsymbol{\beta}_q\right], \tag{7.45}$$

$$\lambda[t|\mathrm{N}(t), \mathbf{Z}(t)] = \lambda_{0q}(t - t_{q-1})\exp\left[\mathbf{Z}(t)'\boldsymbol{\beta}_q\right], \tag{7.46}$$

where $\lambda_{0q}(t)$ is an arbitrary baseline intensity function for each of the intensity models on the repeated event. A primary difference between the PWP models and the conventional stratified proportional hazard model is the specification of $\boldsymbol{\beta}_q$, which represents the stratum-specific coefficient vector on the qth repeated event. Analogous to the AG model, an individual moves to stratum q immediately following the occurrence of the $(q - 1)$th recurrent event and stays there until the occurrence of the qth event or of right censoring. Both Equations (7.45) and (7.46) permit the baseline intensity functions to depend arbitrarily on previous events as well as on other characteristics associated with an individual (Prentice, Williams, and Peterson, 1981). While the total time and the gap time models look similar in certain aspects, there are important conceptual differences between these two perspectives, given different specifications of event times for a repeated event. In the PWP-CP model, the baseline intensity function depends on the total time t, even for later recurrences. On the other hand, the PWP-GT model describes an intensity process from the occurrence of an immediately preceding event, with the gap time defined as $(t - t_{q-1})$; therefore, each survival process defines a different rank order of a specific risk set on the occurrence of a repeated event. Both approaches are conditional models as an individual is not considered in the risk set for the qth event until experiencing the $(q - 1)$th event.

For each of the PWP models, the regression coefficients $\boldsymbol{\beta}_q$ can be estimated by applying the Cox partial likelihood approach. First, let $t_{q0} < t_{q1} < \cdots < t_{qd}$ be the ordered survival times in the repeated event q, where d is the total number of events and $\mathbf{Z}_{iq}(t_{iq})$ is the covariate vector. Then, the partial likelihood function is given by

$$L_p(\boldsymbol{\beta}_q) = \prod_{q \ge 1} \prod_{i=1}^{d_q} \frac{\exp\left[\mathbf{Z}'_{qi}(t_{qi})\boldsymbol{\beta}_q\right]}{\sum_{l \in \mathcal{R}(t_{qi}, q)} \exp\left[\mathbf{Z}'_l(t_{qi})\boldsymbol{\beta}_q\right]}. \tag{7.47}$$

Because $t_{q0} = 0$, the above partial likelihood is the function for the total time model, describing the complete survival process for the occurrence of a series of repeated events. As all risk intervals start at time 0, the event time does not depend on failure times of previous events in the interim.

The gap time model can be specified by adapting the above partial likelihood function. As another type of conditional perspective, stratification in the PWP-GT model is restricted in a way that an individual can contribute at most one event time in a specific stratum. Let $g_{q1} < \cdots < g_{qe_q}$ be the ordered distinct gap times from the immediately preceding failure time and e_q be the total number of failures occurring in stratum q. Then the risk set $\tilde{\mathcal{R}}(g, q)$ in the PWP-GT model is defined with specific regard to those who have experienced the $(q-1)$th event with $t_{q0} = t_{q-1}$. Given these conditions, the partial likelihood function for the gap time model is

$$L_p(\boldsymbol{\beta}_q) = \prod_{q \ge 1} \prod_{i=1}^{e_q} \frac{\exp\left[\mathbf{Z}'_{qi}(t_{qi})\boldsymbol{\beta}_q\right]}{\sum_{l \in \tilde{\mathcal{R}}(t_{qi}, q)} \exp\left[\mathbf{Z}'_l(\tilde{t}_l + g_{qi})\boldsymbol{\beta}_q\right]}, \tag{7.48}$$

where $\tilde{t}_l$ is the last failure time on individual l prior to entry into event q. Notice that in Equation (7.48), the numerator is the same as in Equation (7.47), so its difference from the total time model resides in the risk set that is reordered according to the rank of the gap time $t_{qi} - t_{q-1,i}$ instead of t.

Both of the PWP models can be formulated in terms of the conventional Cox model by redefining the risk interval and the risk set for the recurrences of a specific event. Correspondingly, differences between the total time and the gap time models simply exist in the specification of those two components. With minor modifications, therefore, the PWP-CP and PWP-GT models can be estimated by applying the standard maximization procedures and various testing statistics under the null hypothesis. Additionally, although the PWP models specify event-specific regression coefficients $\boldsymbol{\beta}_q$, the overall estimates $\hat{\boldsymbol{\beta}}$ can be obtained by fitting a single covariate vector $\mathbf{Z}$, in the same fashion as applying the stratified proportional hazard model. In Subsection 7.2.5, I illustrate how to derive both the overall and the event-specific estimates in the PWP models.

The data for estimating the PWP models need to be specially structured for defining the correct risk sets. With respect to the total time model, the data structure is the same as the AG model: an individual with $\mathcal{Q}$ events should be assigned a $(\mathcal{Q}+1) \times 1$ block that contains $(\mathcal{Q}+1)$ observations, with the $(\mathcal{Q}+1)$th observation being a censored case. Here, in addition to the specification of the censoring status variable δ_{iq}, a stratum variable needs to be specified to indicate the rank of the qth interval. For example, for an individual who has experienced two events within a given observation interval, three separate observations should be assigned: $q = 1$, $\delta_1 = 1$ for the first observation, $q = 2$, $\delta_2 = 1$ for the second, and $q = 3$, $\delta_3 = 0$ for the censored observation. Such a specification also applies to the gap time model, except for the definition of a different risk interval. If the risk sets for some later recurrences are extremely small (below 10, say), a maximum number of repeated events needs to be arbitrarily decided for performing an efficient analysis.

Like the Andersen–Gill approach, the PWP models are based on the assumption that recurrent events are conditionally independent given time-dependent covariates. Therefore, the original PWP models are based on the assumption that the joint process $\sqrt{n}\tilde{\boldsymbol{U}}_1(\boldsymbol{\beta}_1, \infty), \ldots, \sqrt{n}\tilde{\boldsymbol{U}}_Q(\boldsymbol{\beta}_Q, \infty)$ can be derived directly from the martingale central limit theorem as local square-integrable martingales. Given this assumption, the inverse of the observed information matrix is used as the valid variance–covariance estimator of the estimated regression coefficients. This strong hypothesis is questionable on many occasions because the effect of dependence cannot always be explained by the effects of observable covariates, thus yielding bias in variance estimates. This type of bias is particular likely in the PWP total time model because it intensifies the intraperson correlation by including gap times of prior events in the risk interval of a later recurrence (Kelly and Lim, 2000). For example, the total time for the third repeated event consists of survival times for both the first and second events and therefore is left truncated. Statistical adjustments are necessary for deriving a robust variance estimator, particularly when an event type recurs frequently and the sample size is small.

7.2.3 The WLW model and extensions

Wei, Lin, and Weissfeld (1989) developed a Cox-type model for repeated events from a different direction, referred to as the WLW model in survival analysis. This approach is based on the underlying assumption that an individual is at risk to all Q events from the beginning of a specific observation period. Given this hypothesis, the WLW model follows a marginal regression perspective applied in longitudinal data analysis, which follows each interval-specific survival process regardless of how many previous events have been experienced for an individual. Consequently, WLW assigns Q strata to each individual, even though many have not experienced any later recurrences yet. The case in the qth risk set without experiencing the $(q-1)$th event is called the *dummy observation*.

Given the marginal design of repeated events, the intensity process for individual i with event q is

$$\lambda_{iq}(t; \boldsymbol{\beta}_q, \mathbf{Z}_{iq}) = Y_{iq}\lambda_{0q}(t)\exp\left[\mathbf{Z}_i'(t)\boldsymbol{\beta}_q\right], \tag{7.49}$$

where $\lambda_{0q}(t)$ is the event-specific baseline intensity function for the qth event and $\boldsymbol{\beta}_q$ is the event-specific vector of regression coefficients.

Given recurrent events data structured in the format of the stratified proportional hazard model, WLW proposes to estimate each event-specific set of regression coefficients, denoted by $\{\boldsymbol{\beta}_1, \ldots, \boldsymbol{\beta}_Q\}$, by maximizing the event-specific partial likelihoods separately. The estimates, represented by $\left\{\hat{\boldsymbol{\beta}}_1, \ldots, \hat{\boldsymbol{\beta}}_Q\right\}$, can be combined to derive an 'average effect' estimator with the smallest asymptotic variance among all linear estimators. While generally dependent given the intraperson correlation, the estimators $\left\{\hat{\boldsymbol{\beta}}_1', \ldots, \hat{\boldsymbol{\beta}}_Q'\right\}$ are considered asymptotically jointly normal with a covariance matrix that can be consistently estimated without assuming a specific correlation structure.

According to WLW, the point estimates of regression coefficients from the Andersen–Gill approach are unbiased, even with strong dependence of failure times. The joint distribution of scores $\sqrt{n}\tilde{\boldsymbol{U}}_1(\boldsymbol{\beta}_1, \infty), \ldots, \sqrt{n}\tilde{\boldsymbol{U}}_q(\boldsymbol{\beta}_q, \infty)$, however, cannot be statistically derived from the martingale central limit theorem for local square-integrable martingales if strong correlation among failure times exists. Because of the predictable covariation process $\langle \mathrm{M}_q, \mathrm{M}_{q'} \rangle \neq 0$ in the presence of intraperson correlation, the martingale central limit theorem does not apply to the series $\{\mathrm{M}_1, \ldots, \mathrm{M}_Q\}$, so the inverse of the observed information matrix $\hat{\boldsymbol{I}}^{-1}(\hat{\boldsymbol{\beta}})$ does not provide an adequate variance estimator of $\hat{\boldsymbol{\beta}}$. Thus, a robust covariance matrix for $\hat{\boldsymbol{\beta}}$ needs to be developed to account for covariance in $\sqrt{n}\tilde{\boldsymbol{U}}_1(\boldsymbol{\beta}_1, \infty), \ldots, \sqrt{n}\tilde{\boldsymbol{U}}_q(\boldsymbol{\beta}_q, \infty)$, thereby satisfying the condition $\sqrt{n}\tilde{\boldsymbol{U}}_q(\boldsymbol{\beta}_q, \infty) \to N[0, \boldsymbol{V}(\boldsymbol{\beta}_q)]$ where $q = 1, \ldots, Q$. Given these concerns, WLW has developed the celebrated robust sandwich variance estimator for addressing intraperson dependence in survival data.

The robust sandwich variance method does not specify the pattern of dependence among correlated failure times; rather, it constructs a robust variance–covariance estimator to account for the intraperson correlation, in the same way as applied by Zeger, Liang, and Albert (1988) in analyzing longitudinal data. Specifically, the asymptotic covariance matrix of an event-specific score statistic is

$$\hat{\boldsymbol{\Sigma}}(\hat{\boldsymbol{\beta}}) = n^{-1} \sum_{i=1}^{n} \tilde{\boldsymbol{U}}_i(\hat{\boldsymbol{\beta}}) \tilde{\boldsymbol{U}}_i(\hat{\boldsymbol{\beta}})', \tag{7.50}$$

where $\hat{\boldsymbol{\Sigma}}$ is the score statistic variance–covariance estimator and $\tilde{\boldsymbol{U}}_i(\boldsymbol{\beta})$ consists of $\{\tilde{\boldsymbol{U}}_{i1}(\boldsymbol{\beta}), \ldots, \tilde{\boldsymbol{U}}_{iQ}(\boldsymbol{\beta})\}$, given by

$$\begin{aligned}\tilde{\boldsymbol{U}}_i(\hat{\boldsymbol{\beta}}) = \delta_i[\mathbf{Z}_i(T_i) - \bar{\mathbf{Z}}(\boldsymbol{\beta}, T_i)] - \sum_{l=1}^{n} \delta_l \frac{\mathrm{Y}_i(T_l)\exp[\mathbf{Z}_i'(T_l)\boldsymbol{\beta}]}{\sum_{l=1}^{n} \mathrm{Y}_l(T_l)\exp[\mathbf{Z}_l'(T_l)\boldsymbol{\beta}]} \\ \times [\mathbf{Z}_i(T_l) - \bar{\mathbf{Z}}(\boldsymbol{\beta}, T_l)].\end{aligned}$$

Then the asymptotic covariance matrix of the estimated regression coefficient is

$$\hat{\boldsymbol{V}}(\hat{\boldsymbol{\beta}}) = \hat{\boldsymbol{I}}^{-1}(\hat{\boldsymbol{\beta}}) \hat{\boldsymbol{\Sigma}}(\hat{\boldsymbol{\beta}}) \hat{\boldsymbol{I}}^{-1}(\hat{\boldsymbol{\beta}}). \tag{7.51}$$

Equation (7.51) is the so-called 'sandwich' variance estimator. As a result of such an adjustment on the dependence of failure times, the random vector $n^{1/2}(\hat{\boldsymbol{\beta}} - \boldsymbol{\beta}^*)$ is asymptotically normal with mean 0 and a covariance matrix that can be estimated by $\hat{\boldsymbol{V}}(\hat{\boldsymbol{\beta}})$ (Lin and Wei, 1989), from which the valid Wald score can be derived for testing the null hypothesis. As both $\hat{\boldsymbol{\beta}}$ and $\boldsymbol{I}(\hat{\boldsymbol{\beta}})$ can be obtained from the standard Cox model, this robust variance estimator does not involve additional statistical inference as long as the underlying risk strata can be identified.

For complex survey designs, a weighted version of the above sandwich estimator needs to be applied. Binder (1992) proposes a straightforward approach to adjust for the original WLW estimator with respect to a complex sampling design. Specifically, weights are incorporated into the robust sandwich variance estimator, given by

$$\hat{V}_w\left(\hat{\boldsymbol{\beta}}\right) = \hat{\boldsymbol{I}}^{-1}\left(\hat{\boldsymbol{\beta}}\right)\left[\sum_{i=1}^{n} w_i^2 \tilde{\boldsymbol{U}}_{iw}\left(\hat{\boldsymbol{\beta}}\right)\tilde{\boldsymbol{U}}_{iw}\left(\hat{\boldsymbol{\beta}}\right)'\right]\hat{\boldsymbol{I}}^{-1}\left(\hat{\boldsymbol{\beta}}\right), \tag{7.52}$$

where w_i is the weight for individual i and

$$\tilde{\boldsymbol{U}}_{iw}\left(\hat{\boldsymbol{\beta}}\right) = \delta_i[\mathbf{Z}_i(T_i) - \bar{\mathbf{Z}}(\boldsymbol{\beta}, T_i)] - \sum_{l=1}^{n} \delta_l \frac{w_l \mathrm{Y}_i(T_l)\exp[\mathbf{Z}_i'(T_l)\boldsymbol{\beta}]}{\sum_{l=1}^{n} \mathrm{Y}_l(T_l)\exp[\mathbf{Z}_l'(T_l)\boldsymbol{\beta}]} \times [\mathbf{Z}_i(T_l) - \bar{\mathbf{Z}}(\boldsymbol{\beta}, T_l)].$$

As a marginal approach, the WLW model estimates the regression coefficients for each event-specific survival process, with one Cox model associated with a separate set of parameters. Each individual is assigned to an equal number of observations no matter how many actual events he or she has experienced. In the presence of an exceptionally high number of repeated events for a sample of individuals, a maximum number of events should be arbitrarily determined for an efficient analysis. For example, if the highest number of repeated events is 10 but only a small portion of individuals have experienced more than five recurrences, setting the maximum number of events at five would be appropriate.

Like the PWP models, the WLW model can be used to estimate both the overall and the event-specific regression coefficients. While the overall estimates $\hat{\boldsymbol{\beta}}$ can be acquired by fitting the single covariate vector $\mathbf{Z}$, the event-specific estimates $\hat{\boldsymbol{\beta}}_q$ are obtained by fitting the model and specifying $\mathbf{Z}_i = (\mathbf{Z}_{i1}, 0, \ldots, 0)'$, $\mathbf{Z}_i = (0, \mathbf{Z}_{i2}, \ldots, 0)'$, $\ldots$, $\mathbf{Z}_i = (0, \ldots, 0, \mathbf{Z}_{iQ})'$, for $q = 1, 2, \ldots, Q$, respectively. The detailed techniques for estimating both the overall and event-specific estimates are illustrated in Subsection 7.2.5.

Given its strong assumption on marginal distributions of repeated events, the WLW model has inevitably encountered some critiques. Although statistically estimable and commonly applied, this method is sometimes considered not to be realistic, thereby causing difficulty in interpreting the results (Kalbfleisch and Prentice, 2002; Kelly and Lim, 2000; Therneau and Grambsch, 2000). It is hard to interpret, for example, how an individual who has experienced just one event can be at risk for the fourth repeated event at time 0. One explanation for the marginal approach is that the assignment of an equal number of observations to all individuals agrees with the working hypothesis on the independence of the repeated events, as applied in longitudinal data analysis. Nevertheless, modeling a time-to-event process differs markedly from modeling the discrete panel data as the length of survival time needs to be taken into account. By including dummy observations in the risk set, there potentially exists a carryover effect of covariates on later recurrences of a repeatable event. This is because the chance of being a dummy observation may be associated with one or more covariates that predict both the intensity rate and the timing of a repeated event. Consequently, the event-specific and common regression coefficients in the WLW model are often found to be severely overestimated (Kalbfleisch and Prentice, 2002; Kelly and Lim, 2000; Therneau and Grambsch, 2000). Additionally, an individual without experiencing the $(q-1)$th event is already known to have a survival rate of one for the occurrence of the qth event within an observation period, so that this person's qth repeated event is left truncated throughout the entire risk interval. Conceptually, the conditional perspective, as specified by the AG and the

PWP models, seems empirically more feasible by excluding all dummy observations from statistical inference. If the Andersen–Gill model is appropriately specified, correlation among failure times can be much mitigated, thereby leading to the condition $\hat{V}(\hat{\beta}) \approx \hat{I}^{-1}(\hat{\beta})$. In such conditions, the use of the sandwich estimator becomes unnecessary.

In spite of the aforementioned arguments, the WLW sandwich variance estimator is widely considered to be highly valuable for deriving a robust variance–covariance matrix in analyzing various types of clustered data (Kalbfleisch and Prentice, 2002; Therneau and Grambsch, 2000). This approach is further discussed in the next subsection and in Chapter 9.

7.2.4 Proportional rate and mean functions of repeated events

The Andersen and Gill model permits repeated events of the same type for an individual by specifying time-dependent variables to reflect the prior history of survival, censoring, and covariates, as formulated by Equation (7.39). Because the dependence of repeated events may not necessarily be entirely reflected by such covariates on many occasions, some statisticians suggest replacing the basic AG model with a more flexible rate function (Lawless and Nadeau, 1995; Lin *et al.*, 2000; Pepe and Cai, 1993).

Specifically, the factor $E\{dN(t)|\mathcal{F}_{t-}\}$ in Equation (7.39) can be more flexibly denoted by $d\mu_Z(t)$, with the equation modified as

$$d\mu_Z(t) = d\mu_0(t)\exp[\mathbf{Z}'(t)\boldsymbol{\beta}_0], \tag{7.53}$$

where $\mu_0(t)$ is an unknown continuous function over t and $\boldsymbol{\beta}_0$ is an $M \times 1$ vector of regression coefficients. The covariate vector $Z(t)$ is defined as consisting of one or more time-dependent variables. Equation (7.53) is called the *proportional rates model*. This rate function is considered more adaptable than Equation (7.39) because it allows arbitrary dependence structures among recurrent events (Lin *et al.*, 2000).

Integrating the rates up to t gives rise to the following cumulative function:

$$\mu_Z(t) = \int_0^t d\mu_0(u)\exp[\mathbf{Z}'(u)\boldsymbol{\beta}_0]. \tag{7.54}$$

Given event repetitions, Equation (7.54) is not conventionally called the 'cumulative hazard' function because the integration of intensity rates from 0 to t is not a cumulative probability function, but it represents a mean function of cumulative counts, with $\mu_z(t)$ allowed to be greater than unity, as indicated in Subsection 7.2.1.

If the vector $\mathbf{Z}$ only contains time-independent covariates, Equation (7.54) reduces to

$$\mu_Z(t) = \mu_0(t)\exp[\mathbf{Z}'(u)\boldsymbol{\beta}_0], \tag{7.55}$$

where the baseline mean function can be expressed as a Nelson–Aalen estimator:

$$\hat{\mu}_0(t) = \int_0^t \frac{d\bar{N}_i(u)}{\sum_{i=1}^{n} Y_i(u)\exp\left[\mathbf{Z}'(u)\hat{\boldsymbol{\beta}}\right]}. \tag{7.56}$$

Equation (7.55) is referred to as the *proportional means model*, given the nature of the outcome variable. The function $\mu_0(t)$ can be understood as the expected number of failures up to time t when all covariates are scaled zero. If **Z** contains covariates centered at the covariate means, $\mu_0(t)$ is the expectation of the mean for a specific population. Correspondingly, $\mu_Z(t)$ is the expectation of the overall intensity rate over the first and the recurrent events, given values of the covariate vector in Z. Because of its cumulative nature, some researchers simply express $\mu_0(t)$ as $\Lambda_0(t)$ and $\mu_Z(t)$ as $\Lambda_Z(t)$ (Kalbfleisch and Prentice, 2002).

A number of statisticians have contributed to statistical inferences and the development of estimating procedures on the proportional rates and mean models. In particular, Pepe and Cai (1993) suggest that the first and recurrent events should be analyzed separately based on the large sample theory, whereas Lawless and Nadeau (1995) propose some Cox-type procedures for discrete failure times, which, theoretically, can be adapted into continuous time processes. More recently, Lin *et al.* (2000) and Nelson (2002) provide refined continuous event time models on the rates and means functions using the counting process formulation. In this text, I focus on the description of the continuous time approaches, given their high applicability.

Given Equation (7.55), the series $\{M_1(t), \ldots, M_n(t)\}$ can be written as

$$dM_i(t) = dN_i(t) - Y_i(t)\exp[\mathbf{Z}_i'(t)\boldsymbol{\beta}_0]d\Lambda_0(t). \tag{7.57}$$

Under Equation (7.55), the $dM_i(t)$ series has expectation 0 at all values of t; therefore unbiased point estimates of $\boldsymbol{\beta}$ can be obtained by developing a score function represented by Equation (7.42). Given violation of the condition $\operatorname{cov}\left(\hat{M}_i, \hat{M}_{i'}\right) = 0$ due to correlation of repeated failure times, however, $\{M_1(\cdot), \ldots, M_n(\cdot)\}$ are not local martingales, so the martingale central limit theorem does not apply. Yet, the asymptotic covariance matrix of the estimated regression coefficients $\hat{\boldsymbol{\beta}}$ can be approximated by using the aforementioned 'sandwich' variance estimator, given by

$$\hat{\boldsymbol{I}}^{-1}\left(\hat{\boldsymbol{\beta}}\right)\sum_{i=1}^{n}\left[\tilde{\boldsymbol{U}}_i\left(\hat{\boldsymbol{\beta}}\right)\tilde{\boldsymbol{U}}_i'\left(\hat{\boldsymbol{\beta}}\right)\right]\hat{\boldsymbol{I}}^{-1}\left(\hat{\boldsymbol{\beta}}\right), \tag{7.58}$$

where

$$\tilde{\boldsymbol{U}}_i(\boldsymbol{\beta}) = \sum_{Q}\delta_{iq}\left[\mathbf{Z}_i(T_{iq}) - \bar{\mathbf{Z}}(\boldsymbol{\beta}, T_{iq})\right] - \sum_{l=1}^{n}\sum_{r}\delta_{lr}\frac{Y_i(T_{lr})\exp[\mathbf{Z}_i'(T_{lr})\boldsymbol{\beta}]}{\sum_{l=1}^{n}Y_l(T_{lr})\exp[\mathbf{Z}_l'(T_{lr})\boldsymbol{\beta}]}$$
$$\times[\mathbf{Z}_i(T_{lr}) - \bar{\mathbf{Z}}(\boldsymbol{\beta}, T_{lr})].$$

Statistically, the specification of the sandwich estimator leads to an asymptotic normal distribution with zero expectation for $\sqrt{n}\left(\hat{\boldsymbol{\beta}} - \boldsymbol{\beta}\right)$ that satisfies $\sqrt{n}\tilde{\boldsymbol{U}}(\boldsymbol{\beta}, \infty) \rightarrow N[0, \boldsymbol{V}(\boldsymbol{\beta})]$, as mentioned previously.

If all covariates are external, $\mu_0(t)$ is the *mean function* when $\mathbf{Z} = \mathbf{0}$. Therefore, given the proportionality assumption, the mean function given a specific covariate vector $\boldsymbol{\Xi}$ can be readily estimated by using Equation (7.56), with $\boldsymbol{\Xi}$ replacing **Z**:

$$\hat{\mu}_{\Xi}(t) = \left[\sum_{i=1}^{n} \sum_{q} \frac{\delta_{iq}}{\sum_{i=1}^{n} Y_{iq}(T_{iq}) \exp\left[\mathbf{Z}'(T_{iq})\hat{\boldsymbol{\beta}}\right]} \right] \exp(\Xi'\boldsymbol{\beta}). \tag{7.59}$$

According to the multivariate central limit theorem, $V(t) \equiv \sqrt{n}\,[\hat{\mu}_{\Xi}(t) - \mu_0(t)]$ converges weakly to a zero-mean Gaussian process with covariance function $\zeta(s, t)$, given by

$$\hat{\zeta}(s,t) \equiv \sqrt{n} \sum_{i=1}^{n} \hat{\boldsymbol{\Psi}}_i(s)\hat{\boldsymbol{\Psi}}_i(t), \tag{7.60}$$

where

$$\boldsymbol{\Psi}_i(t) = \int_0^t \frac{d\hat{M}_i(u)}{\sum_{i=1}^{n} Y_i(u)\exp\left[\mathbf{Z}_i'\hat{\boldsymbol{\beta}}\right]} - H'\left(\hat{\boldsymbol{\beta}}, t\right)\hat{\boldsymbol{I}}_{\Xi}^{-1}$$
$$\int_0^{\tau} \Xi\left(\hat{\boldsymbol{\beta}}, u\right)\left[\mathbf{Z}_i(u) - \bar{\mathbf{Z}}\left(\hat{\boldsymbol{\beta}}, u\right)\right] d\hat{M}_i(u),$$

$$H(\boldsymbol{\beta}, t) = \int_0^t \frac{\bar{\mathbf{Z}}(\boldsymbol{\beta}, u)}{\sum_{i=1}^{n} Y_i(u)\exp\left[\mathbf{Z}'\boldsymbol{\beta}\right]} d\bar{N}(u),$$

and τ is the endpoint of a finite observation interval $[0, \tau]$. Additionally, $\hat{\boldsymbol{I}}_{\Xi}$ is equivalent to the observed information matrix $\hat{\boldsymbol{I}}$ associated with covariate vector Ξ. Then, the variance of the mean function $\hat{\mu}_{\Xi}(t)$ is given by

$$\hat{V}[\hat{\mu}_{\Xi}(t)] = \sum_{i=1}^{n} \left[\frac{1}{n} \hat{\boldsymbol{\Psi}}_i(\Xi, t) \right]. \tag{7.61}$$

The square root of this variance estimator yields an estimate of the standard error for the cumulative mean function $\hat{\mu}_{\Xi}(t)$. Nelson (2002) provides a useful estimator, not presented here, for calculating $\hat{\boldsymbol{\Psi}}_i(t)$ and the variance of $\hat{\mu}_{\Xi}(t)$.

Given the above estimators, the confidence interval for $\hat{\mu}_{\Xi}(t)$ can be calculated. As the cumulative mean function is nonnegative, the calculation is based on the log transformation:

$$\hat{\mu}_{\Xi}(t)\exp\left\{ \pm z_{\alpha/2} \frac{\sqrt{\hat{V}[\hat{\mu}_{\Xi}(t)]}}{\hat{\mu}_{\Xi}(t)} \right\}. \tag{7.62}$$

As it is more useful to evaluate the confidence limits of $\hat{\mu}_{\Xi}(t)$ with respect to the entire region of the process, Lin *et al.* (2000) develop an estimator, not presented in this book, for an approximate $1 - \alpha$ simultaneous confidence bands for all $\hat{\mu}_{\Xi}(t)$ over the time interval $[t_1, t_2]$.

The data structure for analyzing the proportional rates/means model is the same as for the Andersen–Gill method. Analytically, however, the rates or the cumulative mean model uses the sandwich estimator for the covariance matrix estimate, whereas the AG model is based on the inverse of the observed information matrix assuming conditional independence of failure times. As a result, these two models yield exactly the same point estimates of the intensity function, given fixed covariates, but generate different standard errors on most occasions.

7.2.5 Illustration: The effects of a medical treatment on repeated patient visits

This illustration is based on a partly empirical and partly simulated patient dataset for a sample of 255 persons originally diagnosed with PTSD (Posttraumatic Stress Disorder). After diagnosis, those patients were cared for either by a new medical treatment or by a conventional, evidence-based psychotherapy. A patient would pay additional visits to the psychiatrist for further treatment if PTSD symptoms lingered; therefore the frequency of repeated visits and the timing of a recurrent check-in predict the effects of the new medical treatment on the severity of PTSD. In this example, I want to test the null hypothesis that the new treatment does not affect the rate and the number of recurrent visits as compared to the conventional psychotherapy. In this patient data, 116 patients are randomized to receive the new treatment and the remaining 139 persons are in the conventional psychotherapy group. In the data analysis, treatment is a dichotomous variable, named 'Trt,' with 1 = new medical treatment, 0 = conventional psychotherapy. Although the maximum number of visits in the dataset is seven, only a small proportion of those patients have repeated visits beyond the fifth recurrence; therefore, the first four potential repeated visits for each patient are considered in the analysis. Each recurrent time, T1, T2, T3, and T4, is measured from the patient's entry time to the occurrence of the repeated event or to the censored time. A variable 'Count' is created to enumerate the total number of recurrent visits for each patient. Additionally, a variable 'Followup' indicates the endpoint of observation for a patient, defined as the time interval from the entry time to the ending time of observation. For those having more than four visits, the follow-up time is the fifth recurrent time T5. A patient's age and sex are used as the control variables. Appendix C displays this dataset with ten variables.

Given the data of recurrent visits, various survival models on repeated events can be estimated, analyzed, and compared. Given the importance of analyzing repeated events in many disciplines, this illustration applies all of the aforementioned methods and therefore this subsection is lengthy.

There are different ways of programming those repeated events models in SAS. To help the reader learn the standard SAS syntax, I basically follow the programming approach shown in SAS/STAT Example 64.10 in Version 9.2 with contextual modifications. Some researchers use different SAS statements and functions for modeling repeated events that are equally valuable and effective. Therneau and Grambsch (2000), for example, apply some different SAS schemes that supposedly derive exactly the same analytic results.

I begin with estimating the Andersen–Gill intensity rate model on the PTSD patient data, presented in Appendix C, with the following SAS program.

SAS Program 7.3:

```
......

data new1;
  set pclib.chapter7_data;

proc SQL;
  create table new1 as
  select *, age-mean(age) as age_mean,
    sex-mean(sex) as sex_mean
  from new1;
quit;

data PTSD;
  set new1;

  keep ID Visit Status TStart TStop Trt Age_mean Sex_mean;
  retain ID TStart 0;
  array tt T1-T4;

  ID + 1;
  TStart = 0;
  do over tt;
  Visit = _i_;
  if tt = . then do;
    TStop = Followup;
        Status = 0;
  end;
  else do;
    TStop = tt;
        Status = 1;
  end;
  output;
    TStart = TStop;
  end;
  if (TStart < Followup) then delete;
run;

title 'Andersen-Gill Intensity Model';
proc phreg data = PTSD covm;
  model (TStart, TStop) * Status(0) = Trt age_mean sex_mean;
  id id;
  where TStart < TStop;
run;
```

SAS Program 7.3 creates a temporary dataset PTSD for estimating the AG model given a specific data structure. First, the SAS PROC SQL procedure creates two centered covariates as control variables – Age_mean and Sex_mean – and then they are saved into the temporary SAS data file for further analysis. Next, through the SAS programming statements and functions, each patient is assigned four observations, one for each potential recurrence, regardless of how many repeated events have actually occurred. From the original data presented in Appendix C, this SAS program creates several additional variables, including the patient's ID, Visit (the order number of the qth repeated visit), Status (1 = event recurrence, 0 = censored), TStart (time of the immediately preceding event for Count > 1, or 0 if Count = 1, or the follow-up time if the immediately preceding event does not occur), and TStop (time of recurrence if Status = 1 or the follow-up time if Status = 0).

Table 7.1 Observations of the first three patients in the temporary dataset PTSD.

	Trt	Age mean	Sex mean	ID	Tstart	Visit	TStop	Status
1	0	9.537254902	−0.180392157	1	0	1	37	1
2	0	9.537254902	−0.180392157	1	37	2	62	1
3	0	9.537254902	−0.180392157	1	62	3	92	1
4	0	9.537254902	−0.180392157	1	92	4	92	0
5	0	−2.462745098	−0.180392157	2	0	1	54	1
6	0	−2.462745098	−0.180392157	2	54	2	114	1
7	0	−2.462745098	−0.180392157	2	114	3	114	0
8	0	−2.462745098	−0.180392157	2	114	4	114	0
9	0	3.537254902	−0.180392157	3	0	1	0	0
10	0	3.537254902	−0.180392157	3	0	2	0	0
11	0	3.537254902	−0.180392157	3	0	3	0	0
12	0	3.537254902	−0.180392157	3	0	4	0	0

The first three patients in the temporary dataset PTSD are displayed in Table 7.1 in order to help the reader become familiar with the data structure used for estimating the AG model. Table 7.1 displays four observations for each of the first three patients. As the data are sorted by Trt, all three patients are in the conventional psychotherapy group (Trt = 0). For the first person, the variable Status is 1 for the first three observations, indicating that this person has three repeated visits for additional PTSD treatments. The values of Visit, TStart, TStop, and Status for this person are therefore (1, 0, 37, 1), (2, 37, 62, 1), (3, 62, 92, 1), and (4, 92, 92, 1), respectively. As mentioned earlier, (TStop − TStart) defines the time interval for repeated events in the AG model; hence TStop of the immediately preceding event is the TStart of the current risk interval if the preceding event occurs. The Status variable for the second patient, ID = 2, is 1 for the first two observations and 0 for the other two. Therefore, the second patient has two repeated visits, with values of Visit, TStart, TStop, and Status given by (1, 0, 54, 1), (2, 54, 114, 1), (3, 114, 114, 0), and (4, 114, 114, 0), respectively. For the third patient (ID = 3), the value of Status is 0 for each of the four observations, suggesting that this patient has no repeated visits. In the AG model, only the first observation for the third patient is considered in statistical analysis, whereas the first patient has all four and the second patient has three observations to be taken into account.

In the PROC PHREG statement, the COVM option is specified for use of the conventional covariance estimator (the inverse of the observed information matrix), which is in line with the basic specification of the AG model. In the model statement, the counting process formulation is specified: the pair of TStart and TStop is enclosed in parentheses to define an event-specific interval during which the patient is at risk. The value of Status specifies whether TStop is an event time or a censored time. The ID statement specifies the variable for identifying each observation in the input data. Additionally, the WHERE START < TSTOP option deletes potential misspecified cases. The output file of the above SAS program is presented below.

SAS Program Output 7.3:

```
                    Andersen-Gill Intensity Model

                         The PHREG Procedure

                          Model Information

                Data Set                  WORK.PTSD
                Dependent Variable        TStart
                Dependent Variable        TStop
                Censoring Variable        Status
                Censoring Value(s)        0
                Ties Handling             BRESLOW


             Number of Observations Read          430
             Number of Observations Used          430

        Summary of the Number of Event and Censored Values

                                                    Percent
                Total      Event    Censored       Censored

                  430        382          48          11.16


                          Convergence Status

            Convergence criterion (GCONV=1E-8) satisfied.


                        Model Fit Statistics

                                Without           With
             Criterion        Covariates      Covariates

             -2 LOG L           3158.811        3140.887
             AIC                3158.811        3146.887
             SBC                3158.811        3158.724


             Testing Global Null Hypothesis: BETA=0

     Test                 Chi-Square       DF     Pr > ChiSq

     Likelihood Ratio        17.9234        3         0.0005
     Score                   18.5589        3         0.0003
     Wald                    18.3265        3         0.0004
```

Analysis of Maximum Likelihood Estimates

Parameter	DF	Parameter Estimate	Standard Error	Chi-Square	Pr > ChiSq	Hazard Ratio
Trt	1	-0.45518	0.11316	16.1808	<.0001	0.634
age_mean	1	-0.00959	0.00667	2.0676	0.1505	0.990
sex_mean	1	-0.01995	0.13825	0.0208	0.8853	0.980

In SAS Program Output 7.3, the information on the dataset, the dependent variable, the censoring status variable, and the censoring value is reported first. All three tests in the 'Testing Global Null Hypothesis: BETA = 0' section demonstrate that the null hypothesis $\hat{\boldsymbol{\beta}} = \mathbf{0}$ should be rejected.

In the table of 'Analysis of Maximum Likelihood Estimates,' the regression coefficient of 'Trt' is –0.4552 ($SE = 0.1132$), very strongly statistically significant ($\chi^2 = 16.1808$; $p < 0.0001$). The hazard ratio of Trt is 0.634, suggesting that the intensity rate of having a repeated visit is about 37% lower among those receiving the new medical treatment than in the conventional psychotherapy group, other covariates being equal. The regression coefficients of the two control variables are not statistically significant. As indicated earlier, the standard error of Trt estimated for the AG model may be biased due to the use of the conventional variance estimator.

Next, I fit the PWP conditional models, using both total time and gap time. The following SAS program fits the PWP-CP model with event-specific effects.

SAS Program 7.4:

```
......

data PTSD2(drop=LastStatus);
  retain LastStatus;
  set PTSD;
  by ID;
  if first.id then LastStatus = 1;
  if (Status = 0 and LastStatus = 0) then delete;
  LastStatus = Status;
  Gaptime = TStop - TStart;
run;

title 'PWP Total Time Model with Event-specific Effects';
proc phreg data = PTSD2 covm;
  model (TStart, TStop) * Status(0) = Trt1-Trt4 Age_mean1-Age_mean4
                         Sex_mean1-Sex_mean4;
  Trt1 = Trt * (Visit = 1);
  Trt2 = Trt * (Visit = 2);
  Trt3 = Trt * (Visit = 3);
  Trt4 = Trt * (Visit = 4);
  Age_mean1 = Age_mean * (Visit = 1);
  Age_mean2 = Age_mean * (Visit = 2);
  Age_mean3 = Age_mean * (Visit = 3);
```

```
  Age_mean4 = Age_mean * (Visit = 4);
  Sex_mean1 = Sex_mean * (Visit = 1);
  Sex_mean2 = Sex_mean * (Visit = 2);
  Sex_mean3 = Sex_mean * (Visit = 3);
  Sex_mean4 = Sex_mean * (Visit = 4);
  strata Visit;
run;
```

As indicated earlier, the PWP conditional models do not consider individuals who have not experienced the $(q - 1)$th event in the analysis of the qth repeated event. Therefore, given the above SAS program, the data structure for fitting the PWP-CP model differs markedly from the counting process style. As a result, the repeated events data for the first three patients converts to the format shown in Table 7.2, where only the first patient who has three repeated visits has all four observations in the temporary dataset PTSD2, with the last observation being a censored case. The second patient has two repeated events, so this person is a censored observation for the third recurrence and the fourth observation is excluded from the dataset. Patient 3 has no repeated visits at all, and therefore this person only has one censored observation. The last column presents the gap time for each repeated visit.

The PROC PHREG procedure in SAS Program 7.4 specifies the PWP total time model. The variables Trt1 to Trt4 are created for Trt at each repeated visit, so the visit-specific effects can be estimated. Likewise, Age_mean1 to Age_mean4 and Sex_mean1 to Sex_mean4 are the same type of variables serving as visit-specific controls. The COVM option is specified for fitting a typical PWP model using the conventional, or naïve, variance estimator. The STRATA VISIT statement tells SAS that a Cox model is fitted on each repeated visit. The estimated regression coefficients are displayed in SAS Program Output 7.4.

Table 7.2 Observations of the first three patients in the temporary dataset PTSD2.

	Trt	Age mean	Sex mean	ID	TStart	Visit	TStop	Status	Gap
1	0	9.537 254 902	−0.180 392 157	1	0	1	37	1	37
2	0	9.537 254 902	−0.180 392 157	1	37	2	62	1	25
3	0	9.537 254 902	−0.180 392 157	1	62	3	92	1	30
4	0	9.537 254 902	−0.180 392 157	1	92	4	92	0	0
5	0	−2.462 745 098	−0.180 392 157	2	0	1	54	1	54
6	0	−2.462 745 098	−0.180 392 157	2	54	2	114	1	60
7	0	−2.462 745 098	−0.180 392 157	2	114	3	114	0	0
8	0	3.537 254 902	−0.180 392 157	3	0	1	0	0	0

SAS Program Output 7.4:

```
                PWP Total Time Model with Event-specific Effects

                   Analysis of Maximum Likelihood Estimates
```

Parameter	DF	Parameter Estimate	Standard Error	Chi-Square	Pr > ChiSq	Hazard Ratio
Trt1	1	-0.57242	0.17840	10.2954	0.0013	0.564
Trt2	1	-0.17296	0.22876	0.5717	0.4496	0.841
Trt3	1	-0.04893	0.29346	0.0278	0.8676	0.952
Trt4	1	-0.14285	0.35871	0.1586	0.6905	0.867
Age_mean1	1	-0.00177	0.01043	0.0288	0.8653	0.998
Age_mean2	1	-0.02574	0.01337	3.7062	0.0542	0.975
Age_mean3	1	-0.02169	0.01601	1.8371	0.1753	0.979
Age_mean4	1	-0.01179	0.01816	0.4212	0.5163	0.988
Sex_mean1	1	0.03397	0.22143	0.0235	0.8781	1.035
Sex_mean2	1	0.25076	0.25723	0.9503	0.3296	1.285
Sex_mean3	1	0.01853	0.37138	0.0025	0.9602	1.019
Sex_mean4	1	0.15856	0.43934	0.1302	0.7182	1.172

The above table shows that the new treatment has a statistically significant impact on the first repeated visit, with an estimated regression coefficient of −0.5724 ($\chi^2 = 10.2954$; $p = 0.0013$). The hazard ratio of Trt1 is 0.564, suggesting that the patients receiving the new treatment are about half as likely to pay the first repeated visit as those cared for by the conventional psychotherapy. For the subsequent repeated visits, however, the estimated regression coefficients of the new treatment are not statistically significant.

The SAS program for the PWP gap time model is provided below.

SAS Program 7.5:

```
......
title 'PWP Gap Time Model with Event-specific Effects';
proc phreg data = PTSD2 covm;
  model Gaptime * Status(0) = Trt1-Trt4 Age_mean1-Age_mean4
                        Sex_mean1-Sex_mean4;
  Trt1 = Trt * (Visit = 1);
  Trt2 = Trt * (Visit = 2);
  Trt3 = Trt * (Visit = 3);
  Trt4 = Trt * (Visit = 4);
  Age_mean1 = Age_mean * (Visit = 1);
  Age_mean2 = Age_mean * (Visit = 2);
  Age_mean3 = Age_mean * (Visit = 3);
  Age_mean4 = Age_mean * (Visit = 4);
  Sex_mean1 = Sex_mean * (Visit = 1);
  Sex_mean2 = Sex_mean * (Visit = 2);
  Sex_mean3 = Sex_mean * (Visit = 3);
  Sex_mean4 = Sex_mean * (Visit = 4);
  strata Visit;
run;
```

The SAS Program 7.5 is analogous to the previous program except for the specification of the gap time in the MODEL statement. Results of this PWP model are presented below.

SAS Program Output 7.5:

PWP Total Time Model with Event-specific Effects

Analysis of Maximum Likelihood Estimates

Parameter	DF	Parameter Estimate	Standard Error	Chi-Square	Pr > ChiSq	Hazard Ratio
Trt1	1	-0.57242	0.17840	10.2954	0.0013	0.564
Trt2	1	-0.17296	0.22876	0.5717	0.4496	0.841
Trt3	1	-0.04893	0.29346	0.0278	0.8676	0.952
Trt4	1	-0.14285	0.35871	0.1586	0.6905	0.867
Age_mean1	1	-0.00177	0.01043	0.0288	0.8653	0.998
Age_mean2	1	-0.02574	0.01337	3.7062	0.0542	0.975
Age_mean3	1	-0.02169	0.01601	1.8371	0.1753	0.979
Age_mean4	1	-0.01179	0.01816	0.4212	0.5163	0.988
Sex_mean1	1	0.03397	0.22143	0.0235	0.8781	1.035
Sex_mean2	1	0.25076	0.25723	0.9503	0.3296	1.285
Sex_mean3	1	0.01853	0.37138	0.0025	0.9602	1.019
Sex_mean4	1	0.15856	0.43934	0.1302	0.7182	1.172

The statistical results of the PWP gap time model differ somewhat from those of the total time model. While the effects of Trt2 and Trt3 remain statistically insignificant, the estimated regression coefficients of Trt1 and Trt4, −0.5524 and −0.6018, are statistically significant at $\alpha = 0.05$ (χ^2 for Trt1 = 9.7669, $p = 0.0018$; χ^2 for Trt4 = 4.1315, $p = 0.0421$). In general, however, the effect pattern of the new treatment in both PWP models is fairly consistent.

The overall effect of treatment can be estimated by specifying a common effect PWP model combining the four visit-specific covariates of treatment into one. The following SAS program provides codes for both the PWP total time and gap time models with common effects.

SAS Program 7.6:

```
......
title 'PWP Total Time Model with Common Effects';
proc phreg data = PTSD2 covm;
  model (TStart, TStop) * Status(0) = Trt Age_mean Sex_mean;
  strata Visit;
run;

title 'PWP Gap Time Model with Common Effects';
proc phreg data = PTSD2 covm;
  model Gaptime * Status(0) = Trt Age_mean Sex_mean;
  strata Visit;
run;
```

The PWP total time and gap time models with common effects are both nicely fitted (the model fit statistics not presented here), and the overall estimated regression coefficient of Trt in each model is statistically significant, as shown in the following output table.

SAS Program Output 7.6:

PWP Total Time Model with Common Effects

Analysis of Maximum Likelihood Estimates

Parameter	DF	Parameter Estimate	Standard Error	Chi-Square	Pr > ChiSq	Hazard Ratio
Trt	1	-0.31523	0.11893	7.0252	0.0080	0.730
age_mean	1	-0.01465	0.00679	4.6562	0.0309	0.985
sex_mean	1	0.12018	0.14395	0.6970	0.4038	1.128

PWP Gap Time Model with Common Effects

Analysis of Maximum Likelihood Estimates

Parameter	DF	Parameter Estimate	Standard Error	Chi-Square	Pr > ChiSq	Hazard Ratio
Trt	1	-0.40219	0.10977	13.4246	0.0002	0.669
age_mean	1	-0.01739	0.00663	6.8839	0.0087	0.983
sex_mean	1	0.16400	0.13551	1.4648	0.2262	1.178

The two PWP models with common effects derive fairly close point and *SE* estimates of the regression coefficients for Trt. Both estimated regression coefficients, –0.3152 and –0.4022, are associated with very small *p*-values, 0.0080 and 0.0002. As indicated earlier, however, the standard errors of the estimated regression coefficients in the two PWP models are often found to be biased.

The WLW model, as a marginal perspective, uses all four observations for each patient. Though also applying the stratification approach, a major difference of this model from the PWP models is the specification of the robust sandwich variance estimate. The SAS program for the WLW model with visit-specific effects is presented below.

SAS Program 7.7:

```
......
title 'WLW Marginal Model with Event-specific Effects';
proc phreg data = PTSD covs(aggregate);
  model TStop * Status(0) = Trt1-Trt4 Age_mean1-Age_mean4
                            Sex_mean1-Sex_mean4;
  Trt1 = Trt * (Visit = 1);
  Trt2 = Trt * (Visit = 2);
  Trt3 = Trt * (Visit = 3);
  Trt4 = Trt * (Visit = 4);
  Age_mean1 = Age_mean * (Visit = 1);
  Age_mean2 = Age_mean * (Visit = 2);
  Age_mean3 = Age_mean * (Visit = 3);
  Age_mean4 = Age_mean * (Visit = 4);
  Sex_mean1 = Sex_mean * (Visit = 1);
  Sex_mean2 = Sex_mean * (Visit = 2);
  Sex_mean3 = Sex_mean * (Visit = 3);
  Sex_mean4 = Sex_mean * (Visit = 4);
  strata Visit;
  id ID;
  Treatment: test Trt1, Trt2, Trt3, Trt4 / average e;
run;
```

Notice that in SAS Program 7.7, the WLW model uses the temporary dataset PTSD, rather than PTSD2, thus specifying data structure as a counting process style. The COVS(AGGREGATE) option tells SAS that the robust sandwich variance estimator is used for the derivation of the standard error estimates. In the MODEL statement, TSTOP*STATUS(0) specifies a typical marginal perspective for each potential repeated visit. The TREATMENT: TEST statement is specified to perform the global test on the null hypothesis of no treatment effects across all four marginal models ($\beta_{11} = \beta_{12} = \beta_{13} = \beta_{14} = 0$), and the AVERAGE and E options specified for, respectively, testing the common effect of Trt1 to Trt4 and for displaying weights for the common effect. Analytic results of this WLW model are presented below.

SAS Program Output 7.7:

.....

WLW Marginal Model with Event-specific Effects

Summary of the Number of Event and Censored Values

Stratum	Visit	Total	Event	Censored	Percent Censored
1	1	255	155	100	39.22
2	2	255	106	149	58.43
3	3	255	77	178	69.80
4	4	255	55	200	78.43
Total		1020	393	627	61.47

Testing Global Null Hypothesis: BETA=0

Test	Chi-Square	DF	Pr > ChiSq
Likelihood Ratio	39.0611	12	0.0001
Score (Model-Based)	41.5040	12	<.0001
Score (Sandwich)	21.4341	12	0.0444
Wald (Model-Based)	40.1514	12	<.0001
Wald (Sandwich)	17.6280	12	0.1275

Analysis of Maximum Likelihood Estimates

Parameter	DF	Parameter Estimate	Standard Error	StdErr Ratio	Chi-Square	Pr > ChiSq	Hazard Ratio
Trt1	1	-0.55243	0.16302	0.922	11.4834	0.0007	0.576
Trt2	1	-0.66407	0.21244	0.954	9.7712	0.0018	0.515
Trt3	1	-0.72137	0.26291	0.992	7.5285	0.0061	0.486
Trt4	1	-0.96223	0.32454	1.025	8.7906	0.0030	0.382
Age_mean1	1	-0.00306	0.00884	0.854	0.1199	0.7291	0.997
Age_mean2	1	-0.00531	0.01208	0.925	0.1932	0.6602	0.995
Age_mean3	1	-0.01721	0.01394	0.882	1.5246	0.2169	0.983
Age_mean4	1	-0.02059	0.01725	0.931	1.4237	0.2328	0.980
Sex_mean1	1	0.09384	0.24981	1.161	0.1411	0.7072	1.098
Sex_mean2	1	0.13101	0.26899	1.104	0.2372	0.6262	1.140
Sex_mean3	1	-0.19797	0.35978	1.125	0.3028	0.5821	0.820
Sex_mean4	1	-0.42722	0.43915	1.047	0.9464	0.3306	0.652

```
                 Linear Coefficients for Test Treatment

                                                              Average
Parameter        Row 1       Row 2       Row 3       Row 4     Effect

Trt1                 1           0           0           0    1.23308
Trt2                 0           1           0           0   -0.13388
Trt3                 0           0           1           0    0.03212
Trt4                 0           0           0           1   -0.13131
Age_mean1            0           0           0           0    0.00000
Age_mean2            0           0           0           0    0.00000
Age_mean3            0           0           0           0    0.00000
Age_mean4            0           0           0           0    0.00000
Sex_mean1            0           0           0           0    0.00000
Sex_mean2            0           0           0           0    0.00000
Sex_mean3            0           0           0           0    0.00000
Sex_mean4            0           0           0           0    0.00000
CONSTANT             0           0           0           0    0.00000


                      Test Treatment Results

                      Wald
                 Chi-Square      DF     Pr > ChiSq

                    12.8490       4         0.0120


                 Average Effect for Test Treatment

                          Standard
           Estimate          Error       z-Score     Pr > |z|

            -0.4891         0.1587       -3.0810       0.0021
```

SAS Program Output 7.7 demonstrates that out of 255 patients, 155 persons have at least one repeated check-in, 106 make at least two repeated visits, 77 patients have at least three recurrences, and 55 experience all four repeated events. Using the robust sandwich variance estimator, the estimates of all four visit-specific regression coefficients for Trt are statistically significant, with all p-values of the χ^2 statistics smaller than 0.0001. The absolute values of the estimated regression coefficients for Trt2 to Trt4 are considerably higher than those from the AG and the PWP estimates. As discussed earlier, this strong overestimation for later recurrences derives from including too many dummy observations in the risk sets. As those dummies are selected, rather than randomly distributed, into the two treatment groups, there is a strong carryover effect of the new medical treatment on later recurrences, thereby exaggerating the effects of Trt2 to Trt4 on the intensity rate of repeated visits.

The table 'Linear Coefficients for Test Treatment' displays the optimal weights for estimating the common treatment effect: they are 1.233 08, −0.133 88, 0.032 12, and −0.131 31 for Trt1, Trt2, Trt3, and Trt4, respectively. With a total of 1, these estimates, combined, yield a parameter estimate of –0.4891 with the standard error of 0.1587, presented in the table 'Average Effect for Test Treatment.' These estimators indicate the common effect to be statistically significant ($p = 0.0021$). The Wald test, with 4 degrees of freedom, supports the statistical significance of the new treatment effect in any of the four repeated visits ($\chi^2 = 12.8490$; $p = 0.0120$). It is worth noting that, unlike the PWP models, the WLW model has the capability to provide both the visit-specific and the common effects from a single analysis.

The WLW model can also be used to estimate the common effects in the same fashion as do the PWP models. Below is the SAS program for this step.

SAS Program 7.8:

```
......
title 'WLW Marginal Model with Common Effects';
proc phreg data = PTSD covs(aggregate);
  model TStop * Status(0) = Trt Age_mean Sex_mean;
  strata Count;
  id ID;
run;
```

The above SAS program is basically the same as SAS Program 7.7 except for the specification of a set of common covariates. The results are displayed below.

SAS Program Output 7.8:

WLW Marginal Model with Common Effects

Testing Global Null Hypothesis: BETA=0

Test	Chi-Square	DF	Pr > ChiSq
Likelihood Ratio	34.4357	3	<.0001
Score (Model-Based)	36.4119	3	<.0001
Score (Sandwich)	14.2000	3	0.0026
Wald (Model-Based)	35.4420	3	<.0001
Wald (Sandwich)	11.3268	3	0.0101

Analysis of Maximum Likelihood Estimates

Parameter	DF	Parameter Estimate	Standard Error	StdErr Ratio	Chi-Square	Pr > ChiSq	Hazard Ratio
Trt	1	-0.65427	0.19631	1.715	11.1072	0.0009	0.520
age_mean	1	-0.00753	0.01051	1.568	0.5131	0.4738	0.992
sex_mean	1	-0.00545	0.27410	2.023	0.0004	0.9841	0.995

From the WLW model with common effects, the estimated regression coefficient of Trt is –0.6543 with a standard error estimate of 0.1963, very strongly statistically significant ($p = 0.0009$). Compared with those derived from the AG model (–0.4552) and the PWP common effect models (–0.3152 and –0.4022), overestimation of the WLW estimate is sizable. The robust sandwich variance estimator yields a different standard error estimate, which can change the conclusion of a statistical test if the estimated standard error of a regression coefficient is located around the margin of a given acceptance level.

The proportional means model can also be estimated by using the PROC PHREG procedure. For this model, the counting process style for input data is required, with application of the robust sandwich variance–variance estimator for deriving unbiased standard errors of the estimated regression coefficients. The following SAS program is provided for fitting the proportional means model.

SAS Program 7.9:

```
......
data PTSD;
  set pclib.chapter7_PTSD;

......
title 'Cumulative Mean Functions for two Treatment Groups';
proc phreg data = PTSD covs(aggregate) ;
  model (TStart, TStop) * Status(0) = Trt Age_mean Sex_mean;
  id ID;
run;
```

SAS Program 7.9 is analogous to 7.3, except for the specification of the COV(AGGREGATE) option. The following table displays the results.

SAS Program Output 7.9:

Cumulative Mean Functions for two Treatment Groups

......

The PHREG Procedure

Analysis of Maximum Likelihood Estimates

Parameter	DF	Parameter Estimate	Standard Error	StdErr Ratio	Chi-Square	Pr > ChiSq	Hazard Ratio
Trt	1	-0.45518	0.11081	0.979	16.8746	<.0001	0.634
age_mean	1	-0.00959	0.00596	0.894	2.5893	0.1076	0.990
sex_mean	1	-0.01995	0.16850	1.219	0.0140	0.9058	0.980

Not surprisingly, the point estimates of the regression coefficients for Trt and the two control variables are identical to those derived from the Andersen–Gill intensity rate model because both sets of the estimates are obtained by the same partial likelihood score function. As a result, the model fit statistics, not presented in the above output table, are also exactly the same as those from the AG model. The standard error estimates, however, differ slightly between the two models because the proportional means model uses the robust sandwich variance estimator. Such differences are not as sizable as can be anticipated from relevant arguments of various dependence theories, thereby highlighting the high applicability of the Andersen–Gill approach.

As indicated in Chapter 5, statistically significant relative risk may not necessarily translate into strong differences in the hazard rate because differentials in the hazard function also depend on the magnitude of the baseline hazard. Accordingly, it is essential to compare some cumulative lifetime functions between the new treatment and the conventional psychotherapy. In the SAS system, the mean cumulative function (MCF) for the number of events can be well used for such an analysis.

The following SAS program yields a plot of two cumulative mean functions for the two treatment groups, so that the effect of the new medical treatment can be further examined graphically.

SAS Program 7.10:

```
......
data pattern;
  Trt = 0; Age_mean = 0; Sex_mean = 0;
  output;
  Trt = 1; Age_mean = 0; Sex_mean = 0;
  output;
run;

ods graphics on;
ods select MCFPlot;
title 'Cumulative Mean Functions for two Treatment Groups';
proc phreg data = PTSD covs(aggregate) plots(overlay) = MCF;
  model (TStart, TStop) * Status(0) = Trt Age_mean Sex_mean;
  baseline covariates = pattern out = pred1 cmf = _all_ ;
  id ID;
run;
ods graphics off;
```

In SAS Program 7.10, I first create a temporary dataset 'PATTERN' to specify two sets of values for the covariates, used for predicting the two cumulative mean functions (CMFs). As specified, the first pattern represents patients who receive the new treatment and the second designates those in the conventional psychotherapy group, with values of the two control variables fixed at zero (sample means). Using ODS Graphics, the PROC PHREG procedure plots two CMF curves for the two patterns according to the specification saved in the dataset 'PATTERN.' The COV(AGGREGATE) option is specified for computing the sandwich covariance matrix estimate. Similarly, the option PLOTS(OVERPLAY)=MCF tells SAS to overlay both MCF curves in the same plot. The MODEL statement is identical to the preceding program. In the BASELINE statement, the COVARIATES=PATTERN option specifies that the dataset PATTERN contains the set of covariates in the Cox model for the derivation of the two CMF curves. The CMF=_ALL_ option requests that the estimated cumulative function estimates, the standard error estimates, and the lower and upper confidence limits be output into the SAS dataset specified in the OUT=PRED1 option.

The resulting plot is displayed in Figure 7.2, which displays tremendous separation between the two CMF curves, thus highlighting strong effects of the new medical treatment on reducing the intensity rate and the mean number of repeated visits, other covariates being equal. It can confidently be concluded that the hazard ratio of the new treatment, 0.634, is both statistically significant and substantively meaningful after adjusting for the confounders.

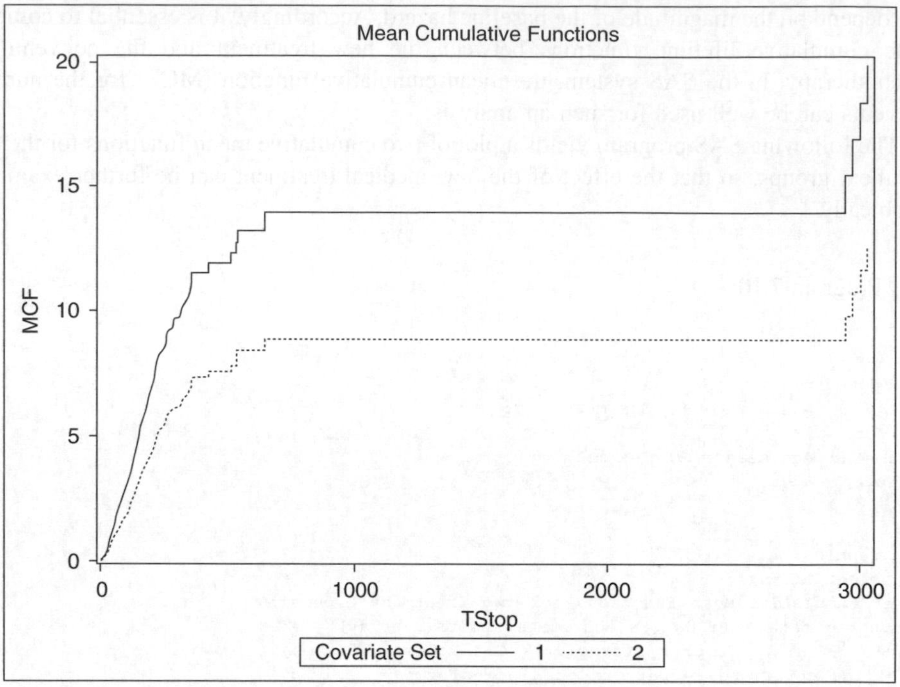

Figure 7.2 Estimated CMF curves for new treatment and conventional psychotherapy groups.

7.3 Summary

In this chapter, several competing risks models are presented with an empirical illustration. All those models, descriptive or analytic, are based on the restrictive assumption that the latent failure time systems of all event types are mutually independent. As the interrelations among different failure modes cannot be statistically tested, the reader needs to keep in mind that those survival models of competing risks should be used under this untestable hypothesis, which cannot be easily justified. I personally believe that various competing risks models described in this chapter are highly applicable if the multiple event types are carefully defined as guided by relevant theories and previous findings. If there is strong theoretical evidence that the competing risks under examination are correlated, great caution must be exercised in using these techniques. If the construction of a competing risks model is necessary, the researcher might want to consider regrouping some theoretically interrelated event types, combining the categories that are most likely to be mutually dependent.

In this chapter, I also delineate and discuss some statistical models for the analysis of survival data with repeated events. Five statistical models in this regard – AG, PWP-CP, PWP-GT, WLW, mean and rate functions – are based on various assumptions and hypotheses, and therefore are often found to yield significantly different parameter estimates. Until now, it remains a topic of debate concerning which model is most suitable for analyzing repeated events.

My personal recommendation is as follows. When the vast majority of subjects in a random sample experience only one or two events and a common baseline function can be justified, the Andersen–Gill model can be applied, given its simplicity and analytic convenience. The AG model is particularly useful in analyzing large-scale survival data, even when clustering does exist. If later recurrences of a given event are frequent, the PWP-GT model combined with the WLW sandwich variance estimator may be the most appropriate perspective for the analysis. Many medical and social events seem to fall into this scenario. The WLW model, though statistically estimable, obviously overestimates the regression coefficients by using the marginal approach, so that it is not highly recommended for empirical analyses. The robust sandwich variance estimator, however, is valuable in handling dependence of clustered survival data, including repeated events and other types of multivariate distribution. In any situation, the event-specific parameters should be estimated first even when there is evidence that regression coefficients for all recurrences do not differ significantly. The total time model should not be applied in any case because its specification carries information of prior events, thus intensifying the intraperson correlation. Finally, for highlighting the importance of an estimated hazard ratio, applying the proportional means model, along with the presentation of a plot with two or more pattern-specific CMF curves, is very informative.

8

Structural hazard rate regression models

8.1 Some thoughts about the structural hazard regression models

In spite of the increased use of life course perspectives in many areas of science, a number of theoretical or specification concerns remain. Prior research has mostly focused on analyzing the effects of covariates on a dynamic event by using a single equation. As these models are not constructed within a theoretical framework, which is often needed as a guide for data analysis in behavioral studies, it is sometimes difficult for researchers and planners to derive constructive implications from them. For example, many studies examine the effects of specific covariates with the presence of other causally related explanatory factors. By doing so, the estimated standard error of a given regression coefficient will be much increased, in turn making the *t*-statistic much smaller (Amemiya, 1985; Liu, 2000). It follows that this coefficient will be much less likely to be statistically significant, in turn possibly yielding erroneous analytic results. These models are statistically estimable on most occasions and might provide information on the direct effect of a given covariate on the hazard rate. The likely insignificance of its regression coefficient, however, can lead to misleading conclusions, particularly because this variable can potentially cause variations in the hazard rate by affecting other covariates that significantly predict the level of hazards.

Indeed, the development of a hazard rate model with strong endogeneity (a term used in Econometrics) should be based on a distinct theoretical framework and should elucidate pathways through which covariates influence the hazard rate. The structural hazard rate model can provide insight into the mechanisms involved in the dynamics of an event history and capture the relative importance of different components of the ecological, economical, and social environment on the occurrences of that event. Hence, an extensive survival analysis with multiple equations is not only important for understanding the structure of covariate interrelationships but it is also useful in fashioning policies and programs.

Survival Analysis: Models and Applications, First Edition. Xian Liu.

So far, there has been limited published work on structural equation models with survival data. There is a rich body of published work, often referred to as the 'medical demography,' in which researchers have developed a variety of hazard rate models for transitions in health status and the distribution of covariates as a cohort ages (Manton and Stallard, 1994; Manton, Stallard, and Singer, 1994; Manton *et al.*, 1994). Additionally, Vermunt (1997) employs latent variable approaches, attempting to explain and address the implications of unobserved heterogeneity or omitted variables in the context of survival analysis. Nevertheless, these statistical models have mainly focused on the description of dynamic processes inherent in a particular event and the general relationship between risk factors and event occurrences. In their systems, much less effort has been devoted to the development of a structural model that specifically concerns the interrelationships among explanatory factors and the decomposition of covariate influences on the occurrences of the event.

The absence of such efforts is perhaps due to the difficulty in linking multiple equations to an integrated estimation process and in specifying various link functions. Specifically, conventional hazard rate models, as described in prior chapters, are generally specified as nonlinear functions in covariates, whereas the prediction of intervening variables can be specified by both linear and nonlinear perspectives. A combination of these linear and nonlinear functions would bring about many specification and prediction problems, because complex transformation and retransformation of data can potentially make the estimation process extremely tedious and complex. In spite of the existence of such difficulties, several researchers have developed useful statistical methods to combine different link functions into a unifying survival model (Asparouhov, Masyn, and Muthen, 2006; Asparouhov and Muthen, 2007; Liu, 2000; Muthen, 1979, 1984, 2002, 2007; Muthen and Masyn, 2005). The following several paragraphs provide some discussions and comments on the structural survival models developed by Muthén and associates, given their increased popularity.

The structural time survival models developed by Muthén and colleagues are a part of their efforts to develop a unifying statistical system to incorporate multilevel models, finite mixture models, and structural equation models into a general and flexible framework (Asparouhov and Muthen, 2007). The purpose of developing those models with latent factors is mainly to reduce measurement error when describing and predicting a time event, as associated with observed explanatory variables in a prespecified structure. In a strict sense, such structural time survival models are not statistical techniques that directly decompose the effects of observed explanatory variables into direct and indirect effects. Given the capability of a multiequation framework, however, these models provide a flexible estimating tool to incorporate intervening variables, either observed or latent, and consequently the analysis of survival time can be formulated as a generalized latent class analysis of survival indicators. The latent class analysis uses covariates and can be combined with the joint modeling of other outcomes such as a continuous survival time or repeated measures for the discrete-time survival process. Here, different link functions are integrated, because each reduced-form equation can be expressed either as a linear regression or a transformed linear regression function; as a result, covariate effects can be decomposed into various components based on parameter estimates on different link functions. More important, potential measurement errors are taken into account under certain assumptions on the distributional function. Because of its unifying capability in handling specifications with complex structures and measurement errors, these time survival models are appealing in some applied disciplines, especially in psychology, sociology, and public health. If empirical data can efficiently support a large number of parameters and parameter estimates for various causal paths are interpretable, the application of those models can solve many specification problems that have concerned scientists for decades. The Mplus software, designed by Muthen and Muthen (2008), includes complex and flexible scenarios and is easy to apply (Plewis, 2001). In general, the tremendous efforts and deep thoughts involved in Muthén *et al.*'s structural equation models are impressive, and undoubtedly these statistical perspectives make a significant contribution to statistical modeling in applied science, including survival analysis.

In spite of increased popularity in psychological and sociological studies, structural equation models on survival data are faced with a number of concerns in their applications. As Muthen (2002) notes, structural equation modeling has so far not been fully accepted in mainstream statistics. Part of the problem might be due to poor applications claiming the establishment of causal models, as structural equation models with different assumptions of causality are often associated with similar or even identical model fit statistics, in turn making the statistical testing on causality extremely difficult (Bollen, 1989). Therefore, structural equation modeling should be viewed as a statistical technique that provides parameter estimates for a well-established theory involving complex pathways; it should not be taken as a statistical tool that tests causal assumptions for a theoretical framework that has yet to be verified. Problems might also arise from strong reliance on latent variables that are often difficult to define and interpret substantively. While the specification of latent variables may be statistically important in overcoming serious measurement error, attempts to explain their substantive connotations can introduce a new type of measurement error because the elements absorbed in a given latent factor are statistically defined without a known metric unit and thus cannot be described accurately with words. Additionally, identification could be a major issue in the presence of a large number of parameters (Bollen, 1989). Strong assumptions and arbitrary restrictions on certain parameters, unavoidable in the process of estimating structural equation models, can produce considerable unrecognizable errors which, combined with specification errors associated with latent variables, can potentially exceed the original measurement error the structural equation modeling is meant to overcome.

Given these concerns regarding applicability, I want to caution the reader that while various structural equation models provide a set of statistical procedures to accommodate multiple equations within an integrated estimating process, the application of these techniques in the analysis of survival data needs additional computational procedures for the interpretation of analytic results. The structural survival models developed by Muthén *et al.* and other experts focus more on the statistical derivation of structural parameter estimates than on the prediction of the outcome variable (Arbuckle, 1999; Bentler, 1995; Bollen, 1989; Joreskog and Sorbom, 1996; Muthen, 1984; Muthen and Muthen, 2008). In a sense, they are techniques about how model parameters are statistically estimated, rather than how they can be appropriately interpreted. From the statistical standpoint, there is no problem with this focus because, in most linear and generalized linear regression models, those parameter estimates can easily translate into interpretable results. In describing survival processes, however, prediction of the hazard or survival rates is frequently needed to compute useful survival effects (e.g., survival curves of different subgroups), so that additional calculation is often required. In a structural hazard rate model involving different link functions, regression coefficients and random errors should be retransformed on the scale of the hazard rate or of the survival function before being translated into interpretable results. Without this additional retransformation procedure, the decomposed effects of variables with different link functions may not provide sufficiently meaningful information for theoretical interpretations.

The parsimony of structural equation modeling with survival data must also be considered. Level of complexity and model coverage does not necessarily act as a criterion for the quality of a statistical model. As indicated in Chapter 1, the purpose of developing a statistical model in survival analysis is to generalize the underlying trends and the related risk factors while overlooking ignorable noises. Although neglect of measurement error sometimes influences the accuracy of parameter estimates, the excessive complication of a statistical model can make the likelihood function unnecessarily flat at the maximum, in effect overparameterizing the model. As also indicated in Chapter 1, the criteria for a good statistical model are relevance to an existing theory, accurate description of empirical data, computational tractability, and generation of interpretable results. If these principles are used to apply various structural time survival models with latent variables, there remain some challenging questions for the researcher to ponder.

In summary, Muthén and colleagues have masterfully established general inferences and estimating procedures of parameters involved in various structural equation models. Yet, caution is suggested when applying those techniques in survival analysis given the complexity inherent in the mechanisms of survival processes. The concrete estimation procedures for Muthén's structural survival models are not described in this book. For more detail, the reader might want to read Asparouhov and Muthen (2007), Muthen (1979, 1984, 2002, 2007), Muthen and Masyn (2005), and Muthen and Muthen (2008).

8.2 Structural hazard rate model with retransformation of random errors

Some research studies, when handling linear or nonlinear regressions, attempt to estimate a structural statistical model from a different direction (Alwin and Hauser, 1975; Winship and Mare, 1983). They argue that, with a well-defined theoretical framework, the direct effect of a given covariate can be obtained by conceptually specifying a full model, which incorporates both exogenous (variables whose causes are not generated from an underlying causal model) and endogenous factors (variables that are partly caused by exogenous variables and thus may transmit a substantial portion of the effect of a specific exogenous variable on the dependent variable of interest). Similarly, they suggest that the total effect of the same covariate can be estimated by specifying a final reduced form that only incorporates exogenous variables. Then an estimate of its indirect effect can be derived by taking the difference between the total and the direct effects. When more than one endogenous variable is involved, a model excluding a specific endogenous factor estimates the direct effect of that covariate plus its indirect influence via the excluded endogenous factor on the dependent variable. This approach is a simple but effective strategy used to decompose a total effect; as long as the underlying theoretical model is correctly specified, the full model is identifiable and the measurement error is ignorable.

The application of this approach on survival data, however, may encounter some prediction problems and additional information is needed for correctly estimating the hazard rate or the survival function. Specifically, for a nonlinear hazard model that generally views log(hazards) as a linear function of covariates and duration, the error term in a reduced-form equation cannot be simply eliminated from the estimation process without conducting some statistical retransformation; otherwise the predicted hazard rate can be substantially biased. The reason is that, if the error term in a generalized linear model is truly normally distributed, the normality of that error term must switch to a lognormally distributed function for correctly predicting the hazard rate. This retransformation implies that the multiplicative effect of that error term is not unity, but some value greater than one (Duan, 1983; Heckman and Singer, 1984; Liu, 2000; Mehran, 1973; Neyman and Scott, 1960; Vermunt, 1997). If the error term in a structural model is not normally distributed, as is often the case in, for example, health transitions (Manning, Duan, and Rogers, 1987), then the estimation of its expected value on the scale of the hazard rate will become more complicated.

I develop a structural hazard rate model that takes into account the interrelationships of covariates and their effects on the hazard rate and the survival function (Liu, 2000). This method is developed by specifying both a full model and a set of sequential reduced-form equations, as an extension of Alwin and Hauser (1975) and Winship and Mare (1983). It focuses on the decomposition of the total effect of a single covariate on the hazard rate into the direct effect and the indirect effects by means of given endogenous variables. In constructing this model, a retransformation approach is used to address bias involved in a conventional reduced-form nonlinear equation. The model has been used in some empirical studies on the mortality of older persons associated with educational attainment and veteran status (Liu *et al.*, 2005; Liu, Hermalin, and Chuang, 1998). The following sections display the procedures of this model and an empirical application of the method.

8.2.1 Model specification

First, I specify a typical causal model involving three types of variables (as can be widely seen in the literature on econometric and sociological research): the exogenous, the endogenous, and the dependent variable. For analytic simplicity and convenience of presenting the method, the model is restricted to block-recursive structures and assumes the absence of measurement error. Figure 8.1 displays a recursive diagram of causal linkages among the

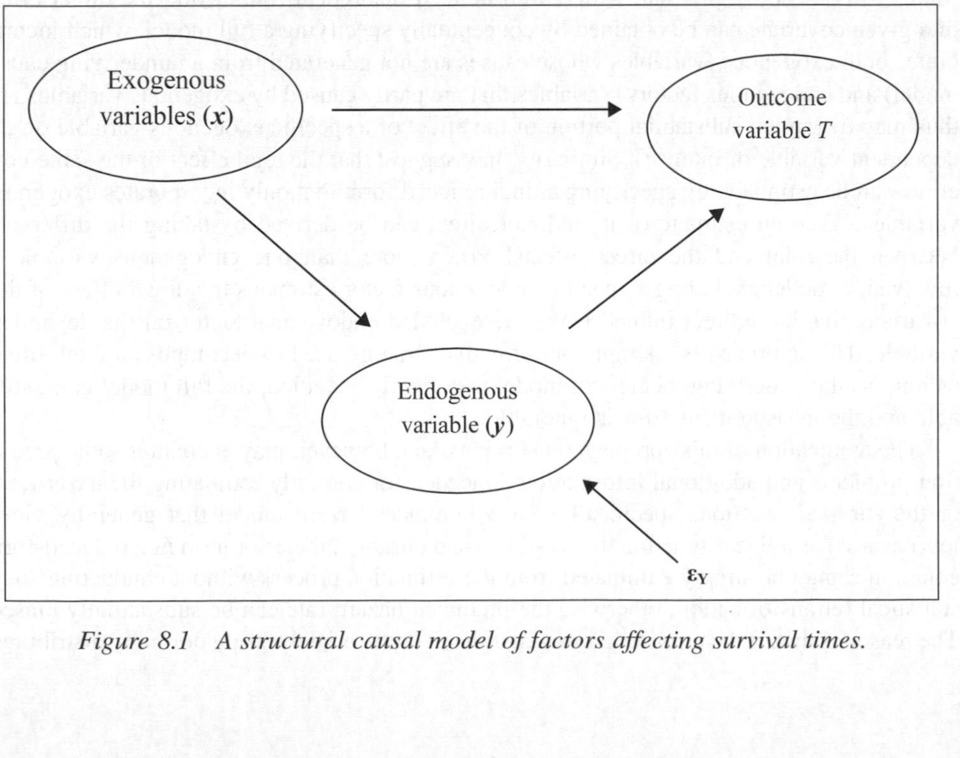

Figure 8.1 A structural causal model of factors affecting survival times.

three types of variables. According to my definition, the exogenous variables, denoted by $\boldsymbol{x}$, a $1 \times M$ vector, are those whose causes are not explicitly generated within the causal model, whereas the endogenous factors, a $1 \times K$ vector and represented by $\boldsymbol{y}$, are dependent on $\boldsymbol{x}$ and some other unidentified factors assumed to be mutually independent. The dependent variable is event time, T, which may be censored. This variable is assumed to follow a specific distribution whose parameters may depend on $\boldsymbol{x}$ and $\boldsymbol{y}$. As indicated in previous chapters, the effect of covariates on the parameters is often modeled using $h(t; \boldsymbol{\theta})$, the hazard rate at time t as a function of a parameter vector $\boldsymbol{\theta}$. As they have an impact on the dependent variable and are also affected by the exogenous variables, the endogenous variables are assumed to transmit a portion of the total effects of the exogenous variables on the hazard rate. Hence, the effects of the exogenous variables on the hazard rate incorporate two components, namely, the direct effects and the indirect effects by means of the endogenous variables.

Each observation under investigation is assumed to be subject to an instantaneous hazard rate, $h(t)$, of experiencing a given event, where $t = 0, 1, \ldots, \omega$, as specified previously. To simplify the analysis, I define an ad hoc structural hazard rate model to operationalize the causal relationships among the three types of variables, depicted in Figure 8.1 and given by

$$h(t|\boldsymbol{x}, \boldsymbol{y}) = h_0(t)\exp(\boldsymbol{x}'\boldsymbol{\beta} + \boldsymbol{y}'\boldsymbol{\alpha}), \tag{8.1a}$$

$$\boldsymbol{y}' = \boldsymbol{x}'\boldsymbol{\gamma} + \boldsymbol{\varepsilon}_y, \tag{8.1b}$$

where $h_0(t)$ denotes a specific (such as Weibull or exponential) or an unspecified baseline hazard function for continuous time T. The parameters, $\boldsymbol{\beta}$, $\boldsymbol{\alpha}$, and $\boldsymbol{\gamma}$, represent three vectors of regression coefficients to be estimated. In the context of structural equation modeling, $\boldsymbol{\beta}$ provides a set of the direct effects of the exogenous variables on the hazard rate and $\boldsymbol{\alpha}$ estimates the effects of the endogenous variables. The term $\boldsymbol{\varepsilon}_y$ is a vector of random errors for Equation (8.1b), hypothesized to be normally distributed with zero expectation and uncorrelated with the exogenous variables. The effects of $\boldsymbol{x}$ and $\boldsymbol{y}$ on the hazard rate are assumed to be multiplicative. Nonmultiplicativity of the effects of given covariates, if it exists, can be captured by the specification of interaction terms, as indicated in Chapters 4 and 5.

Note that, for convenience, the specification of Equation (8.1a) is based on the assumption that all observations with the same $\boldsymbol{x}$ and $\boldsymbol{y}$ values have an equivalent predicted hazard rate; that is, random disturbances for individual observations, given $\boldsymbol{x}$ and $\boldsymbol{y}$, are reflected in the baseline hazard function (Marubini and Valsecchi, 1995). Some researchers contend that the choice of a specific distributional function for random disturbances can influence the estimation of regression coefficients (Heckman and Singer, 1984). Nevertheless, if a structural model is correctly specified, the likelihood function for a full model tends to be flat, so that adding an arbitrarily assumed error term will not significantly improve the quality of parameter estimates, including standard errors, especially for large samples (Andersen and Gill, 1982; Box and Tiao, 1973; Liu, 2000). It has been shown in several empirical examples that covariate effect estimates are robust to misspecification of the distribution, $h_0(t)$ (Marubini and Valsecchi, 1995; Newman and McCulloch, 1984).

The estimation of Equation (8.1b) may be associated with a number of specification problems in empirical research if $\boldsymbol{y}$ includes some dichotomous variables, as is often the case in modeling a life course process. It would be extremely difficult to combine many different link functions within an integrated estimation process, as indicated earlier. However, we can estimate the total and the direct effects of a given covariate on the hazard rate without directly referring to Equation (8.1b), and then take the difference between these two effects as a reasonable estimate of the indirect effect by means of the endogenous variables, as done by Alwin and Hauser (1975) and Winship and Mare (1983). Accordingly, I specify a final reduced-form equation to derive the total effects of exogenous variables. In particular, I insert Equation (8.1b) into (8.1a) to give

$$\begin{aligned} h(t|\boldsymbol{x}, \boldsymbol{y}) &= h_0(t)\exp[\boldsymbol{x}'\boldsymbol{\beta}+(\boldsymbol{x}'\boldsymbol{\gamma}+\boldsymbol{\varepsilon}_y)\boldsymbol{\alpha}] \\ &= h_0(t)\exp(\boldsymbol{x}'\boldsymbol{\beta}+\boldsymbol{x}'\boldsymbol{\gamma\alpha}+\boldsymbol{\varepsilon}_y\boldsymbol{\alpha}) \\ &= h_0(t)\exp[\boldsymbol{x}'(\boldsymbol{\beta}+\boldsymbol{\gamma\alpha})+\boldsymbol{\varepsilon}_y\boldsymbol{\alpha}] \\ &= h_0(t)\exp(\boldsymbol{x}'\boldsymbol{\eta}+\tilde{\boldsymbol{u}}), \end{aligned} \tag{8.2}$$

where $\boldsymbol{\eta} = \boldsymbol{\beta} + \boldsymbol{\gamma\alpha}$ and $\tilde{\boldsymbol{u}} = \boldsymbol{\varepsilon}_y\boldsymbol{\alpha}$. While $\tilde{\boldsymbol{u}}$ is assumed to be uncorrelated with the exogenous variables, this error vector maintains normality if $\boldsymbol{\varepsilon}_y$ has multivariate normality, with $\text{var}(\boldsymbol{\varepsilon}_y\boldsymbol{\alpha}) = \boldsymbol{\alpha}^2\text{var}(\boldsymbol{\varepsilon}_y) = \boldsymbol{\alpha}^2\sigma^2$. I will discuss the specification of $\tilde{\boldsymbol{u}}$ further in Subsection Section 8.2.3.

It is clear that because $\boldsymbol{\eta}$ consists of two components ($\boldsymbol{\beta}$ and $\boldsymbol{\gamma\alpha}$), the regression coefficients in Equation (8.2) measure the total effects of the exogenous variables on the hazard rate given the theoretical framework specified in Figure 8.1.

I can also derive the intermediate effects of the exogenous variables, defined as the direct effects plus the indirect effects by means of the endogenous variable or variables excluded from the full model, by specifying an intermediate reduced-form equation (Alwin and Hauser, 1975; Liu, 2000). Let the vector $\boldsymbol{y}$ be divided into two subvectors: $\boldsymbol{y}_r$, which stands for the vector of the endogenous variables retained in the reduced-reform hazard model, and $\boldsymbol{y}_e$, which contains the endogenous variables excluded. Then the structural hazard model can be written as

$$h(t|\boldsymbol{x}, \boldsymbol{y}_r, \boldsymbol{y}_e) = h_0(t)\exp(\boldsymbol{x}'\boldsymbol{\beta}+\boldsymbol{y}_r'\boldsymbol{\alpha}_r+\boldsymbol{y}_e'\boldsymbol{\alpha}_e), \tag{8.3a}$$

$$\boldsymbol{y}_e' = \boldsymbol{x}'\boldsymbol{\gamma}_e+\boldsymbol{\varepsilon}_e, \tag{8.3b}$$

where $\boldsymbol{\alpha}_r$ and $\boldsymbol{\alpha}_e$ denote, respectively, the vectors of regression coefficients of the endogenous variables *retained in* and *excluded from* the reduced-form model. Similarly, $\boldsymbol{\gamma}_e$ is a vector for the regression coefficients of the exogenous variables on $\boldsymbol{y}_e$. Inserting Equation (8.3b) into (8.3a), we have

$$\begin{aligned} h(t|\boldsymbol{x}, \boldsymbol{y}_r, \boldsymbol{y}_e) &= h_0(t)\exp[\boldsymbol{x}'\boldsymbol{\beta}+\boldsymbol{y}_r'\boldsymbol{\alpha}_r+(\boldsymbol{x}'\boldsymbol{\gamma}_e+\boldsymbol{\varepsilon}_e)\boldsymbol{\alpha}_e] \\ &= h_0(t)\exp(\boldsymbol{x}'\boldsymbol{\beta}+\boldsymbol{y}_r'\boldsymbol{\alpha}_r+\boldsymbol{x}'\boldsymbol{\gamma}_e\boldsymbol{\alpha}_e+\boldsymbol{\varepsilon}_e\boldsymbol{\alpha}_e) \\ &= h_0(t)\exp[\boldsymbol{x}'(\boldsymbol{\beta}+\boldsymbol{\gamma}_e\boldsymbol{\alpha}_e)+\boldsymbol{y}_r'\boldsymbol{\alpha}_r+\boldsymbol{\varepsilon}_e\boldsymbol{\alpha}_e] \\ &= h_0(t)\exp(\boldsymbol{x}'\boldsymbol{\eta}_e+\boldsymbol{y}_r'\boldsymbol{\alpha}_r+\tilde{\boldsymbol{u}}_e), \end{aligned} \tag{8.4}$$

where $\boldsymbol{\eta}_e$ is a vector of the regression coefficients of the exogenous variables in the above intermediate reduced-form hazard model. The error term $\tilde{\boldsymbol{u}}_e$ is assumed to be uncorrelated with both the exogenous and the endogenous variables retained and each element is normally distributed. As $\boldsymbol{\eta}_e$ includes two parts, $\boldsymbol{\beta}$ and $\boldsymbol{\gamma}_e\boldsymbol{\alpha}_e$, it virtually contains the direct effects of the exogenous variables and their indirect effects by means of the endogenous variables excluded on the $h(t)$ function. Hence, we can construct a series of reduced-form equations eliminating the endogenous variables in theoretical sequence; then, from the two successive models, the indirect effects of the exogenous variables by means of a specific mediating factor can be estimated. If two endogenous variables are causally correlated, we are also able to estimate the indirect effects of the two covariates both independently and jointly by changing their orders in the elimination sequence. The application of this method is presented in detail in Subsection Section 8.2.5.

If $\mathbf{y}$ contains one or more binary or nominal variables, Equation (8.3) remains statistically estimable because $\mathbf{y}$ is implied as a latent cluster of covariates in the function. Nevertheless, some elements in $\boldsymbol{\eta}$ may be severely biased given misspecification on $\boldsymbol{\alpha}$. Hence, caution must apply in defining endogenous variables as categorical. A practical approach is to transform a categorical variable into a bounded continuous variable to ease this specification problem.

8.2.2 The estimation of the full model

The estimation of the full model, as represented by Equation (8.1a), is meant to derive the direct effects of the exogenous variables on the hazard rate. The precise definition of regression coefficients in a full model varies among researchers of different disciplines. Given the complexity of life course processes, psychologists, sociologists and other social researchers often perform a regression analysis within the context of a conceptual model, specifying various causal associations in the light of existing theories or specific research interests. The full model, if identified, estimates the effects of the exogenous variables while controlling for the intermediate influences of the endogenous factors; therefore, it is reasonable to view such regression coefficients as the direct effects on the hazard rate, as associated with a well-defined conceptual framework.

First, I define a censoring indicator δ_i for observation i ($i = 1, 2, \ldots, n$), given by

$$\delta_i = \begin{cases} 1 & \text{if } t_i \text{ is not censored,} \\ 0 & \text{if } t_i \text{ is censored,} \end{cases} \qquad i = 1, 2, \ldots, n.$$

As mentioned earlier, I define censoring as the condition that $T_i > t_i$.

The likelihood function for the full model can be written as a joint probability, given by

$$L = \prod_{i=1}^{n} f_i(t|\mathbf{x}_i, \mathbf{y}_i)^{\delta_i} S_i(t_i|\mathbf{x}_i, \mathbf{y}_i)^{1-\delta_i}$$
$$= \prod_{i=1}^{n} [h_0(t)\exp(\mathbf{x}_i'\boldsymbol{\beta} + \mathbf{y}_i'\boldsymbol{\alpha})]^{\delta_i} \exp\left[-\int_0^t h_0(u)\exp(\mathbf{x}_i'\boldsymbol{\beta} + \mathbf{y}_i'\boldsymbol{\alpha})\mathrm{d}u\right], \tag{8.5}$$

where f_i and S_i are, respectively, the probability density and survival functions, as previously specified. Taking log values on both sides of Equation (8.5) yields

$$\log L = \sum_{i=1}^{n} \left\{\delta_i \log[h_0(t)\exp(\mathbf{x}_i'\boldsymbol{\beta} + \mathbf{y}_i'\boldsymbol{\alpha})] - \int_0^t [h_0(u)\exp(\mathbf{x}_i'\boldsymbol{\beta} + \mathbf{y}_i'\boldsymbol{\alpha})]\mathrm{d}u\right\}$$
$$= \sum_{i=1}^{n} \left\{\delta_i [\log h_0(t) + (\mathbf{x}_i'\boldsymbol{\beta} + \mathbf{y}_i'\boldsymbol{\alpha})] - \int_0^t h_0(u)\,\mathrm{d}u \exp(\mathbf{x}_i'\boldsymbol{\beta} + \mathbf{y}_i'\boldsymbol{\alpha})\right\}. \tag{8.6}$$

The log-likelihood function is maximized with respect to an unknown parameter vector, which may contain some functional factors as well as regression coefficients (e.g., $\boldsymbol{\beta}$ and $\boldsymbol{\alpha}$), according to a specific hazard function selected for a particular analysis. For example, if the Weibull model is used to estimate Equation (8.1a), the hazard rate function is given by

$$h(t|\boldsymbol{x}, \boldsymbol{y}) = \lambda_0 \tilde{p}(h_0 t)^{\tilde{p}-1} \exp(\boldsymbol{x}'\boldsymbol{\beta} + \boldsymbol{y}'\boldsymbol{\alpha}), \tag{8.7}$$

where λ_0 is the scale parameter and $\tilde{p}$ is the shape parameter, as defined in Chapter 4. Then the log-likelihood function for the Weibull model is given by

$$\log L_{\text{Weib}} = \sum_{i=1}^{n} \left\{ \delta_i [\log \lambda_0 + \log \tilde{p} + (\tilde{p}-1)\log(\lambda_0 t) + (\boldsymbol{x}_i'\boldsymbol{\beta} + \boldsymbol{y}_i'\boldsymbol{\alpha})] - \left[(\lambda_0 t)^{\tilde{p}} \exp(\boldsymbol{x}_i'\boldsymbol{\beta} + \boldsymbol{y}_i'\boldsymbol{\alpha}) \right] \right\}. \tag{8.8}$$

Maximizing Equation (8.8) requires that this log-likelihood function be differentiated with respect to the parameters of the model λ_0, $\tilde{p}$, $\boldsymbol{\beta}$, and $\boldsymbol{\alpha}$. The concrete estimation procedure for the Weibull function is described in Chapter 4, so I do not elaborate it further in this chapter.

One might suggest that for a linear structural model, equations with both exogenous and endogenous variables included are subject to identification problems. However, the nonlinear restrictions of the full model on regression coefficients can aid in identification (Greene, 2003). Additionally, in many large-scale datasets used by researchers of various disciplines, the correlation coefficients among variables are usually not exceptionally high. As a result, I set forth an important assumption here that there is no exact linear dependence both between $\boldsymbol{x}$ and $\boldsymbol{y}$ and within either the exogenous or the endogenous vectors. I suggest, however, that if any pair-wise correlation coefficient involved in a full model is exceptionally high (over 0.8, say), the researcher needs to be very cautious about the precision of relevant parameter estimates. If the researcher wants to construct an interaction term between two highly correlated covariates, the two variables need to be rescaled so that they are centered at their respective sample means for reducing numeric instability and multicollinearity (Aiken and West, 1991). There are a number of approaches available that can be used to assess the identifiability of a regression model (e.g., see Amemiya, 1985; Greene, 2003).

The reader should keep in mind the fact that a necessary condition for identification of this type of structural regression model is that the number of exogenous variables must be at least as large as the number of endogenous factors included in the full model, referred to as the order condition of identifiability (Amemiya, 1985; Greene, 2003).

8.2.3 The estimation of reduced-form equations

For this step, I begin by estimating a final reduced-form equation that derives the total effects of the exogenous variables on the hazard rate, associated with a specific causal framework. In particular, I intend to find a way to estimate Equation (8.2) given a specific time function of the baseline hazard.

Here the problem in estimating reduced-form equations is how to retransform random disturbances, $\tilde{\boldsymbol{u}}$, for predicting the hazard rate. First, we cannot assume that this error term is zero for each observation, which implies an exact linear dependence of $\boldsymbol{y}$ on $\boldsymbol{x}$, in turn suggesting that the full model is not identified. Second, it is equally misleading to assume that the expected value of the error term is zero when predicting the hazard rate. This condition is due to the necessity of retransforming a normal distribution of random errors to a lognormally distributed function when predicting the hazard rate, as briefly indicated earlier. As a result, the expected value of the error term, after retransformation, is not unity given the properties of a lognormal distribution. Even if the true parameters $\boldsymbol{\eta}$ are known, the function $h_0(t)\exp(\boldsymbol{x}'\boldsymbol{\eta})$ is not the correct estimate of $\mathrm{E}[h(t)]$, such that

$$\mathrm{E}[h(t|\boldsymbol{x})] = h_0(t)\exp(\boldsymbol{x}'\boldsymbol{\eta}+\tilde{u}) \neq h_0(t)\exp(\boldsymbol{x}'\boldsymbol{\eta}).$$

An abundant literature is devoted to the issue of retransforming a transformed linear function to predict an untransformed scale (Bradu and Mundlak, 1970; Duan, 1983; Ebbeler, 1973; Goldberger, 1968; Liu, 2000; Manning, Duan, and Rogers, 1987; Meulenberg, 1965; Mehran, 1973; Neyman and Scott, 1960). The random errors from eliminating an important predictor variable or variables can be understood as the 'frailty' factor (Vaupel, Manton, and Stallard, 1979; Vaupel and Yashin, 1985a, 1985b), which will be introduced extensively in Chapter 9.

If an error term $\tilde{u}$ is normally distributed, then $\exp(\tilde{u})$ represents a multiplicative lognormal disturbance function, with mean

$$\mathrm{E}(\exp[\tilde{u}]) = \exp\left(\tilde{u}+\frac{\sigma^2}{2}\right) = \exp\left(\frac{\sigma^2}{2}\right) \tag{8.9}$$

and variance

$$\begin{aligned}\mathrm{var}(\exp[\tilde{u}]) &= \exp(2\tilde{u})\{\exp[2\sigma^2 - \exp(\sigma^2)]\}\\ &= \exp[2\sigma^2 - \exp(\sigma^2)],\end{aligned} \tag{8.10}$$

where σ^2 is the mean square error. Its mode, median, and moments all have the same functional form (Evans and Shaban, 1974). Whereas the median of $\exp(\tilde{u})$ is simply $e^{\tilde{u}}$, which implies a multiplicative effect of one, the positive skewness of the lognormal distribution mandates that the median lies below the mean, with equality holding if and only if $\sigma^2 = 0$. Clearly, neglect of this error term in estimating any log-linear equation with a reduced form leads to a *median* function, rather than a *mean* function. Consequently, unbiased and consistent quantities on the transformed scale cannot be retransformed into unbiased and consistent quantities on the untransformed scale without considering the retransformation of the error term.

Provided that $\tilde{u}$ is normally distributed and uncorrelated with $h_0(t)$ and $\boldsymbol{x}$, the final reduced-form equation can be written as

$$\begin{aligned}\mathrm{E}[h(t|\boldsymbol{x})] &= h_0(t)\exp\left(\boldsymbol{x}'\boldsymbol{\eta}+\frac{\sigma^2}{2}\right)\\ &= h_0(t)\exp(\boldsymbol{x}'\boldsymbol{\eta})\exp\left(\frac{\sigma^2}{2}\right)\\ &= h_0(t)\exp(\boldsymbol{x}'\boldsymbol{\eta})\varphi,\end{aligned} \tag{8.11}$$

where φ is an adjustment factor in the mean for the retransformation in the reduced-form equation, assuming $\tilde{u}$ to be normally distributed with mean zero and variance σ^2.

There is a variety of approaches to estimate the expected value of random errors for generalized linear models. Perhaps the most popular method is the 'threshold concept' approach (Bock, 1975), also referred to as the latent variable model for dichotomous outcome variables (Long, 1997). This method assumes the existence of a continuous latent variable that underlies the observed dichotomous outcome variable. A threshold determines if the dichotomous response equals 0 or 1. In the case of the logistic regression formulation, the errors are assumed to follow a standard logistic distribution with mean 0 and variance $\pi^2/3$, while for a probit regression random errors are assumed to follow a standard normal distribution with mean 0 and variance 1. The scale of the error is fixed because the continuous response variable is unobserved. This method has been widely applied both in regression modeling of categorical dependent variables (Long, 1997) and in longitudinal and multilevel data analysis (Hedeker and Gibbons, 2006; Merlo *et al.*, 2006). The approach, however, is not practicable for structural hazard rate models because all reduced-form equations, no matter how many endogenous variables are retained or eliminated, would have exactly the same value for the variance of random errors. In the case of structural hazard rate models, with an additional endogenous variable added to or reduced from the hazard rate model, the value of φ should be either decreased or increased. As McCullagh and Nelder (1989) note, the assumption of a continuous latent distribution is a rough model requirement, though providing a useful concept for generalized linear models.

Another approach to obtain the expected value of random errors uses the empirical data. While the actual hazard rate is unobservable, the researcher can recognize the predicted hazard rate derived from the full model as an unbiased and consistent set of h_i to calculate $\hat{\sigma}^2$, a sample estimate for σ^2. In a proportional hazard model, the term φ is theoretically independent of h_0 and $\boldsymbol{x}$ and behaves as a constant multiplicative effect throughout an underlying observation period. If the error term in a well-defined full model is truly ignorable, which I believe is a reasonable presumption, then φ can be estimated using the following equation

$$\hat{\varphi} = \exp\left(\frac{\sum_{i=1}^{n} \left\{ \log\left[\hat{h}_0(t)\exp(\boldsymbol{x}_i'\hat{\boldsymbol{\eta}})\right] - \log\left[\hat{h}_0(t)\exp\left(\boldsymbol{x}_i'\hat{\boldsymbol{\beta}} + \boldsymbol{y}_i'\hat{\boldsymbol{\alpha}}\right)\right]\right\}^2}{2(n-1)} \right)$$

$$= \exp\left(\frac{\sum_{i=1}^{n} \left\{ \log\left[\frac{\hat{h}_0(t)\exp(\boldsymbol{x}_i'\hat{\boldsymbol{\eta}})}{\hat{h}_0(t)\exp\left(\boldsymbol{x}_i'\hat{\boldsymbol{\beta}} + \boldsymbol{y}_i'\hat{\boldsymbol{\alpha}}\right)}\right]\right\}^2}{2(n-1)} \right)$$

$$= \exp\left\{ \frac{\sum_{i=1}^{n} \left[\boldsymbol{x}_i'\left(\hat{\boldsymbol{\eta}} - \hat{\boldsymbol{\beta}}\right) - \boldsymbol{y}_i'\hat{\boldsymbol{\alpha}}\right]^2}{2(n-1)} \right\}. \tag{8.12}$$

From the above equations, φ is constant throughout a specific observation period. In empirical data analyses, a fraction of the errors, obtained from eliminating endogenous variables, might be absorbed into the intercept. As a result, the intercept elements in $\hat{\boldsymbol{\eta}}$ and $\hat{\boldsymbol{\beta}}$ need to be included in calculating φ. Given this requirement for a known estimate of the baseline hazard function, the Cox model and the partial likelihood estimator are not recommended for the estimation of the structural hazard rate model. In certain situations involving complex data structures, a full maximum likelihood estimator is often preferable to predict the natural survival process over the partial likelihood approach (Asparouhov, Masyn, and Muthen, 2006; Johansen, 1983).

Additionally, given the estimate for φ, its variance can be readily derived:

$$\operatorname{var}(\hat{\varphi}) = \exp\left\{\frac{2\sum_{i=1}^{n}\left[\boldsymbol{x}_i'\left(\hat{\boldsymbol{\eta}}-\hat{\boldsymbol{\beta}}\right)-\boldsymbol{y}_i'\hat{\boldsymbol{\alpha}}\right]^2}{n-1} - \exp\left(\frac{\sum_{i=1}^{n}\left[\boldsymbol{x}_i'\left(\hat{\boldsymbol{\eta}}-\hat{\boldsymbol{\beta}}\right)-\boldsymbol{y}_i'\hat{\boldsymbol{\alpha}}\right]^2}{n-1}\right)\right\}. \tag{8.13}$$

The square root of $\operatorname{var}(\hat{\varphi})$ generates the standard error $(\hat{\varphi})$.

When the assumption of normality for $\tilde{u}$ cannot be satisfied, the factor $[\exp(\sigma^2/2)]$ is not the correct adjustment in the mean for the retransformation from the logarithmic scale to the untransformed hazard rate, so this estimator can lead to statistically inconsistent estimates of the hazard rate. In this case, Duan's (1983) retransformation method can be used to estimate Equation (8.2).

First, assuming $\boldsymbol{x}$ to have full rank, we have

$$\begin{aligned}\mathrm{E}[h(t|\boldsymbol{x})] &= \mathrm{E}[h_0(t)\exp(\boldsymbol{x}'\boldsymbol{\eta}+\tilde{u})] \\ &= \int h_0(t)\exp(\boldsymbol{x}'\boldsymbol{\eta}+\tilde{u})\,\mathrm{d}F(\tilde{u}).\end{aligned} \tag{8.14}$$

When the error distribution function F is unknown, I propose to replace this cumulative density function F by its empirical estimate, $\hat{F}_n$, which is referred to as the smearing estimate (Duan, 1983), given by

$$\begin{aligned}\mathrm{E}[h(t|x)] &= \int h_0(t)\exp(\boldsymbol{x}'\boldsymbol{\eta}+\tilde{u})\,\mathrm{d}\hat{F}_n(\tilde{u}) \\ &= \frac{1}{n}\sum_{i=1}^{n} h_0(t)\exp\left(\boldsymbol{x}_i'\boldsymbol{\eta}+\hat{\tilde{\mathrm{u}}}_i\right) \\ &= \left[\hat{h}_0(t)\exp(\boldsymbol{x}'\hat{\boldsymbol{\eta}})\right]n^{-1}\sum_{i=1}^{n}\exp\left(\hat{\tilde{u}}_i\right),\end{aligned} \tag{8.15}$$

where $\hat{\boldsymbol{\eta}}$ can be estimated by employing the maximum likelihood procedure without considering random disturbances given the large-sample theory and the martingale central limit theorem (Andersen and Gill, 1982; Lin *et al.*, 2000). If not confident in the consistency of the variance estimator, $\boldsymbol{\eta}$ can be estimated by taking the estimated residual into consideration, given by

$$\hat{\tilde{u}}_i = \log\left[\hat{h}_i(t|\boldsymbol{x}_i)\right] - \log\left[\hat{h}_i(t|\boldsymbol{x}_i, \boldsymbol{y}_i)\right]$$

or by its standardized form, as a covariate in the final reduced-form equation. I do not, however, expect significant differences between the two sets of the predicted values, as will be discussed further in Chapter 9. For large samples, this smearing estimate for the retransformation in log-linear equations is considered consistent, robust, and efficient (Duan, 1983; Heckman and Singer, 1980; Liu, 2000; Manning, Duan, and Rogers, 1987).

A consistent estimate of the hazard rate for the final reduced-form equation can be given by

$$\mathrm{E}[h(t)] = \hat{h}_0(t)\exp(\boldsymbol{x}'\hat{\boldsymbol{\eta}})\xi, \tag{8.16}$$

where

$$\hat{\xi} = \frac{\sum_{i=1}^{n} \mathrm{e}^{\log \hat{h}(t|x_i) - \log \hat{h}(t|x_i, y_i)}}{n-1} = \frac{\sum_{i=1}^{n} \exp\left[\boldsymbol{x}_i'\left(\hat{\boldsymbol{\eta}} - \hat{\boldsymbol{\beta}}\right) - \boldsymbol{y}_i'\hat{\boldsymbol{\alpha}}\right]}{n-1}. \tag{8.17}$$

Analytically, Equations (8.16) and (8.17) are meant to estimate an unknown error distribution by the empirical c.d.f. of the estimated regression residuals. Specifically, Equation (8.17) takes the desired expectation with respect to the estimated error distribution. Accounting for this 'smearing' effect will not completely eliminate bias when the underlying true specification of the retransformed error is unknown, but the overall prediction bias is negligible if a large sample is used to find a nonparametric distribution.

The aforementioned retransformation methods, either parametric or nonparametric, can be extended to the estimation of intermediate reduced-form equations, which retain a subset of endogenous factors in the estimating process. The smearing effect derived from a given intermediate reduced-form equation, denoted by φ_e or ξ_e, measures the prediction bias in the hazard rate that is incurred by eliminating e endogenous factors from the estimation process.

There are some other approximation approaches in the literature of generalized linear modeling proposed to derive Bayesian-type parameter estimators given random effects (Breslow and Clayton, 1993; Breslow and Lin, 1995; Hedeker and Gibbons, 2006; Stiratelli, Laird, and Ware, 1984; Zeger and Karim, 1991). Specifically, the likelihood function is proposed to be integrated over the random effects incurred from eliminating important predictor variables, and a number of integration techniques, such as the expectation-maximization (EM) and Gaussian quadrature estimators, have been developed for fitting nonlinear maximum likelihood estimates. Given that F is not a cumulative normal function after retransformation, the retransformation of random errors in the reduced-form equations is inevitable for the prediction of hazard or the survival function. For large samples, however, numeric integration of random effects in the likelihood is often shown to be unsuccessful in estimating survival models, as these unobserved random effects tend to be averaged out by the fixed effects of observed covariates. These issues will be revisited in Chapter 9 when I discuss the validity of frailty models.

8.2.4 Decomposition of causal effects on hazard rates and survival functions

As introduced above, the total effect of a given exogenous variable on the hazard rate can be estimated from a final reduced-form equation and its direct effect can be obtained from the full model. Then the difference between the total and the direct effects yields a reasonable estimate for the indirect effect of that variable by means of the endogenous variable or variables considered in an empirical study.

The indirect effect of an exogenous variable through a specific endogenous factor can also be derived from this approach using the same procedure. As indicated earlier, in an intermediate reduced-form model, the vector of regression coefficients, denoted $\boldsymbol{\eta}_e$, virtually includes two components: the direct effects of the exogenous variables on the log(hazard rate) and the indirect effects by means of the endogenous factors excluded from the intermediate reduced-form equation. Hence, the indirect effects of the exogenous variables by means of each endogenous variable can be obtained by constructing a series of ordered reduced-form equations, with each eliminating an endogenous factor from the previous regression. In particular, I define

$$\Delta\boldsymbol{\eta}_e = \boldsymbol{\eta}_e - \boldsymbol{\eta}_{e-1}, \tag{8.18}$$

where $\Delta\boldsymbol{\eta}_e$ is a vector of the indirect effects of the exogenous variables on the hazard rate by means of a specific endogenous factor, and $\boldsymbol{\eta}_e$ and $\boldsymbol{\eta}_{e-1}$ indicate the coefficient vectors of the exogenous variables in two intermediate reduced-form equations eliminating, respectively, e and $e-1$ endogenous factors from the full model. Similarly, the prediction bias caused by eliminating a specific endogenous factor from the previous regression can be estimated by taking the difference between $\hat{\varphi}_e$ and $\hat{\varphi}_{e-1}$ or between $\hat{\xi}_e$ and $\hat{\xi}_{e-1}$.

I propose to test the significance of the indirect effects of the exogenous variables on the hazard rate through the model likelihood ratio test, that is, −2 times the difference of the log likelihood between two consecutive hazard rate models:

$$G_e = -2\times[\log L(\boldsymbol{\eta}_e, \boldsymbol{\alpha}_r; t, \boldsymbol{x}, \boldsymbol{y}_r) - \log L(\boldsymbol{\eta}_{e-1}, \boldsymbol{\alpha}_{r+1}; \mathrm{t}, \boldsymbol{x}, \boldsymbol{y}_{r+1})], \tag{8.19}$$

where G_e is the likelihood ratio statistic for the indirect effect by means of a specific endogenous factor, which is distributed as χ^2 with the degree of freedom being the difference in the number of parameters between the two hazard models. To manage the degree of freedom in this test better, the samples used by the full model and the reduced-form equations must be exactly the same; as a result, the researcher needs to remove missing cases with respect to all covariates involved in a structural equation model before performing the statistical analysis. Consequently, the total, direct, and indirect effects of the exogenous variables on the hazard function can all be statistically estimated and tested without directly referring to Equation (8.1b). By performing this simple procedure, the relative importance of various covariates on the hazard rate can be adequately determined.

This way of decomposition is based on the prediction of log(hazard rate), which behaves as a linear function of both the exogenous and the endogenous variables. In empirical research, the natural logarithm of the hazard rate is often considered meaningful when examining the risk of experiencing a particular event and possesses unique implications. In demographic research, for example, the log(death rate) is an important measure of mortality, used as a useful indicator for simulating human survival (Horiuchi and Coale, 1990). Therefore, interpretation of the decomposed effects on the log(hazard rate) function is similar to that of the unstandardized linear regression coefficients.

Researchers sometimes are interested in using the hazard ratio to demonstrate the multiplicative effect of a given covariate on the hazard function, as described and empirically presented in earlier chapters. Specifically, such effects are informative by displaying the extent to which various multipliers to the hazard rate deviate from unity. Accordingly, the indirect multiplicative effects of the exogenous variables can be measured as follows:

$$\Delta\left[\exp\left(\hat{\boldsymbol{\eta}}_e\right)\right]=\left[\exp\left(\hat{\boldsymbol{\eta}}\right)-\mathbf{1}\right]-\left[\exp\left(\hat{\boldsymbol{\beta}}\right)-\mathbf{1}\right], \tag{8.20}$$

where $\Delta[\exp(\boldsymbol{\eta}_e)]$ denotes a vector of the indirect multiplicative effects of the exogenous variables on the hazard rate by means of K endogenous factors and $\mathbf{1}$ is a unit-vector containing elements of 1's. The indirect multiplicative effects by means of a single endogenous factor can be obtained by taking the difference between two conceptually ordered successive hazard models. Notice that the scale of the exponentiated regression coefficient differs from the scale of the coefficient itself, so that $\Delta[\exp(\boldsymbol{\eta}_e)] \neq \exp(\Delta\boldsymbol{\eta}_K)$.

The decomposition of the additive effects of the exogenous variables on the hazard rate is more complex. Because the hazard rate is specified as a nonlinear function of covariate values as well as of regression coefficients and duration, the additive effects of the exogenous variables on the hazard rate, including the total, direct, and indirect effects, are scale dependent. If such effects are of interest, the researcher can calculate the conditional effects of covariates on the hazard rate with respect to a 'typical' population, as suggested by Fox (1987) and Long (1997). This approach is applied in Chapter 7 in the description of the multinomial logit model; that is, one can calculate the difference between two predicted hazard rates, letting the first be the estimate of the hazard rate when a given covariate is scaled at its sample mean (or 0 in the case of a dichotomous variable) and the second be the estimate when the value of that indexed covariate is one unit greater than its sample mean (or 1 for a dichotomous variable). The difference between the two estimates is the conditional effect of that covariate on the hazard rate. In deriving conditional effects, all other covariates need to be fixed at sample means for representing a typical population. Such 'conditional' effects can then be decomposed from the estimates derived from the full model and those from the reduced-form equations. The standard error of the conditional effect for an exogenous variable can be computed using the delta method (see Appendices A and B) or the standard bootstrapping approach. Theoretically, the conditional effect is sensitive to changes in the value of a covariate, as also indicated in Chapter 7. Within a limited observation period, however, the hazard function usually approximates a straight line, so that such effects do not tend to vary considerably over changes in covariate scales within the zones where most cases are located.

Occasionally, the researcher is interested in comparing survival functions between different treatments or demographic subgroups to highlight the impact of covariates on the sample paths of a lifetime event. The rationale for this presentation is indicated on several occasions in earlier chapters. To reiterate, the baseline hazard rates are not observable in the hazard model, so that statistically significant effects on the hazard rate may not necessarily translate into strong differences in the survival function because such differentials also depend on the magnitude of the baseline hazard rate (Liu, 2000; Teachman and Hayward, 1993). Therefore, it is essential to demonstrate differential survivorship and then decompose the total effects of covariates on the survival function into the direct and the indirect effects.

As indicated earlier, a survival function is intimately related to the hazard function, given by

$$S(t) = \exp\left[-\int_0^t h(u)\mathrm{d}u|\boldsymbol{x}\right] = \exp[-H(t)|\boldsymbol{x}], \tag{8.21}$$

where $H(t)$ is the cumulative hazard from time 0 to time t, as indicated earlier. Equation (8.21) indicates that once we specify a time function for the hazard rate, the survival function can be readily derived from a hazard function. It can be further inferred that the effects of covariates on the hazard rate can also be transformed to different components of effects on the survival function.

There are two approaches that can be applied for demonstrating the effects of covariates on the survival function. The first approach is to predict survival functions for selected subgroups, as applied in Chapter 5. As a survival schedule is specified as a nonlinear function of both covariate values and the regression coefficients, other covariates need to be fixed at sample means for making the comparison effective (Fox, 1987; Long, 1997).

As the next step, group-specific survival curves can be graphically presented, associated both with the full model and with the reduced-form equations, to examine the extent to which those survival curves are separated. Specifically, we let x_m be a specific exogenous variable and $\boldsymbol{x}_r$ be the vector containing other exogenous variables. We may arbitrarily select K values for x_m and present a survival function for each. The survival function for $x_m = k$, as derived from the full model on the hazard rate, is given by

$$\begin{aligned} S[t|x_m = k, \bar{\boldsymbol{x}}_r, \bar{\boldsymbol{y}}] &= \exp\left[-\int_0^t h_0(u)\exp(k\beta_m + \bar{\boldsymbol{x}}_r'\boldsymbol{\beta}_r + \bar{\boldsymbol{y}}'\boldsymbol{\alpha})\mathrm{d}u\right] \\ &= \exp\left[-\int_0^t h_0(u)\mathrm{d}u\exp(k\beta_m + \bar{\boldsymbol{x}}_r'\boldsymbol{\beta}_r + \bar{\boldsymbol{y}}'\boldsymbol{\alpha})\right], \end{aligned} \tag{8.22}$$

where $S[t|x_m = k, \bar{\boldsymbol{x}}_r, \bar{\boldsymbol{y}}]$ is the survival rate at time t for value k with respect to variable x_m with other exogenous and all endogenous variables being fixed at sample means, β_m is the regression coefficient for x_m included in the vector $\boldsymbol{\beta}$, and $\bar{\boldsymbol{x}}_r$ and $\bar{\boldsymbol{y}}$ are vectors containing sample means for the covariates other than x_m.

Similarly, the survival rate for $x_m = k$ can be obtained from the final reduced-form equation:

$$\begin{aligned} S[t|x_m = k, \bar{\boldsymbol{x}}_r, \varphi] &= \exp\left\{-\int_0^t [h_0(u)\exp(kg_z + \bar{\boldsymbol{x}}_r'\boldsymbol{\eta}_r)\varphi]\mathrm{d}u\right\} \\ &= \exp\left[-\varphi\int_0^t h_0(u)\mathrm{d}u\exp(kg_z + \bar{\boldsymbol{x}}_r'\boldsymbol{\eta}_r)\right], \end{aligned} \tag{8.23}$$

where $S[t|x_m = k, \bar{\boldsymbol{x}}_r, \varphi]$ is the survival rate for $x_m = k$ derived from the final reduced-form equation with other covariates fixed at sample means and g_m stands for the regression coefficient of x_m included in vector $\boldsymbol{\eta}$.

If the distribution of $\tilde{u}$, which underlies φ, is not normal, φ needs to be replaced with ξ. The separation of K survival functions can then be assessed with respect both to the full model and to a reduced-form equation; consequently, the indirect effects of the exogenous variables on the survival rate can be effectively evaluated by comparing the two sets of the survival functions.

The second approach concerns the calculation of conditional effects of covariates on the survival rate. In particular, if x_m is a continuous variable, the direct conditional effect of x_m on the survival rate can be calculated as

$$\Delta S(t|\bar{x}_m, \bar{\mathbf{x}}_r, \bar{\mathbf{y}}) = \exp\left\{-\int_0^t h_0(u)\mathrm{d}u \exp[(\bar{x}_m+1)b_z + \bar{\mathbf{x}}_r'\boldsymbol{\beta}_r + \bar{\mathbf{y}}'\boldsymbol{\alpha}]\right\} - \exp\left[-\int_0^t h_0(u)\mathrm{d}u \exp(\bar{x}_m b_z + \bar{\mathbf{x}}_r'\boldsymbol{\beta}_r + \bar{\mathbf{y}}'\boldsymbol{\alpha})\right] \quad (8.24)$$

and the total conditional effect of x_m as (if $\tilde{u} \sim [0, \sigma^2]$)

$$\Delta S(t|\bar{x}_m, \bar{\mathbf{x}}_r, \hat{\varphi}) = \exp\left\{-\hat{\varphi}\int_0^t h_0(u)\mathrm{d}u \exp[(\bar{x}_m+1)g_z + \bar{\mathbf{x}}_r'\boldsymbol{\eta}_r]\right\} - \exp\left[-\hat{\varphi}\int_0^t h_0(u)\mathrm{d}u \exp(\bar{x}_m g_z + \bar{\mathbf{x}}_r'\boldsymbol{\eta}_r)\right], \quad (8.25)$$

where $\Delta S(t|\bar{x}_m, \bar{\mathbf{x}}_r, \bar{\mathbf{y}})$ and $\Delta S(t|\bar{x}_m, \bar{\mathbf{x}}_r, \varphi)$ are defined as the direct and the total conditional effects of x_m on the survival rate, respectively, while other covariates are fixed at sample means (if $\tilde{u}$ is not normally distributed, φ is replaced by ξ).

Similarly, if x_m is a dichotomous variable, the following two equations are used to calculate the direct and the total conditional effects of x_m on the survival rate:

$$\Delta S(t|x_m, \bar{\mathbf{x}}_r, \bar{\mathbf{y}}) = \exp\left[-\int_0^t h_0(u)\mathrm{d}u \exp(\beta_m + \bar{\mathbf{x}}_r'\boldsymbol{\beta}_r + \bar{\mathbf{y}}'\boldsymbol{\alpha})\right] - \exp\left[-\int_0^t h_0(u)\mathrm{d}u \exp(\bar{\mathbf{x}}_r'\boldsymbol{\beta}_r + \bar{\mathbf{y}}'\boldsymbol{\alpha})\right] \quad (8.26)$$

and

$$\Delta S(t|x_m, \bar{\mathbf{x}}_r, \hat{\varphi}) = \exp\left[-\hat{\varphi}\int_0^t h_0(u)\mathrm{d}u \exp(g_z + \bar{\mathbf{x}}_r'\boldsymbol{\eta}_r)\right] - \exp\left[-\hat{\varphi}\int_0^t h_0(u)\mathrm{d}u \exp(\bar{\mathbf{x}}_r'\boldsymbol{\eta}_r)\right]. \quad (8.27)$$

The difference between the total and the direct conditional effects yields an estimate of the indirect conditional effect of x_m on the survival rate. Standard errors of the total, direct, and indirect conditional effects on the survival function can be approximated by applying the delta method.

I would like to emphasize again that the decomposed effects on the survival function is scale dependent. The reader might want to sensitize themselves to the variation in such conditional effects by displaying the effects at different scales using selected values of the control variables.

I also suggest that it is inappropriate to calculate the marginal effect in the survival rate with respect to the instantaneous variation in covariates. As Petersen (1985) notes, the marginal effect of a specific covariate on a probability represents the slope of the probability function with respect to that covariate, which is virtually boundless in value. This specification implicitly violates the necessary condition that the value of a survival rate must range between 0 and 1. Additionally, the marginal effect is not designed to lend substantively meaningful implications and persons not familiar with mathematics or econometrics may have great difficulty in understanding implications of such measures. Consider, for example, the case of dichotomous variables: what does such a marginal change mean to factors taking only two values? The use of qualitative factors taking more than two values as covariates further complicates the interpretability of a covariate's marginal effect on the survival function.

8.2.5 Illustration: The effects of veteran status on the mortality of older Americans and its pathways

In this section, I present an empirical example using the statistical approaches introduced from Subsections 8.2.1 to 8.2.4. With minor modifications, the example is based on a published article by Liu *et al.* (2005). In particular, I examine the mortality differences between American older veterans and nonveterans and the subsequent excess mortality among veterans. The observation range is a four-to-five-year interval from 1993/1994 to the end of 1997. The intervening influences of physical health and mental disorders are taken into account.

8.2.5.1 Conceptual framework

Figure 8.2 presents a structural diagram of the theoretical model to guide the statistical analysis on this subject, where veteran status is viewed as the exogenous variable, with older Americans classified as veterans or nonveterans. Survival time T is the dependent variable, serving as a function of veteran status, physical health conditions, and mental disorders. Not shown in Figure 8.2 are some other exogenous variables such as age, sex, ethnicity, socioeconomic status, and health behaviors, treated as controls in the analysis. Physical and mental health statuses are the endogenous factors that affect the mortality of older veterans (Jonas and Mussolino, 2000; Bullman and Kang, 1994; Fogel, 1993; House *et al.*, 1992). It is hypothesized that, at older ages, veterans have a negative impact on survivorship, once the longstanding effects of prior military service emerge after veterans' health composition becomes comparable to nonveterans. This effect is posited to get increasingly stronger over age according to mortality crossover theories (Hirsch, Liu, and Witten, 2000; Liu and Witten, 1995; the mortality crossover theories are introduced in detail in Chapter 9). The influence of veteran status on old-age mortality is mostly indirect, mediated by physical health conditions and mental disorders. Because they are correlated, physical health conditions and mental disorders not only independently affect the hazard rate but they may modify mortality jointly. It is also hypothesized that veteran status reflects some other factors, as yet unidentified, that mediate its effect on the mortality of older Americans. For this reason, we maintain a residual or direct effect of veteran status on the mortality of older Americans, illustrated as a dotted line in Figure 8.2. This direct effect may also arise from some latent intervening factors for which no suitable measures are currently available, such as social ties, family structure, and the like (Costa, 1993; Fogel, 1993; Wimmer and Fogel, 1991).

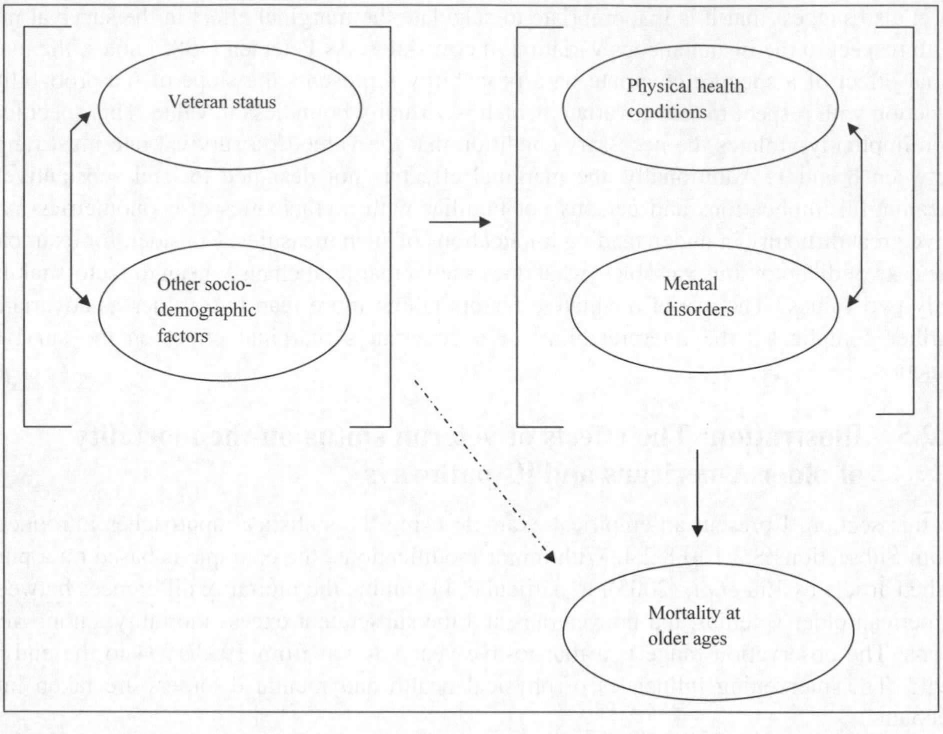

Figure 8.2 Causal model for the association of veteran status with the mortality of older Americans. Source: X. Liu, C.C. Engel, H. Kang and D. Cowan. 2005. The effect of veteran status on mortality among older Americans and its pathways. Population Research and Policy Review *24:573–592.*

8.2.5.2 Data, measures, and models

The data used for this example come from the dataset described in Chapter 1. This illustration employs Wave I data (baseline survey) and the survival information within a four-to-five-year period. Generally, for the convenience of statistical testing on indirect effects, this kind of analysis should use the sample excluding all missing cases with respect to all covariates in the full model, termed the 'effective sample.' This strategy makes an estimation of all equations use the same number of survey respondents, thus facilitating the management of the degree of freedom in the structural equation modeling. The time of death is recorded for those who died between the Wave I interview and December 31, 1997. Of 2000 Wave I respondents in our analysis, 332 are deceased during the interval. For each of the deceased in this four-to-five-year interval, the duration in months from the Wave I interview to the time of death is recorded. As I only use a portion of the original data and change the time range, analytic results from this illustration are not necessarily consistent with those published in the article by Liu *et al.* (2005).

In view of the fact that the application of the Cox hazard rate model is inappropriate for the structural hazard rate modeling, all covariates considered in this analysis are time-independent variables with values fixed at the Wave I survey. The time-independent assumption on some of the covariates (e.g., marital status) might lead to some bias in parameter estimates; however, our main exogenous and intervening variables – veteran status, physical health conditions, and mental disorders – are fairly stable over time among older persons. Veteran status is measured as a dichotomous variable (veteran = 1, nonveteran = 0), named 'VET' in the statistical analysis. Over 90 % of veterans in the dataset served in the military during World War II. Among the control variables, age is defined as the actual years of age reported by respondents at the time of the Wave I survey. As the starting age of the data is 70 years, this variable is rescaled to be centered at age 70 (actual age – 70), termed 'AGE_70' in the analysis, with 0 representing age 70. Given the theoretical hypothesis that the excess mortality among older veterans increases over age, an interaction term is created between Vet and Age_70. Mortality differences at older ages are often viewed as a function of time due to the selection effect, but issues of unobserved heterogeneity in longitudinal data are not the focus in the present illustration. The issue of mortality convergence and crossover is discussed extensively in Chapter 9. Statistically, time-dependent differences in mortality can be addressed by creating an interaction term between a specific covariate and duration, as applied previously; if this interaction is statistically significant, the use of the Weibull or Cox model will generate an adjusted hazard rate function that is actually nonproportional.

In addition to age, three additional theoretically-relevant control variables are specified. Gender is indexed as a dichotomous variable (women = 1, men = 0). Educational attainment, an approximate proxy for socioeconomic status, is measured as the total number of years in school, assuming the influence of education on mortality to be a continuous process (Liu, Hermalin, and Chuang, 1998). Marital status is specified as a dummy variable, with currently married = 1, else = 0. For analytic convenience, these three control variables are all rescaled to be centered at the sample means, termed Female_cnd, Educ_cnd, and Married_cnd, respectively. Empirically, the mean of a dichotomous variable indicates the likelihood or propensity of being in the group coded 1; it can also be understood as the expected proportion in the population the sample represents.

Six variables are used to measure the two dimensions of health status – physical health conditions and mental disorders. An older person's physical health is represented by three variables: serious health conditions, functional limitations, and self-rated health. Serious health conditions are measured as the reported number of five serious illnesses, including cancer, diabetes, heart disease, hypertension, and stroke. Chronic health conditions were not found to add additional information on the mortality of older Americans in the presence of serious health conditions. I measure functional status by a score of activities of daily living (ADL), instrumental activities of daily living (IADL), and other types of functional limitations. This score ranges from 0 (functional independence) to 15 (maximum disability). Self-rated health, regarded as the most commonly used proxy for general health (Idler and Kasl, 1991; Weinberger, Darnell, and Tierney, 1986), is measured with a 5-point scale ranging from 1 (poor) to 5 (excellent). In the analysis, serious health conditions, functional limitations, and self-rated health are all rescaled to be centered at sample means, termed, respectively, Objph1_cnd, Numfunc_cnd, and Subph_cnd.

An older person's mental health is also measured by three variables – mental disorder diagnosis, depression symptoms, and cognitive impairment. The mental disorder diagnosis is a dichotomous variable (yes = 1, no = 0), obtained from a question: 'Have you ever seen a doctor for emotional, nervous, or psychiatric problems?' Because the inclusion of a dichotomous variable can yield seriously biased parameter estimates for intervening factors, as indicated in Subsection Section 8.2.1, I transform this dummy variable into the propensity score by applying the logistic regression. Specifically, using 'diagnosed' or 'not diagnosed' as a dichotomous outcome variable, a logistic regression model is constructed to predict the probability of being diagnosed with mental disorders, with veteran status, age, sex, and some other covariates used as the predictor variables. Then the predicted probability for each individual is saved in the temporary dataset as the propensity score of mental disorders. Depression symptom severity is measured by the Center for Epidemiologic Studies Depression (CES-D) score (Radloff, 1977), an 8-level scale. The 35-item cognitive score (Herzog and Wallace, 1997) is applied to measure an older person's level of cognitive impairment. The three mental health variables are centered at sample means, named Mentalp_cnd, CESD8_cnd, and COG_cnd, respectively.

The following SAS program is used to create the propensity score of psychiatric diagnosis and the centered covariates for the construction of a structural hazard rate model.

SAS Program 8.1:

```
options ps=56;
libname pclib '<local directory>:\Survival Analysis\data\';
options _last_=pclib.chapter8_data;

data new;
 set pclib.chapter8_data;

*Creation of the propensity score of psychiatric diagnosis;
proc logistic data=new descending;
  model mental=vet age female educ married
                           objph1 cesd8 cog;
 output out=new xbeta=xbeta1 p=mentalp;
run;

*Creation of centered covariates;
proc SQL;
 create table new1 as
 select *, age - 70 as age_70,
 female-mean(female) as female_cnd,
 educ-mean(educ) as educ_cnd,
 married-mean(married) as married_cnd,
 numfunc-mean(numfunc) as numfunc_cnd,
 objph1-mean(objph1) as objph1_cnd,
 subph-mean(subph) as subph_cnd,
 mentalp-mean(mentalp) as mentalp_cnd,
 cesd8-mean(cesd8) as cesd8_cnd,
 cog-mean(cog) as cog_cnd
 from new;
quit;
```

In SAS Program 8.1, a temporary SAS data file 'New' is created from the dataset chapter8_data. The SAS PROC LOGISTIC procedure is employed to generate the propensity score of psychiatric diagnosis. The OUTPUT statement updates the SAS data file New by adding the propensity score MENTALP that is predicted for each individual by the logistic regression model. The SAS PROC SQL procedure creates ten centered covariates – four control variables and six endogenous variables – and then they are saved into the new temporary SAS data file 'New1' for further analysis. Table 8.1 displays the mean (or proportions), the standard deviation, and the coding scheme of each original covariate and the variable names of the centered variables, using results generated from SAS Program 8.1.

A hazard rate model is specified to assess the effect of veteran status on the mortality of older Americans. Specifically, a Weibull distribution of the hazard function is defined to model the underlying time function of mortality among older persons. Within the framework of the structural hazard rate model, the application of the Weibull mortality function,

Table 8.1 Means (or proportions), standard deviations, coding schemes of exogenous and endogenous variables: older Americans (N = 2000).

Explanatory variable	Mean or proportion	Standard deviation	Coding scheme	Variable name in analysis
Veteran status	0.19	—	1 = veteran, 0 = nonveteran	Vet
Age (years)	75.79	6.59	Actual number of years from birth	Age_70
Female	0.67	—	1 = yes, 0 = no	Female_cnd
Education	11.11	3.55	Actual years of attending school	Educ_cnd
Currently married	0.55	—	1 = yes, 0 = no	Married_cnd
Functional limitations	2.02	2.57	A 15-level score: 0 = no limitation, 15 = maximum limitation	Numfunc_cnd
Serious physical illnesses	1.14	0.98	A 5-score scale: 0 = no serious illness, 5 = most serious condition	Objph1_cnd
Self-rated health	3.07	1.14	A 5-point scale: 1 = poor, 5 = excellent	Subpj_cnd
Psychiatric problems	0.11	0.07	Propensity score on psychiatric disorder diagnosis	Mentalp_cnd
CES-D score	1.59	1.92	An 8-level score: 0 = no depression, 8 = maximum depression	Cesd8_cnd
Cognitive score	19.99	5.87	A 35-level score: 1 = no impairment, 35 = maximum impairment	Cog_cnd

Note: In analysis, Age_70 = (actual age – 70); the rest of the covariates, except Vet, are mean-centered variables.

a flexible and monotonic model as explained in Chapter 4, is considered most appropriate for the description of mortality processes within a limited time interval, as evidenced by previous work (Liu, 2000; Liu *et al.*, 2006). As shown in Chapter 4, the plot of log[log $S(t)$] versus log (duration) has demonstrated an approximately straight curve, thereby providing some validity of using the Weibull model for this example.

The aforementioned structural hazard rate modeling procedures are applied to estimate the mortality differences between older veterans and nonveterans. First, a full hazard rate model considering all exogenous and endogenous variables is specified. I then specify three reduced-form equations, eliminating the two endogenous factors (each consisting of three variables) from the estimation process in sequence, to estimate the total effect of veteran status on the hazard function and its indirect effects by means of physical health conditions and mental disorders, both individually and jointly. In specifying each of these reduced-form equations, I calculate the mean value of $\hat{\varphi}$ by assuming a normal distribution of transformed random errors. The Weibull model is fitted by employing the SAS PROC LIFEREG procedure given procedures described in Chapter 4. Notice that some of the random effects from eliminating endogenous variables might be absorbed into the estimate of scale or shape parameter, so that their values estimated for the reduced-form equations may vary from the full model. While such a variation can cause some prediction errors, on most occasions differences in the estimates of scale and shape parameters are minor and thus are ignorable. When encountering significant deviations, however, the researcher needs to initialize the scale parameter to the value estimated for the full model, so that unbiased φ estimates can be derived.

As indicated in Chapter 4, SAS LIFEREG does not model the hazard rate and does not produce hazard ratios. Parameter estimates on log(duration), however, can be readily converted to the estimates on the log(hazards) by using SAS software. For example, the SAS Output Delivery System (ODS) can be used for this step, also described in Chapter 4. Consequently, the full hazard rate model (Equation (8.7)) can be fitted using the following SAS code.

SAS Program 8.2:

```
......

ods output Parameterestimates=Weibull_PE;
proc lifereg data=new1 outest=Weibull_outest;
  model duration*followup(0)=vet age_70 vet*age_70
        female_cnd educ_cnd married_cnd numfunc_cnd
        objph1_cnd subph_cnd mentalp_cnd cesd8_cnd
        cog_cnd / dist=weibull;
  run;
ods output close;

* Compute and print corresponding PH estimates and HR *;
data Weibull_PE;
  if _N_=1 then set Weibull_outest(keep=_SCALE_);
  set Weibull_PE;
  string = upcase(trim(Parameter));
  if (string ne 'SCALE') & (string ne 'WEIBULL SHAPE')
     then PH_beta = -1*estimate/_SCALE_;
```

```
  else  if PH_beta=.;
  AFT_beta = estimate;
  HR = exp(PH_beta);
  drop _SCALE_;
options nolabel;

proc print data=Weibull_PE;
  id Parameter;
  var AFT_beta PH_beta HR;
  format PH_beta 8.5 HR 5.3;
  title1 "LIFEREG/Weibull on duration";
  title2 "ParameterEstimate dataset w/ PH_beta & HR computed manually";
  title4 "PH_beta = -1*AFT_beta/scale";
  title6 "HR = exp(PH_beta)";
run;
```

In SAS Program 8.2, the first part estimates the regression coefficients of covariates on log(duration), with parameter estimates saved in the temporary SAS output file Weibull_PE. The second part converts the saved log time coefficients (AFT_beta) into log hazard coefficients (PH_beta) and hazard ratios (HR) using the converting formulas introduced in Chapter 4. Lastly, the third part of the program asks SAS to print three sets of parameter estimates – regression coefficients on log(duration), regression coefficients on log(hazards), and hazard ratios. As discussed in Chapter 4, the converting formulas for standard errors and confidence intervals of the estimated regression coefficients are more complex. In view of the fact that test results of the null hypothesis on log time coefficients also serve as the results of the null hypothesis on log hazard coefficients (Allison, 2010), analytic results of significance tests from the SAS PROC LIFEREG procedure can be borrowed to perform the significance test on regression coefficients in the Weibull hazard rate model.

The reader might readily recognize that the above SAS program is analogous to SAS Program 4.4 and the only difference is that covariates in this illustration are conceptually divided into the exogenous and the endogenous variables within a structural equation modeling framework.

The results from SAS Program 8.2 are presented below.

SAS Program Output 8.1:

```
                    The LIFEREG Procedure

                      Model Information

         Data Set                         WORK.NEW1
         Dependent Variable           Log(duration)
         Censoring Variable                followup
         Censoring Value(s)                       0
         Number of Observations                2000
         Noncensored Values                     332
```

```
              Right Censored Values          1668
              Left Censored Values              0
              Interval Censored Values          0
              Name of Distribution        Weibull
              Log Likelihood         -1047.351285

       Number of Observations Read 2000
       Number of Observations Used 2000

                    Fit Statistics

       -2 Log Likelihood                  2094.703
       AIC (smaller is better)            2122.703
       AICC (smaller is better)           2122.914
       BIC (smaller is better)            2201.115

          Fit Statistics (Unlogged Response)

       -2 Log Likelihood                       4102.464
       Weibull AIC (smaller is better)         4130.464
       Weibull AICC (smaller is better)        4130.675
       Weibull BIC (smaller is better)         4208.876

  Algorithm converged.

              Type III Analysis of Effects

                                   Wald
       Effect          DF    Chi-Square    Pr > ChiSq

       Vet              1        2.9687        0.0849
       Age_70           1        4.7108        0.0300
       Vet*age_70       1        7.9504        0.0048
       Female_cnd       1       13.9445        0.0002
       Educ_cnd         1       12.7219        0.0004
       Married_cnd      1        0.0093        0.9233
       Numfunc_cnd      1       26.4282        <.0001
       Objphl_cnd       1        7.6576        0.0057
```

Subph_cnd	1	6.3456	0.0118
Mentalp_cnd	1	0.2844	0.5938
Cesd8_cnd	1	0.0663	0.7968
Cog_cnd	1	17.7253	<.0001

Analysis of Maximum Likelihood Parameter Estimates

Parameter	DF	Estimate	Standard Error	95% Confidence Limits		Chi-Square	Pr > ChiSq
Intercept	1	5.5387	0.1368	5.2707	5.8068	1639.95	<.0001
Vet	1	0.3279	0.1903	-0.0451	0.7009	2.97	0.0849
Age_70	1	-0.0302	0.0139	-0.0574	-0.0029	4.71	0.0300
Vet*age_70	1	-0.0536	0.0190	-0.0908	-0.0163	7.95	0.0048
Female_cnd	1	0.5226	0.1399	0.2483	0.7969	13.94	0.0002
Educ_cnd	1	-0.0486	0.0136	-0.0752	-0.0219	12.72	0.0004
Married_cnd	1	0.0094	0.0981	-0.1828	0.2017	0.01	0.9233
Numfunc_cnd	1	-0.0836	0.0163	-0.1155	-0.0517	26.43	<.0001
Objph1_cnd	1	-0.1393	0.0503	-0.2380	-0.0406	7.66	0.0057
Subph_cnd	1	0.1164	0.0462	0.0258	0.2069	6.35	0.0118
Mentalp_cnd	1	-0.9204	1.7257	-4.3027	2.4619	0.28	0.5938
Cesd8_cnd	1	-0.0121	0.0470	-0.1043	0.0801	0.07	0.7968
Cog_cnd	1	0.0399	0.0095	0.0213	0.0585	17.73	<.0001
Scale	1	0.7638	0.0401	0.6891	0.8466		
Weibull Shape	1	1.3092	0.0688	1.1812	1.4512		

Parameter	AFT_beta	PH_beta	HR
Intercept	5.53874	-7.25145	0.001
Vet	0.32788	-0.42927	0.651
Age_70	-0.03017	0.03950	1.040
Vet*age_70	-0.05356	0.07013	1.073
Female_cnd	0.52260	-0.68420	0.504
Educ_cnd	-0.04855	0.06357	1.066
Married_cnd	0.00944	-0.01236	0.988
Numfunc_cnd	-0.08363	0.10949	1.116
Objph1_cnd	-0.13931	0.18239	1.200
Subph_cnd	0.11638	-0.15236	0.859
Mentalp_cnd	-0.92038	1.20498	3.337
Cesd8_cnd	-0.01211	0.01586	1.016
Cog_cnd	0.03991	-0.05225	0.949
Scale	0.76381	.	.
Weibull Shape	1.30922	.	.

In SAS Program Output 8.1, the first three sections present the general information that is useful for comparing the goodness of fit between multiple hazard models. In this example, the −2 log likelihood is used to test whether the indirect effects are statistically significant. The 'Type III Analysis of Effects' table displays hypothesis tests for the significance of each of the effects specified in the MODEL statement. The table of parameter estimates demonstrates the LIFEREG estimates on log(duration), derived from the maximum likelihood procedure. As mentioned earlier, the Weibull shape parameter λ for this model is simply the reciprocal of the extreme value scale parameter estimate (1/0.7638 = 1.3092). The last table presents the three sets of parameter estimates – AFT_beta, PH_beta, and HR. As it is a standard output table for a Weibull regression, as described extensively in Section 4.3, I do not make additional interpretations of various statistics and estimators contained in SAS Program Output 8.1.

The SAS program for the reduced-form equations is more complex and lengthy due to the sizable transformation of parameter estimates and the estimation of the parameter φ. The SAS program for the estimation of all four hazard models and the derivation of the φ estimates is provided in Appendix D.

8.2.5.3 Results

The results of the four hazard models are summarized in Table 8.2, which displays the results of four hazard rate models, transformed from analytic results of the corresponding ATF

Table 8.2 Results of four hazard rate models on the mortality of older Americans between 1993 and 1997: Weibull model (n = 2000).

Covariates and other statistics	Model A		Model B		Model C		Model D	
	Coefficient	HR	Coefficient	HR	Coefficient	HR	Coefficient	HR
Vet	−0.429	0.651	−0.446	0.640	−0.343	0.709	−0.241	0.786
Age_70	0.040*	1.040	0.084**	1.088	0.044**	1.045	0.064**	1.066
Vet*age_70	0.070**	1.073	0.064**	1.066	0.057**	1.059	0.046*	1.047
Female_cnd	−0.684**	0.504	−0.807**	0.446	−0.688**	0.503	−0.556**	0.573
Educ_cnd	0.064**	1.066	0.055**	1.056	0.022	1.022	−0.016	0.985
Married_cnd	−0.012	0.988	0.007	1.007	−0.090	0.914	−0.168	0.846
Numfunc_cnd	0.109**	1.116			0.133**	1.142		
Objph1_cnd	0.182**	1.200			0.200**	1.221		
Subph_cnd	−0.152*	0.859			−0.180**	0.836		
Mentalp_cnd	1.205	3.337	6.395**	—				
CESD8_cnd	0.016	1.016	−0.017	0.983				
Cog_cnd	−0.052**	0.949	−0.052**	0.950				
Intercept	−7.252**		−7.359**		−7.213**		−7.092**	
φ	1.000		1.091**		1.041**		1.271**	
Shape	1.309**		1.287**		1.300**		1.265**	
−2 log likelihood	2094.703		2158.787		2121.067		2238.963	

Note: The parameter 'shape' is tested by $(\tilde{p}-1.0)/SE$.
*$0.01 < p < 0.05$;
**$p < 0.01$.

models. As shown in the parenthesis of the table title, the effective sample size, $n = 2000$, is exactly the same as the total sample size, indicating no missing cases with respect to all covariates in the full model. The first regression given in the table is the full model with both exogenous and endogenous variables included, which estimates the direct effect of veteran status on the mortality of older Americans. The following three hazard rate models are the estimates from the reduced-form equations, with each eliminating relevant endogenous variables from a previous regression. The last two columns demonstrate the final reduced-form equation model, providing an estimate for the total effect of veteran status on the log(hazard rate).

The regression coefficients of veteran status in all four models are negative, while those of the interaction term between veteran status and age are all positive, which, combined, suggest a typical pattern of mortality convergence and crossover between older veterans and nonveterans, and the subsequent excess mortality among older veterans. The effects of veteran status on the mortality of older Americans are considered to be statistically significant, given the statistical significance of the interaction terms. Because the absolute value of the main effect for veteran status (−0.241) is greater than that of the interaction term (0.046), veterans are expected to have a death rate that is about 18 % lower than their nonveteran counterparts at age 70 ($e^{-0.241} = 0.823$), other variables being equal. Veterans' mortality, however, is expected to cross with the nonveterans' death rate at the exact age 75.2 years ($70 + |-0.241|/0.046$), and from that age point forward, the excess death rate among older veterans starts and continues to increase steadily over age. The value of $\hat{\varphi}$ for the reduced-form equations ranges from 1.041 to 1.271, all statistically significant, exhibiting the degree of prediction bias in models excluding important predictor variables. As anticipated, the value of $\hat{\varphi}$ in the final reduced-form hazard rate model is considerably greater than the corresponding figures in the two intermediate reduced-form regressions.

The hazard ratio of each regression coefficient (HR) is presented to highlight the multiplicative effects of veteran status on the mortality of older Americans. In Model D, a one-year increase in age would offset the main effect of veteran status by about 7 % of the mortality difference (the multiplicative effect of the interaction), thereby leading to a trend of mortality convergence and mortality crossover between older veterans and nonveterans. The expected value of $\tilde{p}$, the shape parameter, ranges from 1.265 to 1.309, exhibiting a monotonically increasing hazard rate within the interval under investigation. The differences in this estimate over the four Weibull hazard models are regarded as trivial therefore do not affect the quality of the model fit for the present analysis. I would like to emphasize again, however, that if differences in the shape parameter estimate are considerable, the estimated value from the full model should be used to initialize the estimation of this parameter for reduced-form equations; otherwise substantial prediction bias would occur.

Among the endogenous variables, an older person's severity of functional limitations and the number of serious health conditions display positive effects on the mortality of older Americans, as expected. Likewise, self-rated health is negatively linked to old-age mortality, other variables being equal. The effects of all the three physical health variables are statistically significant at $\alpha = 0.05$. The effects of the mental health variables appear much weaker compared to those of physical health conditions. The effects of the psychiatric diagnosis propensity score and the CES-D depression score are not statistically significant in the presence of other covariates. The effect of cognitive impairment is statistically significant on a two-tail test, but it is shown negatively linked to the hazard rate, contrary to my expectation. Nevertheless, the effect of an individual health variable may not be highly meaningful in this analysis because these variables are regarded as components on an integrated health dimension that transmits the effect of veteran status on the hazard function. For example, the inclusion of the CES-D score may 'wash out' some of the key impacts of mental disorder diagnosis on mortality.

With or without the inclusion of mental health variables, the effects of physical health variables remain relatively unchanged, whereas those of the mental health factors vary somewhat when eliminating physical conditions, thereby implying that mental health might affect mortality indirectly by influencing physical health more so than vice versa.

Although signs of the regression coefficients of veteran status are consistent throughout all four models, the mechanisms inherent in these effects may be complicated. For example, the absolute values of veterans' regression coefficients and the veteran × age interaction term in the full model are mostly greater than those in each of the reduced-form hazard models, suggesting that the direct and the indirect effects of veteran status on mortality do not necessarily operate in the same direction. In Table 8.3, the decomposed effects of veteran status on the log (mortality) of older Americans are demonstrated at three exact ages – 70 years, 75 years, and 85 years, given that the veterans' effects on the old-age mortality are age dependent. The right panel of Table 8.3 displays the percentage distribution of the total effects, direct effects, and indirect effects by means of three sources at the three exact ages.

Table 8.3 shows that, when other variables are equal, the direct and indirect effects of veteran status on the hazard rate, all statistically significant given the chi-square test, mostly perform in the opposite direction and that such effects vary enormously over age. For example, at age 70, an older veteran is expected to have a lower death rate than his or her nonveteran counterpart, but the direct and the indirect effects involve disparate mechanisms. About 34 % of the total effect of veteran status comes from the positive indirect effects by means of an older person's health status, especially the combined component of physical health conditions and mental disorders (18.3 %). The direct, or residual, effect at exact age 70 accounts for about 66 % of the total effect, and this effect is negative, opposite to most of the indirect effects. The negative effect among veterans at age 70 is obviously associated with the so-called 'healthy veteran effect' (Kang and Bullman, 1996).

The above pattern is altered dramatically when an older American survives to older ages. First, the negative total effect of veterans on the mortality declines from –0.241 at age 70 to –0.011 at age 75, owing mostly to the increased proportion of the positive indirect effects. At age 85, the total effect rises to 0.449, highlighting considerable excess mortality among veterans. While the two mortality schedules are expected to cross at age 75.2, as mentioned earlier, the excess death rate among older veterans becomes increasingly higher over age as compared to nonveterans. Second, as a cohort ages, the relative importance of the indirect effect varies greatly in causing higher excess mortality among veterans. At age 75, 67.2 % of the total effect of veteran status on the mortality of older Americans is due to the indirect effect, compared to 34.1 % at age 70; then this portion of the veteran effect declines to about 30 % at age 85. In this process, the internal composition of the indirect effects also changes substantially over age. At ages 70 and 75, the indirect effects by means of psychiatric disorders individually and by physical and mental conditions jointly are negative while the effect by means of physical conditions alone is positive. At age 85, only the indirect effect by means of the combined effect of the two health components is negative, suggesting that among the oldest old veterans, it is some unspecified and unknown factors that lead to much higher mortality than among nonveterans.

Table 8.3 Decomposition of total effect of veteran status on log(hazards) into direct and indirect effects: older Americans ($n = 2000$).

Type of effects	Magnitude of effect	Percentage of effect[a]
Age 70		
Direct (residual) effect	−0.429**	65.9 %
Indirect effect	0.188**	34.1
Through physical health condition	−0.017**	2.6
Through mental health condition	0.086**	13.2
Through physical and mental combined	0.119**	18.3
Total effect	−0.241**	100.0 %
Age 75		
Direct (residual) effect	−0.079**	32.8 %
Indirect effect	0.068**	67.2
Through physical health condition	−0.047**	19.5
Through mental health condition	0.021**	8.7
Through physical and mental combined	0.094**	39.0
Total effect	−0.011**	100.0 %
Age 85		
Direct (residual) effect	0.621**	70.5 %
Indirect effect	−0.172**	29.5
Through physical health condition	−0.107**	12.1
Through mental health condition	−0.109**	12.4
Through physical and mental combined	0.044**	5.0
Total effect	0.449**	100.0 %

Note: The significance level of an indirect effect is tested by the likelihood ratio that is distributed as χ^2, that is, −2 times the difference in the values of log likelihood between two models given the same sample size.

[a]The percentage of an effect derived from its absolute value over the absolute sum of all effects.

$^{**}p < 0.01$.

Of the three sources of the indirect effects, the relative importance of veterans' indirect effects on the mortality of older Americans also alters over age. At age 70, the interacted effect of physical health conditions and psychiatric disorders is the dominant intervening factor (18.3 %); physical health alone only plays a very minor role (2.6 %). At age 75, the joint effect of the two health dimensions is still the dominant intervening factor, but the relative importance of physical health alone, accompanied by the increased influence of the indirect effects, increases considerably (from 2.6 % to 19.5 %). At age 85, only 5 % of the total effect of veteran status goes through an older person's physical health conditions and psychiatric disorders jointly, whereas mental disorders alone become a more important intervening factor (12.4 %).

These decomposed effects are based on the scale of log(hazards), serving as a linear function of covariates, and therefore they are easy to compute and interpret. Because all control variables are centered on sample means, only the intercept, values of Vet, and Age_70 and their regression coefficients need to be taken into account when calculating decomposed effects. For example, from Table 8.2, the total effect of veteran status at age 75 is computed simply by the equation $(-0.241 + 0.046 \times 5 = -0.011)$. Similarly, the equation $(-0.429 + 15 \times 0.070 = 0.621)$ gives rise to the estimate of the veteran direct effect at age 85. If the reader is interested in obtaining decomposed effects on the mortality rate itself, the computation becomes more complex and tedious because a covariate effect on the hazard rate is a nonlinear function of time, the regression coefficients, and the values of all covariates. Sometimes, displaying the effects on the hazard rate is important because statistically significant effects on the log(hazards) or hazard ratios may not necessarily translate into meaningful differentials in the hazard rate itself (Liu, 2000; Teachman and Hayward, 1993), as indicated earlier.

Another useful approach to display the effects of veteran status on the mortality of older Americans is to compare the survival functions between older veterans and nonveterans at selected ages, as described and discussed in Section 8.2.4. The Weibull survival rates can be created from parameter estimates on the hazard function and, generally, such survival functions are very close to those derived from the Cox model (Sugisawa, Liang, and Liu, 1994). In particular, the survival rate at time t, given vectors $\boldsymbol{x}_0$ and $\boldsymbol{y}_0$, which contain selected values of the exogenous and endogenous covariates, can be estimated by

$$\hat{S}(t|\tilde{p}, \boldsymbol{x}_0, \boldsymbol{y}_0) = \exp\left[-\exp\left(\boldsymbol{x}_0'\hat{\boldsymbol{\beta}} + \boldsymbol{y}_0'\hat{\boldsymbol{\alpha}}\right)t^{\hat{\tilde{p}}}\right]. \tag{8.28}$$

Similarly, the Weibull survival rate at time t with respect only to $\boldsymbol{x}_0$, the so-called final reduced-form equation, is given by

$$\hat{S}(t|\tilde{p}, \boldsymbol{x}_0, \hat{\varphi}) = \exp\left\{-\exp\left[\boldsymbol{x}_0'\hat{\boldsymbol{\eta}} + \log(\hat{\varphi})\right]t^{\hat{\tilde{p}}}\right\}. \tag{8.29}$$

If the researcher prefers to use the SAS LIFEREG estimates, including the estimated scale factor and the estimated regression coefficients on log(duration), then the corresponding equations are

$$\hat{S}(t|p^*, \boldsymbol{x}_0, \boldsymbol{y}_0) = \exp\left\{-\left[\frac{t}{\exp\left(\boldsymbol{x}_0'\hat{\boldsymbol{\beta}}^* + \boldsymbol{y}_0'\hat{\boldsymbol{\alpha}}^*\right)}\right]^{1/\hat{\lambda}}\right\} \tag{8.30}$$

and

$$\hat{S}(t|p^*, \boldsymbol{x}_0, \hat{\varphi}) = \exp\left\{-\left[\frac{t}{\exp\left(\boldsymbol{x}_0'\hat{\boldsymbol{\eta}}^* + \log(\hat{\varphi})\hat{\lambda}\right)}\right]^{1/\hat{\lambda}}\right\}, \tag{8.31}$$

where $\hat{\boldsymbol{\beta}}^*$, $\hat{\boldsymbol{\alpha}}^*$, $\hat{\boldsymbol{\eta}}^*$, and $\hat{\varphi}$ are the parameter estimates on log(duration), derived from the Weibull accelerated failure time model, described extensively in Chapter 4. The two sets of parameter estimates, hazard or AFT, yield exactly the same survival function estimates.

In the present illustration, I select two sets of survival curves to be calculated, one for older veterans and one for nonveterans, at two exact ages, 70 years and 85 years, based on the parameter estimates derived from the final reduced-form equation (Model D). In estimating these survival curves, the values of covariates other than those of Vet and Age_70 are fixed at sample means, so that the survival functions for older veterans and nonveterans can be compared effectively without being confounded by other predictors. Because they are all centered at sample means, the control variables need not be taken into account when predicting each set of the survival curves.

The survival curves can be easily computed and plotted by various software packages and spreadsheets. First, the reader might want to use the SAS PROC GPLOT to generate the two survival curves at age 70, shown below.

SAS Program 8.3:

```
......
* Calculating survival rates for two groups at age 70 *;

options ls=80 ps=58 nodate;
ods select all;
ods trace off;
ods listing;
title1;
run;

data Weibull_vet;
  do group = 1 to 2;
  do t = 0 to 60;
  if group = 1 then sr = exp(-exp(-7.092 + log(1.271))*(t**1.265));
  if group = 2 then sr = exp(-exp(-7.092 - 0.241 + log(1.271))*(t**1.265));
  output;
  end;
  end;
run;

proc format;
  value group_fmt 1 = 'Nonveterans'
                  2 = 'Veterans';
run;

goptions gsfname = outgraph;
goptions gsfname = outgraph;

Title "Figure 8.3. Survival functions of veterans and nonveterans";

symbol1 c=black i=splines l=1 v=plus;
symbol2 c=red i=splines l=2 v=diamond;

proc gplot data=Weibull_vet;
  format group group_fmt.;
  plot sr*t = group ;
run;;
run;
quit;
```

SAS Program 8.3 generates a clear plot of two survival curves, one for older veterans and one for nonveterans, displayed in Figure 8.3. Corresponding pairs of survival curves at other exact ages can be constructed by inserting the value of Age_70 (actual age – 70), the value of the interaction between age_70 and Vet, and their regression coefficients into the selected equations. Figure 8.3 displays the dominance of the survival function for older veterans at age 70, consistent with the analytic results estimated for the Weibull hazard model.

Sometimes the software spreadsheet is preferable to plot the survival curves if the SAS graphic formatting system is thought of as too restrictive. Use of a software spreadsheet is handy and straightforward, and the format of a survival curve can be constructed according to the researcher's preference. For example, the two survival plots in Figure 8.4, at age 70 and at age 85, respectively, come from Microsoft EXCEL. Figure 8.4 looks more constructive than Figure 8.3. In particular, it plots the evolution of survival functions for older veterans and nonveterans starting at, respectively, age 70 and age 85. The plot highlights the total effect of veteran status on the survival rate of older Americans. Panel A illustrates the two survival functions up to month 60 (five years) starting from exact age 70, whereas Panel B demonstrates the separation of the two survival curves that originate from exact age 85. At each subsequent time point, an older veteran at age 70 is expected to have a slightly higher chance of survival than his or her nonveteran counterpart, but this difference appears small because the two survival curves do not separate noticeably until the end of the observation period. On the other hand, the two survival curves starting from exact age 85 demonstrate a dramatic separation over time, with older veterans subject to much lower survival rates than nonveterans throughout the whole observation interval. The two graphs, combined, highlight the significant effect of being a veteran on the mortality of older Americans and its changing pattern in different age ranges.

The interested reader might want to create and compare more survival functions using the results presented in Table 8.2.

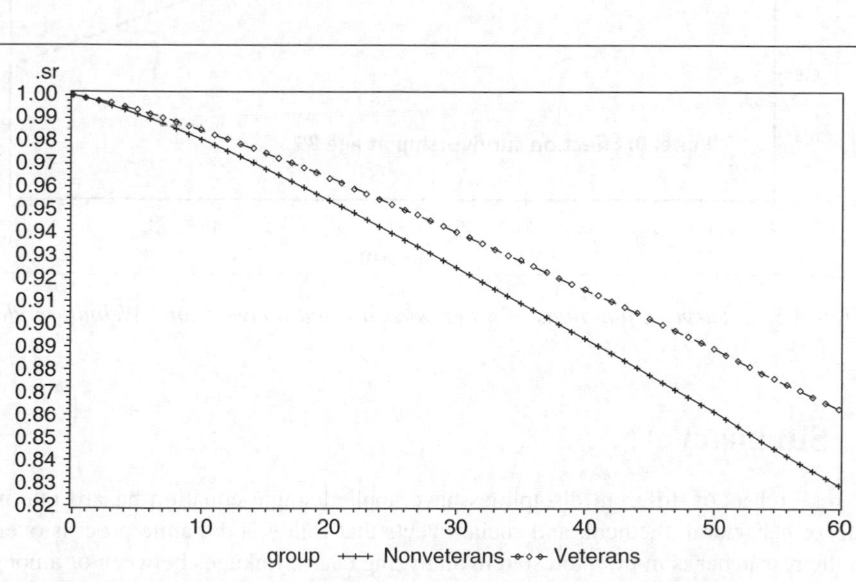

Figure 8.3 Survival functions of veterans and nonveterans.

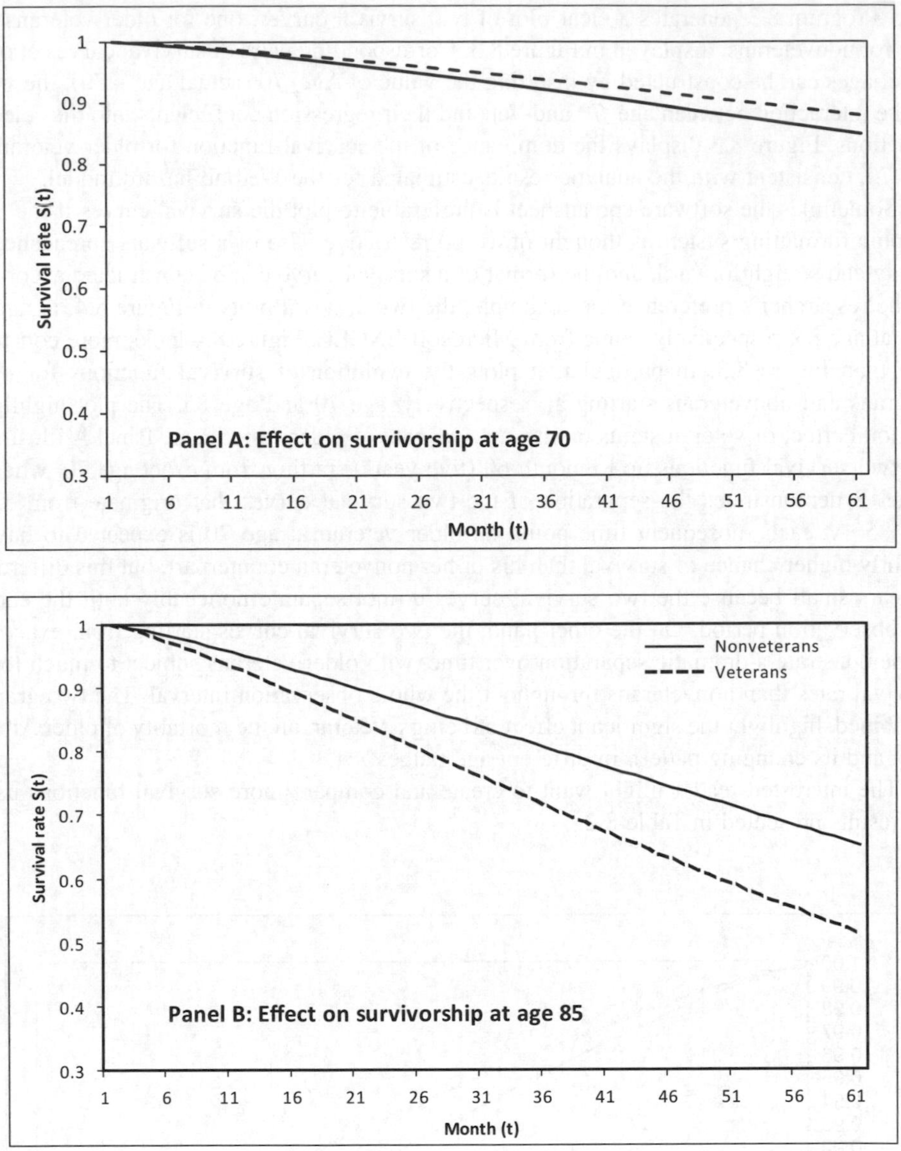

Figure 8.4 Survival functions of older veterans and nonveterans: Weibull model.

8.3 Summary

Many researchers of different disciplines have applied single-equation hazard rate models to analyze behavioral, medical, and social events that follow a dynamic process over time. When the researcher is more interested in analyzing causal linkages between or among a set of conceptual factors, the one-stage survival models are not highly suitable for demonstrating the structure of causality. By involving only a single equation, researchers are sometimes faced with a dilemma in terms of model specification. If they specify a survival model including causally related covariates, the existence of endogeneity will lead to significant bias in the total effects of covariates, although it may absorb more statistical information for predicting an underlying event (Amemiya, 1985). In contrast, a survival model eliminating endogenous variables might reflect the true set of the effects generated by exogenous variables on the stochastic processes; in the meantime, however, a single reduced-form equation can be associated with serious prediction bias, as displayed in this chapter.

In Section 8.1, the merits and the limitations of structural equation models with latent variables are briefly discussed. These methods are intended to address predicaments caused by the existence of measurement error when estimating parameters on a particular event. Given its flexibility and coverage, these structural equation models are promising for assisting in solving many specification and estimation problems. The specification of latent variables in a survival model, however, can make complex statistical models vulnerable to specification errors because the estimation of too many parameters may cause serious identification problems. If time-varying covariates are considered in a statistical model, such vulnerability would become much graver. Additionally, specification of different link functions within a unifying statistical perspective requires complicated transformation and retransformation of parameter estimates and random errors before analytic results become interpretable. While not entirely opposed to adding latent factors or classes as intervening variables, I want to caution the reader that when developing a structural hazard rate model, you need to consider whether including statistically defined factors has any theoretical or practical value to a particular study. A practical strategy is to use both models, with or without latent factors, to decide whether the specification of additional parameters is necessary and interpretable.

In this chapter, I introduce a structural hazard rate model with retransformation of random errors. This method is developed to address some of the concerns existing in structural hazard rate models. A step-by-step illustration is provided to show the interested reader how to apply this approach. Some of the specifications in this model have been theoretically addressed in the work developed by others (Manton, Stallard, and Singer, 1994; Manton *et al.*, 1994; Muthen and Muthen, 2008; Vermunt, 1997). Strictly speaking, because it does not consider the measurement part by assuming the absence of measurement error, this model is virtually an extension of path analysis. Therefore, this retransformation method is considered as a special case of structural equation modeling on survival data (Liu, 2000). Methodologically, it is more suitable for empirical studies where measurements of observed variables are relatively valid.

Questions may be raised about the fact that this structural hazard rate model is based on parameter estimates derived from separate statistical steps, rather than from a unifying estimation process. Such external estimating procedures, however, are not rare in statistical modeling (Liang and Zeger, 1986; Wei, Lin, and Weissfeld, 1989; Zeger, Liang, and Albert, 1988). A unified estimation process with multiple stages, numerous interaction terms, and different link functions can immensely complicate the derivation of parameter estimates, particularly in the presence of an underlying distribution of survival times. Specification of separate statistical models, therefore, can avoid overfitting and overparameterization of a multivariate regression. The unique contribution of this retransformation model is the articulation of procedures for estimating the indirect as well as the direct effects of the exogenous variables that are expressed in terms of the variation in the hazard rate or in the survival probability. If an underlying conceptual framework is assumed correctly and measurement error is ignorable, this estimating system provides reasonable parameter estimates for a two-stage structural hazard rate model.

Like other structural equation modeling techniques, this structural hazard rate model uses a combination of empirical data and qualitative causal assumptions. The model is a statistical approach to estimate values of free parameters on the causal relationships in a dynamic lifetime process. In essence, it is a confirmatory rather than an exploratory perspective, suitable for the verification of a well-accepted theory rather than for theory development. As indicated previously, the limitation of structural equation modeling resides in the fact that the model fit statistics for structural regression models with different presumed causal linkages have often been found to be very close or even identical, thereby making statistical testing very difficult, if not impossible. The retransformation approach is not free of this problem. Given the dynamic nature of survival data, the researcher should be very cautious when applying various structural equation modeling techniques for performing survival analysis.

9

Special topics

9.1 Informative censoring

As discussed in Chapter 1, most survival analyses deal with survival data that are incomplete. In the presence of censored data, survival models described in previous chapters are all based on the assumption that censoring is random and thereby noninformative; that is, censored data are assumed to be independent of survival times of a given population sample, thus viewed as representative of subjects at risk (Kalbfleisch and Prentice, 2002). Given this underlying assumption, censored observations can be integrated in the likelihood function by specifying the probability that lifetime T exceeds censored time C. This independence assumption on censored data is not unreasonable in most situations. In many empirical applications on lifetime events, the true cause of censored cases is often found not to be the response itself but, rather, an unmeasured variable that is only moderately correlated with the response. Failure to account for the cause seems capable of introducing only minor bias (Schafer and Graham, 2002). Little and Rubin (1999) believe that in situations where good covariate information is available and included in the analysis, the missing at-random assumption is a reasonable approximation to reality.

In some particular situations, however, censored data sometimes do not appear random with unusually high or low risk of failure, thereby demonstrating the dependence between survival times and censoring mechanisms. A prominent example is a longitudinal clinical controlled trial, in which a large proportion of dropouts prior to the observation of a given follow-up endpoint are withdrawn because of strong side effects from a specific treatment (Scharfstein *et al.*, 2001). Some medical studies suggest that a small degree of such dependence can have a noticeable effect on the analysis of survival data (Siannis, Copas, and Lu, 2005).

In this section, I describe some analytic techniques for modeling survival data in which event outcomes and censoring times are dependent and hence censoring is informative. To distinguish informative censoring from other types of missing data, I hereby tentatively

Survival Analysis: Models and Applications, First Edition. Xian Liu.

restrict censoring as the loss of follow-up observation on the response variable under investigation. Consequently, only right censoring is discussed. Other types of missing data are less detrimental to the quality of parameter estimates, so that techniques handling those problems are not included in this text. The reader interested in general issues of missing data can read Little and Rubin (2002) and Schafer and Graham (2002).

9.1.1 Selection model

A traditional approach handling informative censoring is to model the censoring process in order to derive unbiased parameter estimates in the presence of nonrandom censoring (Wu and Carroll, 1988). This work is largely motivated by the specification problems encountered in some clinical trials of certain diseases. Specifically, the use of joint modeling, originally developed by Heckman (1979), is proposed for linking the health outcome and censoring by means of a common selection factor. Given the specification of this selection factor, the two responses, survival and censoring, are thought to be conditionally independent; hence more efficient and less-biased parameter estimates can be obtained from this type of statistical modeling.

To expound specifications of the joint modeling approach, here I borrow Heckman's (1979) perspective to exhibit the potential impact of selection bias from informative censoring. To be in line with the tradition of this work, I propose a longitudinal growth model in the form of a random-effects linear regression. For a baseline sample of n individuals and J follow-up time points, I first define, for convenience of analysis, a disease severity score, Y_{ij}, to indicate health status for individual i ($i = 1, 2, \ldots, n$) at time point j ($j = 0, 1, \ldots, J$). In a typical survival analysis, Y_{ij} can be viewed as the log hazard rate for a specific disease. I then assume a hypothetical disease severity score for those who are censored between time point $j - 1$ and time point j, where $j = 1, \ldots, J$. It is further assumed that the hypothetical disease severity score for those censored at time t, denoted by Y_t^c, is greater than or equal to a constant R_t, and the disease severity score among noncensored individuals at t, Y_t^s, are all smaller than this constant R_t. This assumption is based on the belief that informative censoring in a clinical trial often comes from 'inadequate treatment responses' for a specific treatment or from deterioration of other health problems, thus implying higher severity among those who are censored (Collett, 2003; Scharfstein *et al.*, 2001; Wu and Carroll, 1988). As defined, Y_{ij} is a continuous variable.

I begin with two longitudinal random-effects linear regression models, one the complete model that includes all members of the baseline sample and the other a truncated model that consists of noncensored cases only, given by

$$\boldsymbol{Y} = \boldsymbol{X}_1'\boldsymbol{\beta}_1 + \boldsymbol{Z}_1'\boldsymbol{\gamma}_1 + \boldsymbol{\varepsilon}_1, \tag{9.1a}$$

$$(\boldsymbol{Y} \mid \boldsymbol{Y} < \boldsymbol{R}) = \boldsymbol{X}_2'\boldsymbol{\beta}_2 + \boldsymbol{Z}_2'\boldsymbol{\gamma}_2 + \boldsymbol{\varepsilon}_2, \tag{9.1b}$$

where $\boldsymbol{Y}$ represents an $(\boldsymbol{I} \times 1)$ vector of observed outcome data in the context of a block design $[\boldsymbol{I} = n \times (J + 1)]$. The matrix $\boldsymbol{X}$ is an $(\boldsymbol{I} \times M)$ matrix for $M - 1$ independent variables and $\boldsymbol{Z}$ is a $(\boldsymbol{I} \times r)$ design matrix for the between-persons random effects. The matrices $\boldsymbol{\beta}$ and $\boldsymbol{\gamma}$ are parameters for $\boldsymbol{X}$ and $\boldsymbol{Z}$, respectively. The between-persons random effects are assumed to be normally distributed with mean 0 and variance matrix $\boldsymbol{G}$. The $\boldsymbol{\varepsilon}$ terms represent within-persons random effects. The joint distribution of $\boldsymbol{\varepsilon}_1$ $\boldsymbol{\varepsilon}_2$ at a given time is assumed to be a singular distribution with covariance defined as $\boldsymbol{\sigma}_{12}$. While the residual ε_1 is assumed to be normally distributed with mean 0 and variance matrix $\boldsymbol{\sigma}_1^2\mathbf{I}$, it is implausible to assume that elements in $\boldsymbol{\varepsilon}_2$ be normally distributed with zero expectation because the error term in Equation (9.1b) may not be independent of the covariates if informative censoring occurs, as described below.

Because $\boldsymbol{Y}^c$ is not observable, a dichotomous factor δ_{ij} is defined to indicate the censoring status for individual i between time point $(j-1)$ and time point j $(j = 1, \ldots, J)$ and it is used as a proxy for R_j, given by

$$\begin{cases} \delta_{ij} = 0 \text{ if individual } i \text{ is right censored between time points } (j-1) \text{ and } j\,(Y_{ij} \geq R_j), \\ \\ \delta_{ij} = 1 \text{ if individual } i \text{ is not right censored from time points } (j-1) \text{ and } j\,\,(Y_{ij} < R_j). \end{cases}$$

Specifically, I view the disease severity score at time point j as a joint distribution of two sequential events – the likelihood of not being right censored between $(j-1)$ and j and the conditional density function on the disease severity score Y_j among those who are not censored at time point j. Given the aforementioned assumptions, the expected disability severity score for individual i at time point j can be written as

$$\mathrm{E}(Y_{ij}|\boldsymbol{X}_{2i}, \boldsymbol{Z}_{2i}, \delta_{ij}=1) = \Pr(\delta_{ij}=1|\boldsymbol{X}_{1i})\{\boldsymbol{X}_{2i}'\boldsymbol{\beta}_2 + \boldsymbol{Z}_{2i}'\boldsymbol{\gamma}_2 + \mathrm{E}[\boldsymbol{\varepsilon}_{2i}|\boldsymbol{\varepsilon}_{2i} < R_j - (\boldsymbol{X}_{1i}'\boldsymbol{\beta}_1 + \boldsymbol{Z}_{1i}'\boldsymbol{\gamma}_1)]\}. \tag{9.2}$$

Equation (9.2) displays the conditional mean of the disturbance in the noncensored sample as a function of $\boldsymbol{X}_{1i}$ and $\boldsymbol{Z}_{1i}$ if censoring is not random $(Y^c > Y^s)$. If informative censoring exists, the estimation of Equation (9.2) without considering this correlation can lead to inconsistent parameter estimates and some prediction bias. Consequently, the expected value of this disease severity score may not be correctly estimated by a conventional single-equation regression.

According to the above specifications, the existence of informative censoring can be detected by the covariance of the two random error components in the joint modeling. If they are significantly correlated, censoring time C depends on survival time T, thus indicating right censoring to be informative; if they are uncorrelated, censoring is independent of survival and therefore is noninformative. Traditionally, this simple test can be performed by creating a selection model using the probability of not censoring as the dependent variable. At this step, I propose a probit survival model, using the rationale of Heckman's (1979) two-step perspective to estimate the probability of not being censored between time points $(j-1)$ and j. Some empirical studies with joint modeling of longitudinal and survival data have applied other statistical functions to estimate the survival rate, such as the Cox model and logistic regression (Egleston *et al.*, 2006; Kurland and Heagerty, 2005; Leigh, Ward, and Fries, 1993; Pauler, McCoy, and Moinpour, 2003; Ratcliffe, Guo, and Ten Have, 2004). The probit function, however, is used here for convenience of illustration assuming a normal distribution of the survival probability from censoring. Specification of other functions would lead to the same results (Greene, 2003; Kalbfleisch and Prentice, 2002; Wu and Carroll, 1988).

For individual i at time point $(j-1)$ where $j = 1, \ldots, J$, the probability of not being censored up to time point j is given by

$$\Pr(Y_{ij} | \delta_{ij} = 1) = \Phi(X'_{i(j-1)}\boldsymbol{\beta}_p + Z'_{i(j-1)}\boldsymbol{\gamma}_p), \quad j = 1, \ldots, J, \tag{9.3}$$

where $\Phi(\cdot)$ represents the cumulative normal distribution (probit). Notice that the condition $\delta_{ij} = 1$ is equivalent to $Y_{ij} < R_j$. From this equation, the estimated survival rates for each individual in terms of $J - 1$ observation intervals can be obtained. I then save the estimates of $\Phi(\boldsymbol{X'\beta} + \boldsymbol{Z'\gamma})$ for each individual at each follow-up endpoint as an unbiased estimate of the survival rate from right censoring.

Given the assumption on the hypothetical disease severity score for those who are censored between $(j - 1)$ and j, the distribution of survivors' disease severity scores at j is truncated on the right. Accordingly, the inverse Mills ratio for individual i at j can be given by (the inverse Mills ratio is the econometric term of the hazard rate; for more details, read Greene, 2003, and Heckman ,1979)

$$\tilde{\lambda}_{ij} = -\frac{\tilde{\varphi}(X'_{i(j-1)}\boldsymbol{\beta}_p + Z'_{i(j-1)}\boldsymbol{\gamma}_p)}{\Phi(X'_{i(j-1)}\boldsymbol{\beta}_p + Z'_{i(j-1)}\boldsymbol{\gamma}_p)} \quad \text{if } \delta_{ij} = 1\,(Y < R), \tag{9.4a}$$

$$\tilde{\lambda}_{ij} = \frac{\tilde{\varphi}(X'_{i(j-1)}\boldsymbol{\beta}_p + Z'_{i(j-1)}\boldsymbol{\gamma}_p)}{1 - \Phi(X'_{i(j-1)}\boldsymbol{\beta}_p + Z'_{i(j-1)}\boldsymbol{\gamma}_p)} \quad \text{if } \delta_{ij} = 0\,(Y \geq R), \tag{9.4b}$$

where $\tilde{\varphi}(\cdot)$ represents the standard normal density function. The values of $\tilde{\lambda}$ at time 0 (baseline time) is set at zero. As defined, the inverse Mills ratio for censored observations is virtually the hazard rate of not being censored between two successive time points; for those that have not been censored, it stands for the risk of being censored within the observational interval (Greene, 2003).

With the vector $\tilde{\lambda}$ created, I propose a conditionally unbiased truncated random-effects model on the disability severity score at J time points, given by

$$\boldsymbol{Y}(Y | \delta = 1) = X'_2\boldsymbol{\beta}_3 + Z'_2\boldsymbol{\gamma}_3 + \boldsymbol{\sigma}'_{ev}\tilde{\boldsymbol{\lambda}} + \boldsymbol{\varepsilon}_3, \tag{9.5}$$

where σ_{ev} is a vector of covariance between ε_1 and $\boldsymbol{v}$ ($\boldsymbol{v}$ is the latent error vector from Equation (9.3)), specified as the regression coefficients of $\tilde{\boldsymbol{\lambda}}$. As the survival rate and the disease severity score are assumed to be inversely correlated, elements in σ_{ev} are expected to take negative signs except for the first column. With the variable $\tilde{\boldsymbol{\lambda}}$ included in the regression, the error term $\boldsymbol{\varepsilon}_3$ is assumed to have mean 0 and variance $\boldsymbol{\sigma}_3^2\mathbf{I}$ and to be uncorrelated with $\boldsymbol{X}_2$, $\boldsymbol{Z}_2$, and $\tilde{\boldsymbol{\lambda}}$. If all assumptions on error distributions are satisfied, Equation (9.5) generates unbiased and consistent parameter estimates because observations are conditionally independent of each other. Likewise, if elements in σ_{ev} are not statistically significant or the absolute values are trivial, censoring tends to be random and thereby noninformative.

Notice that, in Equation (9.5), the inclusion of $\tilde{\boldsymbol{\lambda}}$ and σ accounts for the covariance between two error terms, $\boldsymbol{\varepsilon}_1$ and $\boldsymbol{v}$, thereby indicating that the joint distribution of two sequential equations, represented by Equation (9.2), is empirically embedded in Equation (9.5).

This two-step parametric joint modeling, however, has been criticized because of considerable dependence on distributional assumptions of the nonignorable dropouts that are impossible to verify (Demirtas, 2004; Hedeker and Gibbons, 2006; Hogan, Roy, and Korkontzelou, 2004; Little and Rubin, 2002, Chapter 17; Liu *et al.*, 2011; Winship and Mare, 1992). In the face of unique characteristics involved in survival processes, the restrictive assumptions of this method on the parametric disturbance function can be readily violated, in turn degrading the quality of parameter estimates and model-based prediction.

9.1.2 Sensitivity analysis models

More recently, Scharfsten and associates propose a series of statistical models for longitudinal and survival data with informative censoring, introducing a sensitivity analysis approach based on latent factors (Scharfstein and Robins, 2002; Scharfstein, Rotnitzky, and Robins, 1999; Scharfstein *et al.*, 2001). Some other researchers follow suit (Siannis, Copas, and Lu, 2005). Rather than fitting an explicit joint distribution of survival time T and censoring time $\boldsymbol{C}$, these models are intended to perform a sensitivity analysis through a bias function and a dependence parameter. In particular, they propose to estimate and compare the treatment-specific distributions of a discrete or a continuous time-to-event variable adjusting for informative censoring due to certain measured prognostic factors. In the meantime, they allow for quantification of the sensitivity of the inference to residual dependence between time to event and censoring due to latent factors. Assuming that n independent and identically distributed (iid) copies are observed, denoted by

$$\{O_i = [Q_i, \tilde{\Delta}_i, \tilde{\Delta}_i Y_i, \bar{V}_i(Q_i)] : i = 1, \ldots, n\},$$

the following equation can be generalized:

$$\boldsymbol{O} = [\boldsymbol{Q}, \tilde{\boldsymbol{\Delta}}, \tilde{\boldsymbol{\Delta}}\boldsymbol{Y}, \bar{\boldsymbol{V}}(\boldsymbol{Q})],$$

where $\boldsymbol{O}$ is the observed data, $\boldsymbol{Q}$ is time to censoring, $\boldsymbol{Y}$ is the outcome variable measured at the fixed end-to-follow-up time j ($j = 1, \ldots, J$), $\tilde{\Delta} = \tilde{I}(Q \geq j : 1, \ldots, J)$ is the censoring indicator, and $\bar{V}_i(t) = [V(u) : 0 \leq u \leq t]$ is the history of all other variables that are recorded through time t in the absence of censoring. Given that $\boldsymbol{Y}$ is observed if and only if $\tilde{\Delta} = 1$, the observed $\boldsymbol{Y}$ $\{Q_i, i = 1, \ldots, n\}$ is marginally distributed. As specified, for those who are not censored out throughout the observation period, the censoring time Q is set as the end of each of the follow-up times.

Given the above specifications, the conditional hazard rate of $\boldsymbol{Q}$, given the history data $[\bar{V}_i(j), \boldsymbol{Y}]$, follows a stratified Cox model:

$$h_Q[j|\bar{\boldsymbol{V}}(j), \boldsymbol{Y}] = h_0[j|\bar{\boldsymbol{V}}(j)]\exp(\tilde{\alpha}_0 \boldsymbol{Y}), \tag{9.6}$$

where $h_Q[j|\bar{V}_i(j), \boldsymbol{Y}]$ is an unrestricted positive function and $\tilde{\alpha}_0$ is an unknown parameter. This equation specifies the hazard of being censored at time point j as depending on the observed history $\bar{V}_i(j)$, the unobserved outcome $\boldsymbol{Y}$, and a dependence parameter $\tilde{\alpha}_0$. If $\tilde{\alpha}_0 = 0$, censoring at j is conditionally independent of the unobserved outcome $\boldsymbol{Y}$ given the observed history $\bar{V}_i(j)$, and therefore being noninformative. In contrast, if $\tilde{\alpha}_0 \neq 0$, censoring is a function of the unobserved outcome $\boldsymbol{Y}$ and thus is informative and nonignorable. Here, the parameter $\tilde{\alpha}_0$ represents the magnitude of selection bias due to informative censoring.

The underlying philosophy of sensitivity analysis for informative censoring is summarized below. Although the magnitude of the selection bias from informative censoring cannot be identified in the absence of further knowledge on unmeasured factors, the law of $\boldsymbol{Y}$, as a function of the selection bias parameter, can be identified through a set of sensible parameterized selection bias functions linked with varying values of $\tilde{\alpha}_0$. Because the data contain no independent evidence about $\tilde{\alpha}_0$, final conclusions would depend on which value or values of $\tilde{\alpha}_0$ are considered plausible. Based on this philosophy, a number of estimation models are developed assuming a range of known $\tilde{\alpha}_0$ values and given relevant link functions and other conditions. Expected values of outcome Y with varying values of $\tilde{\alpha}_0$ can then be compared, evaluated, and interpreted by experts in a relevant subject matter according to prior knowledge about the possible impact censoring yields. Therefore, the so-called sensitivity analysis is a statistical approach that can provide a potentially plausible range for the parameter $\tilde{\alpha}_0$, including its magnitude and direction, rather than a single estimate of a dependence parameter. Substantive inferences largely depend on subjective and empirical feelings about the pattern of variations in the response variable.

9.1.3 Comments on current models handling informative censoring

Unfortunately, none of the currently existing models on informative censoring has so far worked well. The joint modeling approach is based on some very restrictive assumptions, so that parameter estimates can be highly sensitive to minor deviations from its underlying assumptions, such as a lack of normality. Empirically, the degree of its adjustments in longitudinal data analysis is often found to be very limited (Liu *et al.*, 2010). The sensitivity techniques relax some of the restrictions, but they are basically approaches for providing a range of possible alternatives, rather than deriving a single estimate with a confidence interval, thereby displaying its limited usage in survival analysis. As commented by Little and Rubin (1999, pp. 1130) on Scharfstein, Rotnitzky, and Robins (2001), in sensitivity analysis the magnitude of the selection bias cannot be identified, and neither can any functional form of informative censoring mechanisms be determined. As there is no way of knowing the level of dependence between the event time and censoring time, different forms of sensitivity analysis and conclusions derived from them are based on subjective assumptions on possible selection bias mechanisms. As a result, the true impact of informative censoring on the response variable will remain uncertain.

Perhaps due to these problems, SAS survival and hazard model procedures, like most of the other statistical software packages, do not include any algorithm that directly handles informative censoring. If encountering survival data with strong informative censoring, the researcher can program a survival model using an SAS code with some additional parameters addressing censoring mechanisms. The PROC NLMIXED procedure, for example, can be used to create such models (Littell *et al.*, 2006) . Until now, however, there is no consensus regarding whether there is a satisfactory way to compare survival times of two or more groups of individuals in the presence of informative censoring (Collett, 2003). Because one cannot verify or contradict whether or not selection of dropouts is random by simply examining observed data (Demirtas, 2004; Little and Rubin, 2002, Chapter 15), it may be helpful to conduct mathematical simulations on analytic results generated from different statistical models handling various types of censoring. If censoring tends not to be random, caution must be exercised in interpreting the results obtained from a survival model, especially the standard errors and confidence intervals of parameter estimates.

9.2 Bivariate and multivariate survival functions

Most regression models are performed by assuming conditional independence of observations in the presence of specific model parameters. In survival analysis, an individual's event time T is generally assumed to follow a univariate distributional pattern, with heterogeneity of the event's occurrences accounted for by a number of measurable individual or contextual factors, as described extensively in some of the earlier chapters. In certain circumstances, however, failure times are correlated even in the presence of model parameters, so that the independence hypothesis on survival times is violated. Such data with dependence are generally referred to as the *multivariate survival time data*. An individual might experience event repetitions within an observation period, as described in Chapter 7, or some individuals might be clustered by some unknown characteristics, thereby making their failure times correlated. With dependence of failure times in observations, the application of conventional estimating procedures can result in biased parameter estimates and erroneous model-based predictions.

Statisticians, demographers, and other quantitative methodologists have developed a variety of statistical models to handle survival time data with unobserved dependence. In Chapter 7, the statistical structure for repeated events has been described, with association of observations existing within persons. In this section, I introduce statistical conditions and properties for survival time data clustered between persons. First, I present theories and methods dealing with bivariate survival data, an important component of multivariate survival models in the literature. Second, some estimating approaches of multivariate survival models are described. Lastly, I provide a brief discussion on how to analyze bivariate and multivariate survival data using an SAS code.

9.2.1 Inference of the bivariate survival model

The bivariate survival model is developed to deal with survival time data when subjects are paired. Examples of bivariate data structures include twin survival patterns (Holt and Prentice, 1974; Hougaard, Harvald, and Holm, 1992; Oaks, 1989), the occurrence of vision loss in the left and right eyes (Huster, Brookmeyer, and Self, 1989), parental history of a given disease on the incidence in the offspring (Clayton, 1978), and mortality of married couples at older ages (Hougaard, 2000).

Suppose that there are lifetime variables T_1, T_2 associated with a typical pair (e.g., human twin). The survival and the distributional functions can be written as

$$S(t_1,t_2)=\Pr(T_1>t_1,T_2>t_2) \tag{9.7}$$

$$F(t_1,t_2)=\Pr(T_1\le t_1,T_2\le t_2) \tag{9.8}$$

for $t_1 \ge 0$, $t_2 \ge 0$. Given the relationship between survival and density functions, the joint density function for t_1 and t_2 is

$$f(t_1,t_2)=-\frac{\partial^2 S(t_1,t_2)}{\partial t_1 \partial t_2}. \tag{9.9}$$

Given Equation (9.9), the marginal hazard functions for the two members of a given pair are defined by

$$h_1(t)=-\frac{\partial S(t_1,t_2)/\partial t_1}{S(t_1,t_2)}\Big|_{t_1=t_2=t}, \tag{9.10a}$$

$$h_2(t)=-\frac{\partial S(t_1,t_2)/\partial t_2}{S(t_1,t_2)}\Big|_{t_1=t_2=t}. \tag{9.10b}$$

Similarly, the conditional hazard rate function, defined as the hazard rate for one member of a given pair conditional on the survival status of the other, is given by

$$h_{12}(t_1 | t_2) = -\frac{\partial^2 S(t_1, t_2) / \partial t_1 \partial t_2}{S(t_1, t_2) / \partial t_2}, \tag{9.11a}$$

$$h_{21}(t_2 | t_1) = -\frac{\partial^2 S(t_1, t_2) / \partial t_1 \partial t_2}{S(t_1, t_2) / \partial t_1}. \tag{9.11b}$$

The hazard rates for the two members may be associated because they share some genetically common but unobservable characteristic. Therefore, it is reasonable to assume that for those two members, one's failure time predicts that of the other, and so also for the reverse. Given this assumption, the following constant hazard ratio can be assumed (Clayton, 1978):

$$\frac{h_{12}(t_1 | T_2 = t_2)}{h_{12}(t_1 | T_2 > t_2)} = \frac{h_{21}(t_2 | T_1 = t_1)}{h_{21}(t_2 | T_1 > t_1)} = \theta. \tag{9.12}$$

The value of θ denotes the extent to which T_1 and T_2 are associated. If $\theta = 1$, the two marginal hazard rates h_1 and h_2 are independent of each other, thus suggesting the absence of an association between T_1 and T_2. If $\theta > 1$, the failure times for the two members are positively associated and neglect of this term can lead to biased parameter estimates on the hazard rate. When the condition $\theta > 1$ is considered in a statistical model, observations are thought to be conditionally independent, so that more efficient parameter estimates are derived. The scenario $\theta < 1$ is a condition that rarely occurs in reality and therefore it is not discussed in this text.

Given the specification of θ, the bivariate survival function can be mathematically written as

$$S(t_1, t_2) = \int_{t_1}^{\infty} \int_{t_2}^{\infty} f(u, v)\, \mathrm{d}v \mathrm{d}u = \theta \int_{t_1}^{\infty} f(u, t_2)\, \mathrm{d}u \int_{t_2}^{\infty} f(t_1, v)\, \mathrm{d}v. \tag{9.13}$$

In Equation (9.13), the joint survival function is simply expressed as the product of two marginal survival functions and θ, so that the correlation of the two survival times is under control.

Oaks (1982) reparameterizes the above bivariate survival rate as the function of survival, rather than of a combination of the density, marginals, and θ, given by

$$S(t_1, t_2) = \left\{ \left[\frac{1}{S(t_1)} \right]^{\theta - 1} + \left[\frac{1}{S(t_2)} \right]^{\theta - 1} - 1 \right\}^{-1/(\theta - 1)}, \tag{9.14}$$

where $S(t_j)$ is the marginal survival function for member j (j = 1, 2 within pair i), with $S(t_1) = S(t_1, 0)$ and $S(t_2) = S(0, t_2)$. Accordingly, the bivariate hazard function is

$$h(t_1, t_2) = \frac{f(t_1, t_2)}{S(t_1, t_2)} = h_{12}(t_1 | t_2)\, h_{21}(t_2 | t_1) - \frac{\partial^2}{\partial t_1 \partial t_2} [-\log S(t_1, t_2)], \tag{9.15}$$

where the second term on the right of the equation is the second derivative of the bivariate cumulative hazard function. Therefore, the bivariate hazard function is the product of the conditional hazard rates for the two members minus the covariance.

Assuming the association between T_1 and T_2 to be proportional, Equation (9.15) can be rewritten as

$$h(t_1,t_2)=\theta h_{12}(t_1|t_2)h_{21}(t_2|t_1). \tag{9.16}$$

If there is no association between the two failure times, $\theta = 1$ and the bivariate hazard rate is simply the product of the two conditional hazard rates.

The multivariate survival analysis, in which lifetime variables $T_1, \ldots, T_a$ are associated within a specific unit with $n_i \geq 2$, is simply an extension of the bivariate perspective. Other than repeated events described in Chapter 7, one example of the multivariate model is the sibship effect of age at death from a specific disease. The survival and the multivariate density functions are defined as

$$S(t_1,\ldots,t_Q)=\Pr(T_1 \geq t_1,\ldots,T_2 \geq t_Q), \tag{9.17}$$

$$f(t_1,\ldots,t_Q)=-\frac{\partial^Q S(t_1,\ldots,t_Q)}{\partial t_1 \cdots \partial t_Q}. \tag{9.18}$$

In addition to the approach adjusting for the effect of multivariate survival times externally, described in Chapter 7, a general approach for estimating multivariate survival models is to specify independence among observations conditional on a set of latent factors. Given its mathematical complexity and a lack of maturity in empirical applications (Hougaard, 2000), multivariate survival models with latent factors are not further described in this section; some related specifications, however, are described in Section 9.3. The interested reader might want to read Clayton and Cuzick (1985), Hougaard (2000), Hougaard, Harvald, and Holm (1992), and Lawless (2003, Chapter 11).

9.2.2 Estimation of bivariate and multivariate survival models

In estimating a bivariate or a multivariate survival model, the key is to specify a valid and reliable quantity measuring the association between the failure times of matched pairs or clusters. There is a wide array of models proposed to derive efficient parameter estimates for multivariate survival data. Lin (1994) develops a marginal approach formulating the marginal distribution of multivariate failure times with the Cox model. This method does not specify the pattern of dependence among correlated failure times; rather, it constructs robust variance–covariance estimators to account for the intracluster correlation, thus yielding consistent and asymptotically normal parameter estimates. Largely analogous to the method proposed by Liang and Zeger (1986) in longitudinal data analysis, the marginal approach has the advantage that types of dependence need not be specified in yielding reliable and consistent parameter estimates. This is thought to be because the process $n^{1/2}\left(\hat{\boldsymbol{\beta}}-\boldsymbol{\beta}^*\right)$ tends to have an asymptotic normal distribution with mean 0 and a robust variance estimator $n\boldsymbol{I}\left(\hat{\boldsymbol{\beta}}\right)^{-1}\hat{\boldsymbol{\Sigma}}\boldsymbol{I}\left(\hat{\boldsymbol{\beta}}\right)^{-1}$, where $\boldsymbol{I}\left(\hat{\boldsymbol{\beta}}\right)$ is the observed information matrix and $\hat{\boldsymbol{\Sigma}}$ is the score statistic variance estimator. As both $\hat{\boldsymbol{\beta}}$ and $\boldsymbol{I}\left(\hat{\boldsymbol{\beta}}\right)$ can be obtained from the standard Cox model, this robust marginal, external method is relatively simple without involving additional statistical inferences. Though overestimating a covariate's effect on the analysis of repeated events, as indicated in Chapter 7, this sandwich approach fits adequately for analyzing clustered data between persons because left truncation is not an issue with respect to a single event (Kalbfleisch and Prentice, 2002). As it is similar to the WLW sandwich approach introduced in Chapter 7, I do not further describe detailed specifications of this method in this section.

Besides the popular sandwich estimator, some classical estimating approaches for analyzing multivariatc survival data need to be mentioned. Most of those earlier models propose conditional specifications of survival and hazard rate functions for underlying mechanisms of dependence. Holt and Prentice (1974), for example, adapt the Cox proportional hazard model to the context of twins or other matched pairs in which the baseline hazard function $h_0(\cdot)$ is permitted to vary from pair to pair (in the following text, I refer to this method as the Holt–Prentice (HP) model). For member j (j = 1, 2) within the ith pair ($i = 1, \ldots, n'$) with covariate vector $\boldsymbol{x}$, the basic hazard function, denoted by *HP Model I*, is

$$h_{\mathrm{ij}}(t, \boldsymbol{x}_{\mathrm{ij}}) = h_{0i}(t)\exp(\boldsymbol{x}'_{\mathrm{ij}}\boldsymbol{\beta}), \tag{9.19}$$

where $\boldsymbol{\beta}$ is a vector of unknown parameters and the baseline hazard function $h_{0i}(.)$ is constant within pair i but may vary over matched pairs. (Note that the nonitalicized j differs conceptually from the italicized j, as specified in Chapter 5.) Clearly, the underlying assumption of this model is that the two members within a specific pair share exactly the same baseline hazard rate, with variability addressed by different values in $\boldsymbol{x}$.

HP further contend that given the usual small sample size in paired studies, models more restrictive than HP Model I may be developed to increase the precision of $\boldsymbol{\beta}$ estimates. Accordingly, between-pairs properties are assumed to also have multiplicative effects on the hazard rate, in turn permitting the baseline function $h_{0i}(t)$ to vary over a multiplicative constant $\bar{\alpha}_i$. Given this specification, Equation (9.19) becomes

$$h_{\mathrm{ij}}(t, \boldsymbol{x}_{\mathrm{ij}}) = \bar{\alpha}_i h_0(t)\exp(\boldsymbol{x}'_{\mathrm{ij}}\boldsymbol{\beta}). \tag{9.20}$$

Based on this specification, HP consider two additional models, denoted by, respectively, *HP Model II* and *HP Model III*. In particular, HP Model II follows an exponential distribution, given by

$$h_{\mathrm{ij}}(t, \boldsymbol{x}_{\mathrm{ij}}) = \bar{\alpha}_i \exp(\boldsymbol{x}'_{\mathrm{ij}}\boldsymbol{\beta}). \tag{9.21}$$

Correspondingly, HP Model III is a Weibull regression model:

$$h_{\mathrm{ij}}(t, \boldsymbol{x}_{\mathrm{ij}}) = \bar{\alpha}_i t^{\tilde{p}-1}\exp(\boldsymbol{x}'_{\mathrm{ij}}\boldsymbol{\beta}). \tag{9.22}$$

For each of the above three models (HP Models I, II, and III), unknown parameters h_0, $\tilde{p}$, and β are estimated in the form of the maximum marginal likelihood. As defined, $\bar{\alpha}_i$ reflects a cluster or pair effect (Lawless, 2003). In specification of the exponential and Weibull functions, this cluster effect is assumed to be fixed given their parametric nature.

For survival data without censoring, the probability of experiencing a certain event over a pair for Model I is

$$\begin{cases} \Pr(T_{i2} < T_{i2}) = \{\exp[\boldsymbol{\beta}(\boldsymbol{x}_{i1} - \boldsymbol{x}_{i2})] + 1\}^{-1}, \\ \Pr(T_{i1} < T_{i2}) = \{\exp[-\boldsymbol{\beta}(\boldsymbol{x}_{i1} - \boldsymbol{x}_{i2})] + 1\}^{-1}, \end{cases} \quad (9.23a, 9.23b)$$

where T_{i1} and T_{i2} are failure times for members 1 and 2 in the ith pair. As specified above, T_{i1} and T_{i2} for pair i differ only with different values of covariates. The marginal likelihood function for $\boldsymbol{\beta}$ in Model I is proportional to the product of Equations (9.23a) and (9.23b).

Likewise, the marginal likelihood functions for $\boldsymbol{\beta}$ in HP Models II and III are

$$\begin{cases} L_2(\boldsymbol{\beta}) \propto \prod_{i=1}^{n'} \left\{ \exp[\boldsymbol{\beta}(\boldsymbol{x}_{i1} - \boldsymbol{x}_{i2})] \left[1 + \left(\frac{T_{i1}}{T_{i2}} \right) \exp[\boldsymbol{\beta}(\boldsymbol{x}_{i1} - \boldsymbol{x}_{i2})] \right]^{-2} \right\}, & (9.24) \\ L_3(\tilde{p}, \boldsymbol{\beta}) \propto \prod_{i=1}^{n'} \left\{ \tilde{p} \left(\frac{T_{i1}}{T_{i2}} \right)^{\tilde{p}-1} \exp[\boldsymbol{\beta}(\boldsymbol{x}_{i1} - \boldsymbol{x}_{i2})] \left[1 + \left(\frac{T_{i1}}{T_{i2}} \right) \exp[\boldsymbol{\beta}(\boldsymbol{x}_{i1} - \boldsymbol{x}_{i2})] \right]^{-2} \right\}. & (9.25) \end{cases}$$

The log of the ratio (T_{i1}/T_{i2}) from HP Models II and III have logistic density functions. It is believed that if full data are available, efficient estimators of $\boldsymbol{\beta}$ can be obtained from several parametric alternatives, especially the Weibull model (Lawless, 2003; Wild, 1983).

When survival data are censored, however, the invariance arguments used in creating the marginal likelihoods for the exponential and Weibull models break down, and the distribution of the above marginally sufficient statistics generally depends on the censoring times and nuisance parameters (Holt and Prentice, 1974; Wild, 1983). In the presence of censoring, Holt and Prentice (1974) introduce the concept of a doubly censored pair (two members of a pair share the same censoring time) that is marginally sufficient under HP Model I. Then the likelihood function is

$$L_1(\boldsymbol{\beta}) = \prod_{i=1}^{c'} \{\exp[\tilde{\varepsilon}_i \boldsymbol{\beta}(\boldsymbol{x}_{i1} - \boldsymbol{x}_{i2})] + 1\}^{-1}, \quad (9.26)$$

where pairs $i = 1, 2, \ldots, c'$ are uncensored or singly censored, whereas pairs $c' + 1, c' + 2, \ldots, n'$ are doubly censored. The parameter $\tilde{\varepsilon}_i = 1$ if $T_{i2} < T_{i1}$ and $\tilde{\alpha}_i = -1$ if $T_{i1} < T_{i2}$. Thus, consistent estimates of $\boldsymbol{\beta}$ in HP Model I can be based on the likelihood corresponding to the observed portion of the marginally sufficient statistic described above. This result does not hold under HP Models II and III because the ratio T_{i1}/T_{i2}, a required element in likelihood functions (9.24) and (9.25), is not observable with censoring. Given such, HP propose to analyze the survival data of matched pairs using the same rationale for HP Model I; that is, $\boldsymbol{\beta}$ can be estimated exactly by using the observable part of the likelihoods.

Obviously, the HP models are based on several restrictive assumptions so that the quality of parameter estimates derived from the HP approach rely considerably on whether or not those assumptions correspond with reality. Some researchers are concerned with the limitations of those bivariate survival models in the presence of censoring. For example, Wild (1983) raises doubts about the consistency of the above estimators. The use of an observable portion of the aforementioned likelihood functions leads to the omission of doubly censored pairs, and in the case of the exponential function, the assumption that $\boldsymbol{\beta} = 0$ would be biased. Furthermore, the stratified proportional hazard rate model provides an equally efficient but much simpler approach (Lawless, 2003).

Wild (1983) extends the Holt–Prentice approach by treating the cluster or pair effect $\bar{\alpha}_i$ as randomly distributed, independent of $\boldsymbol{x}$. A gamma distribution is assumed for the random term h_{0i}, with the probability density function

$$f(t) = \frac{\lambda(\lambda t)^{\tilde{k}-1} e^{-\lambda t}}{\lambda(\tilde{k})} \quad t > 0, \tag{9.27}$$

where $\tilde{k} > 0$ and $\lambda > 0$ are parameters (λ is a scale parameter and $\tilde{k}$ is a shape parameter, as described in Chapter 3). This parametric distribution includes the exponential function as a special case when $\tilde{k} = 1$.

Let $d_{ij} = 1$ if T_{ij} is a failure time and $d_{ij} = 0$ if otherwise, $d_i = \Sigma_j d_{ij}$, and $d = \Sigma d_i$. Given the condition that $h_{0i} \sim \gamma(\tilde{k}, \lambda)$, the likelihood function with a noninformative right censoring mechanism is given by

$$L(\tilde{k}, \lambda, \tilde{p}, \boldsymbol{\beta}) \propto \prod \left[\frac{\lambda^{\tilde{k}} \Gamma(\tilde{k} + d_i) \tilde{p}^{d_i} \bar{C}_i \bar{B}_i}{\Gamma(\tilde{k})(\lambda + \bar{S}_i)^{\tilde{k}+d_i}} \right], \tag{9.28}$$

where

$$\bar{C}_i = \prod\nolimits_j T_{ij}^{d_{ij}(\tilde{p}-1)},$$

$$\bar{B}_i = \exp\left(\boldsymbol{\beta} \sum\nolimits_j d_{ij} \boldsymbol{x}_{ij}\right),$$

$$\bar{S}_i = \sum\nolimits_j T_{ij}^{\tilde{p}} \exp(\boldsymbol{x}_{ij}' \boldsymbol{\beta}).$$

Given the specification of the parameter d_{ij}, the Wild approach provides more precise estimates of $\boldsymbol{\beta}$ than the exponential or the Weibull model if the cluster size n_i is small and censoring is heavy. As a result, the Wild estimator has seen extensive use in empirical studies with survival data of a bivariate nature.

Sometimes the baseline hazard for pair i, h_{0i}, is viewed as representing a basic but unobserved characteristic of the individuals being studied (e.g., genetic predisposition of human twins). If the important risk factors on the hazard rate are mostly considered in model covariates, including those causing the correlation of matched data, the h_{0i} values would be identically distributed according to a unimodal distribution (Wild, 1983). In biological and medical sciences, however, many potential risk factors are not identifiable or measurable, especially those accounting for between-pair differences. In such situations, observations may be correlated, even in the presence of selected covariates, and therefore statistical structures need to be modified to account for a potential lack of independence. Random-effects survival models are therefore popular in biomedical studies. The theoretical issues and statistical models of survival data with dependence will be further described and discussed in Section 9.3.

9.2.3 Illustration of marginal models handling multivariate survival data

Currently, there are a number of computer software packages that have capabilities to analyze bivariate and multivariate survival data. Among them, the most popular are SAS, STATA, MLwiN, and WinBUGS. Using SAS as the major instrument for computer programming of empirical illustrations, I do not describe other software packages in this text. Kelly (2004) provides a useful overview of features and capabilities for each of the major software packages in this area, so the reader interested in gaining knowledge of other software packages might want to read that article.

As described in Chapter 7, survival data with recurrent events, a unique type of survival data with dependence, can be analyzed by using marginal models (Wei, Lin, and Weissfeld, 1989). Those models, shown to overestimate covariates effects on a repeated event, are perhaps more suitable for analyzing other types of correlated survival data, including data of matched pairs and clustered data structures (Lin, 1994). The marginal model developed by Lin and Wei (1989), boasting the most widely used perspective in this area, estimates regression coefficients in the Cox model by the maximum likelihood estimates, assuming an independent working correlation structure, as extensively introduced in Chapter 7. Specifically, it uses a robust sandwich covariance estimator to account for the intraclusters dependence in survival data. This procedure can be handily programmed in SAS by using the COVS(AGGREGATE) option in the PROC PHREG procedure, given by the following program.

SAS Program 9.1:

```
*Creation of a Cox model with robust sandwich estimate;
proc phreg data=<name of data file> covs(aggregate);
   model time*status(0) = <list of covariates>;
   id = <variable name for cluster id>;
run;
```

In the above SAS program, ID indicates the unit for pairs or clusters and the keyword AGGREGATE enclosed in parentheses requests a summing up of the score residuals for each distinct ID pattern in computation of the robust sandwich covariance estimate. Without the ID statement, the AGGREGATE option has no effect. As this type of marginal models and its application in SAS have been described in Chapter 7, further illustration is not provided.

Random-effects survival models can be programmed by applying the SAS NLMIXED procedure by defining a random-effect latent variable with a known distribution, as described in the next section.

9.3 Frailty models

As mentioned above, the association between two or more members of a matched cluster arises because they share some common characteristics, not because one event influences the other. Without considering the potential impact of this association, unobserved heterogeneity might produce bias to parameter estimates, especially the estimator of standard errors. Some quantitative methodologists attempt to analyze such survival data by defining a quantity termed 'frailty,' a convenient notion used most frequently by mathematical biologists and demographers (Hougaard, 1986; Vaupel, Manton, and Stallard, 1979). Here, frailty may refer to a broad range of dimensions, such as genetic predisposition, physiological senescence parameters, economic capability, family history of diseases, and the like (Hougaard, 1995; Manton *et al.*, 1994; Vaupel, Manton, and Stallard, 1979). Correspondingly, a number of frailty models have been developed to account for correlated survival times thus making observations conditionally independent.

In this section, I introduce several frailty models. First, I briefly describe the frailty theory and the formulations of the survival model with individual frailty, originally developed by Vaupel, Manton, and Stallard (1979) and later advanced and commented on by a number of other scientists (Aalen, 1994; Andersen *et al.*, 1993; Hougaard, 1995, 2000; Lin, 1994). Second, a correlated frailty model, developed by Yashin and associates (Yashin and Iachine, 1995; Yashin, Vaupel, and Iachine, 1995), is briefly introduced. Lastly, I provide an empirical illustration with SAS programs for the application of frailty models.

9.3.1 Hazard models with individual frailty

In the frailty theory, individuals in a random sample have different levels of frailty, and the frailer ones tend to die sooner than the others, other covariates being equal. Because survival is selected systematically by this unobserved frailty factor, the true stochastic process of the hazard function for a population may be masked as a consequence of continued changes in the health composition (Vaupel, Manton, and Stallard, 1979). In particular, selection eliminates less fit individuals from a given cohort as its age increases. Its mortality rate increases less rapidly with age than it would otherwise because the surviving members of the cohort are the ones who are most fit. As a result, the observed hazard function for a population or a population subgroup is often found to rise exponentially at the younger and middle age; then the rate of increase is leveled-off or even declines at older ages. In the frailty theory, this phenomenon is interpreted as the consequence of the reduction in the average 'frailty.'

The existence of an unobserved 'frailty' effect can alter the pattern of mortality differences. There are numerous reports in recent years that age-specific mortality rates of different population subgroups cross in ways that are unanticipated (Hirsch, Liu, and Witten, 2000; Liu and Witten, 1995; Vaupel and Yashin, 1985a). Biological explanations of this crossover phenomenon are based on the frailty theory, assuming the intersecting mortality functions to represent heterogeneous populations that differ in frailty (Manton, Poss, and Wing, 1979; Vaupel, Manton, and Stallard, 1979). A cohort of a genetically or environmentally frail population experiences its youth with a mortality that is greater than that of a genetically or environmentally strong population as their age increases, leading to a greater death rate in the frail population. Gradually, the mortality rate for the frail population increases less rapidly with age because stronger members are more likely to survive. When this selection effect among the frail population becomes strong enough to offset the impact of the initial frailty, the mortality rates for the initially frail and the initially strong populations tend to converge and a mortality crossover may occur.

The original frailty model assumes a heterogeneous lifetime pattern to address the effects of some latent covariates (Aalen, 1994; Hougaard, 1986, 2000; Vaupel, Manton, and Stallard, 1979). Specifically, the unobserved frailty factor can be represented by defining an unobservable random effect, which impacts the baseline hazard function multiplicatively, written by

$$h(t,z,\boldsymbol{x}) = zh_0(t)\exp(\boldsymbol{x}'\boldsymbol{\beta}), \tag{9.29}$$

where z is the frailty factor, with values varying around the grand mean of this variable. As a result, the frailty factor can be modeled as an arbitrarily assumed individual-level random effect. This model has tremendous appeal because the hazard function with the frailty effect can be expressed as the regular proportional hazard model added to a multiplier of random effects. Given the nonnegative nature of the hazard rate, an individual z is also nonnegative, presumed to follow a given parametric distribution. Conditional on this random effect variable z, the failure times are assumed to be independent of each other, so that more efficient estimates of $\boldsymbol{\beta}$ can be derived.

The distribution of this random effect z determines how the specification of a frailty factor affects the expected value of the hazard. Vaupel, Manton, and Stallard (1979) recommend that, given its flexible mathematical properties, a gamma distribution should be used to reflect frailty at birth, with the density function

$$f(t) = \frac{\lambda(\lambda t)^{\tilde{k}-1} e^{-\lambda t}}{\Gamma(\tilde{k})}, \quad t > 0. \tag{9.30}$$

The parameters $\tilde{k}$ and λ in Equation (9.30) have been described previously on several occasions. The mean and variance of the gamma distribution are well defined:

$$\mathrm{E}(z) = \frac{\tilde{k}}{\lambda}, \tag{9.31}$$

$$\mathrm{Var}(z) = \frac{\tilde{k}}{\lambda^2}. \tag{9.32}$$

Given the above specifications, the expected hazard rate with frailty term z following a gamma distribution and covariate vector $\boldsymbol{x}$ can be written as

$$\begin{aligned} \mathrm{E}[h(t,z,\boldsymbol{x})] &= \int zh_0(t)\exp(\boldsymbol{x}'\boldsymbol{\beta})\mathrm{d}F(z) \\ &= \frac{h_0(t)\exp(\boldsymbol{x}'\boldsymbol{\beta})\tilde{k}}{\lambda} \\ &= h_0(t)\exp\left[\boldsymbol{x}'\boldsymbol{\beta} + \log\left(\frac{\tilde{k}}{\lambda}\right)\right], \end{aligned} \tag{9.33}$$

where the error distributional function F is the cumulative density function of z.

For analytic convenience, the mean of z is often set at 1, in turn imposing the conditions that $\lambda = \tilde{k}$ and $\sigma^2 = 1/\tilde{k} = 1/\lambda$. Without these conditions, the estimation of Equation (9.33) would become more complicated due to the addition of model parameters into the estimation of the hazard model. Klein and Moeschberger (2003) recommend the use of an expectation maximization (EM) algorithm for estimating the observable random effect. Specifically, EM is an iterative method that alternates between performing an expectation (E) step and a maximization (M) step and computes parameters maximizing the expected log-likelihood on the E step (Dempster, Laird, and Rubin, 1977). Alternatively, there are some other efficient methods for approximating the integral of the likelihood over the random effects, such as the Gaussian quadrature algorithm. These estimators, however, can sometimes yield different parameter estimates on the hazard function.

Some scientists (Aalen, 1994; Hougaard, 1995, 2000) comment on the use of a gamma distribution for the frailty factor z. Given its mathematical attractiveness with its simple densities, the use of a gamma distribution has several advantages (Vaupel, Manton, and Stallard, 1979). This parametric distribution, however, does have some specification weaknesses (Aalen, 1994; Hougaard, 1995, 2000; Lin, 1994). The basic frailty model, represented by Equation (9.33), cannot be conveniently transformed into a conventional generalized linear regression with a normally distributed error term, thus causing difficulty in interpreting its results. Aalen (1994) suggests that the nature of the frailty effect must be derived from biological knowledge and theoretical assumptions about the known risk factors the frailty factor represents. He provides an example in terms of the effect of blood pressure and serum cholesterol on the incidence of myocardial infarction among middle aged men, contending that both factors are approximately normally distributed with some skewness to the right. It follows that the relative risk due to these factors should be approximately lognormally distributed.

Taking log values on both sides of Equation (9.29) gives rise to

$$\begin{aligned}\log\left[h(t,z,\boldsymbol{x})\right] &= \log\left[h_0(t)\right] + \boldsymbol{x}'\boldsymbol{\beta} + \log(z) \\ &= \log\left[h_0(t)\right] + \boldsymbol{x}'\boldsymbol{\beta} + \varepsilon,\end{aligned} \tag{9.34}$$

where $\log[h_0(t)]$ can be viewed as the intercept and $\varepsilon = \log(z)$. If z is lognormally distributed, then ε is normally distributed with mean 0 and variance σ^2, thereby ushering in a typical generalized linear model with a normally distributed error term.

For a transformed error term with normal distribution, the mean and variance of the frailty factor z are

$$\mathrm{E}(\exp[\varepsilon]) = \exp\left(\varepsilon + \frac{\sigma^2}{2}\right) = \exp\left(\frac{\sigma^2}{2}\right) \tag{9.35}$$

and

$$\begin{aligned}\mathrm{Var}(\exp[\varepsilon]) &= \exp(2u)\left\{\exp\left[2\sigma^2 - \exp(\sigma^2)\right]\right\} \\ &= \exp\left[2\sigma^2 - \exp(\sigma^2)\right].\end{aligned} \tag{9.36}$$

Equations (9.35) and (9.36) are similar to Equations (8.9) and (8.10). Therefore, the random effects in a frailty model can be viewed as those from eliminating statistically important predictor variables, not just from those concerning genetic predisposition. Obviously, the lognormal specification for the frailty factor is a more convenient and parsimonious choice than a gamma distribution. The positive skewness of the lognormal distribution also conforms to the presumption given by the frailty theory. It can be further inferred that if the distribution of random effects does not follow a known function, the nonparametric hazard rate model, described in Chapter 8, can be used to account for unobserved heterogeneity if the sample size is sufficiently large.

Empirically, the application of the above frailty models is not without concerns, especially in the analysis of large-scale survey data. The multiplicative effect of the unobserved frailty factor, independently drawn from a gamma or a lognormal distribution, is assumed to be orthogonal to inferences about other parameters. In reality, an individual's frailty should be closely interacted with many observed factors, and some researchers even use an observable covariate directly as the proxy to measure an individual's level of frailty (Kurland and Heagerty, 2005). If the risk set at a given failure time contains a fairly large number of individuals with covariates scaled at many levels, the unobserved heterogeneity generated from omission of an important latent factor can be easily averaged out by the fixed effects (Arjas, 1988). As commented by Andersen *et al.* (1993), given the process $\sqrt{n}\left(\hat{\boldsymbol{\beta}}-\boldsymbol{\beta}^*\right)\to 0$ as $n \to \infty$, the frailty model, particularly with a gamma distribution, is not statistically supported by the large-sample theory.

Another perspective for modeling the frailty effect is the use of stratification. Equation (9.29) can be extended to the following specification:

$$
\begin{aligned}
h_{ij}(t, z_i, \boldsymbol{x}_{ij}) &= z_i h_0(t)\exp(\boldsymbol{x}_{ij}'\boldsymbol{\beta}) \\
&= h_{0i}(t)\exp(\boldsymbol{x}_{ij}'\boldsymbol{\beta}),
\end{aligned}
\tag{9.37}
$$

where $i = 1, \ldots, n'$ indicates a matched pair or cluster in this context. In Equation (9.37), the frailty model becomes a stratified Cox model. There is evidence that when sample size within each frailty group is at least five, the stratified Cox model fits as well as a frailty model with a gamma distribution (Hosmer, Lemeshow, and May, 2008). The application of the stratification approach, however, has its disadvantages (Hougaard, 2000). First, it is very difficult, if not impossible, to examine the effects of variables common within the group, including the strata differences. Second, the use of the stratification approach loses estimating power, sometimes massively, because stratification reduces the number of events involved in the estimation process. This disadvantage is particularly serious for the analysis of clinical data of a small sample size.

The effect of the frailty factor can also be addressed empirically in survey data analysis. The inherent effect of unobserved heterogeneity may gradually mitigate the effects of some observed covariates on the relative risk, even if the observed and unobserved factors are mutually independent (Hougaard, 1995; Vaupel, Manton, and Stallard, 1979). When the researcher is aware of a specific covariate whose effects on the hazard rate are confounded by selection bias, then an interaction between this covariate and time (or age) can be created to account for the unobserved selection effect indirectly. Conditional on this interaction term, the effect of the unobservable frailty factor can be largely 'washed out' by the fixed effects of observable variables, particularly by that of the interaction term. In such cases, the application of a standard proportional hazard model is efficient and robust for reducing or even eliminating the bias in parameter estimates. In Subsection 9.3.3, these issues will be further discussed given the analytic results of an empirical illustration.

Dependence of survival data also exists because the occurrence of one event can change the risk for future events, referred to as *event-related dependence* (Hougaard, 2000). One prominent example is the change in death rate after marital bereavement. Here, the dependence of survival times is not linked to a latent association factor like genetic frailty but to the occurrence of a previous event. This type of dependence is thought to be due to some nongenetic factors, such as psychological effects, change in environment, or a lack of help from the late person and his or her significant others (Hougaard, 2000). Frailty models are not particularly designed to account for the mechanisms involved in this type of dependence. While statistical modeling of event-related dependence is not covered by this text, the interested reader is referred to Hougaard (2000, Chapter 6) for a more detailed description on this topic.

9.3.2 The correlated frailty model

In Clayton's (1978) bivariate model, survival times of a matched pair are assumed to share a common relative risk. This model is also referred to as the *shared 'frailty'* model (Clayton and Cuzick, 1985; Hougaard, 2000; Yashin and Iachine, 1995; Yashin, Vaupel, and Iachine, 1995) because the shared relative risk can be considered the shared frailty representing unobserved heterogeneity. The concept is sometimes extended to the multivariate case in which more than two individuals in a cluster can share the same frailty level (Hougaard, 2000). In this model, the frailty variable is associated with a pair or a group of individuals, rather than with one individual. It is believed that accounting for this shared frailty in a survival model can lead to conditional independence of survival times, in turn deriving unbiased parameter estimates.

Conceptually, the notion of the shared frailty differs from the individual frailty defined by Vaupel, Manton, and Stallard (1979). In the shared frailty model, two or more members in a specific unit have exactly the same quantity representing frailty and thus the impact of the frailty factor is completely addressed through the between-units random effects. As a result, the within-persons component of variance in random errors is ignored.

To highlight the difference between the hazard model with individual frailty and the shared frailty model, I reformulate Equation (9.34) in the context of a mixed linear regression. Let $\log[h_{ij}(t, z_i, \boldsymbol{x}_{ij})]$ be Y_{ij} and the baseline hazard rate $\log[h_{0i}(t)]$ be β_{0i}, where ij indicates the jth individual associated with the ith pair or cluster. It follows that Equation (9.34) can be rewritten as

$$\begin{aligned} Y_{ij} &= \log[h_{0i}(t)] + \boldsymbol{x}'_{ij}\boldsymbol{\beta} + \log(z_{ij}) \\ &= \beta_{0i} + \boldsymbol{x}'_{ij}\boldsymbol{\beta} + \varepsilon_{ij}. \end{aligned} \tag{9.38}$$

As theoretically specified in the shared frailty model, the baseline hazard rate varies across n' pairs or clusters, given by

$$\beta_{0i} = \gamma_{00} + u_{0i}, \quad \text{where} \quad \tilde{u}_{0i} \sim N(0, \tau_{00}), \tag{9.39}$$

where γ_{00} is the intercept of the cluster-specific baseline hazard rate, $\tilde{u}_{0i}$ represents the cluster-level random effects for the intercept, and τ_{00} is the between-clusters variance. For analytic simplicity, only β_0 is assumed to be random and all parameters contained in the vector $\boldsymbol{\beta}$ are fixed. Then, combining the above two equations gives rise to the following equation

$$Y_{ij} = \gamma_{00} + \boldsymbol{x}'_{ij}\boldsymbol{\beta} + u_{0i} + \varepsilon_{ij}. \tag{9.40}$$

This simple multilevel derivation suggests that for survival data with matched pairs or clusters, two types of random errors can be specified – between-clusters random errors and within-clusters random errors; that is, the frailty factor z can be decomposed into two components. The first error term $\tilde{u}_{0i}$ indicates that the covariance is τ_{00} for any two individuals within the same pair or cluster, whereas the second error term ε_{ij} specifies that individuals are independent of each other conditional on $\boldsymbol{\beta}$ and $\tilde{u}_{0i}$. Consequently, the intraclusters correlation can be calculated by

$$Corr(Y_{ij}, Y_{ij'}) = \frac{\tau_{00}}{\tau_{00} + \sigma^2}. \tag{9.41}$$

A high value of the intraclusters correlation suggests that survival times of members within a given pair or cluster tend to be correlated. In the shared frailty model, clearly the intraclusters correlation is perfect because it does not specify an individual-level random effect.

Yashin and Iachine (1995) and Yashin, Vaupel, and Iachine (1995) discuss the rationale of the shared frailty model by referring to genetic differences between monozygotic (MZ) and dizygotic (DZ) twins. In given circumstances, the shared frailty model cannot satisfy the condition in which unshared components of frailty exist within a specific cluster. For example, within the construct of the shared frailty model the underlying hazard function for any MZ and DZ twins is assumed to be identical, therefore failing to account for the variation within twins. Accordingly, Yashin and associates develop a correlated frailty model seeking to analyze the bivariate survival data in a more efficient and flexible fashion.

In the correlated frailty model, the association of survival times is designed to be captured by the correlation between individual frailties. The bivariate distribution of frailty is constructed by using three independent gamma-distributed random variables. Let T_{ij} and z_{ij}, where j = 1, 2, be the event time and the frailty for individual j within a matched pair i. The individual hazard rate can be expressed by a familiar proportional hazard model with frailty factor z:

$$h(t, z_j, \boldsymbol{x}_j) = z_j h_0(t) \exp(\boldsymbol{x}_j' \boldsymbol{\beta}), \quad j = 1, 2. \tag{9.42}$$

Within the pair, the two frailties differ by the equations

$$z_1 = \tilde{Y}_0 + \tilde{Y}_1, \tag{9.43a}$$

$$z_2 = \tilde{Y}_0 + \tilde{Y}_2, \tag{9.43b}$$

where $\tilde{Y}_0$, $\tilde{Y}_1$, and $\tilde{Y}_2$ are independent nonnegative gamma-distributed random variables with parameters $\tilde{k}_m$, λ_m (m = 0, 1, 2). For analytic convenience, the scale parameters λ_0, λ_1, λ_2 of the gamma-distributed random variables Y_0, Y_1, Y_2 are assumed to be identical. It is also assumed that two shape parameters, $\tilde{k}_1$, $\tilde{k}_2$ for the distribution of Y_1 and Y_2 are the same. With these assumptions, the frailties z_1 and z_2 are gamma-distributed and correlated random variables. Given known variances $V(Y_0)$ and $V(z_j)$, the correlation coefficient ρ is given by

$$\rho_z = \frac{V(Y_0)}{\sqrt{V(z_1)V(z_2)}}. \tag{9.44}$$

Given the definition of a gamma-distributed function, $V(Y_0)$ and $V(z_j)$ can be written as

$$V(Y_0)=\frac{\tilde{k}_0}{\lambda^2}, \tag{9.45a}$$

$$V(z_j)=\frac{\tilde{k}_0+\tilde{k}_1}{\lambda^2}=\sigma_z^2, \quad j=1,2. \tag{9.45b}$$

Inserting Equations (9.45a) and (9.45b) into Equation (9.44), the correlation coefficient can be obtained by

$$\rho_z=\frac{\tilde{k}_0}{\tilde{k}_0+\tilde{k}_1}. \tag{9.46}$$

In creating the correlated frailty model, Yashin and associates continue to assume the mean frailty of individuals to be unity, thereby imposing the condition $(\tilde{k}_0+\tilde{k})/\lambda=1$. Given the specification of z_1 and z_2, the survival times T_1 and T_2 are assumed to be conditionally independent, thereby yielding efficient parameter estimates.

Given the above assumptions and after much algebra, the marginal bivariate survival function can be written as

$$S(t_1,t_2)=\frac{S(t_1)^{1-\rho_z}\,S(t_2)^{1-\rho_z}}{\left[S(t_1)^{-\sigma_z^2}+S(t_2)^{-\sigma_z^2}-1\right]^{\rho_z/\rho_z^2}}. \tag{9.47}$$

The derivation of the bivariate probability density function is not presented in this text. When $\rho_z=1$, the correlated frailty survival and probability density functions reduce to those specified by the shared frailty model.

Compared to the shared frailty model, the correlated frailty model is based on a number of additional restrictive assumptions. The method is particularly valuable for analyzing biologically relevant survival data with a high correlation between subjects. For example, correlations of failure times within monozygotic (MZ) twins and within dizygotic (DZ) twins are very likely to differ, so using the shared frailty model can result in biased parameter estimates. Under such circumstances, the use of the correlated frailty model provides a more flexible perspective. This model is also applicable for the analysis of large-scale vital registration data in which suitable measures for particular predictor variables of interest are often not available. For analyzing large-scale survey data, however, this model can be subject to overfitting and overparameterization given the consideration of covariates.

9.3.3 Illustration of frailty models: The effect of veteran status on the mortality of older Americans revisited

In this illustrative subsection, I revisit the empirical example presented in Subsection 8.2.5. The previous example examines the mortality difference between American older veterans and nonveterans and its changing pattern over time. The observation interval is a four–five-year interval from 1993/1994 to the end of 1997. Because frailty models are meant to parameterize random effects arising from eliminating important predictor variables, in this illustration I focus on reanalyzing the final reduced-form equation specified in Subsection 8.2.5, adding a single term of random effects. As described in Subsection 8.2.5, the final reduced-form equation includes six predictor variables: Vet (veteran status; veteran = 1, nonveteran = 0), Age_70 (actual age at baseline – 70), Vet × Age_70, Female_cnd (centered variable), Educ_cnd (centered variable), and Married_cnd (centered variable). Specifications and basic statistics of these covariates are presented in Table 8.1.

As mentioned in Subsection 8.2.5, removal of six intervening variables from the full hazard model guarantees that strong unobserved heterogeneity exists in the regression analysis thus necessitates the consideration and estimation of random effects. Therefore, in this illustration I apply frailty models to account for such disturbances. A common feature of various frailty models is to parameterize the random effect in the hazard model for accomplishing conditional independence among observations. I continue to use the Weibull hazard model, adding a term of the random effect, in order to be in line with the analysis displayed in Subsection 8.2.5. The adjusted Weibull model is then given by

$$h(t|\boldsymbol{x},z) = \lambda_0 \tilde{p}(h_0 t)^{\tilde{p}-1} \exp[\boldsymbol{x}'\boldsymbol{\beta} + \log(z)], \tag{9.48}$$

where, as indicated previously, λ_0 is the scale parameter, $\tilde{p}$ is the shape parameter, and z is the frailty factor, or random effects. The matrix $\boldsymbol{x}$, defined as a matrix of exogenous variables in Chapter 8, contains six predictor variables. Notice that with the addition of a random-effects term, this adjusted Weibull hazard function does not have proportional and monotonic properties, and individually the distribution would fall off from a typical Weibull distribution. Nevertheless, in this illustration I am more concerned with the quality of parameter estimates and the potential impact the presumed random effect might yield, rather than with the shape of a baseline survival function.

The crucial part of creating a frailty model is to select a specific distributional function for the frailty effect z. The most widely used distribution for frailties is a lognormal or a gamma distribution, as described in Subsection 9.3.1. Statistically, fitting a hazard model with individual frailty requires integrating the likelihood over the random effect. Generally, all estimation processes with an added random term are complex and intractable, so that selection of a random-effects distributional function must be based on underlying theories concerning, among other things, the distribution of the frailty factor.

In SAS, there is currently no specific code to fit a frailty model either using the Cox proportional or applying the accelerated failure time procedures. The SAS PROC NLMIXED procedure, however, can be applied to fit a Cox or an AFT frailty model with an arbitrarily assumed error term (Collett, 2003; Kelly, 2004), as this procedure can handle nonlinear mixed models with a single random effect. By using this software, frailty models can be fitted by maximizing an approximation to the likelihood integrated over the random effect. A number of integration techniques, such as Gaussian quadrature, can be used for fitting nonlinear maximum likelihood estimates, both fixed and random. Specifically, an n-point Gaussian quadrature rule provides an approximation of the definite integral of a distributional function, usually stated as a weighted sum of functional values at specified points within the domain of integration.

In this illustration, I propose to fit two Weibull regression models with individual-level random effects integrated into the estimation of the maximum likelihood: (1) the Weibull hazard model with the random variable z assumed to be lognormally distributed (normal in the linear predictor with mean 0 and variance σ^2) and (2) the Weibull hazard model with z assumed to have a gamma distribution (log gamma distributed in the linear predictor). I compare three sets of parameter estimates derived, respectively, from the final reduced-form equation model presented in Subsection 8.2.5 (using the smearing estimate approach), the hazard model with a lognormal-distributed random term, and the hazard model with a gamma distribution. In particula, I am interested in examining the model fit for each of these hazard models because a significant improvement in the overall model fit is the prerequisite for evaluating statistically the modifications in parameter estimates with an added random-effects term (Gelman *et al.*, 2004). First, I want to analyze whether the integration over random effects is statistically necessary in fitting the Weibull model, using the model chi-square criterion. Next, I want to know whether the gamma-distributed random effect fits the data significantly better than the model with a lognormal distribution, also using the model chi-square criterion. Useful theoretical implications can be derived by deviations of the parameter estimates and the model fit statistics. Empirically, I want to test the null hypothesis that integration of individual-level random effects in the estimation of the Weibull regression model, either lognormally or gamma distributed, does not contribute significantly to the quality of the estimation.

I use the SAS NLMIXED procedure to derive AFT parameter estimates that can be easily converted to the hazard coefficients and the hazard ratios by using the SAS Output Delivery System (ODS). First, I use the following SAS program to fit the frailty model with a log-normal random effect.

SAS Program 9.2:

```
......
* Estimate the frailty model with lognormal random effect *;
ods output ParameterEstimates=Frailty_est;
proc nlmixed data=new1;
  parms logsig = 0 lambda=1.265 b0=5.61 b1=0.19 b2=-0.05
       b3=-0.04 b4=0.44 b5=0.01 b6=0.13;
  bounds lambda > 0;
  linp = b0 + b1*vet + b2*age_70 + b3*vetage_70 + b4*female_cnd
       + b5*educ_cnd + b6*married_cnd + b_i;
  alpha = exp(-linp);
  G_t = exp(-(alpha*duration)**lambda);
  g = lambda*alpha*((alpha*duration)**(lambda-1))*G_t;
  ll = (censor = 0)*log(g) + (censor = 1)*log(G_t);
  model duration □ general(ll);
  random b_i □ normal(0, exp(2*logsig)) subject=subject out=EB;
  predict 1-G_t out=cdf;
  run;
ods output close;

data _null_;
  set Frailty_est;
  if parameter = 'lambda' then call symput("lambda", estimate);
run;
```

```
*Compute and print corresponding PH estimates and HR *;
data Frailty_est;
  set Frailty_est;
  string = upcase(trim(Parameter));
  if (string ne 'LAMBDA') & (string ne 'ALPHA')
      then PH_beta = -1*estimate/(1/&lambda);
  else if PH_beta = .;
  AFT_beta = estimate;
  HR = exp(PH_beta);
  drop _Lambda_;
options nolabel;

proc print data=Frailty_est;
  id Parameter;
  var AFT_beta PH_beta HR;
  format PH_beta 8.5 HR 5.3;
  title1 "LIFEREG/Weibull on duration";
  title2 "ParameterEstimate dataset w/ PH_beta & HR computed manually";
  title4 "PH_beta = -1*AFT_beta/scale";
  title6 "HR = exp(PH_beta)";
run;
```

In SAS Program 9.2, a Weibull AFT model is fitted with the addition of a lognormally distributed individual-level random effect. The first part estimates the regression coefficients of covariates on log(duration), with parameter estimates saved in the temporary SAS output file Frailty_est. The error term b_i indicates the transformed random variable z on the log(duration), which is normally distributed with zero expectation. The PARMS statement specifies starting values of parameter estimates, obtained from results of the final reduced-form equation presented in Table 8.2. If the PARMS statement is not given, the NLMIXED procedure assigns the default value of 1.0. Notice that if starting values are too far away from final estimated values, numerical integration techniques will not perform well given the usual complexity of a nonlinear regression. Therefore, before running the NLMIXED procedure, starting values should be chosen from a model fitted without the random effect by running the PROC LIFEREG procedure. Without the RANDOM statement adding the term b_i to the linear predictor, parameter estimates and their standard errors derived from Program 9.2 would be identical to those obtained from the LIFEREG procedure except model fit statistics.

The second part in SAS Program 9.2 converts the saved log time coefficients (AFT_beta) into the log hazard coefficients (PH_beta) and the corresponding hazard ratios (HR), as also displayed in Subsection 8.2.5. The third part of the program asks SAS to print three sets of parameter estimates – the regression coefficients on log(duration), the regression coefficients on log(hazards), and the hazard ratios. I borrow analytic results on AFT parameters to perform the significance test on the regression coefficients in the Weibull hazard rate model. The results from SAS Program 9.2 are presented below.

SAS Program Output 9.1:

The NLMIXED Procedure

Specifications

Data Set	WORK.NEW1
Dependent Variable	duration
Distribution for Dependent Variable	General
Random Effects	b_i
Distribution for Random Effects	Normal
Subject Variable	subject
Optimization Technique	Dual Quasi-Newton
Integration Method	Adaptive Gaussian Quadrature

Dimensions

Observations Used	2000
Observations Not Used	0
Total Observations	2000
Subjects	2000
Max Obs Per Subject	1
Parameters	9
Quadrature Points	7

Parameters

logsig	lambda	b0	b1	b2	b3	b4	b5	b6	NegLogLike
0	1.265	5.61	0.19	-0.05	-0.04	0.44	0.01	0.13	2165.64065

Iteration History

Iter	Calls	NegLogLike	Diff	MaxGrad	Slope

1	4	2148.88601	16.75464	227.7063	-14990.4
2	6	2141.11817	7.767848	222.4395	-280.334
3	7	2131.65578	9.462387	237.2747	-435.854
4	9	2131.32633	0.329454	200.0567	-17.1397
5	11	2125.71081	5.615515	31.73061	-38.6567
6	13	2125.29582	0.414991	15.40665	-0.47479
7	14	2125.17567	0.120153	110.3093	-0.4068
8	16	2124.69307	0.4826	29.4505	-1.04307
9	17	2124.40097	0.292102	52.42622	-0.30436
10	18	2124.03926	0.361703	27.71011	-0.55291
11	21	2123.93734	0.101918	68.22913	-0.1339
12	22	2123.78693	0.150419	9.897491	-0.22878
13	23	2123.62815	0.158771	88.74776	-0.13748
14	25	2123.5293	0.098851	6.65051	-0.14546
15	27	2123.47594	0.05336	30.45955	-0.04363
16	29	2123.44543	0.030513	19.06074	-0.06534
17	30	2123.40922	0.036213	30.40652	-0.05016
18	32	2123.39129	0.017924	7.390543	-0.02594
19	33	2123.37863	0.01266	21.81052	-0.01192
20	35	2123.37084	0.007792	2.747508	-0.0131
21	37	2123.3673	0.003543	2.332511	-0.00206
22	38	2123.36626	0.001039	6.461833	-0.00309
23	40	2123.36335	0.002914	2.70996	-0.00478
24	42	2123.36256	0.000786	2.243333	-0.00065
25	44	2123.36227	0.000291	0.870772	-0.00041
26	45	2123.36205	0.000213	0.601767	-0.0001
27	47	2123.36192	0.000138	0.126985	-0.00019
28	49	2123.36188	0.000034	0.196741	-0.00003
29	51	2123.36187	0.000018	0.16801	-0.00002

NOTE: GCONV convergence criterion satisfied.

Fit Statistics

-2 Log Likelihood	4246.7
AIC (smaller is better)	4264.7
AICC (smaller is better)	4264.8
BIC (smaller is better)	4315.1

Parameter Estimates

Parameter	Estimate	Standard Error	DF	t Value	Pr > |t|	Alpha	Lower	Upper	Gradient
logsig	-5.9990	126.25	1999	-0.05	0.9621	0.05	-253.59	241.59	0.000031
lambda	1.2653	0.06745	1999	18.76	<.0001	0.05	1.1330	1.3975	0.003484
b0	5.6053	0.1271	1999	44.09	<.0001	0.05	5.3559	5.8546	0.010157
b1	0.1904	0.1928	1999	0.99	0.3236	0.05	-0.1878	0.5686	-0.01554
b2	-0.05071	0.008222	1999	-6.17	<.0001	0.05	-0.06683	-0.03458	0.16801
b3	-0.03661	0.01922	1999	-1.90	0.0570	0.05	-0.07430	0.001087	-0.1183
b4	0.4395	0.1177	1999	3.73	0.0002	0.05	0.2086	0.6704	0.00765
b5	0.01230	0.01195	1999	1.03	0.3034	0.05	-0.01113	0.03573	-0.01586
b6	0.1326	0.1013	1999	1.31	0.1908	0.05	-0.06612	0.3313	-0.0061

```
                    PH_beta = -1*AFT_beta/scale

                        HR = exp(PH_beta)

      Parameter      AFT_beta       PH_beta          HR

       logsig        -5.99898       7.59031        1979
       lambda         1.26527        .              .
       b0             5.60526      -7.09215        0.001
       b1             0.19041      -0.24092        0.786
       b2            -0.05071       0.06416        1.066
       b3            -0.03661       0.04632        1.047
       b4             0.43952      -0.55611        0.573
       b5             0.01230      -0.01556        0.985
       b6             0.13258      -0.16774        0.846
```

In SAS Program Output 9.1, the 'Specification' table displays the integration that is computed by the adaptive Gaussian quadrature due to the presence of the random effect. This approximation uses the empirical Bayes estimates of random effects as the central point for the quadrature, and it updates them for every iterative step. The 'Dimension' table reports seven quadrature points used to integrate over random effects. The section 'Parameter' prints the starting values given for the derivation of model parameters. As displayed, the procedure converges after 29 iterations. The value of the $-2\log$ likelihood, used to compute the model chi-square for testing the statistical significance of the random effect, is almost identical to the figure in the model without the arbitrarily assumed random effect. Consequently, the addition of the random effect does not improve the model significantly in this example.

In the 'Parameter Estimates' section, the random effect is not statistically significant ($t = -0.05$, $p = 0.96$). Values of the other parameter estimates are identical to those derived from the model without the random effect (the final reduced-form equation model in Subsection 8.2.5). Accordingly, the PH_beta and HR values, presented in the last part, are analogous to those reported in the last two columns of Table 8.2. The standard errors of AFT parameters, not displayed here, are also exactly the same. The variance of the normal random effect is $\exp(-2 \times 5.9990) = 0.000\,006$, so that the mean frailty with a lognormal distribution is $\exp(0.000\,006/2) = 1.000\,003$. Obviously, in this example the estimation of parameters is not sensitive at all to the addition of a lognormally distributed random effect.

Next, I fit a Weibull regression model with a gamma distribution to estimate the model parameters in Equation (9.48). To perform this analysis in SAS, some additional conditions need to be specified. Let $\bar{\theta}_1$ and $\bar{\theta}_2$ are variances of the parameters $\tilde{k}$ and λ. Then the density function of the gamma distribution becomes

$$f\left(z_i \middle| \bar{\theta}_1, \bar{\theta}_2\right) = \frac{z_i^{1/\bar{\theta}_1 - 1} \exp\left(-z_i / \bar{\theta}_2\right)}{\Gamma\left(1/\bar{\theta}_1\right) \bar{\theta}_2^{1/\bar{\theta}_1}}. \tag{9.49}$$

For analytic convenience and consideration of identifiability, the mean of z values is set at 1, given the conditions that $\lambda = \tilde{k}$ and thus $\bar{\theta}_2 = \bar{\theta}_1 = 1/\tilde{k}$. It follows that Equation (9.49) reduces to

$$f\left(z_i \middle| \bar{\theta}_1\right) = \frac{z_i^{1/\bar{\theta}_1 - 1} \exp\left(-z_i / \bar{\theta}_1\right)}{\Gamma\left(1/\bar{\theta}_1\right) \bar{\theta}_1^{1/\bar{\theta}_1}}. \tag{9.50}$$

The parameter $\bar{\theta}_1$ indicates the extent to which observations within a cluster are dependent in the presence of covariates, with greater values of $\bar{\theta}_1$ highlighting higher intracluster correlation.

As the PROC NLMIXED procedure in SAS only allows a single random effect with a normal distribution, I adapt the method of the probability integral transformation, recommended by Nelson *et al.* (2006) to fit the model with a gamma distributed random effect. Specifically, when using PROC NLMIXED, the gamma random effect z_i can be obtained from a set of transformations: (1) $\alpha_i \sim N(0, 1)$, (2) $p_i = \Phi(\alpha_i)$, (3) $z_{i2} = F_{\bar{\theta}_1}^{-1}(p_i)$, and (4) $z_i = \bar{\theta}\, z_{i21}$, where $F_{\bar{\theta}_1}^{-1}(\cdot)$ is the inverse c.d.f. of the gamma distribution and $\Phi(.)$ is the standard normal c.d.f. (the probit function). Given these specifications of transformation, a Weibull AFT model with a gamma distribution can be estimated using the following SAS program.

SAS Program 9.3:

```
......
* Compute frailty model with gamma random effect *;
ods output ParameterEstimates=Frailty_est;
proc nlmixed data=new1 method=GAUSS NOAD fd qpoints=30;
 parms theta_1=1 lambda=1.265 b0=5.61 b1=0.19 b2=-0.05
      b3=-0.04 b4=0.44 b5=0.01 b6=0.13;
 bounds lambda > 0;
 p_i = CDF('NORMAL',a_i);
 if (p_i > 0.999999) then p_i = 0.999999;
 g_i2 = quantile('GAMMA',p_i,1/theta_1);
 g_i = theta_1*g_i2;
 linp = b0 + b1*vet + b2*age_70 + b3*vetage_70 + b4*female_cnd
      + b5*educ_cnd + b6*married_cnd + log(g_i);
 alpha = exp(-linp);
 G_t = exp(-(alpha*duration)**lambda);
 g = lambda*alpha*((alpha*duration)**(lambda-1))*G_t;
 ll = (censor = 0)*log(g) + (censor = 1)*log(G_t);
 model duration ~ general(ll);
 random a_i ~ normal(0, 1) subject=subject;
 predict 1-G_t out=cdf;
 run;
ods output close;

data _null_;
 set Frailty_est;
 if parameter = 'lambda' then call symput("lambda", estimate);
run;

*Compute and print corresponding PH estimates and HR *;
data Frailty_est;
 set Frailty_est;
 string = upcase(trim(Parameter));
 if (string ne 'LAMBDA') & (string ne 'ALPHA')
      then PH_beta = -1*estimate/(1/&lambda);
 else if PH_beta = .;
 AFT_beta = estimate;
```

```
  HR = exp(PH_beta);
  drop _Lambda_;
options nolabel;

proc print data=Frailty_est;
  id Parameter;
  var AFT_beta PH_beta HR;
  format PH_beta 8.5 HR 5.3;
  title1 "LIFEREG/Weibull on duration";
  title2 "ParameterEstimate dataset w/ PH_beta & HR computed manually";
  title4 "PH_beta = -1*AFT_beta/scale";
  title6 "HR = exp(PH_beta)";
run;
```

In SAS Program 9.3, the syntax remains the same as Program 9.2 except the part specifying steps for a gamma distributed random effect. In the PROC NLMIXED statement, the MTHOD=GAUSS option calls for the application of the Gaussian quadrature, NOAD requests that the Gaussian quadrature be nonadaptive, FD specifies that all derivatives be computed using finite difference approximations, and qpoints=30 tells SAS that 30 quadrature points be used in each dimension of the random effects. Here the number of quadrature points can be increased or decreased as desired. In principle, a higher number of quadrature points improve the accuracy of the approximation but in the meantime, however, it increases the computational burden.

Also, in the above program, the starting values for parameters remain the same except for the addition of $\bar{\theta}_1 = 1$. The procedures for transforming the parameter estimates on log(duration) to those on log(hazard) are the same. The output of the program, not displayed here, displays a statistically significant estimate of $\bar{\theta}_1$ (0.6421; $t = 10.80$, $p < 0.0001$). Compared to the frailty model with a lognormal distribution, however, the statistical model generates no gain in the model chi-square because the difference in the value of $-2 \times$ (log likelihood) is negative (4246.7 versus 4250.9). According to the statistical criterion that less is better with regard to the value of −2(LLR), the frailty model with a gamma distribution loses important statistical information and therefore is not statistically efficient compared to the model with only fixed effects and the model with a lognormal random effect. There are some distinct variations in the values of other parameter estimates.

Table 9.1 summarizes the results derived from the three hazard rate models. In Table 9.1, the first hazard rate model is the regression that specifies a number of fixed effects and a random term, assumed to be lognormally distributed and estimated externally from the smearing estimate approach. It is equivalent to the final reduced-form equation model described in Subsection 8.2.5, reproduced by running the PROC NLMIXED procedure. The next two hazard models are the Weibull functions fitted by maximizing an approximation to the likelihood integrated over unobserved random effects, distributed either as lognormal or as gamma. The maximum likelihood estimates of regression coefficients based on the first two models are almost identical, with trivial differences observed only in some of the standard error estimates and p values. As indicated earlier, the mean of frailties for the second model (the multiplicative random effect, defined as $\exp[\sigma^2/2]$) is 1.000003, which is not statistically significant.

Compared to the first two models, the third Weibull model with a gamma distributed random effect derives different parameter estimates. First, the random effect parameter

Table 9.1 Results of hazard rate models on the mortality of older persons between 1993 and 1997: fixed-effects and frailty models (***n*** = 2000).

Covariates and other statistics	Fixed effects model		Lognormal frailty model		Gamma frailty model	
	Coefficient	*HR*	Coefficient	*HR*	Coefficient	*HR*
Vet	−0.241	0.786	−0.241	0.786	−0.392	0.676
Age_70	0.064***	1.066	0.064***	1.066	0.101***	1.106
Vet*age_70	0.046**	1.047	0.046*	1.047	0.082*	1.085
Female_cnd	−0.556***	0.573	−0.556***	0.573	−0.911***	0.402
Educ_cnd	−0.016	0.985	−0.016	0.985	−0.027	0.973
Married_cnd	−0.168	0.846	−0.168	0.846	−0.286	0.751
Intercept	−7.092***		−7.092***		−11.493***	
Mean frailty	1.271***		1.000		1.000	
Shape	1.265***		1.265***		1.915***	
−2 log likelihood	4246.70		4246.7		4250.9	

Note: The parameter 'shape' is tested by $(\tilde{p}-1.0)$/SE.
*0.05 < p < 0.10;
**0.01 < p < 0.05;
***p < 0.01.

$\bar{\theta}_1$ (0.6421; $t = 10.80$, $p < 0.0001$) is statistically significant. Second, the estimate of the Weibull shape factor is considerably increased, 1.915, compared to 1.265 obtained from the first two models. Third, the absolute values of the regression coefficients on log(hazard rate) are much elevated, obviously due to the increased amount of the shape parameter. However, these changes do not affect the consistence of the analytic results. In all three models, the regression coefficient of veteran status is negative, while that of the interaction term between veteran status and age is positive, which, combined, suggest a typical pattern of mortality convergence and crossover between older veterans and nonveterans, and the subsequent excess mortality among older veterans. The effect of veteran status on the mortality of older Americans is considered statistically significant given the significance of the interaction term. Because the absolute value of the main effect for veteran status is greater than that of the interaction term, veterans are expected to have mortality considerably lower than their nonveteran counterparts at age 70, other variables being equal.

Because of the elevated value of −2(LLR) estimated for the model with a gamma distributed random effect, I cannot reject the null hypothesis that the integration of a random effect does not significantly improve the estimating quality of the hazard model. Clearly, the specification of the interaction between veteran status and age accounts significantly for the impact of selection in survival processes, so that adding an arbitrarily assumed error term does not contribute further to the estimation of model parameters and the overall model fit statistics. The application of the smearing estimate approach, described in Chapter 8, might be a more appropriate technique for capturing prediction bias in analyzing survival data of large samples.

I would like to emphasize that the results shown here do not necessarily suggest that frailty models, particularly the model with a gamma distribution, are not useful. The results presented above only demonstrate that for this particular example with this particular dataset, the application of frailty models is not shown to significantly improve the quality of parameter estimates and the model fit statistics. In applied fields, particularly in social science, empirical studies are often based on large-scale observational surveys, from which a large quantity of variables are generally available to allow for the specification of complex conceptual models. If a theoretical model is correctly specified for guiding the analysis of survival data, the impact of random effects on various parameter estimates can be largely absorbed by other well-specified parameters (Andersen *et al.*, 1993; Arjas, 1988). This advantage is often not available in biological and medical research. For example, in a clinical trial theoretically relevant explanatory factors are often not measurable, and the use of survival data with a small sample size does not permit for the specification of a complex causal framework. In large-scale vital registration data, usable explanatory information is usually restricted by a few demographic variables, thereby making the specification of a causal model difficult. Under those circumstances, the frailty theory and its attaching statistical models are highly valuable to account for the potential lack of independence in observations, thus deriving more efficient parameter estimates.

In survival analysis, there is always a trade-off between the accuracy of approximation and the parsimony of a statistical model. The researcher might construct several hazard models at the same time, with or without specification of random effects, either a normal or a gamma distribution, and then they can compare the model fit statistics in those regression models using various statistical criteria. If the model fit statistics do not deviate significantly, the simplest and the most parsimonious model should always be the first choice.

9.4 Mortality crossovers and the maximum life span

No matter how valid and practical the frailty theory is, there is an increasing skepticism concerning constant mortality differentials throughout the life course. Some human research studies have reported mortality crossovers in later life using empirical data (Liu and Witten, 1995; Vaupel, Manton, and Stallard, 1979). These findings have led to controversies on this crossover phenomenon, in turn leading to two schools of thought on the issue (Nam, 1994; Olshansky, 1995). Some researchers use the notion of 'survival of the fittest' to explain the crossover of two mortality schedules (Manton, Poss, and Wing, 1979; Vaupel, Manton, and Stallard, 1979), as discussed previously when describing the frailty theory. Some other researchers cast doubts on the validity of the theoretical hypothesis of mortality crossovers (Coale and Kisker, 1986; Elo and Preston, 1994). They contend that there are substantial influences of age misreporting among the oldest old in datasets, thus displaying a mortality crossover.

I am inclined to accept the demographic reality of mortality crossovers and the scientific value inherent in their occurrence. Mortality crossovers have not only been reported with socioeconomic status like race (Manton, Poss, and Wing, 1979) but also by some genetic population subgroups such as women versus men (Liu and Witten, 1995). It is unlikely that all these reports are in serious error. Most significantly, such crossovers have been observed in carefully controlled laboratory populations of nonhuman animals (Carey and Liedo, 1995; Heller *et al.*, 1998), among whom age misreporting is not relevant.

Further examination of this issue cast additional doubts on the validity of the hypothesis on proportional mortality differences throughout the life course. Consider the following example. If the mortality rates for two population subgroups (e.g., white versus black, men versus women) differ proportionally over the entire life course, the mortality differences would follow a divergent pattern over age, given the steady increase in general mortality. As a consequence, the 'disadvantaged' persons would eventually die out much faster than do the 'advantaged.' The dynamics of this dying out process would be governed by the value of the constant ratio of the two group mortalities. It follows then that, beyond a certain age, all of the survivors would be those who are initially 'advantaged.' Consequently, the population would have become homogeneous with respect to its survival advantage. This survival pattern is obviously not observable in human populations. In Japan, where more reliable registration data are available for older persons, centenarians include not only the socioeconomically advantaged but the socioeconomically disadvantaged as well (TMIG, 1973).

Additionally, the proportionality of mortality differences over the entire life course would automatically imply that the maximum length of human life potential, often referred to as the maximum life span (Eakin and Witten, 1995), is a function of the external environment. This implication conflicts with the generally held belief that the human maximum life span is, at least partially, genetically predetermined (Arking, 1987; Olshansky and Carnes, 1994; Ratten, 1995; Rose and Graves, 1990). From the biological standpoint, mortality among older survivors may depend more on the natural exhaustion of the organism through the life history and into age (Gavrilov and Gavrilov, 2004; Hirsch, 1994; Kirkwood, 1992; Lints, 1989). With the possible existence of a biologically mandated upper bound on the human maximum life span, a valid initial assumption, two subgroup mortalities within a population may cross in later life if the two subgroups are initially subject to two levels of mortality. This relationship is a consequence of the fact that the two survival curves associated with the two subgroups must converge at a given point of time in later life. Consequently, the group initially having the lower level of mortality would sooner or later experience faster mortality acceleration in order to complete this convergence. This 'acceleration' (Liu and Witten, 1995; Witten, 1989) will eventually lead to a higher mortality schedule for the advantaged persons.

It may be further inferred that mortality crossovers can also occur even if the human maximum life span differs across subgroups of a population. When the disparity in the maximum life span between two particular subgroups is considerably smaller than what the proportionality in mortality would suggest, mortality for the advantaged group would eventually have to accelerate faster than for the disadvantaged, thereby fostering the possible occurrence of a mortality crossover, though this crossover is most likely to occur at a very old age.

These theoretical issues on the changing pattern of mortality differentials lead to a number of important implications for future studies of human mortality and the distribution of health status. First, the occurrence of a mortality crossover calls for both a faster pace of mortality acceleration and, at a later life stage, a higher absolute increase in the mortality rate of the advantaged group, as compared with the disadvantaged. The phenomenon of mortality crossover virtually reflects a long-standing process of variations in differential mortality. Consequently, the level of differential mortality, at least at some very older ages, would be a function of the life stage. Second, as the existence of a predetermined human maximum life span can force the convergence of initially different survival functions, this relationship is independent of any other exogenous factors. For example, if two different frailty subgroups are subject to a common maximum life span, the two mortality schedules may tend to converge asymptotically due to the dragging force of survival convergence, thus possibly leading to a mortality crossover. Lastly, application of the basic survival function must be consistent with the underlying pattern that mortality differentials are convergent, rather than divergent, over age (Antonovsky, 1967; Coale and Demeny, 1966; Gavrilov and Gavrilov, 1991; Liu and Witten, 1995).

In this section, I describe basic specifications about mortality differences and the impact of the existence of a common maximum life span. As this topic has been discussed dominantly in biology, I describe the related concepts and functions using the mathematical terminology generally applied by mathematical biologists. First, I portray changes in the survival curves for two hypothetical population subgroups and the resulting changes in differential mortality, given a genetically predetermined human maximum life span. Then I discuss the possibility of a mortality crossover in the absence of a common maximum life span. Lastly, mathematical conditions about the relationship between a predetermined maximum human life span and a mortality crossover are formulated.

9.4.1 Basic specifications

I begin by introducing the familiar survival function, defined here as the proportion of a birth cohort surviving to exact age 'a' and denoted by $S(a)$. As a mortality crossover concerns a phenomenon that occurs at a specific age, in this section I describe survival and other lifetime processes as related to exact age a, rather than to time t.

The instantaneous death rate at age a, often referred to as the force of mortality in demography and noted as $h(a)$, is closely related to the survival function:

$$h(a) = -\frac{\mathrm{d}\log S(a)}{\mathrm{d}a}. \tag{9.51}$$

In empirical studies, the age-dependent survival process $S(a)$ is often specified as discontinuous at the observed age of death for analytic convenience (Kalbfleisch and Prentice, 2002). Assuming that the infinitesimal change in population size, denoted $\mathrm{d}N(a)$, in an infinitesimal age interval $\mathrm{d}a$ is proportional to $N(a)$, then the hazard rate, or the force of mortality, can be written by

$$h(a) = -\frac{1}{S(a)}\frac{\mathrm{d}S(a)}{\mathrm{d}a} = -\frac{1}{N(a)}\frac{\mathrm{d}N(a)}{\mathrm{d}a}, \tag{9.52}$$

where $N(a)$ represents the number of individuals at age a. As a survival function is monotonically decreasing, the hazard rate $h(a)$ is nonnegative, but not necessarily smaller than or equal to one, as also discussed in Chapter 1.

Beyond a certain age (around 30 years of age), the mortality rate for human populations has been demonstrated to follow approximately an exponential mortality schedule, particularly over the range 40–80 years, which can be approximated by the Gompertz function (Eakin and Witten, 1995; Finch, Pike, and Witten, 1990; Hirsch, Liu, and Witten, 2000; Liu and Witten, 1995; Riggs, 1990). The classical Gompertzian survival curve, as described in Chapter 3, is

$$S(a) = \exp\left[\frac{h_0}{r}(1 - e^{ra})\right]. \tag{9.53}$$

Accordingly, the hazard rate is given by

$$h(a) = h_0 e^{ra}, \tag{9.54}$$

where the positive parameter h_0 is often referred to as the age-independent hazard rate coefficient and the positive parameter r is the age-dependent mortality rate coefficient in biological and demographic studies.

As noted in the previous section, some empirical data have suggested that, at advanced ages, the rate of increase slows down and, as a consequence, the trajectory of mortality falls off from an exponential curve (Carey *et al.*, 1992; Vaupel, Manton, and Stallard, 1979). Here, however, I use the exponential mortality function (the so-called Gompertz law) for setting up basic specifications because of its simplicity of illustration. The presentations shown below do not depend on the validity of the Gompertz law, and any other more flexible mortality function would lead to the same results for the demonstration of a relative risk.

The absolute change per unit of time in the hazard rate may be expressed as the derivative of Equation (9.54). Based on the Gompertz function, this mortality indicator is given by

$$\tilde{\eta}(a) = \frac{dh(a)}{da} = h_0 r e^{ra}, \tag{9.55}$$

where $\tilde{\eta}(a)$ represents the absolute change in the hazard rate at exact age a. If $\tilde{\eta}(a)$ is positive, the force of mortality is increasing; likewise, if it is negative, the rate of mortality is declining. A constant rate of mortality rate over age would imply $\tilde{\eta}(a) \equiv 0$, which gives rise to an exponential survival function.

While the value of $\tilde{\eta}(a)$ has been observed to be continuously positive after age 10 (Coale and Demeny, 1966), mathematical biologists and demographers are also concerned with whether the rate of change in $\tilde{\eta}$ increases or decreases over age, because this rate describes the trend of mortality evolution. An appropriate measure of this sort can be obtained from the second derivative of the hazard rate, given by

$$\tilde{v}(a) = \frac{d^2 h(a)}{da^2} = h_0 r^2 e^{ra}, \tag{9.56}$$

where $\tilde{v}(a)$ is defined as the indicator displaying mortality acceleration given a Gompertz function.

With the existence of a predetermined upper bound for an individual life span, denoted by ω, I impose the conditions that $S(\omega) = 0$ and $h(\omega) = \infty$. By definition, a Gompertz survival function is not associated with a biological upper bound on the life span. As a result, $S(a)$ in Equation (9.53) has the properties that $S(\omega) > 0$ and $h(\omega) \neq \infty$. To adjust for this discordance, the Gompertz survival function needs to be truncated, thus generating the adjusted survival rate, the mortality rate, the mortality change per unit of time, and the mortality acceleration. Rccognizing the proportional distribution of the Gompertz survival function, the truncated survival function S^* can be written as

$$S^*(a) = \left\{ \begin{array}{ll} \dfrac{S(a) - S(\omega)}{1 - S(\omega)}, & a \leq \omega \\ 0, & a > \omega \end{array} \right\}, \tag{9.57}$$

where $S^*(a)$ refers to the adjusted value of $S(a)$.

Accordingly, in the construct of the Gompertzian distribution, the adjusted value of the mortality rate at age a, denoted by $h^*(a)$, is

$$h^*(a) = \frac{\mathrm{d}\log\left[S^*(a)\right]}{\mathrm{d}a} = \frac{h_0 e^{ra}}{\left[1 - \dfrac{S(\omega)}{S(a)}\right]}. \tag{9.58}$$

Likewise, the adjusted measures of $\tilde{\eta}(a)$ and $\tilde{v}(a)$, for the truncated Gompertzian, are defined by

$$\tilde{\eta}^*(a) = \frac{\mathrm{d}h^*(a)}{\mathrm{d}a} = h^*(a)\left[r + h^*(a)\frac{S(\omega)}{S(a)}\right] \tag{9.59}$$

and

$$\begin{aligned} \tilde{v}^*(a) &= \frac{\mathrm{d}^2 h^*(a)}{\mathrm{d}a^2} \\ &= h^*(a)\left\{r^2 + 3rh^*(a)\tilde{\Phi}(a) + h^*(a)^2\tilde{\Phi}(a)\left[1 + \tilde{\Phi}(a)\right]\right\}, \end{aligned} \tag{9.60a}$$

where $\tilde{\eta}^*(a)$ and $\tilde{v}^*(a)$ are, respectively, the adjusted mortality change per unit of time at age a and the adjusted mortality acceleration at age a, and $\tilde{\Phi}(a)$ is

$$\tilde{\Phi}(a) = \frac{S(\omega)}{S(a)}. \tag{9.60b}$$

The indicator $\tilde{v}^*(a)$, which I refer to as the *index of absolute mortality acceleration*, denotes the shape of a mortality schedule. If $\tilde{v}^*(a)$ is zero, the absolute change in the hazard rate is constant; hence there is no acceleration or deceleration in the force of mortality. The mortality curve associated with this condition is a straight line. If $\tilde{v}^*(a)$ is negative, the mortality rate might still increase over age, but the rate of such positive changes is declining. The condition that $\tilde{v}^*(a)<0$ indicates a process of mortality deceleration, with the shape of the mortality function being globally concave. Correspondingly, $\tilde{v}^*(a)>0$ reflects a monotonically increasing trend in the rate of change in the force of mortality. Given this condition, the curve of mortality rate with all $\tilde{v}^*(a)>0$ is globally convex.

The above truncation leads to the mathematical conditions that $S^*(\omega) = 0$ and $h^*(\omega) = \infty$. For human populations, the values of $S^*(a)$, $h^*(a)$, $\tilde{\eta}^*(a)$, and $\tilde{v}^*(a)$ are identical to the original Gompertz functions, except those at some oldest ages, given a considerably long human maximum life span. This approach, however, is meaningful for other more short-lived species.

9.4.2 Relative acceleration of the hazard rate and timing of mortality crossing

For the purpose of analytic simplicity and convenience and without loss of generality, I now propose a number of additional axioms regarding mortality differences. First, I assume that there are two groups in a birth cohort, with each described by a different survival function. I term Group I (G_1) as the 'advantaged' group and term Group II (G_2) as the 'disadvantaged' group. Accordingly, Group I has a lower mortality rate initially than does Group II because of the favorable early life conditions. As previously noted, a predetermined maximum human lifespan ω is assumed to exist. Individuals within each group, however, do not necessarily have the same maximum length of life potential. Lastly, I hypothesize that, although they would eventually converge given the existence of a common maximum life span ω, the two survival curves would never cross.

Making use of Equations (9.58), (9.59), and (9.60), one can easily calculate the relative change in mortality, the relative rate of mortality change, and the index of relative mortality acceleration, at each exact age. The relative change in mortality, denoted by $\delta h^*(a)$, is simply the difference in the hazard rate at exact age a between G_1 and G_2, namely $[h_1^*(a)-h_2^*(a)]$. Similarly, the relative rate of mortality change, denoted by $\delta\tilde{\eta}^*(a)$, is the difference in the absolute changes in mortality between G_1 and G_2: $[\tilde{\eta}_1^*(a)-\tilde{\eta}_2^*(a)]$. The index of relative mortality acceleration, represented by $\delta\tilde{v}^*(a)$, is the difference between $\tilde{v}_1^*(a)$ and $\tilde{v}_2^*(a)$. As G_1 initially has the lower mortality rate, the value of $\delta h^*(a)$ is negative at the outset of the life course. The other two relative indicators, $\delta\tilde{\eta}^*(a)$ and $\delta\tilde{v}^*(a)$, are not necessarily negative at the beginning of the life course because their signs depend on the shapes of the survival curves for G_1 and G_2, respectively.

As the absolute mortality rates vary massively over age, the above three indicators of mortality differences may not necessarily reflect the extent to which the two mortality schedules deviate. To make these indicators comparable throughout all ages, I create three standardized measures of mortality differences between G_1 and G_2: *the standardized deviation of mortality rate*, *the standardized deviation of the rate of mortality change*, and *the standardized deviation of mortality acceleration*, denoted by, respectively, $\delta D_{h^*}(a)$, $\delta D_{\tilde{\eta}^*}(a)$, and $\delta D_{\tilde{v}^*}(a)$.

First, $\delta D_{h^*}(a)$ is mathematically defined as

$$\delta D_{h^*}(a)=\frac{\mathrm{d}\log\left[\delta h^*(a)\right]}{\mathrm{d}a}=\frac{\mathrm{d}\delta h^*(a)/\mathrm{d}a}{\delta h^*(a)}=\frac{\delta\tilde{\eta}^*(a)}{\delta h^*(a)}. \tag{9.61}$$

The second standardized measure, the standardized deviation of the rate of mortality change, is

$$\delta D_{\eta^*}(a) = \frac{\mathrm{d}\log\left[\delta\tilde{\eta}^*(a)\right]}{\mathrm{d}a} = \frac{\delta\tilde{v}^*(a)}{\delta\tilde{\eta}^*(a)}. \tag{9.62}$$

Finally, the third measure, the standardized deviation of mortality acceleration, is given by

$$\delta D_{\tilde{v}^*}(a) = \frac{\mathrm{d}\log\left[\delta\tilde{v}^*(a)\right]}{\mathrm{d}a} = \frac{\kappa_1^*(a) - \kappa_2^*(a)}{\delta\tilde{v}^*(a)}, \tag{9.63}$$

where $\kappa_k^*(a) = \mathrm{d}\,\tilde{v}_k^*(a)/\mathrm{d}a$ and its mathematical derivation is presented in Appendix E. The combination of these three standardized measures demonstrates the dynamic processes over the life course in terms of mortality differences between the two population subgroups, as relative to the risk of death.

As indicated above, values of $h_1^*(a)$ and $h_2^*(a)$ may cross at some exact age point given a predetermined maximum life span ω. If both $\delta\tilde{\eta}^*(0)$ and $\delta\tilde{v}^*(0)$ are negative, the functions $\tilde{\eta}_1^*(a)$ and $\tilde{\eta}_2^*(a)$ or $\tilde{v}_1^*(a)$ and $\tilde{v}_2^*(a)$ will have to experience crossovers as well if a mortality crossover eventually occurs. Conceivably, given the conditions that $\tilde{\eta}_1^*(0) < \tilde{\eta}_2^*(0)$ and $\tilde{v}_1^*(0) < \tilde{v}_2^*(0)$, beyond the exact age at which $\delta\tilde{v}^* = 0$, the mortality rate for G_1 would accelerate at an increasingly faster pace than for G_2. Subsequently, the time point a' at which $\delta\tilde{\eta}^* = 0$ would indicate the advent of the phase in which the absolute increase in mortality rate for G_1 exceeds the increase for G_2. Finally, the exact age a'' at which $\delta h^* = 0$ would denote the exact age point for a mortality crossover and the beginning of higher mortality for the advantaged group.

Within the construct of the Gompertzian survival function, the crossing points for the force of mortality, the absolute change per unit of time, and the mortality acceleration between G_1 and G_2 are well defined, given the occurrence of a mortality crossover, given by

$$a_h = \frac{1}{r_2 - r_1}\ln\left[\frac{h_0^{(1)}}{h_0^{(2)}}\right], \tag{9.64}$$

$$a_{\tilde{\eta}} = \frac{1}{r_2 - r_1}\ln\left[\frac{h_0^{(1)} r_1}{h_0^{(2)} r_2}\right], \tag{9.65}$$

and

$$a_{\tilde{v}} = \frac{1}{r_2 - r_1}\ln\left[\frac{h_0^{(1)} r_1^2}{h_0^{(2)} r_2^2}\right], \tag{9.66}$$

where a_h, $a_{\tilde{\eta}}$, and $a_{\tilde{v}}$ represent, respectively, the crossing age of the hazard rate, of the absolute change, and of the mortality acceleration, and $h_0^{(k)}$ and r_k are the Gompertzian parameters h_0 and r for group k (k = 1, 2).

In the definition of a truncated survival function, there is no analytic solution for those crossing points. These age points, however, can be easily identified using a simple approximation approach. Basically, the crossing points of the adjusted mortality indicators are very close to those of the original Gompertzian function because $S(\omega)$ tends to be a very small value. Given the truncated survival functions, the crossing ages for the hazard rate, the absolute change, and the mortality acceleration are denoted by, respectively, a_h^*, $a_{\tilde{\eta}}^*$, and $a_{\tilde{v}}^*$, as will be used below.

As $h_1^*(0) < h_2^*(0)$, the occurrence of a mortality crossover calls for a higher absolute increase in mortality for G_1 as its precondition. Furthermore, providing $\tilde{v}_1^*(0) < \tilde{v}_2^*(0)$ and $\tilde{\eta}_1^*(0) < \tilde{\eta}_2^*(0)$, the crossover of the rate of mortality acceleration must predate the crossing of the absolute increase in the hazard rate. Therefore, it can be inferred that $a_h^* > a_{\tilde{\eta}}^* > a_{\tilde{v}}^*$ under the conditions that $r_1 \neq r_2$ and that a mortality crossover eventually occurs in later life. In fact, the existence of a predetermined maximum life span may intrinsically highlight crossovers of three interrelated mortality functions.

Neither the crossover of $\tilde{\eta}^*(a)$ nor the crossover of $\tilde{v}^*(a)$, however, is a necessary or a sufficient condition for the occurrence of a mortality crossover. If $\tilde{\eta}_1^*(0) > \tilde{\eta}_2^*(0)$ or $\tilde{v}_1^*(0) > \tilde{v}_2^*(0)$, there can be no crossovers at all between $\tilde{\eta}_1^*(a)$ and $\tilde{\eta}_2^*(a)$ or between $\tilde{v}_1^*(a)$ and $\tilde{v}_2^*(a)$ because the rate of absolute increase or the rate of acceleration for G_1 may be higher than for G_2 throughout the whole life course (Doubal and Klemera, 1990; Liu and Witten, 1995). It is conceivable that, as the intrinsic mortality crossover requires consistent acceleration of mortality for the advantaged persons, $\delta\tilde{v}^*(a) < 0$ could never exist. In terms of the truncated Gompertzian survival function, whether the crossover between $\tilde{\eta}_1^*(a)$ and $\tilde{\eta}_2^*(a)$ or between $\tilde{v}_1^*(0)$ and $\tilde{v}_2^*(0)\alpha_1^*(a)$ occurs depends on the values of h_0 and r for the two groups.

9.4.3 Mathematical conditions for maximum life span and mortality crossover

In an earlier article on mortality crossovers (Liu and Witten, 1995), my coauthor and I examined a class of continuous survival functions in which the existence of a maximum life span requires a crossover in the mortality functions of advantaged and disadvantaged subpopulations. Specifically, we considered the implication of a predetermined maximum life span on two distinct population subgroups: one group environmentally advantaged, the other group disadvantaged. By illustrations via some simulated examples, we showed that the existence of a genetically predetermined maximum life span might impose the condition that the two subgroup mortality rates cross in later life. We further observed that proportional mortality differences are associated with a divergent trend over the life course that is generally not observable among older persons. Furthermore, we demonstrated the occurrence of a possible mortality crossover in the absence of a common maximum life span for the two subpopulations, thereby implying that the existence of a genetically predetermined maximum life span is not a necessary condition for mortality crossovers.

Results in another piece of our work on this issue (Hirsch, Liu, and Witten, 2000) further indicated that if the survival functions are discontinuous, proportional mortality differences can be consistent with survival functions having a maximum life span. This relationship suggests that although crossovers of different mortality schedules are highly possible, the existence of a common maximum life span between two population subgroups is not a sufficient condition for a mortality crossover. In large human populations, $S(\omega)$ tends to be very small, and the truncated survival and mortality functions differ slightly from the extended forms. The truncation transformation, formulated by Equation (9.57), effectively stretches the ordinate of the survival function. If $S(\omega)$ is small, then the degree of stretch is small. The transformation, however, produces a qualitative change in the shape of the mortality function. In terms of the truncated Gompertz function, the truncated mortality rate $h^*(\omega)$, obtained from the truncated survival function $S^*(\omega)$, becomes infinite due to the singularity introduced in the denominator of Equation (9.58). The mortality rate in rectangular coordinates may approach a vertical asymptote hyperbolically at the maximum life span given a discontinuous step function of survival.

An approximate discrete form of the mortality function, $h^{*\Delta}(\omega)$, is defined by replacing the differentials dS^* and da in Equation (9.52) with finite differences:

$$h^{*\Delta}(a) = -\frac{1}{S^*(a)}\frac{\Delta S^*(a)}{\Delta a}, \tag{9.67}$$

where

$$\Delta S^*(a) = S^*(a) - S^*(\omega) \tag{9.68}$$

and

$$\Delta a = a - \omega. \tag{9.69}$$

With the use of Equation (9.57), $S^*(\omega) = 0$, and, from Equation (9.68), $\Delta S^*(a) = S^*(a)$. Simultaneous solution of Equations (9.67) to (9.69) then yields

$$h^{*\Delta}(a) = -\frac{1}{\omega - a}. \tag{9.70}$$

Thus, the approximate form of the mortality rate is hyperbolic. The corresponding survival function, $S^{*\Delta}$, is linear:

$$S^{*\Delta}(a) = 1 - \frac{a}{\omega}. \tag{9.71}$$

The relation between Equations (9.70) and (9.71) can be verified by substitution of the derivative of Equation (9.71) into Equation (9.52). Notice that the only approximation used to obtain Equation (9.70) is the substitution of finite differences for differentials.

The above equations, together with some empirical examples, illustrate the general result that theoretically the existence of a common predetermined maximum life span does not necessarily imply a mortality crossover between the advantaged and disadvantaged subpopulations if the mortality functions approach infinity at the maximum life span. In particular, mortality functions of two different population subgroups may be proportional throughout the life course and may therefore fail to cross if the survival functions of these groups are discontinuous.

9.5 Survival convergence and the preceding mortality crossover

As discussed in Section 9.4, a common maximum life span for two population subgroups is neither a necessary nor a sufficient condition for the occurrence of a mortality crossover in later life. Hirsch, Liu, and Witten (2000) and Wilmoth (1997) both state that the mortality rate must approach infinity as age approaches the maximum life span, as also described in Chapter 1. The approach to infinity occurs in both the accelerated-mortality and sudden-death models (Hirsch, Liu, and Witten, 2000) but not in the scenarios examined by Liu and Witten (1995), where survival functions are continuous. This inference prompts the introduction of another interesting theoretical question regarding the mortality crossover between two population subgroups: If two survival curves converge before all members die out, then will the two mortality schedules have to cross at some age point before ω?

My answer to this theoretical question is a firm 'yes.' As discussed earlier, survival functions for two population subgroups, one environmentally advantaged and one disadvantaged, tend to converge in later life no matter how much they are separated at younger ages. Consequently, the group initially having the lower level of mortality will sooner or later experience faster mortality acceleration to complete the convergence of the two survival functions (Hirsch, Liu, and Witten, 2000; Liu *et al.*, 2008; Liu and Witten, 1995). Such mortality acceleration will eventually usher in a higher mortality rate for the advantaged group before the two survival curves converge at a given age point. This relationship can be readily identified from distinct changes in the shapes of two group survival curves and can be mathematically proved. It follows that survival convergence implies a mortality crossover to be a frequently occurring demographic event, closely associated with the dynamic process of survival convergence.

In this section, I first provide mathematical proofs for the relationship between survival convergence and the occurrence of a mortality crossover. Then some simulations are illustrated. The section is concluded with several explanations on the occurrence of survival convergence and the preceding mortality crossover.

9.5.1 Mathematical proofs for survival convergence and mortality crossovers

I follow the basic specifications and the additional axioms concerning mortality differences described in Subsections 9.4.1 and 9.4.2. Here, I seek to mathematically prove that convergence of two survival functions implies the preceding occurrence of a mortality crossover. Theoretically, as emphasized in Chapter 1, the survival and the hazard functions are simply two profiles of a single demographic phenomenon. The reason I view the mortality rate as the function of its affiliated survival probability is twofold. First, it is much easier to capture the changing pattern of differences between two survival functions, as they both start at one and end at zero. Second, the convergence of two survival curves is a widely accepted phenomenon among demographers and biologists, and many view survival convergence as a natural consequence of human longevity. In Fries' (1980) theory on compression of morbidity, for example, new medical treatments for diseases and environmental improvements rectangularize the survival function, but it remains bounded at its theoretical upper end.

Suppose that for two population subgroups G_1 and G_2 with continuous hazard functions, the hazard rate of G_1, the advantaged, is initially lower than that of G_2, the disadvantaged, denoted by $h_1(0) < h_2(0)$, but the two survival curves, S_1 and S_2, converge at exact age $a^* > 0$, given by

$$S_1(a^*) = S_2(a^*). \tag{9.72}$$

Given this convergence, I further specify the proposition that given the condition $S_1(a^*) = S_2(a^*)$, there must exist an interval $(\acute{l}, \acute{u}) \subset (0, a^*)$ where $h_1(a) > h_2(a)$ for $a \in (\acute{l}, \acute{u})$. Below, I provide two mathematical proofs for this proposition.

Proof 1:
By contradiction, suppose $h_1(a) < h_2(a)$ for all $a \in (0, a^*)$, given by

$$\int_0^{a^*} h_1(a)\mathrm{d}a < \int_0^{a^*} h_2(a)\mathrm{d}a. \tag{9.73}$$

This inequality is strict because $h_1(0) < h_2(0)$ and both $h_1(a)$ and $h_2(a)$ are continuous. It follows that

$$S_1(a^*) = \exp\left(-\int_0^{a^*} h_1(a)\,\mathrm{d}a\right) > \exp\left[-\int_0^{a^*} h_2(a)\,\mathrm{d}a\right] = S_2(a^*). \tag{9.74}$$

Obviously, Equation (9.74) contradicts the condition that $S_1(a^*) = S_2(a^*)$. Therefore, there must exist at least one point $\hat{a}$ between 0 and a^* at which $h_1(\hat{a}) > h_2(\hat{a})$. The continuity of the hazard function ensures that $h_1(a) > h_2(a)$ holds in an age interval around $\hat{a}$.

Proof 2:
Given the specification

$$S(a) = \exp\left(-\int_0^{a} h(u)\,\mathrm{d}u\right) = \exp[-H(a)],$$

Equation (9.72) can be expressed as

$$\exp\left(-\int_0^{a^*} h_1(a)\,\mathrm{d}a\right) = \exp\left[-\int_0^{a^*} h_2(a)\,\mathrm{d}a\right] \tag{9.75a}$$

or

$$\exp[-H_1(a^*)] = \exp[-H_2(a^*)]. \tag{9.75b}$$

As defined in Chapter 1, $H(a)$ is the cumulative hazard rate at age a. Mathematically, Equation (9.75b) can reduce further to

$$H_1(a^*) = H_2(a^*). \tag{9.76}$$

As the cumulative mortality rate at age a^* is simply the sum of all hazard rates from age 0 to age a^*, there must exist an age range, older than $\acute{l}$, where the death rates of G_1 are higher than those of G_2, to satisfy the condition imposed by Equation (9.76). This relationship implies that the occurrence of the mortality crossover must precede the survival convergence given the continuity of the hazard function.

The above equations verify that as long as the mortality rates for two population subgroups differ initially and their survival functions converge at an older age before all group members die out, a mortality crossover must occur prior to the convergence of the two survival curves. Therefore, mortality crossovers among population subgroups are a highly observable demographic event, just as the survival convergence is a frequently observed phenomenon. If survival convergence occurs for two population subgroups, the overall mortality for both subpopulations must be identical at the age of convergence, as shown by Equation (9.76). This relationship suggests that for a specific population subgroup, a sizable relative reduction in mortality at younger ages must be complemented by a substantial mortality increase in later life as long as its survival curve converges asymptotically with those for other population subgroups. Advantaged persons can benefit from such a survival pattern because their average life is extended, but the timing for them to die out tends to be the same as for their disadvantaged counterparts. Consequently, individuals who are environmentally advantaged have to die faster in later life, given a greater force of mortality. Rejection of the occurrence of a mortality crossover as a realistic demographic phenomenon, therefore, implicitly leads to the proposition that, of numerous survival curves for a species, none would converge with any of the others throughout the entire life course. Obviously, this pattern contradicts what is usually observed in the real world.

Notice that while it is a sufficient condition, survival convergence is not a necessary condition for the occurrence of a mortality crossover because mortality crossovers can take place without survival convergence. This property is discussed in Section 9.4 and is empirically demonstrated in the following simulations.

9.5.2 Simulations

In this subsection, I present the results of two simulations to strengthen empirically the argument on the relationship between survival convergence and the preceding mortality crossover. Data used for the simulations primarily come from several Japanese life tables in the period 1987–1990 (Japanese Ministry of Education (Ed.), *Abridged Life Tables, 1987–1990*, Health and Welfare Statistics Association, Tokyo). At present, Japan has the longest life expectancy in the world and boasts a highly reliable vital registration system. Therefore, it is appropriate to make use of these data for empirical illustrations on the association between survival convergence and a mortality crossover in later life.

The classic Gompertzian survival function is applied for the simulations. Here, I consider the convergence of the survival functions for two population cohorts that can happen at any age in the life course. In particular, two patterns of differential mortality are examined: (1) the occurrence of a mortality crossover and its timing in conjunction with the convergence of two group survival functions and (2) the occurrence of a mortality crossover and its timing without survival convergence.

9.5.2.1 Scenario I

Scenario I illustrates the process of survival convergence and the preceding mortality crossover between G_1 and G_2, hypothesized to follow two different Gompertzian survival functions. The values of $h_0^{(1)}$, $h_0^{(2)}$, r_1, and r_2, required to fit the two survival curves and the corresponding mortality rates, are derived from the empirical survival data of two Japanese life tables, using Equation (9.53). (Note that because only the life tables by gender are available, I select the 1987 male life table to represent the survival function for an environmentally disadvantaged group, and the 1990 female life table as the advantaged group.) The method of nonlinear least squares regression is employed to generate these estimates, using data of proportions surviving at age 15 through 85. The SAS PROC NLIN procedure is used to derive the parameter estimates – $h_0^{(1)}$, $h_0^{(2)}$, r_1, and r_2. Below is the SAS program for the derivation of the parameter estimates of h_0 and r for the 'disadvantaged' group (G_2).

SAS Program 9.4:

```
......

data Gompertz;
  input age survival@@;
cards;
15 .99044 16 .99008 17 .98956 18 .98888 19 .98809
20 .98726 21 .98646 22 .98567 23 .98492 24 .98419
25 .98346 26 .98271 27 .98194 28 .98115 29 .98036
30 .97957 31 .97879 32 .97798 33 .97712 34 .97621
35 .97525 36 .97422 37 .97311 38 .97188 39 .97053
40 .96905 41 .96741 42 .96563 43 .96368 44 .96153
45 .95915 46 .95655 47 .95371 48 .95061 49 .94721
50 .94344 51 .93924 52 .93452 53 .92920 54 .92323
55 .91664 56 .90949 57 .90186 58 .89377 59 .88519
60 .87609 61 .86642 62 .85610 63 .84504 64 .83312
65 .82037 66 .80672 67 .79211 68 .77635 69 .75922
70 .74061 71 .72049 72 .69884 73 .67560 74 .65057
75 .62361 76 .59453 77 .56332 78 .53004 79 .49493
80 .45839 81 .42092 82 .38285 83 .34466 84 .30683
85 .26985
;

proc nlin data=Gompertz maxiter=50 converge=0.00001;
  model survival = exp(h0/r*(1-exp(age*r)));
  parms h0 = 0.00016, r = 0.10;
run;
```

The SAS temporary dataset Gompertz contains two variables Age (exact age) and Survival (survival rate). The double trailing at sign @@ in the INPUT statement tells SAS that observations are input from each line until all of the values are read. The DATA = option specifies that the SAS dataset Gompertz be used in the analysis. The MAXITER = option specifies the number of iterations PROC NLIN performs before it gives up trying to converge. The CONVERGE option informs SAS of the convergence criteria for PROC NLIN. I do not specify the METHOD option because the default METHOD = GAUSS is used. The MODEL statement specifies the classical Gompertzian survival model specified by Equation (9.53). The PARMS statement specifies the parameters and their initial values. The parameter initial values are obtained from results of previous studies. Alternatively, the researcher can specify a range of values for any parameter.

The parameter estimates from PROC NLIN are displayed in the following SAS output.

SAS Program Output 9.2:

The NLIN Procedure
Dependent Variable survival
Method: Gauss-Newton

Iterative Phase

Iter	h0	r	Sum of Squares
0	0.000160	0.1000	6.6988
1	0.000550	0.0266	2.1841
2	0.000298	0.0419	1.8033
3	0.000122	0.0605	1.4075
4	0.000035	0.0879	0.4612
5	0.000057	0.0874	0.0201
6	0.000050	0.0906	0.00741
7	0.000050	0.0907	0.00731
8	0.000050	0.0907	0.00731
9	0.000050	0.0907	0.00731

NOTE: Convergence criterion met.

Estimation Summary

Method	Gauss-Newton
Iterations	9
Subiterations	4
Average Subiterations	0.444444
R	2.902E-6
PPC(h0)	1.542E-6
RPC(h0)	0.00002
Object	1.748E-9
Objective	0.007312
Observations Read	71
Observations Used	71
Observations Missing	0

NOTE: An intercept was not specified for this model.

Source	DF	Sum of Squares	Mean Square	F Value	Approx Pr > F
Model	2	53.3427	26.6714	251677	<.0001
Error	69	0.00731	0.000106		
Uncorrected Total	71	53.3500			

Parameter	Estimate	Approx Std Error	Approximate 95% Confidence Limits	
h0	0.000050	3.263E-6	0.000043	0.000056
r	0.0907	0.000995	0.0887	0.0927

In SAS Program Output 9.2, the first section displays the iteration history. Specifically, when the relative measure is less than 10^{-5}, the convergence is declared. The second section, Estimation Summary, presents a summary of the estimation including several convergence measures – R, PPC, RPC, and Object. In particular, R is a relative offset convergence measure and the PPC value (1.542E-6) shows that the parameter h_0 would change by that relative amount if PROC NLIN takes an additional iteration step. Likewise, the RPC value indicates a change by 0.00002, relative to its value in the last iteration. The third section displays the least-squares summary statistics for the Gompertzian model, including the degrees of freedom sums of squares and mean squares. Not surprisingly, the Gompertzian model fits the data extremely well, with the value of R^2 very close to 1. The last section displays the estimates for each parameter, the asymptotic standard error, and the upper and lower values for the 95 % confidence interval. PROC NLIN also calculates the asymptotic correlation between the estimated parameters, not presented in this illustration.

The parameter estimates of h_0 and r for the 'advantaged' group (G_1) can be derived using the same PROC NLIN procedure, inputting its survival rates at each age from 15 to 85. Because the differences in survival rates between male and female may not be separated enough to highlight the mortality differences between two socioeconomic groups, I use the upper points of $h_0^{(1)}$ and r_1, on the basis of the 95 % confidence interval, as the estimates for the advantaged group. The four measures are estimated as follows: $h_0^{(1)} = 0.000\,015$, $h_0^{(2)} = 0.000\,050$, $r_1 = 0.1043$, and $r_2 = 0.0907$. Given these values of Gompertzian parameters, I let 110 years be the exact age at which S_1 and S_2 are assumed to converge. For analytic convenience, it is further assumed that no one in G_1 and G_2 would survive beyond age 110. As a consequence, the truncated values of the Gompertzian survival function and the adjusted mortality measures, described in Section 9.4, are calculated, which, except for the values at several oldest ages, are identical to those derived from the original Gompertzian model. The SAS program computing those truncated mortality indicators is presented below.

SAS Program 9.5:

```
......

data Crossover;

r1 = 0.1043;
r2 = 0.0907;
h0_1 = 0.000015;
h0_2 = 0.000050;

w1 = 110;
w2 = 110;
lastage = 110;

do age=15 to lastage by 5;

exp1 = exp(r1 * age);
exp2 = exp(r2 * age);

hx1 = h0_1 * exp1;
hx2 = h0_2 * exp2;
```

```
sw1 = exp((h0_1 / r1) * (1 - exp(r1*w1)));
sw2 = exp((h0_2 / r2) * (1 - exp(r2*w2)));

sx1 = exp((h0_1 / r1) * (1 - exp1));
sx2 = exp((h0_2 / r2) * (1 - exp2));

etax1 = hx1 * r1;
etax2 = hx2 * r2;

alpha1 = etax1 * r1;
alpha2 = etax2 * r2;

sx1_star = (sx1 - sw1) / (1 - sw1);
sx2_star = (sx2 - sw2) / (1 - sw2);

phi1 = sw1 / sx1;
phi2 = sw2 / sx2;

hx1_star = hx1 (1 - phi1);
hx2_star = hx2 / (1 - phi2);

etax1_star = hx1_star * (r1 + hx1_star * phi1);
etax2_star = hx2_star * (r2 + hx2_star * phi2);

psi1_star = (r1**2) + (3*r1*hx1_star*phi1) + ((hx1_star**2*phi1)
           * (1 + phi1));
psi2_star = (r2**2) + (3*r2*hx2_star*phi2) + ((hx2_star**2*phi2)
           * (1 + phi2));

alphax1_star = hx1_star * psi1_star;
alphax2_star = hx2_star * psi2_star;

kappa1_star = (psi1_star*etax1_star) + hx1_star*((hx1_star**2)*(1+2*phi1)
    *(hx1_star*phi1)*(1-phi1)+(phi1*(1+phi1)*2*hx1_star*etax1_star)
    + (3*r1*phi1)*(etax1_star+(hx1_star*hx1_star*(1-phi1))));
kappa2_star = (psi2_star*etax2_star) + hx2_star*((hx2_star**2)*(1+2*phi2)
    *(hx2_star*phi2)*(1-phi2)+(phi2*(1+phi2)*2*hx2_star*etax2_star)
    + (3*r2*phi2)*(etax2_star+(hx2_star*hx2_star*(1-phi2))));

dhstar = hx1_star - hx2_star;
detastar = etax1_star - etax2_star;
dalphastar = alphax1_star - alphax2_star;
dkappastar = kappa1_star - kappa2_star;

dhstar_std = detastar / dhstar;
detastar_std = dalphastar - detastar;
dalphastar_std = dkappastar / dalphastar;

xh = (1/(r2-r1)) * log(h0_1/h0_2);
xeta = (1/(r2-r1)) * log((h0_1*r1)/(h0_2*r2));
xalpha = (1/(r2-r1)) * log((h0_1*(r1**2))/(h0_2*(r2**2)));

output;
end;

proc print data=crossover;
 var age-xalpha;
run;
```

SAS Program 9.5 yields a data file displaying outcomes for all survival and mortality indicators specified in Subsection 9.4.1. Given its large amount of information, I select a portion of the output to demonstrate the results, shown in Table 9.2, which displays the estimates of survival and mortality for G_1 and G_2, given the aforementioned conditions. Consistent with general circumstances, the initial survival is substantially higher for G_1 because of the favorable environment for members of this subgroup. Such differentials are observed to widen until the population approaches 80 years of age and thereafter it gradually decreases to the eventual convergence of the two survival curves. Accordingly, the initial mortality rates of G_1 are much lower than those of G_2. The absolute change over age in differential mortality is shown by differences between h_1 and h_2. While absolute differences may not necessarily reflect the degree of the relative change, the value of δD_{h^*}, the standardized deviation of mortality rates, demonstrates the trend of mortality convergence and crossover. At age 15, the estimate of δD_{h^*} is 0.082 78, and then its absolute value declines steadily until age 85 years. The two mortality schedules cross at age 88.53 years (this crossing point is almost identical to the estimate calculated from the original Gompertzian function). Immediately after this crossing age, the mortality rate of G_1 starts to be greater than that of G_2 and the absolute difference between h_1 and h_2 diverges over age. The value of δD_{h^*} is much increased right after the mortality crossover, but then starts decreasing. As expected, the crossing for the absolute change per unit of time and of the mortality acceleration occurs much earlier than for the hazard rate. The values of $a_{\bar{\eta}}^*$ and $a_{\bar{\nu}}^*$, not presented in Table 9.2, are 78.25 and 67.98 years of age, respectively.

Figure 9.1 plots the evolution of the two survival curves and the two corresponding mortality schedules from age 15 to age 110. Panel A displays the gradual process of convergence between S_1 and S_2, whereas Panel B shows the convergence and the crossover between h_1 and h_2. These two graphs together demonstrate steady changes in the slopes of the two survival curves, the mortality acceleration of the 'advantaged' persons, and the crossing of the two mortality schedules. They also suggest that although survival convergence and the mortality crossover occur at some very older ages, the underlying process of mortality convergence, in accordance with survival convergence, starts at a much earlier age.

9.5.2.2 Scenario II

Scenario II displays a possible mortality crossover in the absence of survival convergence between G_1 and G_2. In this step, the survival and mortality functions of G_2 are assumed to remain the same, whereas those of G_1 are modified such that no one survives beyond the exact age of 120 years, so the two survival curves would never converge. Accordingly, the value of $h_0^{(1)}$ is adjusted as 0.000 013. Table 9.3 presents the results of this simulation.

In Scenario II, the pattern of mortality differences appears fairly close to that in Scenario I. As the baseline hazard rate of G_1 is lowered, the initial survival for this subgroup is somewhat higher than in Scenario I. Accordingly, the mortality rate at age 15 for G_1 is lower than previously reported, in turn elevating the mortality differences at younger ages. Compared to mortality differences in Scenario I, the mortality rate of G_1 in Scenario II is shown to accelerate less sharply at older ages, given the absence of survival convergence. Nevertheless, as G_1 maintains faster mortality acceleration at older ages than G_2, a mortality crossover

Table 9.2 Survival probabilities and mortality rates for G_1 and G_2: Scenario I ($h_0^{(1)} = 0.000015$, $h_0^{(2)} = 0.000050$, $r_1 = 0.104300$, and $r_2 = 0.090700$).

Age	Survival (S)		Mortality Rate and Relative Change			
(a)	S_1	S_2	h_1	h_2	δh	δD_{h^*}
15	0.99946	0.99840	0.00007	0.00019	−0.00012	0.08278
20	0.99899	0.99717	0.00012	0.00031	−0.00019	0.08187
25	0.99819	0.99524	0.00020	0.00048	−0.00028	0.08079
30	0.99686	0.99220	0.00034	0.00076	−0.00042	0.07952
35	0.99462	0.98745	0.00058	0.00120	−0.00062	0.07800
40	0.99086	0.98001	0.00097	0.00188	−0.00091	0.07615
45	0.98455	0.96841	0.00164	0.00296	−0.00132	0.07386
50	0.97402	0.95043	0.00276	0.00466	−0.00190	0.07095
55	0.95654	0.92281	0.00465	0.00734	−0.00269	0.06716
60	0.92779	0.88096	0.00783	0.01155	−0.00371	0.06201
65	0.88130	0.81891	0.01319	0.01817	−0.00498	0.05464
70	0.80819	0.72998	0.02223	0.02860	−0.00637	0.04324
75	0.69849	0.60918	0.03744	0.04501	−0.00756	0.02337
80	0.54630	0.45824	0.06307	0.07083	−0.00776	−0.01988
85	0.36112	0.29274	0.10625	0.11147	−0.00522	−0.18587
90	0.17980	0.14461	0.17898	0.17544	0.00354	0.77769
95	0.05554	0.04766	0.30151	0.27614	0.02537	0.25195
100	0.00768	0.00830	0.50797	0.43490	0.07307	0.18351
105	0.00027	0.00052	0.85872	0.69303	0.16569	0.13908
110	0.00000	0.00000	—	—	—	—
a_h			88.53			

Source: Japanese Ministry of Health (ed.) (1991) *Abridged Life Tables 1987–1990.*

still occurs, though at an older age. As indicated in Table 9.3, the mortality crossover between G_1 and G_2 takes place at age 99.09 years, about 11 years before all disadvantaged persons die out. Figure 9.2 visually displays the dynamic process of this mortality crossover given Scenario II.

The simulation of Scenario II provides strong evidence that a mortality crossover can take place in the absence of survival convergence. If two distinct survival curves get closer at older ages, the mortality rate among advantaged persons tends to accelerate at a faster pace, thereby leading to a possible mortality crossover.

9.5.3 Explanations for survival convergence and the preceding mortality crossover

Researchers in survival analysis and differential mortality have exploited a number of explanations for the mechanisms involved in the occurrence of survival convergence and the preceding mortality crossover.

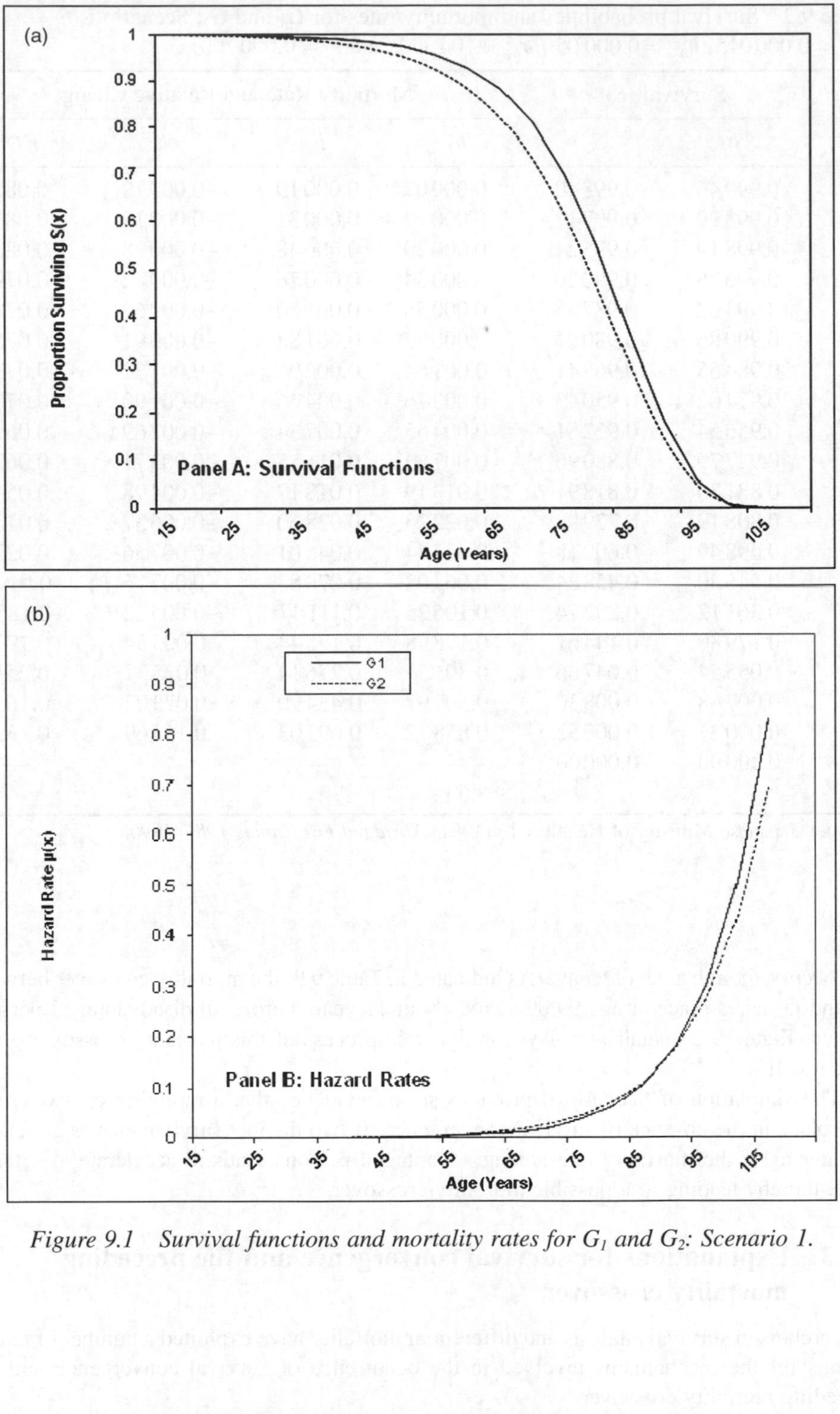

Figure 9.1 Survival functions and mortality rates for G_1 and G_2: Scenario 1.

Table 9.3 Survival probabilities and mortality rates for G_1 and G_2: Scenario II ($h_0^{(1)} = 0.000\,013$, $h_0^{(2)} = 0.000\,050$, $r_1 = 0.104\,300$, and $r_2 = 0.090\,700$).

Age	Survival (S)		Mortality rate and relative change			
(a)	S_1	S_2	h_1	h_2	δh	δD_{h^*}
15	0.99953	0.99840	0.00006	0.00019	−0.00013	0.08433
20	0.99912	0.99717	0.00010	0.00031	−0.00020	0.08365
25	0.99844	0.99524	0.00018	0.00048	−0.00031	0.08287
30	0.99728	0.99220	0.00030	0.00076	−0.00046	0.08197
35	0.99534	0.98745	0.00050	0.00120	−0.00070	0.08091
40	0.99207	0.98001	0.00084	0.00188	−0.00104	0.07966
45	0.98660	0.96841	0.00142	0.00296	−0.00154	0.07817
50	0.97745	0.95043	0.00239	0.00466	−0.00227	0.07636
55	0.96222	0.92281	0.00403	0.00734	−0.00331	0.07412
60	0.93711	0.88096	0.00679	0.01155	−0.00476	0.07129
65	0.89627	0.81891	0.01144	0.01817	−0.00674	0.06761
70	0.83147	0.72998	0.01926	0.02860	−0.00933	0.06263
75	0.73272	0.60918	0.03245	0.04501	−0.01256	0.05555
80	0.59216	0.45824	0.05466	0.07083	−0.01617	0.04472
85	0.41365	0.29274	0.09208	0.11147	−0.01939	0.02613
90	0.22602	0.14461	0.15512	0.17544	−0.02032	−0.01303
95	0.08166	0.04766	0.26131	0.27614	−0.01484	−0.14809
100	0.01470	0.00830	0.44018	0.43490	0.00529	1.19304
105	0.00082	0.00052	0.74151	0.69303	0.04849	0.16780
110	0.00001	0.00000	1.24912	—	—	—
a_h			99.09			

One plausible hypothesis is the ‘frailty’ theory (Vaupel, 1990; Vaupel, Manton, and Stallard, 1979), described extensively in Section 9.3. This theory concerns the change over age in population health composition because the process of human survival selects out more relatively frail persons among the environmentally disadvantaged. When such a compositional change exerts a strong negative effect on survivorship, thus offsetting the positive impact of a favorable environment among advantaged persons, its mortality rate starts accelerating faster than would be anticipated, in turn leading to the occurrence of a mortality crossover. This explanation, however, should be linked with sustained convergence between two mortality schedules arising from the dynamic ‘selection of the fittest’ process (Liu and Witten, 1995). Increased excess mortality among initially advantaged persons may indicate that other factors contribute more significantly to mortality differences in later life than the ‘frailty’ factor.

Some researchers argue that changes in mortality differentials over the life cycle do not necessarily arise from the impact the ‘frailty’ factor has on population health composition (Khazaeli, Xiu, and Curtsinger, 1995). Changes in an individual’s behavior and physiological

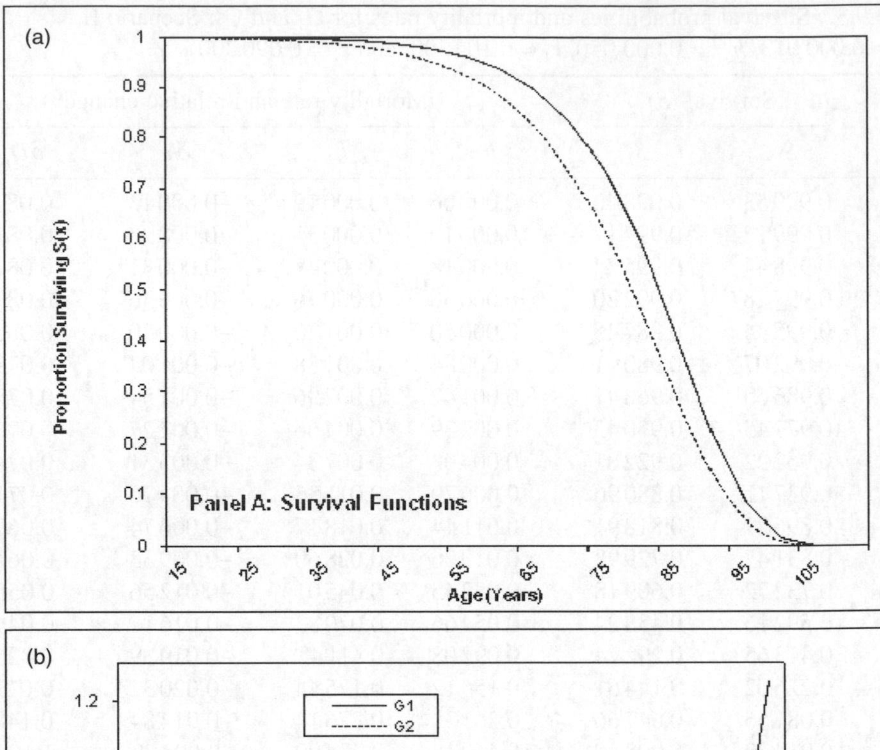

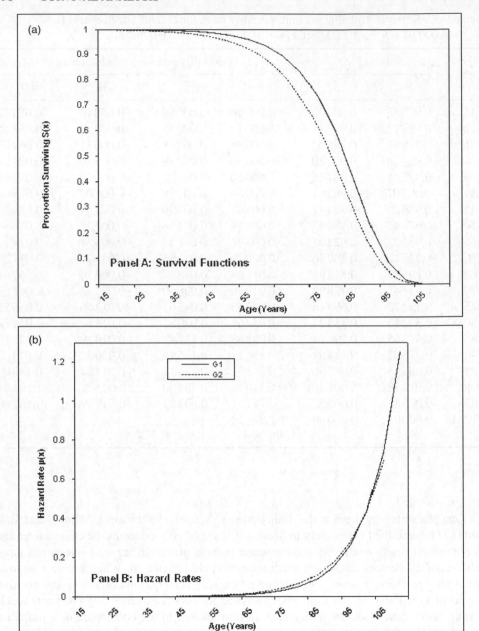

Figure 9.2 Survival functions and mortality rates for G_1 and G_2: Scenario II.

functions, and economic, social, and medical developments in a society can also contribute substantially to mortality crossovers at older ages (Horiuchi, 1989; Horiuchi and Wilmoth, 1998). It is possible that in the long-standing process of mortality evolution, a variety of social and economic factors can usher in dramatic structural changes in differential mortality (Liu, Hermalin, and Chuang, 1998; Preston, 1990). Extensive family support for older persons, for example, may distinctively mitigate mortality differences by socioeconomic status.

A third hypothesis links survival convergence and mortality crossover to the existence of a predetermined maximum life span, beyond which no member of a given species survives (Hirsch, Liu, and Witten, 2000; Liu and Witten, 1995). Given a biologically mandated upper bound on the human maximum life span, the survival curves for two population subgroups, separate in early life, would converge asymptotically late in the life course toward a common maximum life span. This trend leads to faster mortality acceleration in advantaged persons, thus fostering the occurrence of a mortality crossover, by means of whatever channel the process goes through. This theory also explains well why the two mortality schedules often diverge after a crossover. I personally believe that the frequently observed convergence of survival curves in later life should be mandated by an invisible hand – the existence of a potential upper bound for human species. As Wilmoth (1997) comments, however, it is difficult to find sufficient data to find a maximum life span, thus making it a difficult hypothesis to test. Moreover, theoretically a mortality crossover does not necessarily occur if the two survival curves do not converge until the maximum exact age, where the hazard rate is infinitive (Hirsch, Liu, and Witten, 2000; Wilmoth, 1997).

Each of the above explanations can lead to a mortality crossover between any two population subgroups. I hold, however, that, in reality, survival convergence and the preceding mortality crossover should result from combined influences of more than one factor. The formation of a greater force of mortality among the 'advantaged' persons must operate through some specific observable factors, such as the worsening of average health, lack of appropriate social support, and the like. My analysis on the mortality crossover between older veterans and nonveterans has suggested that the selection of the fittest and the long-term health impact of military service both contribute significantly to the long-standing process of mortality convergence, mortality crossover, and the subsequent excess death rate among older veterans (Liu *et al.*, 2006). It has also been found in the same analysis that many of the changes in mortality differences between older veterans and nonveterans are not captured by variations in health status, especially among the oldest old. The mechanisms inherent in the occurrence of a mortality crossover can be far more complex than we currently understand.

Further knowledge of these theoretical issues is important for both researchers and policy makers. For researchers, clarifying the relationship between survival convergence and a mortality crossover expands understanding of the mechanisms involved in human longevity and the pattern of differential mortality. Statisticians, demographers, and biologists would become more attuned to the fact that, in modeling and analyzing mortality processes, there exist some unknown and intractable factors that can substantially modify the direction and magnitude of mortality differentials over the life course. For planners and policy makers, extensive knowledge of the association between survival convergence and the occurrence of a mortality crossover allows for a deeper understanding of structural changes in the distribution of health status among older persons, thus facilitating a more appropriate allocation of social and economic resources.

9.6 Sample size required and power analysis

Statistics is science of inference. It comprises a set of rules and procedures for collecting, describing, analyzing, and interpreting numerical data. In most scientific studies, data of an entire population under investigation are not available, either because the population is too large or because the process of data collection is too costly. Frequently, researchers collect data from a portion of a target population selected randomly by following some rigorous sampling procedures. From such sampled data, they compute certain statistics or quantities to examine characteristics of the population.

While using data of a random sample for estimating population statistics, researchers are faced with two basic issues concerning the quality of data. First, they need to know how to determine the appropriate sample size required for the derivation of reliable and valid population estimates. Second, they should ascertain whether a quantity or an estimate derived from a random sample with a given sample size is statistically meaningful for the entire population. In statistics, power analysis deals with those issues, involving a wide array of well-developed techniques. Conventionally, the power of a statistical test is defined as the probability that yields statistically significant results (Cohen, 1988). Increased power indicates the decrease in the chance of a Type II error, specified as the false negative rate and mathematically denoted by the nonitalicized symbol β. Thus, statistically power is equal to $1 - \beta$. In most empirical studies, the desired statistical power is set at 0.8 ($\beta = 0.20$). The significance level of α, the Type I error, is another key element used to calculate statistical power.

In survival analysis, data are sometimes obtained from large-scale sample surveys, with needed information collected by responses to numerous well-designed questions from selected individuals or their proxies. Because the cost is relatively low, the sample size for an observational survey is usually large enough to warrant high statistical power for the estimation of model parameters, in turn providing reliable population estimates and model-based prediction. In biomedical research, however, survival data are generally collected by clinical trials or other types of experimental design. Such studies are often aimed at comparing population means or rates between two or more alternative treatments in order to assess the effectiveness of a new treatment or a new medicine. Accordingly, they usually involve repeated measurements of certain medical biomarkers or health care indicators for selected patients or other types of subjects in treatments. Because patients selected for a clinical trial need to be observed and tested intensively and repeatedly, the measurement process is expensive and time-consuming. As a result, sample size in biomedical research is generally much smaller than in observational studies. Hence, power analysis and calculation of sample size required is essential in medical and biological settings. Without such preliminary analyses, sample size may be too high or too low. If sample size is too low, the experiment will lack the precision to describe the characteristics for a particular population; if it is too high, time and resources will be unnecessarily wasted.

In this section, I describe a popular statistical technique for calculating the sample size required in survival analysis, with specific regard to a clinical trial design. Though including the PROC POWER and PROC GLMPOWER procedures for general power and sample size computations, the SAS software package has limited capability in performing power analysis on survival data of a clinical trial design. If needed, however, the computational procedure can be easily programmed, as displayed below.

9.6.1 Calculation of sample size required

In this text, I describe formulas to calculate the sample size required specifically for proportional hazard models. The perspective is originally developed by Schoenfeld (1983) and later summarized and advanced with mathematical derivations by some other scientists (Barthel *et al.*, 2006; Collett, 2003; Shih, 1995). These formulas have been widely used for clinical trials and have been referenced in several textbooks on survival analysis (e.g., Collett, 2003; Hosmer, Lemeshow, and May, 2008). The calculation is based on the logrank score test, a hypothesis test used to compare survival functions of two samples, as described in Chapter 2. For detailed mathematical derivations of these formulas, the interested reader is referred to Collett (2003).

Suppose that there are two treatments in a study, denoted by A and B. The proportional hazard model specifies a constant hazard ratio θ for a patient given treatment B to the same person given treatment A. For analytic convenience, the outcome health measure is given as the risk of death. As specified in earlier chapters, this constant hazard ratio is independent of time and the patient's characteristics, reflecting the multiplicative effect of a given treatment. If the hazard ratio is greater than 1, treatment B has a positive effect on the mortality rate; if it is smaller than 1, the effect is negative. The calculation of the sample size required depends on the condition that the hazard ratio is significantly different from unity given a significance level α (0.05 or 0.01, say), a probability of $1 - \beta$ (e.g., 0.80), and an expected value of the hazard ratio.

The calculation procedure starts with the required number of deaths, denoted by d, which can be obtained from the following equation:

$$d = \frac{4(z_{\alpha/2} + z_{\beta})^2}{\psi \theta_R^2}, \tag{9.77}$$

where $z_{\alpha/2}$ and z_{β} are the upper $\alpha/2$ and upper β-points of the standard normal distribution (z-scores), obtainable from a table of standard normal distribution, θ_R is the log hazard ratio assumed to be distributed normally with mean 0 and variance σ^2, and ψ is the probability of not being censored by the end of the trial.

The above equation is valid only for balanced data (each treatment is assigned the same number of patients). If the two treatments have different numbers of assignment, as required by some randomized clinical controlled trials, Equation (9.77) needs to be adjusted by

$$d = \frac{(z_{\alpha/2} + z_{\beta})^2}{\pi(1-\pi)\psi \theta_R^2}, \tag{9.78}$$

where π is the proportion of patients allocated to Group A. Both Equations (9.77) and (9.78) are easy to apply. For example, let $\alpha = 0.05$, $1 - \beta$ (power) $= 0.80$, $\theta_R = -0.69$ ($HR = 0.50$), $\psi = 0.80$, and $\pi = 0.50$. Then the required number of deaths can be written as

$$d = \frac{4 \times (1.96 + 0.842)^2}{0.80 \times (0.69)^2} \approx 82.$$

Given the required number of deaths and the probability of dying over a specific observation period, the minimum sample size required for a clinical trial is

$$\hat{n} = \frac{d}{\mathrm{Prob}(\mathrm{death})}, \tag{9.79}$$

where $\hat{n}$ is the sample size required.

The next step is to calculate the probability of death within an observation interval. Suppose that there is a given length of the recruitment period, denoted by $\hat{a}$, and an additional length of the follow-up period, denoted by $\hat{f}$. Schoenfeld (1983) generates a formula to calculate the approximate probability of dying. For treatment A, it is given by

$$\mathrm{Prob}(\mathrm{death,A}) = 1 - \frac{1}{6}\left[S_{\mathrm{A}}(\hat{f}) + 4S_{\mathrm{A}}(\hat{f} + 0.5\hat{a}) + S_{\mathrm{A}}(\hat{a} + \hat{f})\right], \tag{9.80}$$

where $S_{\mathrm{A}}(t)$ is the survival rate at time t for treatment A. Similarly, the probability for treatment B is

$$\mathrm{Prob}(\mathrm{death,B}) = 1 - \frac{1}{6}\left[S_{\mathrm{B}}(\hat{f}) + 4S_{\mathrm{B}}(\hat{f} + 0.5\hat{a}) + S_{\mathrm{B}}(\hat{a} + \hat{f})\right]. \tag{9.81}$$

Given a constant hazard ratio θ, the estimate of $S_{\mathrm{B}}(t)$ can also be written by

$$\hat{S}_{\mathrm{B}}(t) = \left[\hat{S}_{\mathrm{A}}(t)\right]^{\exp(\theta)}.$$

Therefore, Equation (9.81) can be rewritten by

$$\mathrm{Prob}(\mathrm{death,B}) = 1 - \frac{1}{6}\left[S_{\mathrm{A}}(\hat{f})^{\exp(\theta)} + 4S_{\mathrm{A}}(\hat{f} + 0.5\hat{a})^{\exp(\theta)} + S_{\mathrm{A}}(\hat{a} + \hat{f})^{\exp(\theta)}\right]. \tag{9.82}$$

For a balanced design, the overall probability of death is given by

$$\mathrm{Prob}(\mathrm{death}) = 1 - \frac{1}{6}\left[\bar{S}(\hat{f}) + 4\bar{S}(\hat{f} + 0.5\hat{a}) + \bar{S}(\hat{a} + \hat{f})\right], \tag{9.83}$$

where

$$\bar{S}(t) = \frac{S_{\mathrm{A}}(t) + S_{\mathrm{B}}(t)}{2}.$$

If individuals are not equally allocated to the two treatments, the overall probability of death is

$$\text{Prob}(\text{death}) = \pi \text{Prob}(\text{death, A}) + (1-\pi)\text{Prob}(\text{death, B}). \tag{9.84}$$

Notice that the above formulas on the sample size required are based on the proportional hazards assumption, valid only when the multiplicative effect of treatment is constant throughout the entire observation period.

More recently, some researchers extend the calculation of sample size required to more complicated survey designs, such as clinical trials involving three or more treatments, non-proportional hazards, treatment crossovers, and delayed entry. In some sense, these advances are simply the extensions of the two-sample and proportional techniques. The reader interested in those advanced techniques might want to read Ahnn and Anderson (1998), Barthel *et al.* (2006), Halabi and Singh (2004), and Shih (1995). Additionally, there are specific formulas in reliability analysis for the calculation of the sample size required, and for this literature the interested reader might want to read Meeker and Escobar (1998).

9.6.2 Illustration: Calculating sample size required

In this illustration, I present an example to calculate the minimum sample size required for a clinical trial involving two treatments, A and B. First, I assume several preconditions depending on the results of some empirical analyses. In the randomization process, patients are recruited to the study over a 6-month period ($\hat{a} = 6$), and the subsequent follow-up observation period takes another 18 months ($\hat{f} = 18$). Recruited patients are evenly allocated to treatment A and treatment B. Additionally, the survival rates at 18 months ($\hat{f}$), 21 months ($\hat{f} + 0.5\hat{a}$), and 24 months ($\hat{a} + \hat{f}$) are expected to be 0.80, 0.76, and 0.70, respectively, and the probability of not being censored by the end of the trial (ψ) is 0.80. The significance level is set at $\alpha = 0.05$ ($\alpha/2 = 0.025$).

I give a series of values for the expected hazard ratio, ranging from 0.35 to 0.75 with an interval of 0.05, and a series of values for β (power = 1 – β), ranging from 0.10 to 0.30 with an interval of 0.05. With these specifications, I aim to provide a range of the sample size required, associated with nine hazard ratio values, five levels of statistical power, and the aforementioned preconditions. Using formulas provided in Subsection 9.6.1, a unifying equation for the sample size required is

$$\hat{n} = \frac{4\left(z_{0.025} + z_{\beta}\right)^2}{0.80 \times [\log(\theta)]^2 \left\langle 1 - \frac{1}{6}\left\{\frac{\left[0.80 + 0.80^{\exp(\theta)}\right]}{2} + 4\frac{\left[0.76 + 0.76^{\exp(\theta)}\right]}{2} + \frac{\left[0.70 + 0.70^{\exp(\theta)}\right]}{2}\right\}\right\rangle}.$$

With the above unifying equation, I create the following SAS TABULATE program to generate a table of the sample size required, given the above-mentioned data of recruitment period, follow-up length of time, survival rates at three time points, the significance level, the probability of not being censored, and selected values of θ and β.

SAS Program 9.6:

```
......

* Calculating the sample size required *;

Options pagesize = 60 linesize = 90 nodate;
```

```
Data Sample_size;
  do theta=0.35 to 0.75 by 0.05;
    do beta= 0.10 to 0.30 by 0.05;
    n =  (4*(probit(1-0.025)+probit(1-beta))**2)/(0.80*((log(theta))**2))/(1- 1/6)
         *((0.80+(0.80)**exp(theta))/2+4*(0.76+(0.76)**exp(theta))/2
         +(0.70+(0.70)**exp(theta))/2));
    output;
    end;
  end;

ODS RTF file='<subdirectory to save this table>\table_9.RTF';

Proc Tabulate format = 5.0;
  class beta theta;
  var n;
  Table beta,theta*n /rts = 9 box = 'Sample Size Estimate' condense;
  Label theta = 'Hazard Ratio';
  Keylabel sum = ' ';
  Title 'Sample size estimates for survival analysis';
Run;

ODS RTF CLOSE;
```

In SAS Program 9.6, a series of the sample size required is calculated with the significance level at $\alpha = 0.05$, $S(18) = 0.80$, $S(21) = 0.76$, and $S(24) = 0.70$. Setting these preconditions, the program provides 45 numbers of the sample size required, associated with five β (0.10 to 0.30) and nine θ values (0.35 to 0.75). The first part of the program specifies the mathematical formula to calculate the sample size required and the repeated computational process with varying values of β and θ. In the equation of the DATA statement, the probit(p) function calculates the *p*th quantile of the *z*-score for a standard normal distribution.

The second part of the program specifies the format of a table containing the computational results from the first part, using the PROC TABULATE procedure. The ODS RTF statement is used to route the table to a Microsoft-WORD document. The KEYLABEL statement asks SAS to remove the cells with the word ‘SUM.’ The table created by SAS Program 9.6 is displayed in Table 9.4, which provides a wide range of numbers of the sample size required for the researcher to select according to his or her criteria or interest with regard to the quality of a clinical trial with a balanced design. As the reader can recognize from the above table, the sample size required is larger if the expected hazard ratio is closer to unity or the predetermined value of β is lower (increased power). Likewise, the sample size required is smaller if the value of β is increased (decreased power) or the hazard ratio is expected to be more distant from 1. Such associations indicate that if the researcher expects the hazard ratio to be closer to 1 (a small difference in the hazard rate) or wants to achieve greater power for the estimates of model parameters, then he or she needs to increase the sample size.

The reader can readily revise SAS Program 9.6 by modifying input data as desired. For example, for certain experimental studies the period of recruitment may take longer than six months, or the researcher wants to observe the effectiveness of a new treatment for three years instead of 18 months. Additionally, for different diseases, the survival rate at time *t* varies greatly, and the researcher might want to consider more appropriate

Table 9.4 Sample size estimates for survival analysis.

Sample size estimate	Hazard ratio								
	0.35	0.4	0.45	0.5	0.55	0.6	0.65	0.7	0.75
	n	*n*	*n*	*n*	*n*	*n*	*n*	*n*	*n*
Beta									
0.1	167	215	276	358	470	628	863	1229	1845
0.15	143	183	236	306	401	537	737	1050	1576
0.2	125	160	206	267	351	469	644	918	1378
0.25	111	142	182	236	310	415	570	812	1219
0.3	98	126	162	210	276	369	507	722	1084

survival rates accordingly. Input data are usually obtainable from the results of previous empirical studies, or they can be simply simulated according to the researcher's interest. Sometimes, the hazard ratio is expected to be more deviant from 1, so that a new set of hazard ratios needs to be specified. Whatever the modification, computation of the sample size required is simple and straightforward, particularly with the availability of the above SAS program. Just plug in new values you desire into the above SAS program. Then you will obtain a new table of the sample size required containing a new range of estimates for you to select.

9.7 Summary

The purpose of this chapter is to describe some advanced techniques related to several special topics. Some of those topics represent the new developments in survival analysis, posing unique challenges to statisticians, demographers, and other quantitative methodologists. Empirically, most approaches described in this chapter are more suitable for medical or biological studies because of restrictions of sample size, unavailability of measurable variables, and the existence of unobserved genetic heterogeneity. For example, the application of frailty models is highly useful in biomedical research, particularly since sample size is generally small and many potentially important risk factors on the occurrence of a particular medical or biological event are not identifiable or measurable. In those situations, the specification of a survival model with random effects is highly valuable. In social science, on the other hand, survival data are often obtained from large-scale observational surveys, and the potential effects of latent genetic or physical predisposition can be considerably 'washed out' by the fixed effects of observable covariates; therefore adding an arbitrarily assigned error term may be unnecessary and redundant.

The reader might want to bear in mind that selection of an appropriate survival model cannot be dictated by the level of statistical complexity and coverage; rather, it should be based on relevance to an existing theory, the accurate description of empirical data, computational tractability, and generation of interpretable results. The application of the survival techniques introduced in this chapter, however statistically advanced, should also follow those primary principles. Here, to conclude this book, I want to review with the reader Box's (1976) celebrated remarks on statistical modeling: All models are wrong, and the scientists cannot obtain a "correct" one by excessive elaboration; nevertheless, if a statistical model correctly describes the essence and the trend of a phenomenon while overlooking ignorable noises, it is a useful perspective for the scientist to apply.

Appendix A

The delta method

The delta method is a statistical approach to derive an approximate probability distribution for a function of an asymptotically normal estimator using the Taylor series approximation.

Let X be a random variable asymptotically distributed as $N(\mu, \sigma^2)$ with p.d.f. $f(x)$ and g(X) be a single-valued function. If the integral $\int_{-\infty}^{+\infty} g(x)\mathrm{d}F$ exists, it is called the mathematical expectation of g(X), denoted by E[g(X)]. The mean and variance of g(X) of the random variable X may not be readily obtainable. If X has the standard normal density, the integral corresponding to E[g(X)] does not have a tractable expression. In these situations, approximate mean and variance for g(X) can be obtained by taking a linear approximation of g(X) in the neighborhood of μ. With μ = E(X) and g(X) being continuous, the Taylor series expansion of the function g(X) about μ is given by

$$g(X) = g(\mu) + g'(\mu)(X - \mu) + g''(\mu)\frac{(X-\mu)^2}{2!} + \cdots, \tag{A.1}$$

where the higher-order terms can be dropped to yield the approximation

$$g(X) \approx g(\mu) + g'(\mu)(X - \mu). \tag{A.2}$$

Let g(X) = y about μ; the g(X) can be expressed as

$$y = g(X) \approx g(\mu) + g'(\mu)(X - \mu). \tag{A.3}$$

Taking the variance of both sides of (A.3) yields

$$V(Y) = V[g(X)] \approx [g'(X)]^2 V(X). \tag{A.4}$$

Survival Analysis: Models and Applications, First Edition. Xian Liu.

Therefore, if Y, or $g(X)$, is any function of a random variable X, only the variance of X and the first derivative of the function need to be considered in calculating the approximate for the variance of $g(X)$.

The delta method for the multivariate case is simply the extension of the above specifications. Suppose that $\boldsymbol{X} = (X_1, \ldots, X_M)'$ is a random vector with mean $\boldsymbol{\mu}$ and variance–covariance matrix $\Sigma(\boldsymbol{X})$ and $g(\boldsymbol{X})$ is a vector-valued transform of $\boldsymbol{X}$ where g is the link function. Let $\hat{\boldsymbol{X}} = \left(\hat{X}_1, \ldots, \hat{X}_M\right)$ and $g\left(\hat{\boldsymbol{X}}\right)$ be the estimates of $\boldsymbol{X}$ and $g(\boldsymbol{X})$, respectively. Then, the first-order Taylor series expansion of $g\left(\hat{\boldsymbol{X}}\right)$ yields the approximation of mean

$$\mathrm{E}\left[g\left(\hat{\boldsymbol{X}}\right)\right] \approx g(\boldsymbol{\mu}). \tag{A.5}$$

and the variance–covariance matrix of $\boldsymbol{V}\left[g\left(\hat{\boldsymbol{X}}\right)\right]$ is

$$\boldsymbol{V}\left[g\left(\hat{\boldsymbol{X}}\right)\right] \approx \left[\frac{\partial g\left(\hat{\boldsymbol{X}}\right)}{\partial \hat{\boldsymbol{X}}}\bigg| \hat{\boldsymbol{X}} = \boldsymbol{\mu}\right]' \boldsymbol{\Sigma}\left(\hat{\boldsymbol{X}}\right)\left[\frac{\partial g\left(\hat{\boldsymbol{X}}\right)}{\partial \hat{\boldsymbol{X}}}\bigg| \hat{\boldsymbol{X}} = \boldsymbol{\mu}\right]. \tag{A.6}$$

where

$$\frac{\partial g(\boldsymbol{X})}{\partial \boldsymbol{X}} = \left[\frac{\partial g_1(\boldsymbol{X})}{\partial \boldsymbol{X}}, \frac{\partial g_2(\boldsymbol{X})}{\partial \boldsymbol{X}}, \ldots\right]$$

and

$$\boldsymbol{\Sigma}\left(\hat{\boldsymbol{X}}\right) \begin{pmatrix} V\left(\hat{X}_1\right) & \mathrm{Cov}\left(\hat{X}_1, \hat{X}_2\right) & \cdots & \mathrm{Cov}\left(\hat{X}_1, \hat{X}_M\right) \\ & V\left(\hat{X}_2\right) & \cdots & \mathrm{Cov}\left(\hat{X}_2, \hat{X}_M\right) \\ & & \ddots & \\ & & & V\left(\hat{X}_M\right) \end{pmatrix}.$$

The delta method depends on the validity of the Taylor series approximation, so some caution must be exercised when using it before its adequacy is verified by simulation.

Appendix B

Approximation of the variance–covariance matrix for the predicted probabilities from results of the multinomial logit model

Suppose $\hat{\boldsymbol{L}}$ is a random vector of predicted logits $\left(\hat{\boldsymbol{L}} = \hat{L}_1, \hat{L}_2, \ldots, \hat{L}_K\right)$ from Equation (7.28) with mean μ and variance matrix $\boldsymbol{\Sigma}\left(\hat{\boldsymbol{L}}\right)$, and $\hat{\boldsymbol{P}} = g\left(\hat{\boldsymbol{L}}\right)$ is a transform of $\hat{\boldsymbol{L}}$ where g is the link function defined by Equation (7.26). The first-order Taylor series expansion of $g\left(\hat{\boldsymbol{L}}\right)$ yields the approximation of mean

$$\mathrm{E}\left[g\left(\hat{\boldsymbol{L}}\right)\right] \approx g(\boldsymbol{\mu}). \tag{B.1}$$

and the variance–covariance matrix $\hat{\boldsymbol{V}}\left(\hat{\boldsymbol{P}}\right)$

$$\boldsymbol{V}\left[g\left(\hat{\boldsymbol{L}}\right)\right] \approx \left[\left.\frac{\partial g\left(\hat{\boldsymbol{L}}\right)}{\partial \hat{\boldsymbol{L}}}\right| \hat{\boldsymbol{L}} = \boldsymbol{\mu}\right] \boldsymbol{\Sigma}\left(\hat{\boldsymbol{L}}\right) \left[\left.\frac{\partial g\left(\hat{\boldsymbol{L}}\right)}{\partial \hat{\boldsymbol{L}}}\right| \hat{\boldsymbol{L}} = \boldsymbol{\mu}\right]. \tag{B.2}$$

Suppose $\hat{\boldsymbol{L}} = \left(\hat{L}_1, \hat{L}_2, \hat{L}_3\right)'$ and $\hat{\boldsymbol{P}} = \left(\hat{P}_1, \hat{P}_2, \hat{P}_3\right)'$ are defined as

$$\hat{P}_1 = \left[1 + \sum_{k=1}^{3} \exp\left(\hat{L}_k\right)\right]^{-1} \exp\left(\hat{L}_1\right), \tag{B.3}$$

$$\hat{P}_2 = \left[1 + \sum_{k=1}^{3} \exp\left(\hat{L}_k\right)\right]^{-1} \exp\left(\hat{L}_2\right), \tag{B.4}$$

Survival Analysis: Models and Applications, First Edition. Xian Liu.

$$\hat{P}_3 = \left[1 + \sum_{k=1}^{3} \exp\left(\hat{L}_k\right) \right]^{-1} \exp\left(\hat{L}_3\right). \tag{B.5}$$

The calculation of the partial derivatives is based on a basic formula in calculus for the derivation of a ratio of two one-dimensional functions:

$$\frac{\mathrm{d}}{\mathrm{d}X}\left[\frac{a(X)}{b(X)}\right] = \frac{a'(X)b(X) - a(X)b'(X)}{[b(X)]^2},$$

where $a'(X)$ is the derivative of a with respect to X.

Then the partial derivatives defined in (B.2) can be readily calculated. Let us start with respect to $\hat{P}_1$:

$$\frac{\partial \hat{P}_1}{\partial \hat{L}_1} = \left\{ \left[1 + \sum_{k=1}^{3} \exp\left(\hat{L}_k\right) \right]^2 \right\}^{-1} \exp\left(\hat{L}_1\right)\left[1 + \exp\left(\hat{L}_2\right) + \exp\left(\hat{L}_3\right)\right] = B_{11}, \tag{B.6}$$

$$\frac{\partial \hat{P}_1}{\partial \hat{L}_2} = \left\{ \left[1 + \sum_{k=1}^{3} \exp\left(\hat{L}_k\right) \right]^2 \right\}^{-1} \left[-\exp\left(\hat{L}_1\right)\exp\left(\hat{L}_2\right)\right] = B_{12}, \tag{B.7}$$

$$\frac{\partial \hat{P}_1}{\partial \hat{L}_3} = \left\{ \left[1 + \sum_{k=1}^{3} \exp\left(\hat{L}_k\right) \right]^2 \right\}^{-1} \left[-\exp\left(\hat{L}_1\right)\exp\left(\hat{L}_3\right)\right] = B_{13}. \tag{B.8}$$

With respect to $\hat{P}_2$, the partial derivatives are

$$\frac{\partial \hat{P}_2}{\partial \hat{L}_1} = \left\{ \left[1 + \sum_{k=1}^{3} \exp\left(\hat{L}_k\right) \right]^2 \right\}^{-1} \left[-\exp\left(\hat{L}_1\right)\exp\left(\hat{L}_2\right)\right] = B_{21}, \tag{B.9}$$

$$\frac{\partial \hat{P}_2}{\partial \hat{L}_2} = \left\{ \left[1 + \sum_{k=1}^{3} \exp\left(\hat{L}_k\right) \right]^2 \right\}^{-1} \exp\left(\hat{L}_2\right)\left[1 + \exp\left(\hat{L}_1\right) + \exp\left(\hat{L}_3\right)\right] = B_{22}, \tag{B.10}$$

$$\frac{\partial \hat{P}_2}{\partial \hat{L}_3} = \left\{ \left[1 + \sum_{k=1}^{3} \exp\left(\hat{L}_k\right) \right]^2 \right\}^{-1} \left[-\exp\left(\hat{L}_2\right)\exp\left(\hat{L}_3\right)\right] = B_{23}. \tag{B.11}$$

Similarly, with regard to $\hat{P}_3$,

$$\frac{\partial \hat{P}_3}{\partial \hat{L}_1} = \left\{ \left[1 + \sum_{k=1}^{3} \exp\left(\hat{L}_k\right) \right]^2 \right\}^{-1} \left[-\exp\left(\hat{L}_1\right)\exp\left(\hat{L}_3\right)\right] = B_{31}, \tag{B.12}$$

$$\frac{\partial \hat{P}_3}{\partial \hat{L}_2} = \left\{ \left[1 + \sum_{k=1}^{3} \exp\left(\hat{L}_k\right) \right]^2 \right\}^{-1} \left[-\exp\left(\hat{L}_2\right)\exp\left(\hat{L}_3\right)\right] = B_{32}, \tag{B.13}$$

$$\frac{\partial \hat{P}_3}{\partial \hat{L}_3} = \left\{ \left[1 + \sum_{k=1}^{3} \exp\left(\hat{L}_k\right) \right]^2 \right\}^{-1} \exp\left(\hat{L}_3\right)\left[1 + \exp\left(\hat{L}_1\right) + \exp\left(\hat{L}_2\right)\right] = B_{33}. \tag{B.14}$$

Therefore,

$$\left[\left. \frac{\partial g\left(\hat{\boldsymbol{L}}\right)}{\partial \hat{\boldsymbol{L}}} \right|_{\hat{L}=\mu} \right] = \boldsymbol{B},$$

where

$$\boldsymbol{B} = \begin{pmatrix} B_{11} & B_{12} & B_{13} \\ B_{21} & B_{22} & B_{23} \\ B_{31} & B_{32} & B_{33} \end{pmatrix}. \tag{B.15}$$

The variance–covariance matrix of the predicted probabilities $\hat{P}_1$, $\hat{P}_2$, and $\hat{P}_3$ can be approximated by

$$\boldsymbol{V}\left(\hat{\boldsymbol{P}}\right) \approx \boldsymbol{B}\boldsymbol{\Sigma}\boldsymbol{B}', \tag{B.16}$$

where

$$\boldsymbol{\Sigma} = \begin{pmatrix} \sigma_1^2 & \sigma_{12} & \sigma_{13} \\ \sigma_{21} & \sigma_2^2 & \sigma_{23} \\ \sigma_{31} & \sigma_{32} & \sigma_3^2 \end{pmatrix}$$

is the varianc–covariance matrix of $\left(\hat{L}_1, \hat{L}_2, \hat{L}_3\right)$, which can be approximated by the variance–covariance matrix of the intercepts when covariates are centered or fixed at selected values.

Appendix C

Simulated patient data on treatment of PTSD (n = 255)

Pclib.Chapter7_data

	Trt	Age	Sex	Count	T1	T2	T3	T4	Followup
1	0	39	0	3	37	62	92	.	92
2	0	27	0	2	54	114	.	.	114
3	0	33	0	0	.	.	.	.	0
4	0	27	1	2	29	25	.	.	25
5	0	38	0	0	.	.	.	.	1
6	0	32	0	0	.	.	.	.	1
7	0	24	1	0	.	.	.	.	0
8	0	19	0	0	.	.	.	.	2
9	0	34	0	1	8	.	.	.	9
10	0	22	0	0	.	.	.	.	0
11	0	34	0	0	.	.	.	.	0
12	0	32	0	0	.	.	.	.	0
13	0	23	0	1	7	.	.	.	7
14	0	38	0	0	.	.	.	.	0
15	0	20	0	1	14	.	.	.	14
16	0	29	1	1	28	.	.	.	28
17	0	28	0	4	14	31	51	70	79
18	0	29	0	1	4	.	.	.	4
19	0	33	0	2	6	38	.	.	38
20	0	24	0	1	57	.	.	.	57
21	0	28	0	0	.	.	.	.	0
22	0	28	1	1	8	.	.	.	8
23	0	23	0	1	49	.	.	.	51

Survival Analysis: Models and Applications, First Edition. Xian Liu.

	Trt	Age	Sex	Count	T1	T2	T3	T4	Followup
24	0	34	0	0	.	.	.	.	0
25	0	35	0	2	41	117	.	.	117
26	0	22	0	1	16	.	.	.	16
27	0	37	0	4	34	62	86	114	141
28	0	37	0	4	34	62	89	119	161
29	0	24	0	0	.	.	.	.	0
30	0	23	0	3	34	68	113	.	115
31	0	42	0	0	.	.	.	.	0
32	0	22	0	0	.	.	.	.	0
33	0	30	0	1	15	.	.	.	17
34	0	59	1	0	.	.	.	.	0
35	0	23	0	0	.	.	.	.	0
36	0	44	0	0	.	.	.	.	2
37	0	36	0	4	42	70	142	154	154
38	0	20	0	4	54	93	131	198	198
39	0	26	0	4	5	12	20	27	28
40	0	25	0	3	152	194	220	.	220
41	0	22	0	2	60	95	.	.	95
42	0	19	0	1	51	.	.	.	51
43	0	37	0	4	29	56	85	115	161
44	0	20	0	1	78	.	.	.	78
45	0	24	0	2	34	70	.	.	71
46	0	22	0	4	0	0	0	0	0
47	0	22	0	0	.	.	.	.	0
48	0	19	0	1	87	.	.	.	88
49	0	20	0	0	.	.	.	.	0
50	0	21	1	0	.	.	.	.	0
51	0	19	0	0	.	.	.	.	0
52	0	30	0	4	26	66	106	135	135
53	0	21	0	1	14	.	.	.	14
54	0	18	0	0	.	.	.	.	0
55	0	26	0	0	.	.	.	.	0
56	0	23	0	0	.	.	.	.	2
57	0	28	0	0	.	.	.	.	0
58	0	27	0	0	.	.	.	.	30
59	0	21	0	1	30	.	.	.	30
60	0	31	0	0	.	.	.	.	2
61	0	21	0	0	.	.	.	.	0
62	0	21	0	0	.	.	.	.	0
63	0	34	0	1	116	.	.	.	116
64	0	28	0	0	.	.	.	.	0
65	0	42	0	3	39	79	115	.	116
66	0	19	1	0	.	.	.	.	0

(*continued overleaf*)

	Trt	Age	Sex	Count	T1	T2	T3	T4	Followup
67	0	22	0	4	30	58	62	78	111
68	0	19	0	0	.	.	.	.	50
69	0	23	0	1	50	.	.	.	50
70	0	37	0	1	30	.	.	.	30
71	0	31	0	4	32	67	109	134	134
72	0	26	0	1	34	.	.	.	35
73	0	38	0	0	.	.	.	.	0
74	0	38	0	0	.	.	.	.	0
75	0	35	0	4	26	61	119	154	189
76	0	42	0	0	.	.	.	.	0
77	0	26	0	0	.	.	.	.	0
78	0	24	1	2	86	124	.	.	125
79	0	42	0	4	32	70	112	148	173
80	0	22	0	0	.	.	.	.	0
81	0	42	0	0	.	.	.	.	0
82	0	18	0	0	.	.	.	.	0
83	0	44	0	4	32	111	150	181	215
84	0	32	0	0	.	.	.	.	2
85	0	21	1	0	.	.	.	.	0
86	0	22	0	4	8	11	16	17	17
87	0	42	0	0	.	.	.	.	2
88	0	59	0	0	.	.	.	.	2
89	0	22	0	0	.	.	.	.	0
90	0	21	0	4	15	62	78	135	198
91	0	24	0	0	.	.	.	.	0
92	0	19	0	0	.	.	.	.	0
93	0	49	0	1	37	.	.	.	38
94	0	39	1	0	.	.	.	.	0
95	0	44	0	2	45	41	.	.	43
96	0	18	1	0	.	.	.	.	2
97	0	34	1	2	20	43	.	.	43
98	0	19	1	3	28	63	90	.	90
99	0	20	0	1	36	.	.	.	36
100	0	44	0	0	.	.	.	.	0
101	0	29	0	1	49	.	.	.	51
102	0	20	0	1	27	.	.	.	27
103	0	25	0	1	25	.	.	.	25
104	0	47	0	4	35	63	93	119	148
105	0	23	0	1	46	.	.	.	46
106	0	38	0	1	42	.	.	.	42
107	0	21	1	0	.	.	.	.	0
108	0	33	0	0	.	.	.	.	2
109	0	20	1	0	.	.	.	.	0
110	0	24	0	0	.	.	.	.	2
111	0	20	0	0	.	.	.	.	0

	Trt	Age	Sex	Count	T1	T2	T3	T4	Followup
112	0	50	0	1	37	.	.	.	37
113	0	42	0	0	.	.	.	.	0
114	0	20	0	0	.	.	.	.	0
115	0	20	0	2	28	55	.	.	55
116	0	32	1	0	.	.	.	.	0
117	0	42	0	4	45	122	214	269	269
118	0	42	0	0	.	.	.	.	0
119	0	42	0	4	6	28	62	96	96
120	0	24	0	1	51	.	.	.	51
121	0	36	0	0	.	.	.	.	0
122	0	38	0	0	.	.	.	.	0
123	0	28	0	0	.	.	.	.	0
124	0	39	0	2	38	72	.	.	72
125	0	20	1	4	26	53	87	115	145
126	0	29	0	1	20	.	.	.	20
127	0	32	0	0	.	.	.	.	1
128	0	54	1	0	.	.	.	.	0
129	0	25	0	2	7	23	.	.	23
130	0	40	0	1	35	.	.	.	35
131	0	33	0	0	.	.	.	.	0
132	0	18	0	4	28	61	91	118	152
133	0	26	0	1	42	.	.	.	42
134	0	24	0	0	.	.	.	.	0
135	0	34	0	0	.	.	.	.	1
136	0	21	0	0	.	.	.	.	0
137	0	24	0	3	45	77	104	.	104
138	0	30	0	0	.	.	.	.	0
139	0	37	0	3	51	112	122	.	122
140	1	25	1	4	8	38	69	99	130
141	1	20	0	4	34	59	90	118	118
142	1	42	0	3	62	118	160	.	160
143	1	25	1	2	31	61	.	.	61
144	1	44	0	4	7	52	113	163	191
145	1	36	0	4	33	69	91	0	161
146	1	26	0	1	41	.	.	.	41
147	1	25	0	0	.	.	.	.	0
148	1	23	1	4	28	56	91	121	122
149	1	39	0	2	28	67	.	.	67
150	1	22	0	2	31	84	.	.	84
151	1	32	1	0	.	.	.	.	0
152	1	36	0	0	.	.	.	.	0
153	1	38	1	2	38	72	.	.	72
154	1	24	0	0	.	.	.	.	0

(*continued overleaf*)

	Trt	Age	Sex	Count	T1	T2	T3	T4	Followup
155	1	21	1	2	16	77	.	.	77
156	1	22	0	1	26	.	.	.	26
157	1	22	0	4	29	33	72	83	83
158	1	20	0	4	27	56	84	112	167
159	1	30	0	0	.	.	.	.	0
160	1	42	0	3	71	104	125	.	126
161	1	21	0	4	27	54	82	104	132
162	1	49	0	0	.	.	.	.	0
163	1	24	0	2	42	70	.	.	70
164	1	36	0	2	28	57	.	.	58
165	1	42	0	4	35	66	97	144	186
166	1	24	0	0	.	.	.	.	2
167	1	44	0	0	.	.	.	.	0
168	1	24	1	3	30	56	85	.	85
169	1	27	0	0	.	.	.	.	1
170	1	20	0	3	34	59	84	.	84
171	1	38	1	2	33	68	.	.	69
172	1	25	0	1	64	.	.	.	64
173	1	22	1	1	24	.	.	.	24
174	1	22	0	4	23	54	83	112	139
175	1	19	0	4	97	133	177	212	214
176	1	25	0	4	44	77	112	136	165
177	1	35	0	0	.	.	.	.	0
178	1	21	0	4	69	111	139	187	187
179	1	36	0	1	35	.	.	.	35
180	1	41	0	0	.	.	.	.	0
181	1	23	1	4	31	61	92	122	0
182	1	24	0	3	35	76	119	.	119
183	1	24	0	0	.	.	.	.	1
184	1	22	0	4	2939	2967	2996	3025	3027
185	1	19	0	1	33	.	.	.	33
186	1	23	0	1	32	.	.	.	32
187	1	29	0	0	.	.	.	.	0
188	1	37	0	0	.	.	.	.	0
189	1	29	0	4	118	157	187	218	218
190	1	21	1	1	0	.	.	.	0
191	1	39	1	0	.	.	.	.	0
192	1	42	0	1	48	.	.	.	48
193	1	39	1	2	35	70	.	.	71
194	1	40	0	3	356	423	510	.	635
195	1	36	1	2	37	76	.	.	76
196	1	24	0	2	37	69	.	.	69
197	1	27	0	4	115	356	540	645	650
198	1	38	0	4	56	156	189	256	270
199	1	21	0	0	.	.	.	.	0

	Trt	Age	Sex	Count	T1	T2	T3	T4	Followup
200	1	20	0	4	148	177	214	253	284
201	1	42	0	0	.	.	.	.	1
202	1	25	0	1	36	.	.	.	36
203	1	32	0	4	128	155	191	217	245
204	1	27	0	2	32	74	.	.	74
205	1	23	0	1	33	.	.	.	33
206	1	24	1	3	25	63	96	.	96
207	1	33	1	3	0	0	0	.	0
208	1	36	0	0	.	.	.	.	0
209	1	20	1	3	25	36	127	.	127
210	1	25	0	3	35	56	84	.	84
211	1	29	0	4	132	167	226	317	319
212	1	30	1	4	140	147	156	217	279
213	1	19	1	2	42	72	.	.	72
214	1	24	0	2	37	72	.	.	72
215	1	26	0	4	133	165	185	224	225
216	1	27	0	3	129	156	190	.	190
217	1	42	0	1	59	.	.	.	59
218	1	33	0	4	56	145	174	211	244
219	1	24	0	0	.	.	.	.	0
220	1	37	1	4	145	161	181	223	242
221	1	19	0	1	39	.	.	.	39
222	1	33	0	2	33	62	.	.	62
223	1	31	0	0	.	.	.	.	0
224	1	41	1	4	148	205	230	261	293
225	1	28	0	3	245	287	330	.	332
226	1	27	0	4	138	157	171	533	563
227	1	36	0	4	28	59	98	126	154
228	1	23	0	1	37	.	.	.	38
229	1	27	0	4	128	152	190	218	218
230	1	23	0	0	.	.	.	.	0
231	1	25	0	0	.	.	.	.	0
232	1	36	0	4	129	158	257	284	284
233	1	37	0	4	38	187	220	250	250
234	1	26	1	0	.	.	.	.	0
235	1	23	0	2	22	48	.	.	50
236	1	22	0	0	.	.	.	.	0
237	1	26	1	0	.	.	.	.	0
238	1	26	0	0	.	.	.	.	2
239	1	26	0	0	.	.	.	.	0
240	1	32	0	4	22	54	82	106	118
241	1	26	0	4	127	155	183	211	239
242	1	33	0	1	23	.	.	.	23

(*continued overleaf*)

	Trt	Age	Sex	Count	T1	T2	T3	T4	Followup
243	1	38	0	0	.	.	.	.	0
244	1	30	1	3	192	314	348	.	348
245	1	43	0	4	76	133	171	203	203
246	1	25	0	0	.	.	.	.	2
247	1	25	0	3	134	159	193	.	195
248	1	26	1	1	70	.	.	.	71
249	1	33	0	3	29	97	127	.	129
250	1	51	0	0	.	.	.	.	1
251	1	22	1	2	112	154	.	.	154
252	1	21	0	0	.	.	.	.	0
253	1	33	0	0	.	.	.	.	0
254	1	38	0	1	7	.	.	.	8
255	1	40	1	1	15	.	.	.	16

Appendix D

SAS code for derivation of φ estimates in reduced-form equations

```
options ps=56;
libname pclib 'c:\Survival Analysis\data\';
options _last_=pclib.chapter8_data;

data new;
 set pclib.chapter8_data;

if z107=. then death=0;
 else if z107>1997 then death=0;
 else death=1;

if death=0 then d_time=.;
 else d_time=z107*12+z105;

e_time=1997*12+12;

if death=0 then time=e_time-DOI;
 else time=d_time-DOI;

if time>-1 then duration=time+0.5;
 else duration=0.5;

followup=0;
if death=1 then followup=1;
```

Survival Analysis: Models and Applications, First Edition. Xian Liu.

```
proc logistic data=new descending;
   model mental=vet age female educ married
   objph1 cesd8 cog;
     output out=new xbeta=xbeta1 p=mentalp;
run;


proc SQL;
  create table new1 as
  select *, age-70 as age_70,
  vet*age-vet*70 as vetage_70,
  female-mean(female) as female_cnd,
  educ-mean(educ) as educ_cnd,
  married-mean(married) as married_cnd,
  numfunc-mean(numfunc) as numfunc_cnd,
  objph1-mean(objph1) as objph1_cnd,
  subph-mean(subph) as subph_cnd,
  mentalp-mean(mentalp) as mentalp_cnd,
  cesd8-mean(cesd8) as cesd8_cnd,
  cog-mean(cog) as cog_cnd
  from new;
quit;


* Compute xbeta estimates from the full model *;
proc lifereg data=new1 outest=Weibull_outest1;
  model duration*followup(0)=vet age_70 vetage_70
       female_cnd educ_cnd married_cnd numfunc_cnd
       objph1_cnd subph_cnd mentalp_cnd cesd8_cnd
       cog_cnd / dist=weibull;
  run;


proc SQL;
  create table Weibull_outest1 as
  select _name_, _type_,
  -1*intercept as intercept,
  -1*vet/_SCALE_ as vet,
  -1*age_70/_SCALE_ as age_70,
  -1*vetage_70/_SCALE_ as vetage_70,
  -1*female_cnd/_SCALE_ as female_cnd,
  -1*educ_cnd/_SCALE_ as educ_cnd,
  -1*married_cnd/_SCALE_ as married_cnd,
  -1*numfunc_cnd/_SCALE_ as numfunc_cnd,
  -1*objph1_cnd/_SCALE_ as objph1_cnd,
  -1*subph_cnd/_SCALE_ as subph_cnd,
  -1*mentalp_cnd/_SCALE_ as mentalp_cnd,
  -1*cesd8_cnd/_SCALE_ as cesd8_cnd,
  -1*cog_cnd/_SCALE_ as cog_cnd,
  1/_SCALE_ as shape
  from Weibull_outest1;
quit;
run;
```

```
proc score data=new1 score=Weibull_outest1 out=new1 type=parms;
  var vet age_70 vetage_70 female_cnd educ_cnd married_cnd
     numfunc_cnd objph1_cnd subph_cnd mentalp_cnd cesd8_cnd
     cog_cnd;
run;

* Compute xbeta estimates from Model B *;
proc lifereg data=new1 outest=Weibull_outest2;
  model duration*followup(0)=vet age_70 vetage_70 female_cnd
       educ_cnd married_cnd mentalp_cnd cesd8_cnd cog_cnd
       / dist=weibull;
  run;

proc SQL;
  create table Weibull_outest2 as
  select _name_, _type_,
  -1*intercept as intercept,
  -1*vet/_SCALE_ as vet,
  -1*age_70/_SCALE_ as age_70,
  -1*vetage_70/_SCALE_ as vetage_70,
  -1*female_cnd/_SCALE_ as female_cnd,
  -1*educ_cnd/_SCALE_ as educ_cnd,
  -1*married_cnd/_SCALE_ as married_cnd,
  -1*mentalp_cnd/_SCALE_ as mentalp_cnd,
  -1*cesd8_cnd/_SCALE_ as cesd8_cnd,
  -1*cog_cnd/_SCALE_ as cog_cnd,
  1/_SCALE_ as shape
  from Weibull_outest2;
quit;
run;

proc score data=new1 score=Weibull_outest2 out=new1 type=parms;
  var vet age_70 vetage_70 female_cnd educ_cnd married_cnd
     mentalp_cnd cesd8_cnd cog_cnd;
run;

* Compute xbeta estimates from Model C *;
proc lifereg data=new1 outest=Weibull_outest3;
  model duration*followup(0)=vet age_70 vetage_70
       female_cnd educ_cnd married_cnd numfunc_cnd
       objph1_cnd subph_cnd / dist=weibull;
  run;

proc SQL;
  create table Weibull_outest3 as
  select _name_, _type_,
  -1*intercept as intercept,
  -1*vet/_SCALE_ as vet,
  -1*age_70/_SCALE_ as age_70,
  -1*vetage_70/_SCALE_ as vetage_70,
  -1*female_cnd/_SCALE_ as female_cnd,
  -1*educ_cnd/_SCALE_ as educ_cnd,
  -1*married_cnd/_SCALE_ as married_cnd,
```

```
  -1*numfunc_cnd/_SCALE_ as numfunc_cnd,
  -1*objph1_cnd/_SCALE_ as objph1_cnd,
  -1*subph_cnd/_SCALE_ as subph_cnd,
  1/_SCALE_ as shape
  from Weibull_outest3;
quit;
run;

proc score data=new1 score=Weibull_outest3 out=new1 type=parms;
  var vet age_70 vetage_70 female_cnd educ_cnd married_cnd
      numfunc_cnd objph1_cnd subph_cnd;
run;

* Compute xbeta estimates from Model D *;
proc lifereg data=new1 outest=Weibull_outest4;
  model duration*followup(0)=vet age_70 vetage_70 female_cnd
        educ_cnd married_cnd / dist=weibull;
  run;

proc SQL;
  create table Weibull_outest4 as
  select _name_, _type_,
  -1*intercept as intercept,
  -1*vet/_SCALE_ as vet,
  -1*age_70/_SCALE_ as age_70,
  -1*vetage_70/_SCALE_ as vetage_70,
  -1*female_cnd/_SCALE_ as female_cnd,
  -1*educ_cnd/_SCALE_ as educ_cnd,
  -1*married_cnd/_SCALE_ as married_cnd,
  1/_SCALE_ as shape
  from Weibull_outest4;
quit;
run;

proc score data=new1 score=Weibull_outest4 out=new1 type=parms;
  var vet age_70 vetage_70 female_cnd educ_cnd married_cnd;
run;

* Calculation of mean square errors in reduced-form euqations *;
data errors;
  set new1;

error1 = 0;
error2 = (duration2 - duration3)**2;
error3 = (duration2 - duration4)**2;
error4 = (duration2 - duration5)**2;

proc SQL;
  create table mean_errors as
  select mean(error1) as error1_mean,
        mean(error2) as error2_mean,
        mean(error3) as error3_mean,
            mean(error4) as error4_mean
  from errors;
quit;
```

```
* Calculation of phi estimates in reduced-form euqations *;
data Phi;
  set mean_errors;

  n = 2000;

  PhiA = 1.0000;

  PhiB = exp(error2_mean*n / (2*(n-1)));

  PhiC = exp(error3_mean*n / (2*(n-1)));

  PhiD = exp(error4_mean*n / (2*(n-1)));

  PhiA_SD = 0;

  PhiB_SD = exp(2*(error2_mean*n)/(n-1) - exp(error2_mean*n/(n-1)));

  PhiC_SD = exp(2*(error3_mean*n)/(n-1) - exp(error3_mean*n/(n-1)));

  PhiD_SD = exp(2*(error4_mean*n)/(n-1) - exp(error4_mean*n/(n-1)));

run;

proc print data=Phi noobs;
  var error1_mean error2_mean error3_mean error4_mean PhiA PhiB PhiC
      PhiD PhiA_SD PhiB_SD PhiC_SD PhiD_SD;
run;
```

Appendix E

The analytic result of $\kappa^*(x)$

In Subsection 9.4.2, the indicator $\kappa^*(x)$ is given by

$$\kappa^*(x) = \frac{\mathrm{d}\alpha^*(x)}{\mathrm{d}x}, \tag{E.1}$$

where $\alpha^*(x)$ is the adjusted indicator for mortality acceleration. For the truncated Gompertzian function, $\alpha^*(x)$ is defined to be

$$\alpha^*(x) = h^*(x)\left\{r^2 + 3rh^*(x)\Phi(x) + h^*(x)^2\Phi(x)[1+\Phi(x)]\right\}, \tag{E.2}$$

where $h^*(x)$ is the adjusted indicator for the force of mortality, r refers to the age-dependent mortality rate coefficient in a Gompertz function, and $\Phi(x)$ is as specified in Equation (9.60b). Substituting (E.2) into (E.1), we have

$$\kappa^*(x) = \frac{\mathrm{d}}{\mathrm{d}x}\left[h^*(x)\psi(x)\right], \tag{E.3a}$$

where

$$\psi(x) = r^2 + 3rh^*(x)\Phi(x) + h^*(x)^2\Phi(x)[1+\Phi(x)]. \tag{E.3b}$$

Now we have

$$\begin{aligned}\kappa^*(x) &= \psi(x)\frac{\mathrm{d}h^*(x)}{\mathrm{d}x} + h^*(x)\frac{\mathrm{d}\psi(x)}{\mathrm{d}x} \\ &= \psi(x)\eta^*(x) + h^*(x)\frac{\mathrm{d}\psi(x)}{\mathrm{d}x},\end{aligned} \tag{E.4}$$

Survival Analysis: Models and Applications, First Edition. Xian Liu.

where $\eta^*(x)$ is defined as the adjusted indicator for mortality change per unit of time at x. After much algebra, we find that $\kappa^*(x)$ is given by the following equation:

$$\kappa^*(x)=\psi(x)\eta^*(x)+h^*(x)\Big\{\big[h^*(x)^2(1+2\Phi(x))\big]\big[h^*(x)\Phi(x)(1-\Phi(x))\big] \\ +\Phi(x)[1+\Phi(x)]2h^*(x)\eta^*(x)+3r\Phi(x)\big[\eta^*(x)+h^*(x)^2(1-\Phi(x))\big]\Big\}. \quad \text{(E.5)}$$

References

Aalen, O.O. (1975) Statistical inference for a family of counting processes. Ph.D. Dissertation, University of California, Berkeley.

Aalen, O.O. (1978) Nonparametric inference for a family of counting processes. *Annals of Statistics*, **6**, 534–545.

Aalen, O.O. (1994) Effects of frailty in survival analysis. *Statistical Methods in Medical Research*, **3**, 227–243.

Ahnn, S. and Anderson, S.J. (1998) Sample size determination in complex clinical trials comparing more than two groups for survival endpoints. *Statistics in Medicine*, **17**, 2525–2534.

Aiken, L.S. and West, S.G. (1991) *Multiple Regression: Testing and Interpreting Interactions*, Sage Publications, Beverly Hills, CA.

Allison, P.D. (1984) *Event History Analysis*, Sage Publications, Beverly Hills, CA.

Allison, P.D. (2010) *Survival Analysis Using the SAS System: A Practical Guide*, 2nd edn, SAS Institute Inc., Cary, NC.

Alwin, D.F. and Hauser, R.M. (1975) The decomposition of effects in path analysis. *American Sociological Review*, **40**, 37–47.

Amemiya, T. (1981) Qualitative response models: a survey. *Journal of Economic Literature*, **19**, 1483–1536.

Amemiya, T. (1985) *Advanced Econometrics*, Harvard University Press, Cambridge, MA.

Andersen, P.K. (1982) Testing goodness of fit of Cox's regression and life model. *Biometrics*, **38**, 67–77.

Andersen, P.K., Bentzon, M.W., and Klein, J.P. (1996) Estimating the survival function in the proportional hazards regression model: a study of the small sample size properties. *Scandinavian Journal of Statistics*, **23**, 1–12.

Andersen, P.K. and Gill, R.D. (1982) Cox's regression model for counting processes: a large sample study. *The Annals of Statistics*, **10**, 1100–1120.

Survival Analysis: Models and Applications, First Edition. Xian Liu.

Andersen, P.K., Borgan, Ø., Gill, R.D., and Keiding, N. (1982) Linear nonparametric tests for comparison of counting processes, with application to censored survival data. *International Statistical Review*, **50**, 219–258.

Andersen, P.K., Borgan, Ø., Gill, R.D., and Keiding, N. (1993) *Statistical Models Based on Counting Processes*, Springer, New York.

Antonovsky, A. (1967) Social class, life expectancy and overall mortality. *Milbank Memorial Fund Quarterly*, **45**, 31–73.

Arbuckle, J.L. (1999) *Amos 4.0 User's Guide*, SPSS, Chicago, IL.

Arjas, E. (1988) A graphical method for assessing goodness of fit in Cox's proportional hazards model. *Journal of the American Statistical Association*, **83**, 204–212.

Arking, R. (1987) Successful selection for increased longevity in Drosophila: analysis of survival data and presentation of a hypothesis on the genetic regulation of longevity. *Experimental Gerontology*, **22**, 199–220.

Asparouhov, T., Masyn, K., and Muthen, B. (2006) Continuous time survival in latent variable models, in Proceedings of the Joint Statistical Meeting, Seattle, August 2006. ASA Section on Biometrics, pp. 180–187.

Asparouhov, T. and Muthen, B. (2007) Multilevel mixture models, in *Advances in Latent Variable Mixture Models* (eds G.R. Hancock and K.M. Samuelsen), Information Age Publishing, Inc., Charlotte, NC, pp. 27–51.

Barlow, W.E. and Prentice, R.L. (1988) Residuals for relative risk regression. *Biometrika*, **75**, 65–74.

Barthel, F.M.-S., Babiker, A., Royston, P., and Parmer, M.K.B. (2006) Evaluation of sample size and power for multi-arm survival trials allowing for non-uniform accrual, non-proportional hazards, loss to follow-up and cross-over. *Statistics in Medicine*, **25**, 2521–2542.

Bentler, P.M. (1995) *EQS: Structural Equations Program Manual*, Multivariate Software, Inc., Los Angeles, CA.

Binder, D.A. (1992) Fitting Cox's proportional hazards models from survey data. *Biometrika*, **79**, 139–147.

Bock, R.D. (1975) *Multivariate Statistical Methods in Behavioral Research*, McGraw-Hill, New York.

Bollen, K.A. (1989) *Structural Equations with Latent Variables*, John Wiley & Sons, Inc., New York.

Borgan, Ø. and Liestøl, K. (1990) A note on confidence intervals and bands for the survival function based on transformation. *Scandinavian Journal of Statistics*, **17**, 35–41.

Box, G.E.P. (1976) Science and statistics. *Journal of the American Statistical Association*, **71**, 791–799.

Box, G.E.P. and Cox, D.R. (1964) An analysis of transformation. *Journal of the Royal Statistical Society*, **B26**, 211–252.

Box, G.E.P. and Tiao, G.C. (1973) *Bayesian Inference in Statistical Analysis*, John Wiley & Sons, Inc., New York.

Bradu, D. and Mundlak, Y. (1970) Estimation in lognormal linear models. *Journal of the American Statistical Association*, **65**, 198–211.

Breslow, N.E. (1970) A generalized Kruskal–Wallis test for comparing K samples subject to unequal patterns of censorship. *Biometrika*, **57**, 579–594.

Breslow, N.E. (1972) Discussion of paper by D.R. Cox. *Journal of the Royal Statistical Society*, **B34**, 216–217.

Breslow, N.E. (1974) Covariance analysis of censored survival data. *Biometrics*, **30**, 89–99.

Breslow, N.R. and Clayton, D.G. (1993) Approximate inference in generalized linear mixed models. *Journal of the American Statistical Association*, **88**, 9–25.

Breslow, N.R. and Lin, X. (1995) Bias correction in generalized linear mixed models with a single component of dispersion. *Biometrika*, **82**, 81–91.

Bullman, T.A. and Kang, H.K. (1994) The effects of mustard gas, ionizing radiation, herbicides, trauma, and oil smoke on US military personnel: the results of veteran studies. *Annual Review of Public Health*, **15**, 69–90.

Cain, K.C. and Lange, N.T. (1984) Approximate case influence for the proportional hazards regression model with censored data. *Biometrics*, **40**, 493–499.

Carey, J.R. and Liedo, D. (1995) Sex-specific life table aging rates in large medfly cohorts. *Experimental Gerontology*, **30**, 315–325.

Carey, J.R., Liedo, D., Orozco, D., and Vaupel, J.W. (1992) Slowing on mortality rates at older ages in large medfly cohorts. *Science*, **258**, 457–461.

Chhikara, R.S. and Folks, J.L. (1989) *The Inverse Gaussian Distribution: Theory, Methodology, and Applications*, Dekker, New York.

Clayton, D.G. (1978) A model for association in bivariate life tables and its application in epidemiological studies of familial tendency in chronic disease incidence. *Biometrika*, **65**, 141–151.

Clayton, D.G. and Cuzick, J. (1985) Multivariate generalizations of the proportional hazards model. *Journal of the Royal Statistical Society*, **A148**, 82–117.

Coale, A.J. and Demeny, P. (1966) *Regional Model Life Tables and Stable Populations*, Princeton University Press, Princeton, NJ.

Coale, A.J. and Kisker, E.E. (1986) Mortality crossovers: reality or bad data? *Population Studies*, **40**, 389–401.

Cohen, J. (1988) *Statistical Power Analysis for the Behavioral Sciences*, 2nd edn, Lawrence Erlbaum Associates, Hillsdale, NJ.

Coles, S. (2001) *An Introduction to Statistical Modeling of Extreme Values*, Springer, London.

Collett, D. (2003) *Modeling Survival Data in Medical Research*, 2nd edn, Chapman Hall, London.

Cook, R.D. (1986) Assessment of local influence. *Journal of the Royal Statistical Society*, **B48**, 133–169.

Costa, D.L. (1993) Height, weight, wartime stress, and old age mortality: evidence from the union army records. *Explorations in Economic History*, **30**, 424–449.

Cox, D.R. (1972) Regression models and life tables (with discussion). *Journal of the Royal Statistical Society*, **B34**, 187–220.

Cox, D.R. and Miller, H.D. (1978) *The Theory of Stochastic Processes*, 2nd edn, Chapman & Hall, New York.

Cox, D.R. and Snell, E.J. (1968) A general definition of residuals (with discussion). *Journal of the Royal Statistical Society*, **B30**, 248–275.

Crimmins, E.M., Hayward, M.D., and Saito, Y. (1996) Differentials in active life expectancy in the older population of the United States. *Journal of Gerontology: Social Sciences*, **51B**, S111–S120.

David, H.A. (1974) Parametric approaches to the theory of competing risks, in *Reliability and Biometry: Statistical Analysis of Lifelength* (eds F. Proschan and R.J. Serfling), SIAM, Philadelphia, PA, pp. 275–290.

Davis, M.J. (2010) Contrast coding in multiple regression analysis: strengths, weaknesses, and utility of popular coding structures. *Journal of Data Science*, **8**, 61–73.

Demirtas, H. (2004) Modeling incomplete longitudinal data. *Journal of Modern Applied Statistical Methods*, **3**, 305–321.

Dempster, A.P., Laird, N.M., and Rubin, D.B. (1977) Maximum likelihood from incomplete data via the EM algorithm. *Journal of the Royal Statistical Society*, **B39**, 1–38.

Doubal, S. and Klemera, P. (1990) Influence of aging rate change on mortality curves. *Mechanisms of Aging and Development*, **54**, 75–85.

Duan, N. (1983) Smearing estimate: a nonparametric retransformation method. *Journal of the American Statistical Association*, **78**, 605–610.

Eakin, T. and Witten, T.M. (1995) How square is the survival curve of a given species? *Experimental Gerontology*, **30**, 33–64.

Ebbeler, D.H. (1973) A note on large-sample approximation in lognormal linear models. *Journal of the American Statistical Association*, **68**, 231.

Efron, B. (1977) The efficiency of Cox's likelihood function for censored data. *Journal of the American Statistical Association*, **72**, 557–565.

Efron, B. and Tibshirani, R.J. (1993) *An Introduction to the Bootstrap*, Chapman & Hall, New York.

Egleston, B.L., Scharfstein, D.O., Freeman, E.E., and West, S.K. (2006) Causal inference for non-mortality outcomes in the presence of death. *Biostatistics*, **8**, 526–545.

Elo, I.T. and Preston, S.H. (1994) Estimating African-American mortality from inaccurate data. *Demography*, **31**, 427–458.

Evans, I.G. and Shaban, S.A. (1974) A note on estimation in lognormal models. *Journal of the American Statistical Association*, **69**, 779–781.

Finch, C.E., Pike, M.C., and Witten, T.M. (1990) Slow mortality rate acceleration during aging in some animals approximate that of humans. *Science*, **249**, 902–905.

Fisher, L.D. and Lin, D.Y. (1999) Time-dependent covariates in the Cox proportional-hazards regression model. *Annual Review of Public Health*, **20**, 145–157.

Fleming, T.R. and Harrington, D.P. (1991) *Counting Processes and Survival Analysis*, John Wiley & Sons, Inc., New York.

Fogel, R.W. (1993) New sources and new techniques for the study of secular trends in nutritional status, health, mortality, and the process of aging. *Historical Methods*, **26**, 5–43.

Fox, J. (1987) Effect displays for generalized linear models. *Sociological Methodology*, **17**, 347–361.

Fox, J. (1991) *Regression Diagnostics*, Sage, Newbury Park, CA.

Fries, J.F. (1980) Aging, natural death, and the compression of morbidity. *The New England Journal of Medicine*, **303**, 130–135.

Gavrilov, L. and Gavrilov, N. (1991) *The Biology of Lifespan*, Harwood, Chur, Switzerland.

Gavrilov, L. and Gavrilov, N. (2004) Why we fall apart? Spectrum Online. http://www.spectrum.ieee.org/WEBONLY/publicfeature/sep04/0904age.html (4 September 2004).

Gehan, E.A. (1967) A generalized Wilcoxon test for comparing arbitrarily single singly censored samples. *Biometrica*, **52**, 203–223.

Gehan, E.A. (1969) Estimating survival functions from the life table. *Journal of Chronic Diseases*, **21**, 629–644.

Gelman, A., Carlin, J.B., Stern, H.S., and Rubin, D.B. (2004). *Bayesian Data Analysis*. 2nd edn. Chapman & Hall/CRC, Boca Raton, Florida.

Gill, R. and Schumacher, M. (1987) A simple test of the proportional hazards assumption. *Biometrika*, **74**, 289–300.

Goldberger, A.S. (1968) The interpretation and estimation of Cobb–Douglas functions. *Econometrica*, **35**, 464–472.

Gompertz, B. (1820) A sketch on the analysis and the notation applicable to the value of life contingencies. *Philosophical Transactions of the Royal Society*, **110**, 214–294.

Gompertz, B. (1825) On the nature of the function expressive of the law of human mortality and on a new model of determining the value of life contingencies. *Philosophical Transactions of the Royal Society*, **115**, 513–585.

Grambsch, P.M. and Therneau, T.M. (1994) Proportional hazards tests and diagnostics based on weighted residuals. *Biometrica*, **81**, 515–526.

Graunt, J. (1939) *Natural and Political Observations Made upon the Bills of Mortality*, Johns Hopkins Press, Baltimore, MD (original edition 1662).

Greene, W.H. (2003) *Econometric Analysis*, 5th edn, Prentice, New Jersey.

Greenwood, M. (1926) The natural duration of cancer, in *Reports on Public Health and Medical Subjects*, vol. 33, Her Majesty's Stationary Office, London, pp. 1–26.

Halabi, S. and Singh, B. (2004) Sample size determination for comparing survival curves with unequal allocations. *Statistics in Medicine*, **23**, 1793–1815.

Hall, W.J. and Wellner, J.A. (1980) Confidence bands for a survival curve from censored data. *Biometrica*, **67**, 133–143.

Hardy, M. and Reynolds, J. (2004) Incorporating categorical information into regression models: the utility of dummy variables, in *Handbook of Data Analysis* (eds M. Hardy and A. Bryman), Sage, London, pp. 209–236.

Hayward, M.D. and Grady, W.R. (1990) Work and retirement among a cohort of older men in the United States: 1966–1983. *Demography*, **27**, 337–356.

Heckman, J.J. (1979) Sample selection bias as a specification error. *Annals of Econometrica*, **47**, 153–161.

Heckman, J.J. and Singer, B. (1980) The identification problem in econometric models for duration data, Chapter 2 in *Advances in Econometrics: Proceedings of World Meetings of the Econometric Society* (ed. W. Hildenbrand), Cambridge University Press, Cambridge, MA, pp. 39–77.

Heckman, J.J. and Singer, B. (1984) A method for minimizing the impact of distributional assumptions in econometric models for duration data. *Econometrica*, **52**, 271–320.

Hedeker, D. and Gibbons, R.D. (2006) *Longitudinal Data Analysis*, John Wiley & Sons, Inc., Hoboken, NJ.

Heller, D.A., Ahern, F.M., Stout, J.T., and McClearn, J.E. (1998) Mortality and biomarkers of aging in heterogeneous stocks (HS) mice. *Journal of Gerontology: Biological Sciences*, **53A**, B217–B230.

Hertz-Picciotto, I. and Rockhill, B. (1997) Validity and efficiency of approximation methods for tied survival times in Cox regression. *Biometrics*, **53**, 1151–1156.

Herzog, A.R. and Wallace, R.B. (1997) Measures of cognitive functioning in the AHEAD study. *The Journal of Gerontology Series B*, **52B**, 37–48.

Hirsch, H.R. (1994) Can an improved environment cause maximum lifespan to decrease? Comments on lifespan criteria and longitudinal Gompertzian analysis. *Experimental Gerontology*, **29**, 119–137.

Hirsch, H.R., Liu, X., and Witten, T.M. (2000) Mortality-rate crossovers and maximum lifespan in advantaged and disadvantaged populations: accelerated-mortality and sudden-death models. *Journal of Theoretical Biology*, **205**, 171–180.

Hoem, J.M. and Jensen, U.F. (1982) Multistate life table methodology: a probabilistic critique, in *Multidimensional Mathematical Demography* (eds K.C. Land and A. Rogers), Academic Press, New York, pp. 155–264.

Hogan, J.W., Roy, J., and Korkontzelou, C. (2004) Tutorial in biostatistics: handling drop-out in longitudinal studies. *Statistics in Medicine*, **23**, 1455–1497.

Holt, J.D. and Prentice, R.L. (1974) Survival analysis in twin studies and matched pair experiments. *Biometrika*, **61**, 17–30.

Horiuchi, S. (1989) Some methodological issues in the assessment of the deceleration of the mortality decline, in *Differential Mortality: Methodological Issues and Biosocial Factors* (eds L. Ruzicka, G. Wunsch, and P. Kane), Clarendon Press, Oxford, England, pp. 64–78.

Horiuchi, S. and Coale, A.J. (1990) Age patterns of mortality for older women: an analysis using the age specific rate of mortality change with age. *Mathematical Population Studies*, **2**, 245–267.

Horiuchi, S. and Wilmoth, J.R. (1998) Deceleration in the age pattern of mortality at older ages. *Demography*, **35**, 391–412.

Hosmer, D.W., Lemeshow, S., and May, S. (2008) *Applied Survival Analysis: Regression Modeling of Time-to-Event Data*, 2nd edn, John Wiley & Sons, Inc., Hoboken, NJ.

Hougaard, P. (1986) Survival models for heterogeneous populations derived from stable distributions. *Biometrika*, **73**, 387–396.

Hougaard, P. (1995) Frailty models for survival data. *Lifetime Data Analysis*, **1**, 255–273.

Hougaard, P. (2000) *Analysis of Multivariate Survival Data*, Springer, New York.

Hougaard, P., Harvald, B., and Holm, N.V. (1992) Measuring the similarities between the lifetimes of adult Danish twins born between 1881–1930. *Journal of the American Statistical Association*, **87**, 17–24.

House, J.S., Kessler, R.C., Herzog, A.R., *et al.* (1992) Social stratification, age, and health, in *Aging, Health Behavior, and Health Outcomes* (eds K.W. Shaie, D. Blazer, and J.S. House), Erlbaum, Hillsdale, NJ, pp. 1–32.

Huster, W.J., Brookmeyer, R., and Self, S.G. (1989) Modeling paired survival data with covariates. *Biometrics*, **45**, 145–156.

Idler, E.L. and Kasl, S. (1991) Health perceptions and survival: do global evaluations of health status really predict mortality? *Journal of Gerontology: Social Sciences*, **46**, S55–S65.

Johansen, S. (1983) An extension of Cox's regression model. *International Statistical Review*, **51**, 165–174.

Jonas, B.S. and Mussolino, M.E. (2000) Symptoms of depression as a prospective risk factor for stroke. *Psychosomatic Medicine*, **62**, 463–471.

Joreskog, K.G. and Sorbom, D. (1996) *LISREL 8: User's Reference Guide*, Scientific Software International, Chicago, IL.

Kalbfleisch, J.D. and Prentice, R.L. (1973) Marginal likelihoods based on Cox's regression and life model. *Biometrika*, **60**, 267–278.

Kalbfleisch, J.D. and Prentice, R.L. (2002) *The Statistical Analysis of Failure Time Data*, 2nd edn, John Wiley & Sons, Inc., New York.

Kang, H.K. and Bullman, T.A. (1996) Mortality among U.S. veterans of the Persian Gulf War. *New England Journal of Medicine*, **335**, 1498–1504.

Kaplan, E.L. and Meier, P. (1958) Nonparametric estimation from incomplete observations. *Journal of the American Statistical Association*, **53**, 457–481.

Kelly, P.J. (2004) A review of software packages for analyzing correlated survival data. *The American Statistician*, **58**, 337–342.

Kelly, P.J. and Lim, L.L. (2000) Survival analysis for recurrent event data: an application to childhood infectious disease. *Statistics in Medicine*, **19**, 13–33.

Keyfitz, N. (1985) *Applied Mathematical Demography*, Springer-Verlag, New York.

Khazaeli, A.A., Xiu, L., and Curtsinger, J.W. (1995) Stress experiments as means of investigating age-specific mortality in *Drosophila melanogaster*. *Experimental Gerontology*, **30**, 177–184.

Kirkwood, T.B.L. (1992) Comparative lifespans of species: why do species have the lifespans they do? *American Journal of Clinical Nutrition*, **55**, 1191S–1195S.

Klein, J.P. and Moeschberger, M.L. (2003) *Survival Analysis: Techniques for Censored and Truncated Data*, 2nd edn, Springer.

Kurland, B.F. and Heagerty, P.J. (2005) Directly parameterized regression conditioning on being alive: analysis of longitudinal data truncated by death. *Biostatistics*, **6**, 241–258.

Lagakos, S.W. and Schoenfeld, D.A. (1984) Properties of proportional-hazard score tests under misspecified regression models. *Biometrics*, **40**, 1037–1048.

Land, K.C., Guralnik, J.M., and Blazer, D.J. (1994) Estimating increment–decrement life tables with multiple covariates from panel data: the case of active life expectancy. *Demography*, **31**, 297–319.

Land, K.C. and Schoen, R. (1982) Statistical methods for Markov-generated increment–decrement life tables with polynomial gross flow functions, in *Multidimensional Mathematical Demography* (eds K.C. Land and A. Rogers), Academic Press, New York, pp. 265–346.

Lawless, J.F. (2003) *Statistical Models and Methods for Lifetime Data*, 2nd edn, John Wiley & Sons, Inc., New York.

Lawless, J.F. and Nadeau, C. (1995) Some simple robust methods for the analysis of recurrent events. *Technometrics*, **37**, 158–168.

Lee, E.W., Wei, L.J., and Amato, D.A. (1992) Cox-type regression analysis for large numbers of small groups of correlated failure time observations, in *Survival Analysis: State of Art* (eds J.P. Klein and P.K. Goel), Kluwer Academic Publisher, Dordrecht, pp. 237–247.

Leigh, J.P., Ward, M.M., and Fries, J.F. (1993) Reducing attrition bias with an instrumental variable in a regression model: results from a panel of rheumatoid arthritis patients. *Statistics in Medicine*, **12**, 1005–1018.

Liang, K.Y. and Zeger, S.L. (1986) Longitudinal data analysis using generalized linear models. *Biometrika*, **73**, 13–22.

Liang, J., Liu, X., Tu, E.J., and Whitelaw, N. (1993) Patterns of health care utilization in the U.S., in *Social Security and Aging in Taiwan* (ed. G.Y. Wong), Institute of Social Welfare, Chung Cheng University, Taiwan, pp. 155–178.

Liang, J., Liu, X., Tu, E.J., and Whitelaw, N. (1996) Probability and lifetime durations of short-stay hospital and nursing home utilization in the U.S., 1985. *Medical Care*, **34**, 1018–1036.

Liao, T.F. (1994) *Interpreting Probability Models: Logit, Probit, and Other Generalized Linear Models*, Quantitative Applications in the Social Sciences Series 101, SAGE Publications, Thousand Oaks, CA.

Liestol, K. and Andersen, P.K. (2002) Updating of covariates and choice of time origin in survival analysis: problems with vaguely defined disease states. *Statistics in Medicine*, **21**, 3701–3714.

Lin, D.Y. (1994) Cox regression analysis of multivariate failure time data: the marginal approach. *Statistics in Medicine*, **13**, 2233–2247.

Lin, D.Y. and Wei, L.J. (1989) The robust inference for the Cox proportional hazards model. *Journal of the American Statistical Association*, **84**, 1074–1078.

Lin, D.Y., Wei, L.J., and Ying, Z. (1993) Checking the Cox model with cumulative sums of martingale-based residuals. *Biometrika*, **80**, 557–572.

Lin, D.Y., Wei, L.J., Yang, I., and Ying, Z. (2000) Semiparametric regression for the mean and rate functions of recurrent events. *Journal of the Royal Statistical Society*, **B62**, 711–730.

Lints, F.A. (1989) Rate of living theory revisited. *The Gerontologist*, **35**, 36–57.

Littell, R.C., Milliken, G.A., Stroup, W.W., *et al.* (2006) *SAS for Mixed Models*, 2nd edn, SAS Institute, Inc, Gary, NC.

Little, R.J.A. and Rubin, D.B. (1999) Comment on D.O. Scharfstein, A. Rotnitzky, and J.M. Robins, Adjusting for nonignorable drop-out using semiparametric nonresponse models. *Journal of the American Statistical Association*, **94**, 1130–1132.

Little, R.J.A. and Rubin, D.B. (2002) *Statistical Analysis with Missing Data*, 2nd edn, John Wiley & Sons, Inc., New York.

Liu, X. (2000) Development of a structural hazard rate model in sociological research. *Sociological Methods and Research*, **29**, 77–177.

Liu, X., Hermalin, A.I., and Chuang, Y.L. (1998) The effect of education on mortality among older Taiwanese and its pathways. *The Journal of Gerontology: Social Sciences*, **53B**, S71–S82.

Liu, X. and Witten, T.M. (1995) A biologically based explanation for mortality crossover in human populations. *The Gerontologist*, **35**, 609–615.

Liu, X., Liang, J., Muramatsu, N., and Sugisawa, H. (1995) Transitions in functional status and active life expectancy among older people in Japan. *Journal of Gerontology: Social Sciences*, **50B**, S383–S394.

Liu, X., Liang, J., Tu, E.J., and Whitelaw, N. (1997) Modeling multidimensional transitions in health care. *Sociological Methods and Research*, **25**, 284–317.

Liu, X., Engel Jr., C.C., Kang, H., and Cowan, D. (2005) The effect of veteran status on mortality among older Americans and its pathways. *Population Research and Policy Review*, **24**, 573–592.

Liu, X., Engel Jr., C.C., Kang, H., and Armstrong, D.W. (2006) Veterans and functional status transitions in older Americans. *Military Medicine*, **171**, 943–949.

Liu, X., Engel Jr., C.C., Armstrong, D.W., and Kang, H. (2008) Survival convergence and the preceding mortality crossover for two population subgroups. *Population Research and Policy Review*, **27**, 293–306.

Liu, X., Engel Jr., C.C., Kang, H., and Gore, K. (2010) Reducing selection bias in analyzing longitudinal health data with high mortality rates. *Journal of Modern Applied Statistical Methods*, **9**, 403–413.

Long, J.S. (1997) *Regression Models for Categorical and Limited Dependent Variables*, Sage Publications, Thousand Oaks, CA.

McCullagh, P. and Nelder, J.A. (1989) *Generalized Linear Models*, 2nd edn, Chapman and Hall, New York.

Maddala, G.S. (1983) *Limited-Dependent and Qualitative Variables in Econometrics*, Cambridge University Press, Cambridge.

Makeham, W.M. (1867) On the law of mortality and the construction of annuity tables. *Journal of Industrial Actuaries and Insurance*, **8**, 301–310.

Manning, W.G., Duan, N., and Rogers, W.H. (1987) Monte Carlo evidence on the choice between sample selection and two-part models. *Journal of Econometrics*, **35**, 59–82.

Mantel, N. and Haenszel, W. (1959) Statistical aspects of the analysis of data from retrospective studies of disease. *Journal of the National Cancer Institute*, **22**, 719–748.

Manton, K.G., Poss, S.S. and Wing, S. (1979) The black/white mortality crossover: investigation from the perspective of components of aging. *The Gerontologist*, **19**, 291–300.

Manton, K.G. and Stallard, E. (1979) Maximum likelihood estimation of a stochastic compartment model of lung cancer mortality among white females in the U.S. *Computer and Biomedical Research*, **12**, 313–325.

Manton, K.G. and Stallard, E. (1994) Medical demography: interaction of disability dynamics and mortality, in *Demography of Aging* (eds L.G. Martin and S.H. Preston), National Academy Press, Washington, D.C., pp. 217–278.

Manton, K.G., Stallard, E. and Singer, B.H. (1994) Methods of projecting the future size and health status of the U.S. elderly population, in *Studies in the Economics of Aging* (ed. D.A. Wise), The University of Chicago Press, Chicago, IL, pp. 41–77.

Manton, K.G., Stallard, E., Woodbury, M.A. and Dowd, J.E. (1994) Time-varying covariates in models of human mortality and aging: multidimensional generalizations of the Gompertz. *Journal of Gerontology: Biological Sciences*, **49**, B169–BB190.

Marubini, E. and Valsecchi, M.G. (1995) *Analyzing Survival Data from Clinical Trials and Observational Studies*, John Wiley & Sons, Inc., New York.

Meeker, W.Q. and Escobar, L.A. (1998) *Statistical Models for Reliability Data*, John Wiley & Sons, Inc., New York.

Mehran, F. (1973) Variance of the MVUE for the lognormal mean. *Journal of the American Statistical Association*, **68**, 726–727.

Merlo, J., Chaix, B., Ohlsson, H., *et al.* (2006) A brief conceptual tutorial of multilevel analysis in social epidemiology: using measures if clustering in multilevel logistic regression to investigate contextual phenomena. *Journal of Epidemiology and Community Health*, **60**, 290–297.

Meulenberg, M.T.G. (1965) On the estimation of an exponential function. *Econometrica*, **33**, 863–868.

Muthen, B. (1979) A structural probit model with latent variables. *Journal of the American Statistical Association*, **74**, 807–811.

Muthen, B. (1984) A general structural equation model with dichotomous, ordered categorical, and continuous latent variable indicators. *Psychometrika*, **49**, 115–132.

Muthen, B. (2002) Beyond SEM: general latent variable modeling. *Behaviormetrika*, **29**, 81–117.

Muthen, B. (2007) Latent variable hybrids: overview of old and new models, in *Advances in Latent Variable Mixture Models* (eds G.R. Hancock and K.M. Samuelsen), Information Age Publishing, Inc, Charlotte, NC, pp. 1–24.

Muthen, B. and Masyn, K. (2005) Discrete-time survival mixture analysis. *Journal of Education and Behavioral Statistics*, **30**, 27–58.

Muthen, L. and Muthen, B. (2008) *Mplus User's Guide*, Muthen and Muthen, Los Angeles, CA.

Nair, V.N. (1984) Confidence bands for survival functions with censored data: a comparative study. *Technometrics*, **26**, 265–275.

Nam, C.B. (1994) Another look at mortality crossovers. *Social Biology*, **42**, 133–142.

Namboodiri, K. and Suchindran, C.M. (1987) *Life Table Techniques and Their Applications*, Academic Press, New York.

Nelson, W. (1972) Theory and applications of hazard plotting for censored failure data. *Technometrics*, **14**, 945–965.

Nelson, W. (2002) Recurrent Events Data Analysis for Product Repairs, Disease Recurrences, and Other Applications. ASA-SIAM Series on Statistics and Applied Probability.

Nelson, K.P., Lipsitz, S.R., Fitzmaurice, G.M., *et al.* (2006) Use of the probability integral transformation to fit nonlinear mixed-effects models with nonnormal random effects. *Journal of Computational and Graphical Statistics*, **15**, 39–57.

Newman, J.L. and McCulloch, C.E. (1984) A hazard rate approach to the timing of births. *Econometrica*, **52**, 939–961.

Neyman, J. and Scott, E.L. (1960) Correction for bias introduced by a transformation of variables. *Annals of Mathematical Statistics*, **31**, 643–655.

Oaks, D. (1982) A model for association in bivariate survival data. *Journal of the Royal Statistical Society*, **B44**, 414–422.

Oaks, D. (1989) Bivariate survival models induced by frailties. *Journal of the American Statistical Association*, **84**, 487–493.

Olshansky, S.J. (1995) Mortality crossovers and selective survival in human and nonhuman populations. *The Gerontologist*, **35**, 583–587.

Olshansky, S.J. and Carnes, B.A. (1994) Demographic perspectives on human senescence. *Population and Development Review*, **20**, 57–80.

Pattitt, A.N. and Bin Raud, I. (1989) Case-weighted measures of influence for proportional hazards regression. *Applied Statistics*, **38**, 51–67.

Pauler, D.K., McCoy, S., and Moinpour, C. (2003) Pattern mixture models for longitudinal quality of life studies in advanced stage disease. *Statistics in Medicine*, **22**, 795–809.

Pepe, M.S. and Cai, J. (1993) Some graphical displays and marginal regression analyses for recurrent failure times and time dependent covariates. *Journal of the American Statistical Association*, **88**, 811–820.

Petersen, T. (1985) A comment on presenting results from logit and probit models. *American Sociological Review*, **50**, 130–131.

Peto, R. and Peto, J. (1972) Asymptotically efficient rank invariant procedures. *Journal of the Royal Statistical Society*, **A135**, 185–207.

Peto, R., Pike, M.C., Armitage, P., *et al.* (1977) Design and analysis of randomized clinical trials requiring prolonged observation of each patient. *British Journal of Cancer*, **35**, 1–39.

Plewis, I. (2001) Using Mplus for multilevel modeling. *Multilevel Modeling Newsletter*, **13**, 13–15.

Prentice, R.L. (1978) Linear rank tests with right censored data. *Biometrika*, **65**, 167–179.

Prentice, R.L. and Marek, P. (1979) A qualitative discrepancy between censored data rank tests. *Biometrics*, **35**, 861–867.

Prentice, R.L., Williams, B.J., and Peterson, A.V. (1981) On the regression analysis of multivariate failure time data. *Biometrika*, **68**, 373–379.

Prentice, R.L., Kalbfleisch, J.D., Peterson, A.V., *et al.* (1978) The analysis of failure times in the presence of competing risks. *Biometrics*, **34**, 541–554.

Preston, S.H. (1990) Sources of variation in vital rates: an overview, in *Convergent Issues in Genetics and Demography* (eds J. Adams, A.I. Hermalin, D. Lam, and P. Smouse), Oxford University Press, New York, pp. 335–350.

Radloff, L.S. (1977) The CES-D scale: a self-report depression scale for research in the general population. *Applied Psychological Measurement*, **1**, 385–401.

Ratcliffe, S.J., Guo, W. and Ten Have, T.R. (2004) Joint modeling of longitudinal and survival data via a common frailty. *Biometrics*, **60**, 892–899.

Ratten, S.I.S. (1995) Gerontogenes: real or virtual? *Federation of the American Societies of Experimental Biology Journal*, **50**, 284–285.

Rebolledo, R. (1980) Central limit theorem for local martingales. *Zeitschrift fur Wahrscheinlichkeitstheory und Verw. Gebiete*, **51**, 269–286.

Riggs, J.E. (1990) Longitudinal Gomperzian analysis of adult human mortality in the U.S., 1900–1986. *Mechanisms of Aging and Development*, **54**, 235–247.

Rogers, A. (1975) *Introduction to Multiregional Mathematical Demography*, John Wiley & Sons, Inc., New York.

Rogers, A., Rogers, R.G., and Belanger, A. (1990) Longer life but worse health? Measurement and dynamics. *The Gerontologist*, **30**, 640–649.

Rose, M.R. and Graves, J.L. (1990) Revolution of aging. *Review of Biological Research*, **4**, 3–14.

Sakia, R.M. (1992) The box-Cox transformation technique: a overview. *The Statistician*, **41**, 169–178.

Sampson, R.J., Raudenbush, S.W., and Earls, F. (1997) Neighborhoods and violent crime: a multilevel study of collective efficacy. *Science*, **277**, 918–924.

SAS (2009) *SAS/STAT 9.2: User's Guide*, 2nd edn, SAS Institute Inc, Cary, NC.

Schafer, J.L. and Graham, J.W. (2002) Missing data: our view of the state of the art. *Psychological Methods*, **7**, 147–177.

Scharfstein, D.O. and Robins, J.M. (2002) Estimation of the failure time distribution in the presence of informative censoring. *Biometrika*, **89**, 617–634.

Scharfstein, D.O., Rotnitzky, A., and Robins, J.M. (1999) Adjusting for nonignorable drop-out using semiparametric nonresponse models (with discussion). *Journal of the American Statistical Association*, **94**, 1096–1146.

Scharfstein, D.O., Robins, J.M., Eddings, W., and Rotnitzky, A. (2001) Inference in randomized studies with informative censoring and discrete time-to-event endpoints. *Biometrics*, **57**, 404–413.

Schoen, R. (1988) *Modeling Multigroup Populations*, Plenum Press, New York.

Schoen, R. and Land, K.C. (1979) A general algorithm for estimating a Markov-generated increment–decrement life table with application to marital-status patterns. *Journal of the American Statistical Association*, **74**, 761–776.

Schoenfeld, D.A. (1982) Partial residuals for the proportional hazards regression model. *Biometrika*, **69**, 239–341.

Schoenfeld, D.A. (1983) Sample-size formula for the proportional-hazards regression model. *Biostatistics*, **39**, 499–503.

Shih, J.H. (1995) Sample size calculation for complex clinical trials with survival endpoints. *Controlled Clinical Trials*, **16**, 396–407.

Siannis, F., Copas, J., and Lu, G. (2005) Sentivity analysis for informative censoring in parametric survival models. *Biostatistics*, **6**, 77–91.

Siegel, J.S. and Swanson, D.A. (eds) (2004) *Methods and Materials of Demography*, 2nd edn, Academic Press, New York.

Stiratelli, R., Laird, N., and Ware, J.H. (1984) Random-effects models for series observations with binary response. *Biometrics*, **40**, 961–971.

Steele, F., Goldstein, H., and Browne, W.J. (2004) A general multistate competing risks model for event history data, with an application to a study of contraceptive use dynamics. *Statistical Modeling*, **4**, 145–159.

Storer, B.E. and Crowley, J. (1985) A diagnostic for Cox regression and general conditional likelihoods. *Journal of the American Statistical Association*, **80**, 139–147.

Struthers, C.A. and Kalbfleisch, J.D. (1986) Misspecified proportional hazard models. *Biometrika*, **73**, 363–369.

Sugisawa, H., Liang, J., and Liu, X. (1994) Social networks, social support, and mortality among older people in Japan. *Journal of Gerontology: Social Sciences*, **49**, S3–S13.

Sullivan, D.F. (1971) A single index of mortality and morbidity. *HSMHA Health Reports*, **54**, 1063–1070.

Tarone, R.E. and Ware, J.H. (1977) On distribution-free tests for equality for survival distributions. *Biometrika*, **64**, 156–160.

Teachman, J.D. (1983b) Analyzing social processes: life tables and proportional hazards models. *Social Science Research*, **12**, 263–301.

Teachman, J.D. and Hayward, M.D. (1993) Interpreting hazard rate models. *Sociological Methods and Research*, **21**, 340–371.

Therneau, T.M. and Grambsch, P.M. (2000) *Modeling Survival Data: Extending the Cox Model*, Springer-Verlag, New York.

Therneau, T.M., Grambsch, P.M., and Fleming, T.R. (1990) Martingale-based residuals for survival models. *Biometrika*, **77**, 147–160.

Tokyo Metropolitan Institute of Gerontology (TMIG) (1973) *Project Report on Centenarians*, TMIG, Tokyo, Japan (in Japanese).

Tsiatis, A. (1975) A nonidentifiability aspect of the problem of competing risks. *Proceedings of the National Academy of Science*, **72**, 20–22.

Turnbull, B.W. (1974) Nonparametric estimation of a survivorship function with doubly censored data. *Journal of the American Statistical Association*, **69**, 290–295.

U.S. Census Bureau Public Information Office (2002) U.S. Census Bureau facts and features, Veteran Day 2002: November 11. http://www.census.gov/newsroom/releases/archives/facts_for_features_special_editions/cb10-ff21.html (accessed 01 March 2012)

Vaupel, J.W. (1990) Kindred lifetimes: frailty models in population genetics, in *Convergent Issues in Genetics and Demography* (eds J. Adams, A.I. Hermalin, D. Lam, and P. Smouse), Oxford University Press, New York, pp. 155–170.

Vaupel, J.W., Manton, K.G., and Stallard, E. (1979) The impact of heterogeneity in individual frailty on the dynamics of mortality. *Demography*, **16**, 439–454.

Vaupel, J.W. and Yashin, A.I. (1985a) The deviant dynamics of death in heterogeneous populations, in *Sociological Methodology 1985* (ed. N.B. Tuma), Jossey-Bass, San Francisco, CA, pp. 179–211.

Vaupel, J.W. and Yashin, A.I. (1985b) Heterogeneity ruses: some surprising effects of selection on population dynamics. *The American Statistician*, **39**, 176–185.

Vermunt, J.K. (1997) *Log-Linear Models for Event Histories. Advanced Quantitative Techniques in the Social Sciences Series*, vol. 8, SAGE Publications, Thousand Oaks, CA.

Ware, J.H. and DeMets, D.L. (1976) Reanalysis of some baboon descent data. *Biometrics*, **32**, 459–463.

Wei, L.J., Lin, D.Y., and Weissfeld, L. (1989) Regression analysis of multivariate incomplete failure time data by modeling marginal distributions. *Journal of the American Statistical Association*, **84**, 1065–1073.

Weinberger, M., Darnell, J.C., and Tierney, W.M. (1986) Self-rated health as a predictor of hospital admission and nursing home placement in elderly public housing tenants. *American Journal of Public Health*, **76**, 457–459.

Wilcoxon, F. (1945) Individual comparisons by ranking methods. *Biometrics*, **1**, 80–83.

Wild, C.J. (1983) Failure time models with matched data. *Biometrika*, **70**, 633–641.

Wilmoth, J.R. (1997) In search of limit, in *Between Zeus and the Salmon* (eds K.W. Wachter and C.E. Finch), National Academy Press, Washington, D.C., pp. 38–64.

Wilson, E.B. (1927) Probable inference, the law of succession, and statistical inference. *Journal of the American Statistical Association*, **22**, 209–212.

Wimmer, L.T. and Fogel, R.W. (1991) Aging of union army men: a longitudinal study, 1830–1940. *Journal of the American Statistical Association, Proceedings of the Government Statistical Section*, 56–61.

Winship, C. and Mare, R.D. (1983) Structural equations and path analysis for discrete data. *American Journal of Sociology*, **89**, 54–110.

Winship, C. and Mare, R.D. (1992) Models for sample selection bias. *Annual Reviews of Sociology*, **18**, 327–350.

Witten, T.M. (1989) Quantifying the concepts of rate and acceleration/deceleration of aging. *Growth, Development, and Aging*, **53**, 7–16.

Wu, M.C. and Carroll, R.J. (1988) Estimation and comparison of changes in the presence of informative censoring by modeling the censoring process. *Biometrics*, **44**, 175–188.

Yashin, A.I. and Iachine, I.A. (1995) Genetic analysis of duration: correlated frailty model applied to survival of Danish twins. *Genetic Epidemiology*, **12**, 529–538.

Yashin, A.I., Vaupel, J.W., and Iachine, I.A. (1994) A duality in aging: the equivalence of mortality models based on radically different concepts. *Mechanisms of Aging and Development*, **74**, 1–14.

Yashin, A.I., Vaupel, J.W., and Iachine, I.A. (1995) Correlated individual frailty: an advantageous approach to survival analysis of bivariate data. *Mathematical Population Studies*, **5**, 145–159.

Zeger, S.L. and Karim, M.R. (1991) Generalized linear models with random effects: a Gibbs sampling approach. *Journal of the American Statistical Association*, **86**, 79–86.

Zeger, S.L., Liang, K., and Albert, P.S. (1988) Models for longitudinal data: a generalized estimating equation approach. *Biometrics*, **44**, 1049–1060.

Further reading

Allison, P.D. (1982) Discrete-time methods for the analysis of event histories, in *Sociological Methodology 1982* (ed. S. Leinhardt), Jossey-Bass, San Francisco, CA, pp. 61–98.

Amemiya, T. and Nold, F. (1975) A modified logit model. *Review of Economics and Statistics*, **57**, 255–257.

Blossfeld, H.-P., Golsch, K., and Rohwer, G. (2007) *Event History Analysis with Stata*. Lawrence Erlbaum, New York, New York.

Clayton, D.G. (1988) The analysis of event history data: a review of progress and outstanding problems. *Statistics in Medicine*, **7**, 819–841.

Clayton, D.G. (1994) Some approaches to the analysis of recurrent event data. *Statistical Methods in Medical Research*, **3**, 244–262.

DeLong, D.M., Guirguis, G.H., and So, Y.C. (1994) Efficient computation of subset selection probabilities with application to Cox regression. *Biometrika*, **81**, 607–611.

Eakin, T., Shouman, R., Qi, Y., *et al.* (1995) Estimating parametric survival model parameters in gerontological aging studies: methodological problems and insights. *Journal of Gerontology: Biological Sciences*, **50A**, B166–B176.

Heckman, J.J. and Singer, B. (1982) Population heterogeneity in demographic models, in *Multidimensional Mathematical Demography* (eds K.C. Land and A. Rogers), Academic Press, New York, pp. 567–599.

Guo, G. and Rodriguez, G. (1992) Estimating a multivariate proportional hazards model for clustered data using the EM algorithm, with an application to child survival in Guatemala. *Journal of the American Statistical Association*, **87**, 969–976.

Mantel, N. (1966) Evaluation of survival data and two new rank order statistics arising in its consideration. *Cancer Chemotherapy Reports*, **50**, 163–170.

Myers, G.C. (1989) Mortality and health dynamics at older ages, in *Differential Mortality: Methodological Issues and Biosocial Factors* (eds L. Ruzicka, G. Wunsch, and P. Kane), Clarendon Press, Oxford, England, pp. 189–214.

Land, K.C., Nagin, D.S., and McCall, P.L. (2001) Discrete-time hazard regression models with hidden heterogeneity: The semiparametric mixed Poisson regression approach. *Sociological Methods & Research*, **29**, 342–373.

Lillard, L.A. (1993) Simultaneous equations for hazards: Marriage duration and fertility timing. *Journal of Econometrics*, **56**, 189–217.

Preston, S.H. and Taubman, P. (1994) Socioeconomic differences in adult mortality and health status, in *Demography of Aging* (eds L.G. Martin and S.H. Preston), National Academy Press, Washington, D.C., pp. 279–318.

Ramanathan, R. (1993) *Statistical Methods in Econometrics*, Academic Press, San Diego, CA.

Schoenfeld, D.A. (1981) The asymptotic properties of nonparametric tests for comparing survival distributions. *Biometrika*, **68**, 316–319.

Steele, F., Goldstein, H., and Browne, W.J. (2002). A general multistate competing risks model for event history data, with an application to a study of contraceptive use dynamics. *Statistical Modeling*, **4**, 145–159.

Teachman, J.D. (1983a) Early marriage, premarital fertility, and marital dissolution: results from whites and blacks. *Journal of Family Issues*, **4**, 105–126.

Tuma, N.B. and Hannan, M.T. (1984) *Social Dynamics–Models and Methods*, Academic Press, Orlando, FL.

Weibull, W. (1951) A statistical distribution function of wide applicability. *Journal of Applied Mechanics*, **18**, 293–297.

Wu, L.L. (1990) Simple graphical goodness-of-fit tests for hazard rate models, in *Event History Analysis in Life Course Research* (eds K.U. Mayer and N.B. Tuma), University of Wisconsin Press, Madison, WI, pp. 184–199.

Yamaguchi, K. (1991) *Event History Analysis*, SAGE Publications, Newbury Park, CA.

Index

Survival Analysis: Models and Applications, First Edition. Xian Liu.